Foundations of Exercise Psychology

Foundations of Exercise Psychology

Second Edition

Bonnie G. Berger, Ed.D.
Bowling Green State University

David Pargman, Ph.D.
Florida State University

Robert S. Weinberg, Ph.D.
Miami University of Ohio

Fitness Information Technology
A Division of the International Center for Performance Excellence
262 Coliseum, WVU-PE, PO Box 6116
Morgantown, WV 26506-6116

Library of Congress Card Catalog Number: 2006927660

ISBN: 978-1-885693-69-3

Copyeditors: Corey Madsen, Danielle Costello, Katherine Kline
Cover Design: Bellerophon Productions
Production Editor: Corey Madsen
Typesetter: Bellerophon Productions
Proofreader: Maria denBoer
Indexer: Maria denBoer
Cover photos: Woman on exercise bike courtesy of © Bongarts/Sports Chrome.
          Refer to pp. 245 & 353 for other photo credits

Printed by Sheridan Books
10   9   8   7   6   5   4

Fitness Information Technology
A Division of the International Center for Performance Excellence
262 Coliseum, WVU-PE
PO Box 6116
Morgantown, WV 26506-6116
800.477.4348 toll free
304.293.6888 phone
304.293.6658 fax
Email: fitcustomerservice@mail.wvu.edu
Website: www.fitinfotech.com

DEDICATION

With love and affection

- To my family, who contribute so much to my life—my mom, Mildred Berger, my dad and his wife, Bernard and Helen Berger, and my son and his wife, Stephen and Natasha Casher; and

- To my friends, mentors, and colleagues who have encouraged me to follow my dreams.

  —BGB

- To Marsha, Deena, and Michelle—three women who believe in the need for regular exercise and conduct their lives accordingly.

  —DP

- To my family, the most important part of my life.

  —RSW

CONTENTS

DETAILED CONTENTS

SECTION C: Motivation to Exercise

SECTION D: Exercise and Specific Populations

FOREWORD

Stuart J. H. Biddle
Professor of Exercise & Sport Psychology and Head
School of Sport & Exercise Science
Loughborough University
Loughborough, UK

It is strange to think that when I was a student in the United States in the late 1970s, few people outside academia took seriously the public health benefits of physical activity and exercise. Governmental agencies focused on competitive sport, as far as activity was concerned, or on nutrition and smoking as the key public health issues. Ken Powell and colleagues' paper on CHD and exercise (Powell, Thompson, Caspersen, & Kendrick, 1987) was the first to suggest that inactivity might be causally related to CHD—less than 20 years ago as I write! When I was a member of the UK Government's "Physical Activity Task Force" in the mid-1990s, it was "touch and go" whether physical activity would even feature in the "Health of the Nation" strategy.

Even in academia much of the emphasis for undergraduates has been on sport, with psychology often centered on performance and acquisition of skills. If you tell someone at a party that you are a psychologist in a kinesiology/sport and exercise science department, they will assume you are a "sport" psychologist interested in elite performance. An "exercise psychologist" seems incomprehensible to many.

Things have changed. We now have a body of evidence, expertly summarized and crafted in this second edition, on health-related aspects of physical activity from a behavioral and psychological viewpoint—"exercise psychology." While the field is not new, it is only quite recently that textbooks have emerged. Even governments are now interested and there is talk of inter-agency collaboration across the social and behavioral sciences in attempting behavior change.

I am particularly pleased to write this foreword for a text written by Americans. As a British academic who studied in the United States, I have huge respect for the contributions emanating from the American system. There are differences in approach between some European and American researchers, but essentially we face the same issues across most, if not all, of the industrialized western world as far as physical activity is concerned. In fact, I was first introduced to what is "exercise psychology" when I was at Penn State University in 1978. The late Dorothy V. Harris taught me a variety of concepts featured in her 1973 textbook *Involvement in Sport* (probably incorrectly titled, with reference only to sport in today's climate, as it included much excellent material on sport and exercise psychology). Topics included motivation for physical activity, body image, and obesity (Harris, 1973). Not bad for 1973!

Things have moved on considerably, though, as reflected in this excellent text, *Foundations of Exercise Psychology*. The authors are commended for excellent coverage of important topics, such as the role of exercise in quality of life, enhanced self-perceptions, mood, and stress reduction, as well as innovative coverage of new topics, such as the personal meaning of exercise. Moreover, motivation to exercise is key, and rightly the authors devote considerably coverage to topics such as theories, determinants, and strategies. This provides an excellent foundation for the study of specific populations differing by gender and age, topics often missing from other texts in this field. Ever mindful of application, Bonnie and colleagues provide most useful guidelines for optimizing the exercise experience. I commend the authors, also, for excellent coverage of Professional Practice of Exercise Psychology, not covered in many other texts, and Exercise Design and Application, thus bridging the gap between behavioral theory and practice.

This area is so important. Whoever said "it's not rocket science—it's more complex than that!" was absolutely right. Exercise psychology is a vital cog in the wheel of understanding current destructive behaviours associated with lifestyle. Enjoy an excellent and important read! I congratulate Bonnie, David, and Bob for creating this successful text and bringing forth a second edition that will, no doubt, help shape the field over the next decade.

References

Harris, D. V. (1973). *Involvement in sport: A somatopsychic rationale for physical activity*. Philadelphia: Lea & Febiger.

Powell, K. E., Thompson, P. D., Caspersen, C. J., & Kendrick, J. S. (1987). Physical activity and the incidence of coronary heart disease. *Annual Review of Public Health, 8*, 253–287.

PREFACE

Physical activity in the form of exercise is an important and complex aspect of human behavior. Exercise is integrally tied to our health—its physical, psychological, and spiritual components. Exercise is complex because it includes diverse activity modes, which are performed at various levels of intensity, duration, and frequency in a variety of settings by a broad spectrum of participants. This text focuses on the interrelationships between exercise and psychology and how the integration of the two can help us understand and adopt more healthy and positive behaviors.

Foundations of Exercise Psychology will help you examine the psychological factors related to exercise and well-being. It is written for upper level undergraduate students and graduate students who want to better understand the implications of exercise. This text is also directed toward health and exercise professionals such as physical educators, health educators, coaches, athletic trainers, personal trainers, and fitness instructors, as well as interested exercisers who have no professional ties to physical activity. The text is designed as a beginning tool for students who wish to become exercise or sport psychologists. Regardless of your interests, *Foundations of Exercise Psychology* will provide you with information about exercise, factors that influence exercise participation, and aspects of psychological well-being that are influenced by physical activity.

Biomedical and Health Enhancement Models

The text begins with the utilitarian biomedical model of exercise and later introduces an emancipatory model that fosters body/mind integration. We first define exercise and how it differs from play and sport. We examine why some people enjoy exercise and others do not, and explore what determines personal preferences for specific types of exercise.

Desirable and Undesirable Psychological Changes

Some of the potential psychological benefits examined throughout *Foundations of Exercise Psychology* include mood alteration, stress management, enhanced self-concept and self-esteem, increased motivation, and enhanced quality of life. Additional benefits that habitual participation in exercise can provide are opportunities for increased self-awareness and for peak moments, including peak experiences and flow.

We also examine some of the undesirable aspects of exercise including exercise dependence, exercise-related injury, eating disorders, and substance abuse. Similar to most activities, exercise in moderation is highly desirable. However, both too little and too much exercise can detract from our overall quality of life.

Encouraging Exercise Participation

Despite the benefits of exercise, a relatively small portion of the population exercises across the lifespan sufficiently to establish high levels of health. To assist professionals working in exercise-related areas to enhance exercise participation, we present the latest information on helping motivate clients and students to exercise.

Knowledge about various models of exercise behavior, such as the health belief model, theory of reasoned action, transtheoretical model, theory of planned behavior, and the social-cognitive theory of exercise behavior, help you examine the complexities of exercise behavior. In addition to providing the basic components of these theories, we also present a broad picture of motivational determinants in the general categories of personal, environmental, programmatic, and characteristics of the activity itself that seem to boost exercise adherence. Since exercise motivation is related to various personal meanings such as fun and enjoyment, time away, communing with nature, and searching for spirituality, we explore this underdeveloped area.

There is little doubt that exercise has specific meaning, implications, motives, and benefits for specific populations. To begin to examine these population-related issues, we have focused on three sub-populations of exercisers. These include the women and men exercisers and gender issues, children and youth and exercise participation implications, and older individuals and quality of life.

Professional Practice and Exercise Program Design

Finally, to explore the paradoxical psychological changes, both desirable and undesirable, that can be associated with exercise, it is necessary to examine the role of exercise components in facilitating these changes. Exercise enjoyment, type or mode of exercise, and the training characteristics of intensity, duration, and frequency are important considerations when designing an exercise program. These exercise components seem to influence the direction and extent of the psychological changes. They may also influence participant motivation, the personal meanings within exercise experiences, and opportunities for self-awareness and understanding.

Let Us Hear From You

As you finish reading this text, let's hear from you. We are exceedingly interested in hearing your thoughts, reactions, and comments about the book.

We wrote *Foundations of Exercise Psychology* for you, and thus you are in an ideal position to provide feedback so that we can better meet your needs—and those of future students.

We hope that you enjoy learning about exercise psychology as much as we have throughout our careers. We have enjoyed our visit with you, and hope that we have provided exercise information that is useful to you as you embark on your journey to become an exercise/movement professional and a well-informed exercise participant.

Bonnie G. Berger, bberger@bgnet.bgsu.edu

David Pargman, dpargman@edres.fsu.edu

Robert S. Weinberg, weinber@muohio.edu

Acknowledgments

As I wrote my chapters, I realized that I owe so much to many individuals for their support—former teachers, colleagues, friends, graduate students, and coauthors. I greatly appreciate the Teachers College, Columbia University faculty who have become mentors: Larry Locke, Ann Gentile, Bill Anderson, and Marlin M. MacKenzie. Thanks for showing me the way.

I value my many colleagues and friends, especially Kate Hays, Dawne Larkin, Elizabeth Rose, Mark Andersen, Dan Kirschenbaum, Andy Meyer, Bill Morgan, David Owen, Michael Sachs, Bob Singer, Waneen Spirduso, Jerry Thomas, Michael Wade, and my colleagues at Bowling Green State University for encouraging me to forge ahead and to be kind to myself.

To my friends of many years, Elaine Foster, Jan Jelinek, Brenda Newman, Gil Videau, and Jerry Winter: Thanks for your belief in my finishing this second edition! You helped keep me sane through the process.

This edition would not have been written without the assistance of numerous graduate students with whom it has been a privilege to work. I would like to extend special thanks to John Wasinski, Megan Valentine, Ginenne Lanese, and Brendan Rokke at Bowling Green State University for facilitating my thinking and for their endless library searches and editing tasks. I am eternally grateful to you all!

I would like to say to my coauthors, David and Bob, I have truly enjoyed working together on this second edition, a most rewarding project. Finally, I must acknowledge the staff at Fitness Information Technology, especially Corey Madsen, for making the writing of this book more manageable and Andy Ostrow for his guidance on the book's conception and evolution.

—BGB

I offer my most sincere expression of gratitude to my graduate research assistant, Kimberlee Bethany, who has been of invaluable assistance in the preparation of my portion of the book. There has never been a reference that she was incapable of tracking down. Also, my warmest thanks to Bonnie and Bob, my competent and knowledgeable coauthors, with whom it was a pleasure to collaborate.

—DP

I'd like to thank many people for supporting me during the writing of this text. But rather than name names (and probably forget some), I'd just like to dedicate this text to my close friends and family who have been a constant source of comfort and support, not only during the process of writing for this text, but throughout my life. These, of course, include my sport/exercise psychology colleagues from whom I have learned a great deal over the years (many of whom have become dear friends).

Of course, let me thank David and Bonnie for asking me to join their team and be a part of this endeavor. You have always been great colleagues and I have enjoyed working with both of you. A special thanks to Bonnie who has really been the key person bringing all the minutia and details together as well as keeping us on track.

—RSW

CHAPTER 1

EXERCISE PSYCHOLOGY: WHAT IS IT?

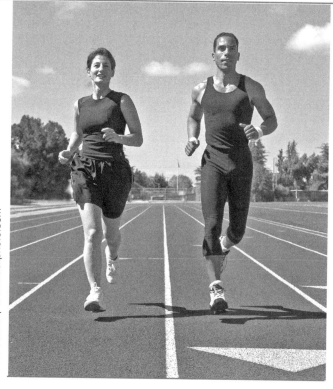

Photo courtesy of © iStockphoto.com

After reading this chapter, you should be able to

- Define the terms *exercise*, *play*, and *sport*,

- Compare the *humanistic model* of exercise with the *medical model* of exercise,

- Distinguish between *exercise psychology* and *sport psychology*,

- Describe the key areas of interest within *exercise psychology*,

- Identify the areas of interest within *health psychology*, *performance enhancement*, and *social psychology*, and

- Elaborate on the professional competencies required of *educational*, *clinical*, and *research exercise psychologists*.

Introduction to Exercise Psychology

Exercise is a term that is all encompassing and widely used. Because of its common use in daily conversation, the term *exercise* has many different, and occasionally conflicting, definitions. *Exercise* is a noun that sometimes refers to all types of large muscle activity, especially to fitness activities such as sit-ups or riding a stationary bicycle. Other times, *exercise* is a verb that refers to performing large muscle activities, often for purposes of health.

Exercise is surprisingly difficult to define. The Latin root of exercise is *exercitium*, meaning "to train," and the dictionary defines the word *exercise (*noun) as "regular or repeated use of a faculty or bodily organ," or "bodily exertion for the sake of developing and maintaining physical fitness" (*Merriam-Webster's Collegiate Dictionary*, 2003, p. 437). *Exercise* also can be used as a verb, and then is defined as "to use repeatedly in order to strengthen or develop < ~ a muscle >" (*Merriam-Webster's Collegiate Dictionary*, 2003, p. 437). According to the American College of Sports Medicine, "Exercise, a type of physical activity, is defined as planned, structured, and repetitive bodily movement done to improve or maintain one or more components of physical fitness" (ACSM, 2006, p. 3). Combining and expanding upon the above definitions, *exercise* can be defined as

- Large muscle activity,
- Planned, structured, and purposeful physical activity,
- Muscle activity that often includes repetitive bodily movements, and
- An activity with health, physical fitness, skill, and/or competitive foci.

Exercise participants focus on such unique goals as improving physical fitness, losing weight, enhancing their appearance, engaging in friendly competition, improving their skill levels, enjoying social interaction, altering their mood, reducing stress, and "feeling good."

In summary, exercise is a motor activity that employs the large muscles of the body to increase skill or fitness through practice and performance. This broad definition of exercise includes diverse types of physical activity. These types include the usual exercise activities such as walking, jogging, swimming, and hatha yoga as well as competitive recreational physical activity of basketball, tennis, racquetball, and rugby.

The specialization of *exercise psychology* includes diverse psychological issues, theories, and general information related to exercise. Specialists in exercise psychology focus on the contributions of exercise to psychological well-being and mental health as illustrated in Figure 1.1. Possible contributions of exercise to mental health include the use of exercise for mood alteration, stress management, treatment of psychological disorders, enhanced self-concept and self-

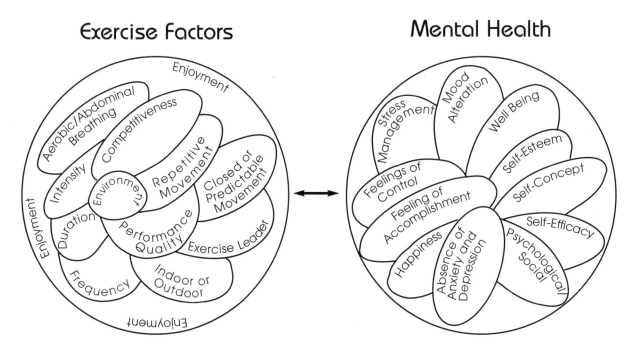

Figure 1.1. Interrelationships between exercise factors and mental health.

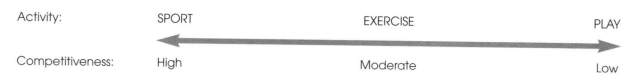

Figure 1.2. A physical activity continuum based on competitiveness.

efficacy, and increased personal fulfillment. (See the circle on the right side of the figure for an illustration of some of the mental health benefits.) Specialists in exercise psychology also examine exercise-specific factors such as intensity, duration, and program characteristics as illustrated by the circle on the left side of Figure 1.1. These exercise factors and others may influence psychological well-being and mental health. Specific exercise factors also contribute to exercise adoption and adherence.

Illustrating the bi-directional relationship between exercise participation and psychological well-being as depicted in Figure 1.1, exercise psychologists also investigate the relationship between psychological well-being and exercise participation. For example, people who are stressed or depressed may be more likely to exercise than those who are not. Additional areas of investigation within exercise psychology include the influences of specific exercise characteristics on exercise enjoyment, the underlying mechanisms that mediate the exercise-mental health relationship, ways to enhance flow states, and factors that might lead to exercise addiction.

To better understand exercise psychology as a field of study and as a profession, initially you will explore a physical activity continuum based on the degree of competitiveness and the interrelationships of exercise, play, and sport. In the latter portion of this introductory chapter, you will examine three possible ways of viewing the content of exercise and sport psychology.

A Physical Activity Continuum: Exercise, Play, and Sport

Physical activity is an umbrella term that includes all forms of human movement—especially exercise, play, and sport. This section highlights the major characteristics of physical activity and particularly those of exercise to provide an overview of the role of exercise within the context of physical activity.

Not all physical activity is the same, and the differences have implications for exercise and sport psychologists. For example, the specific physical activities of exercise, sport, and play can be arranged along various continua, such as exercise intensity, exercise duration, and competitive intensity along with the accompanying focus on winning. Sport and play anchor the two ends of the competition continuum, which ranges from high

to low levels of competition (see Figure 1.2). Play generally is less competitive than exercise, and exercise is less competitive than sport.

Placing specific physical activities along this competitiveness continuum illustrates the difficulty of determining "average" levels of competition for participants in different types of physical activity. In addition, once an "average" level of competition seems to be clear, there are individual exceptions. As suggested in Figure 1.3, amateur, international, and professional sport athletes tend to be highly competitive. Some athletes in professional sport, however, may consciously decrease their competitiveness to prolong their professional careers. Despite such individual variation, professional athletes generally are more competitive than average runners in the NYC marathon. A marathoner, even a recreational one, tends to be more competitive than someone hiking in the country.

As you examine the placement of activities in Figure 1.3, you personally may NOT agree with all of the activity placements along the continuum. Don't be disturbed by your lack of agreement. Such differences in opinion reflect the complexity of differentiating between play, exercise, and sport. The continuum in Figure 1.3 simply illustrates one of many ways to distinguish between these three types of activities. In the following sections, we will examine the main characteristics of exercise, play, and sport and related models in order to better understand these diverse activities that often include physical activity.

Exercise

Exercise is the focus of this book, and it constitutes the midsection of the competition continuum. Exercise tends to be more structured and competitive than play, but less structured and competitive than sport. In most situations, exercisers have no coach giving them directions, and they are free to do whatever they choose. One of the joys of exercise is that the participant can do what "feels good" or "appropriate" at the time, and can focus on enjoying the movement.

Two models of exercise: The medical model and the humanistic model. Too often, exercisers focus excessively on exercise outcomes or benefits, such as skilled performance, body toning, cardiorespiratory fitness, or victory in a tennis match, rather than on the process. Participants who focus on exercise outcomes are following the ***medical model of exercise***. According to this

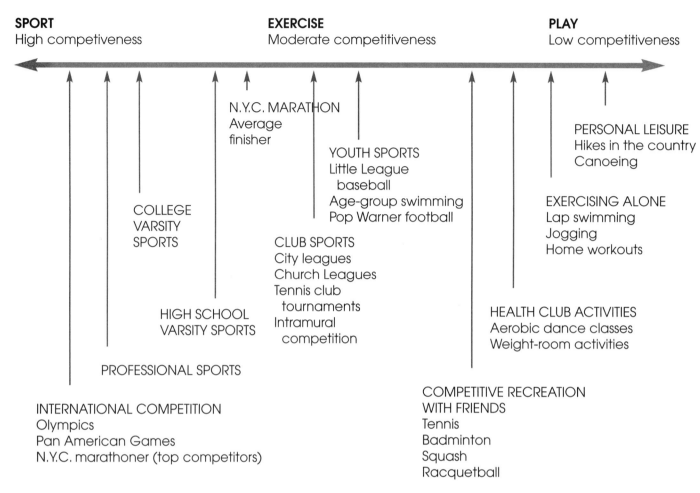

Figure 1.3. Activities along the physical activity continuum.

model, exercise is the treatment or medicine (e.g., something to be tolerated), and the outcomes are the benefits. However, exercisers do not need to follow a formula or prescription and actually can freely choose to regulate the intensity, duration, and extent of their participation on a daily or even moment-to-moment basis. Participants in a structured exercise class may have less of a choice in how they are exercising. Of course, they choose whether or not to participate in a particular class and can leave prior to completing the class session.

The humanistic model of exercise, in contrast to the *medical model*, merges scientific physiological and psychological information with the personal preferences of the participants. The humanistic model emphasizes freedom of choice when exercising. It also accentuates the joy of effort and aids in establishing lifetime participation in exercise. The humanistic model of exercise is a unifying tenet of this text.

The humanistic model as summarized in Table 1.1 stresses the importance of tailoring exercise programs to the individualized preferences of participants. The model also emphasizes that exercisers have the valuable option of "listening to their bodies" and exercising accordingly. Some exercisers, however, choose to follow—perhaps too strictly—the medical model of exercise. The medical model depicted in Table 1.1 incorporates specific ways of exercising based on the physical training guidelines established by scientists in exercise physiology. These exercisers and the terms *exercise prescription* and *exercise dose* are key components of the medical model of exercise. The terms *prescription* and *dose* tend to reinforce the false impression that only a specific amount of exercise will enhance health and is analogous to the "correct amount of medicine" as denoted by a physician's prescription.

In conclusion, exercise includes physical exertion; it is process oriented, as well as directed toward a goal or end product. Common exercise goals include muscle toning and body sculpting, weight loss, cardiovascular fitness, and "feeling better." Less common exercise goals are mood enhancement, stress reduction, and social interaction. Even less common goals of exercisers include experiencing flow and peak moments, creating a period of peace and quiet, searching for an exercise "high," communing with nature, and enhancing spirituality. Many people desire these exercise results, but a relatively small proportion of the

Table 1.1
Models of Exercise

Humanistic Model	Medical Model
Merges scientific information with *personal preferences*	Uses scientific information to determine an *exercise prescription*
Emphasizes freedom to choose exercise, intensity, duration, and frequency	Outlines the necessary exercise *dose*
Encourages exercisers to listen to their bodies to plan an exercise session	Encourages exercisers to listen to exercise or medical experts as well as their bodies to plan a session
Results in a flexible exercise program	Results in a prescribed exercise program that *should* be followed
Focuses on the exercise *process*, e.g., the joy of movement	Focuses on exercise *outcomes* and *health benefits*
Can result in low, moderate, or high levels of fitness	Often results in high levels of fitness and sport performance
Tends to promote lifetime exercise patterns of continuous, but varied, exercise at different stages of life	Tends to promote sporadic exercise patterns of starting and stopping

American population exercises appropriately to reap these benefits (see Chapter 11). A major focus throughout this text is the examination of the psychological changes associated with specific types of exercise. Ultimately, this information can assist people in reaching their exercise goals and in incorporating exercise into their lives.

A small portion of the population is physically active. Despite the psychological, social, physical, and spiritual benefits of physical activity, the proportion of the population who participate in regular, sustained physical activity is surprisingly small. In several different studies, approximately 22% of the American population was observed to participate in light- to moderate-intensity physical activity for 30 minutes per day in their leisure time (USDHHS, 1996). The proportion of the adult population who participate in regular, vigorous physical activity is even smaller— approximately 15% of the American population (USDHHS, 1996). Researchers consistently report gender differences in exercise populations, with more men than women being physically active. The male to female ratio is approximately 1.1 to 1.3. The likelihood of regular, sustained physical activity also tends to decrease with age. Specifically, habitual exercise is higher among 18- to 29-year-olds than among other adult age groups. It also is higher among whites than among blacks and Hispanics (USDHHS, 1996).

Exercise: The health benefits. The relatively small number of people who exercise regularly is surprising because habitual exercise provides participants with multiple health benefits. Despite the desirability of the health benefits, many people are physically inactive and need the assistance of an exercise psychologist. One of many benefits is that exercise facilitates energy expenditure and counterbalances weight gains through food intake. In addition, exercise and caloric restriction together often are more successful in promoting weight loss than caloric restriction alone (Lohman & Wright, 2004). Another exercise health benefit, especially if the exercise activity is weight-bearing, is the enhancement of bone mineral mass and strength and the delay of the onset and progression of osteoporosis. Exercise also has an inverse relationship with resting blood pressure. The more a person exercises, the lower his or her resting blood pressure tends to be; habitual physical activity may protect against an age-associated increase in blood pressure. See the USDHHS (1996) chapter, "The Effects of Physical Activity on Health and Disease," for additional descriptions of the multiple health benefits of exercise.

In another review examining the health benefits of

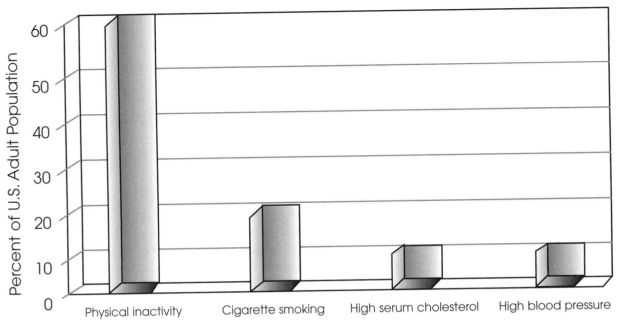

Figure 1.4. Prevalence of risk factors for coronary heart disease in the general U.S. population for the years 1980–1987. *Note:* From "Biological Aspects of the Active Living Concept," by C. Bouchard, In J. E. Curtis, & S. J. Russell (Eds.), *Physical Activity in Human Experience: Interdisciplinary perspectives,* p. 37, 1997, Champaign, IL: Human Kinetics. Copyright 1997 by Canadian Fitness and Lifestyle Research Institute. Adapted with permission.

exercise, Claude Bouchard (1997) suggests that habitual physical activity is beneficial in the prevention and treatment of coronary heart disease, stroke, and diabetes; for the general functioning of the immune system; and for age-related decreases in physical capacity. With physical benefits as important and as broad as these, it is amazing that such a small percentage of the U.S. population is sufficiently physically active to reap such benefits. See Figure 1.4 for the percentages of the U.S. adult population who have specific risk factors for coronary heart disease. The 60% prevalence rate of physical inactivity for the U.S. population of adults is considerably higher than the approximately 10% prevalence rate of high blood pressure (or hypertension) and high cholesterol levels. As emphasized in Figure 1.4, physical inactivity is prevalent in the adult population and has major implications for the development of coronary heart disease.

A low aerobic fitness level or physical inactivity is a leading contributor not only to heart disease, but to death from all causes including cancer and cardiovascular disease (see Figure 1.5). As emphasized by Steve Blair and colleagues (1996) in their classic study, low aerobic fitness when measured by VO_2 max (oxygen consumed per kilogram of body weight per minute) is even more highly related to death than are common health concerns. These include high cholesterol (CHOL), cigarette smoking, body mass index (BMI) or obesity, and hypertension as indicated by a systolic blood pressure (SBP) reading of more than 140

mmHg. This study by Steve Blair and colleagues included a large sample size of 7,080 women and 25,341 men who ranged in age from 20 to 88 years at baseline and completed a preventive medical examination including a maximal exercise test on a treadmill.

As noted in Figure 1.5, the effect of aerobic fitness on risk of death was greater for women than for men. Women who scored in the lowest fitness category died at a rate that was 55% higher than women in the moderately fit category. For all of the fitness categories combined, women's fitness-related risk of death from all causes was 2.23, as adjusted for age and examination year. For the least fit men, the relative risk of death from all causes was 41% higher than the rate for those in the moderately fit category. The men's fitness-related risk of death was 2.03 over all fitness categories combined. A conclusion from the study was that low aerobic fitness is an important precursor of mortality, and that mortality rates greatly decrease with a moderate level of fitness. In addition, the protective effect of fitness was evidenced in smokers and nonsmokers, and those with and without elevated cholesterol levels or blood pressure. Based on figures such as those in Figure 1.5, there clearly is a need for exercise psychologists to work with diverse members of the population to assist them in adopting and continuing exercise programs throughout their lives.

An exercise dilemma: Working out versus playing. It seems that too many people view exercise as work, rather than as play or as an enjoyable activity. *Work*

Adjusted Relative Risk for All-cause Mortality

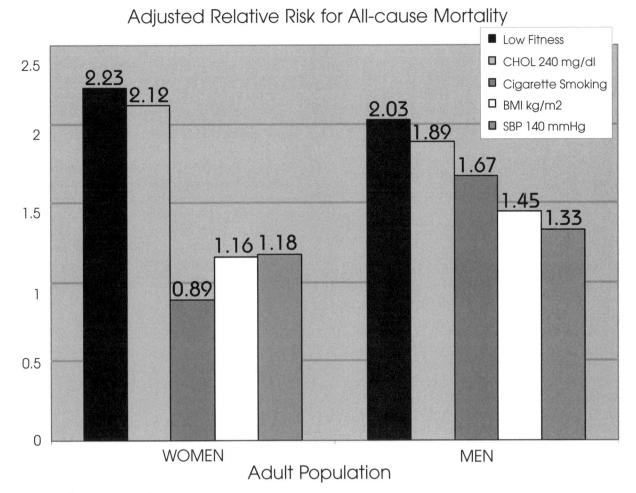

Figure 1.5. Adjusted[1] relative risk of death from selected mortality predictors including low fitness, or lack of physical activity. Graph from W. W. Spirduso, K. L. Francis, & P. G. MacRae, *Physical Dimensions of Aging*, p. 23, 2005, Champaign, IL: Human Kinetics. Based on data from "Influences of cardiorespiratory fitness and other precursors on cardiovascular disease and all-cause mortality in men and women," by S. N. Blair et al., p. 207, 1996, *Journal of American Medical Association*, 276.

connotes drudgery, unpleasantness, and even pain from exertion. To combat this negative view of exercise, Dean Ornish (1990), a respected cardiologist and researcher, has suggested that the term *workout* be replaced by *playout*. This change in terminology has not occurred. However, decreased use of the term "workout" would allow diverse exercise professionals such as physical education teachers, coaches, exercise psychologists, and physical therapists—who encourage people to be physically active—to emphasize the pleasurable and enjoyable aspects of exercise. If the term *playout* seems inappropriate for the people you work with, you simply may try to avoid using both the terms *playout* and *workout*. Obviously, the "no pain, no gain" ethic is inappropriate for encouraging widespread participation in physical activity.

Although we may not be consciously aware of the effects of terminology, it influences unconscious perceptions, emotional responses, and, ultimately, behavior. Most individuals need encouragement to view their exercise sessions as a pleasurable, personally meaningful activity that includes elements of fun and personal fulfillment. Throughout this text, we will emphasize the need to value the entire *process* of exercise, as well as the final *product* of exercise and the specific benefits we seek.

Lifelong participants in physical activity who prefer the humanistic model of exercise often include a playful element in their exercise programs. A playful, less "serious" approach facilitates creating a personal exercise program based on physical and psychological needs, goals, and preferences. Playfulness in exercise tends to increase enjoyment and to decrease tedium.

As illustrated by the depiction of the interrelation-

---

[1]Adjusted for age and examination year.

ships of exercise, play, and sport in Figure 1.6, play *can* be an integral component of both exercise and sport. But it can also include more than that, thus extending beyond the two circles in the figure. The pie-shaped slice in the circles illustrates that a portion of exercise also is play and that an even smaller portion of sport is play. Some people may include the element of play considerably more than others do in their exercise and sport activities. Play can cut across both exercise and sport and includes elements of spontaneity, diversion from everyday activities, and freedom.

The smaller, more specialized circle of sport within the larger, more encompassing exercise circle in Figure 1.6 illustrates the necessity of exercise conditioning and the exercise components included within sport. Although exercise is a part of all sport, sport is not a part of all exercise. Sport is more specialized than exercise and focuses on physical conditioning, while emphasizing high-level skilled movement, competition, and winning.

Many types of exercise such as friendly recreational games of tennis and golf include elements of both sport and play. As emphasized in Figure 1.6, exercise, play, and sport are not always separate entities. Sheehan (1978), a sport and exercise philosopher, has captured the need to include the element of play in all physical activity as he observes

> *Exercise that is not play accentuates rather than heals the split between body and spirit. Exercise that is drudgery, labor; something done only for the final result is a waste of time.*
>
> *What, then, should you do? Run only if you must. If running is an imperative that comes from inside you and not from your doctor. Otherwise, heed the inner calling to your own play* [italics added]. Listen if you can to the person you were and are and

can be. Then do what you do best and feel best at. Something you would do for nothing. Something that gives you security and self-acceptance and a feeling of completion; even moments when you are fused with your universe and your Creator.

> *There is no better test for play than the desire to be doing it when you die* [italics added]. (pp. 76–77)

Exercising needs to be much more than a job or a task that we "should" perform. Rather than work, exercise can be viewed as a treat to ourselves. Exercise is an opportunity to integrate mind and body, a reward for a hard day's work, and a special time for ourselves. Focusing on the positive elements within exercise such as fun, enjoyment, and play seems likely to increase the number of the Americans who exercise on a regular basis (see Chapters 12 and 13).

Play

Play often includes physical activity, as illustrated in Figure 1.6. It can be a valuable, meaningful human activity for adults as well as children.

For adults, as well as children. Fink (1979) captured the value of play as he commented on both its importance and significance for adults:

> When philosophers and poets stress the *power and meaning of play as a profound human reality* [italics added], perhaps we should remember the words that warn us that we will not enter into the kingdom of heaven unless we become like little children. (p. 83)

Breaking through the triviality barrier. Exercise psychologists need to be familiar with the work of researchers in anthropology, sport sociology, and development psychology who have carefully investigated the meaning of play and playful meanings, especially as they relate to sport and exercise (e.g., Drewe, 2003; Dunning & Rojek, 1992; Holowchak, 2002). As a result, researchers in the area of play are beginning to break through the "triviality barrier" of play to investigate the values, expectations, and organization within play (Power, 2000). Breaking the triviality barrier removes the "lack of time" excuse and the impression that play is a waste of time.

The section in this chapter on play captures only a small portion of the available research and emphasizes the multidisciplinary base of exercise psychology. Exercise psychology is a multidisciplinary specialty that incorporates relevant information from a variety of academic areas such as cultural anthro-

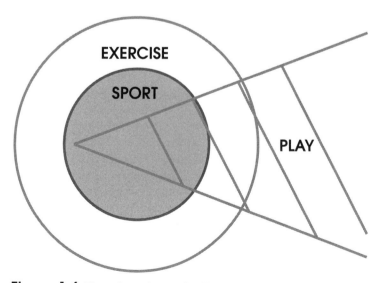

Figure 1.6. The play element within exercise and sport.

pology, sociology, philosophy of sport, exercise physiology, and numerous areas within the parent disciplines of psychology, physiology, sociology, and anthropology.

Play can be an integral component of exercise. As previously emphasized, exercise, play, and sport have different foci, but are not mutually exclusive. To understand play and its relationship to exercise, it is helpful to describe some of its characteristics that Drewe (2003) recently reviewed and explored in her book, *Why Sport: An Introduction to the Philosophy of Sport.* Play is

- Voluntary on the part of participants;
- Fun and has no real goals or purpose and stands outside of immediate wants;
- A stepping out of ordinary life;
- A temporary sphere of activity that occurs within agreed upon limits of time and space;
- Relatively low in competitiveness (play is at one extreme side of the physical activity continuum in Figures 1.2 and 1.3 as determined by its non-competitive nature); and
- Spontaneous and self-directed (play is enjoyed for its own sake—e.g., it is an autotelic activity).

All these characteristics of play are dependent on its context and environment, and are not absolute (Dunning & Rojek, 1992).

Exercise can be a part of play. Although exercise can be a part of play, exercise is not absolutely essential to play. Children play games of tag, which include an exercise component. However, children also play "school," which usually includes low levels of physical activity. Complicating efforts to distinguish among play, exercise, and sport is the everyday use of the term *play.* For example, athletes describe themselves as "football players" and "tennis players." Many participants in these physical activities, however, find it difficult to maintain the critical elements of play such as spontaneity, fun, and a lack of seriousness. Based on this observation, some participants should not be called football "players" because they may not be playing the game of football.

Diversion from the ordinary. The word *play* can also suggest diversion from everyday activities, suspension of the ordinary, childlike qualities, and a source of fun (Huizinga, 1955). In fact, play ceases when one is no longer having fun (Figler & Whitaker, 1991). Emphasizing the inherent fun and suspension of the ordinary world, Schmitz (1979) suggests that there are four different styles of play that are listed below. The last two of these can include physical activity:

- Simple spontaneous frolic,
- Make-believe or pretend play,

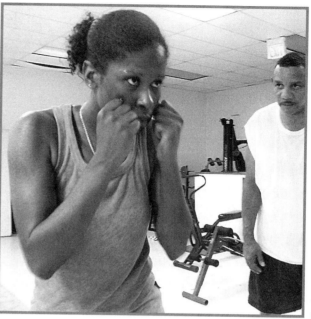

Photo by Sgt. Jerron Barnett, courtesy of USAF

- Physical skills such as surfing and mountain climbing, and
- Games.

Implicit rather than explicit rules. Explicit rules are nearly absent in play, and that absence is another way to distinguish some of the differences among play, exercise, and sport. Although play has few, if any, *explicit,* or clear, rules governing participation, it does have *implicit* or suggested rules, such as the need for fairness, as indicated by the phrase *fair play.* Other implicit rules within play are that quitting is unacceptable (even if the participant does not get his or her way) and that cheating is not tolerated. See Table 1.2 for a summary of the characteristics of play, exercise, and sport.

"Freedom from" and "freedom to." Play, separated from ordinary life and related to a sense of freedom, can be an important, enjoyable activity for people of all ages. Too often, play is regarded as trivial, designed exclusively for children. Play (and the accompanying time-out from daily routine) represents "freedom from" social expectations and personal responsibilities. Play provides opportunities for fun in one's day and enables participants to gain fresh perspectives on daily concerns upon returning to their regular everyday activities.

Play also provides an opportunity for "freedom to." Participants have the freedom to do whatever they might want to do within certain parameters. Playful exercise activities provide the freedom to exercise in any manner a person chooses (e.g., to be in nature, or to be with friends).

Fink (1979) observed that people tend to devalue play and see it as a trivial waste of time. More than 20 years after this observation, play is still undervalued—

Table 1.2
Characteristics of Exercise, Play, and Sport

Exercise

- Choice of training parameters
- Enjoyment
- Focus on psychological well-being
- Moderately structured
- Self-directed
- Time-out of daily activities

- Diverse personal meanings
- Fitness
- Goal-directed: Health, appearance, weight loss, etc.
- Recreational competition
- Stress management

Sport

- Coach-directed
- Complex motor skills
- Exhilaration
- Goal-directed: winning, etc.
- Spectators
- Structured team approach

- Competition
- Exclusionary environment
- Explicit rules
- Physical prowess
- Stress creating

Play

- Absorbing
- Fun
- Not for personal gain
- Relatively noncompetitive
- Separate from ordinary life
- Time out from daily activities

- Few explicit rules; some implicit rules
- Lack of seriousness
- Personal freedom
- Self-directed
- Spontaneous
- Voluntary

---

despite its contributions to daily enjoyment and the overall quality of life. As noted by Fink:

> By force of habit we limit play by contrasting it to the seriousness of life, to an attitude of moral commitment, to work—to all of the prosaic things of reality. We identify it with frolic, with flight toward the regions of imagination, away from the hard realities of life to dreams and utopia. *It exists just to keep man from succumbing to the modern world of work, from forgetting how to laugh amid moral rigorism, from becoming the prisoner to duty. Analysts of civilization recommend play to ward off disasters. It takes on a therapeutic value against the ills of the soul* [italics added]. (p. 74)

Sport

Sport is another type of physical activity and is located at the high end of the competitiveness continuum for physical activity as depicted in Figure 1.2.

High-levels of physical skill and competition. As emphasized by Drewe (2003, pp. 9–13), the two major characteristics of sport are as follows:

- The requirement of physical skill and
- An emphasis on competition. *Com-petitio* means *striving together* and thus requires another individual to strive with to produce maximum performance in the pursuit of excellence.

Com-petitio or competition negates the possibility of competing against one's self or a force of nature such as a mountain (Drewe, 2003, pp. 10–11). Competing against one's self may be pursuing excellence, but it is not considered to be true competition. For a more in-depth philosophical discussion of competition, see Drewe (2003). *Sport* is highly competitive, and focuses on *agon*, the Greek word for contest. Sport embodies the spirit of rivalry and competition and the accompanying pursuit of honor, fame, and glory (Slowikowski & Loy, 1993).

Explicit rules and team structure. Sport also has formal structure, as reflected by a set of rules, and involves a high level of complex motor skills. Although the motor skills necessary in specific sports differ, formal sport activities share specific common characteristics. Sport includes structured team practices and a body of rules that enable as well as constrain. Most forms of sport include coaches, strategy, and competitors who are somewhat evenly matched. Outcome in sport determines winners and losers. In contrast to the sports of the Middle Ages, modern organized sport is

- Secular and not religious,
- Egalitarian—theoretically, teammates are chosen on the basis of personal ability, and the rules are the same for all participants—and
- Quantitative with a focus on scores, even an obsession with records as observed for some spectator sports (Guttmann, 1988).

An element of play in sport. Ideally, sport includes the element of play and is pursued for its own sake. "One becomes involved in sport—in theory—not for extrinsic rewards (parental approval, academic credit, cardiovascular fitness, or take-home pay) but for the intrinsic pleasures of the activity" (Guttmann, 1988, p. 1). Some of the intrinsic pleasures or reasons for participating include

- The development of physical skills,
- A sense of mastery over one's body,
- The joy of movement,
- The stimulation of meeting challenges, and
- Social interaction.

As illustrated in Figure 1.6, the spontaneous, creative freedom of play is possible in sport, but it is not essential. The portion of sport that includes play often is rather small. In fact, many athletes participate in sport without maintaining a playful sense of freedom, fun, and absorption. It is the unusual athlete who is able to maintain a sense of playfulness when practicing and competing. Sport and play both share exhilaration, immediacy, and uncertainty of outcome (Schmitz, 1979). The intensity of these aspects, however, varies greatly between and within sport and play activities.

A focus on winning. Winning is a major goal of sport participants. As noted in the philosophical examination of *A Whole New Ballgame*, competition is a central element in all sport (Guttmann, 1988). Most athletes want to perfect their physical sport skills and develop maximal fitness to achieve their goals of winning. Most athletes also have a coach who helps them win and perfect their physical abilities. Winning is a major focus of most athletes and coaches who emphasize that "Winning isn't everything: It's the only thing!" This emphasis on winning can usurp intrinsic reasons for participating, such as enjoyment and fun, and become all-consuming (Figler & Whitaker, 1991).

Meaning of the word "athlete." When exploring the definition of sport, it helps to clarify the meaning of the word *athlete*. Generally, most sport participants are considered to be athletes.

Take a moment to answer the following questions about athletes to begin to clarify the meaning of the word:

- What is your personal definition of an athlete?
- Can exercisers be athletes?
- Do you consider yourself to be an athlete?

You may have discovered when answering the questions that defining the word *athlete* is surprisingly difficult. John Leonard (1977) searched for a definition of the ultimate athlete throughout his book, *The Ultimate Athlete*. Leonard philosophically concluded that ALL of life, the period between birth and death, is a game. From this perspective, life is the Game of Games.

The "Ultimate Athlete" then, according to Leonard, is a dancer in exercise and sport as well as in the broader game of life. Although the Ultimate Athlete is a dancer, not every dancer is the Ultimate Athlete. Dancers embody fluidity of movement and concentrate on breathing, strength, and specific motor skills. Dancers also develop psychological as well as mental and physical endurance, agility, and balance at higher levels than athletes in many other types of physical activity. These physical and psychological abilities are important in exercise as well as in our daily lives, and they provide mental and physical endurance, agility, and balance that help prepare us to become an Ultimate Athlete.

According to Leonard, everyone on earth is a potential athlete. An Ultimate Athlete embodies the following attitudes described by Leonard as well as the stereotypical physical attributes and skills:

> For me, then—and this may be purely arbitrary—an athlete in the Game of Games is one who plays life intensely, with heightened awareness of this endeavor. An athlete is one who can perceive discord and harmony both, who can accept contradiction as the very stuff of play while not losing sight of the ultimate harmony. An athlete in this Game . . . plays voluntarily and wholeheartedly, even while realizing that this Game is not all there is . . . This athlete contends in a game for a prize and the prize is play itself, a life fully experienced and examined. (p. 189)

Returning to our earlier question, how do you define the word *athlete*?

- Some people might define an athlete as a dancer.
- Others would select another type of elite, highly skilled sport participant as an example of an athlete. For example, participants in the Olympic Games are athletes.
- Still other people might consider *fitness buffs* to be athletes.

A broad definition of an *athlete* is anyone who is a member of an organized sport team that has a coach directing them. However, as noted by Kleiber and Kirshnit (1991), membership on a sports team is not requisite to the definition of an athlete. Being an athlete seems to include more than being a member of a team and having a coach. Athletes are personally committed to developing excellence in motor skills and enthusiastically exhibit maximal sport performance as emphasized in the following description of athletes:

"Young athletes" (among 10- to 12-year-olds) may be so labeled because of the aspiration of coaches and program leaders, and this may be a misnomer with respect to commitment. When sport involvement does not reflect a child's personal preference, when he or she is forced to "play" by parents, or when a gifted adolescent betrays his or her recalcitrance in half-hearted efforts, the label of athlete is inappropriate. (p. 200)

Athletes are ultimate strivers, competitors who never cease their quest to obtain optimal performance in sport and exercise. Athletes in the game of life are striving in work, personal relationships, or hobbies. Regardless of the definition adopted, athletes engage in training programs to be the "best" that they can be in specific activities.

Differences and Similarities Among Exercise, Play, and Sport: Concluding Observations

During a 20-year running career, a philosopher of running named George Sheehan (1992b) emphasized the need to analyze *play*, *exercise*, and *sport*. He came to distinguish these three types of physical movement this way:

I learned something I always knew but did not remember: the difference between exercise and play and sports. Each is a separate and distinct entity, each with its own function, each essential and fundamental to our nature. Each fulfills in some way our need to demonstrate who we are. Each makes us feel better about ourselves and the lives we lead.

For too long people have tended to use the words interchangeably . . . We need all three activities. *Exercise* is a science. *Play* is an art. *Sport* is both [italics added]. Exercise is mechanical. Play is free flowing. Sport is exercise with rules and a reckoning at the finish. (pp. 144–145)

As previously emphasized, exercise, play, and sport have different foci and are not mutually exclusive. Depending on the individual and the situation, these

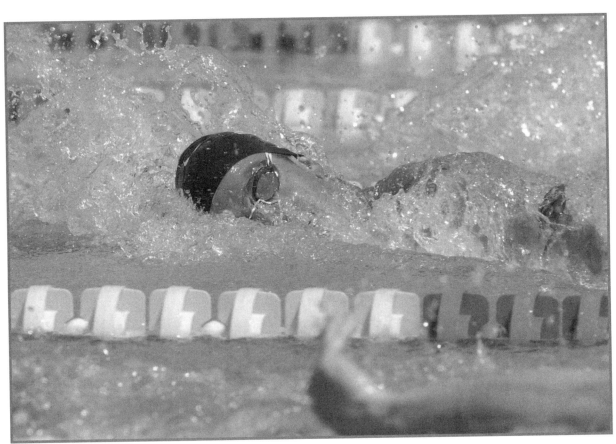

Photo courtesy of US Army

activities can overlap along the competitiveness continuum. Again, refer to Figure 1.2 and to Table 1.2. Ideally, *play* is an integral component of both exercise and sport as illustrated by the pie-shaped wedge in Figure 1.6. *Exercise* is goal directed, more structured than play, and associated with health, stress management, and fitness benefits. Exercise is a major component of sport and often of play. Play is a relatively noncompetitive, spontaneous activity with few rules. It is absorbing and fun. *Sport* is highly competitive, and participants concentrate on developing complex motor skills and physical prowess.

Playing while exercising facilitates reaching one's exercise goals. Similarly, sport, which concentrates on performance excellence and competitiveness, can be carried out within the spirit of play. Playfulness is one of the more important elements in determining the quality of one's life and thus deserves careful attention. In a delightful philosophical discussion of sport and play, Kenneth L. Schmitz (1979) cautions that the pleasurable elements of play, and thus play itself, is destroyed in exercise and sport by the following three common abuses:

- Needing to win at all costs,
- Overvaluing efficiency and technical competence at the cost of human considerations, and
- Focusing on the presence of spectators, who change a sport into a commercial venture with an entertainment or gladiatorial focus.

Now that the distinctions between play, exercise, and sport are clear, take a moment once again to examine the activities in Figure 1.3. Professional sport athletes are the most competitive of all athletes, although there always are individual exceptions. Some people may consider Olympic and college athletes more competitive than professional athletes, who may pace themselves and be less "competitive" in order to avoid overuse injuries and thus extend their professional careers. The average professional athlete tends to be more competitive, or more focused on winning, than does the average runner in a marathon who has no plans for placing within the top 10 finishers. Most marathoners are competing against the clock and against their own previous performances. Based on the information about competition and play, exercise, and sport just reviewed, design your own arrangement of the activities listed in Figure 1.3.

In conclusion, exercise and sport have both different as well as similar characteristics. Thus, it is not surprising that exercise psychology and sport psychology are two separate areas of study that have overlapping areas of interest. The next section of this chapter describes the following three systems for organizing the content within exercise and sport psychology. The systems emphasize the diverse content and areas of professional expertise within exercise and sport psychology. The three systems include the following:

1. Exercise and sport psychology,
2. Health psychology, performance enhancement, and social psychology, and
3. Educational, clinical, and research psychology in exercise and sport.

Pay particular attention to the first of the three systems, because it is the one employed in this book with its emphasis on exercise psychology.

The Field of Exercise and Sport Psychology

Professional organizations in exercise psychology have defined sport psychology very broadly, and it often includes both exercise and sport psychology. According to the European Federation of Sport Psychology (FEPSAC), for example, *sport* "includes all kinds of exercise, sport, and physically active pursuits" (European Federation of Sport Psychology, 1996, p. 221). In response to the question "What is sport psychology?" FEPSAC has offered the following definition:

> Sport psychology is concerned with the psychological foundations, processes, and consequences of the psychological regulation of sport-related activities of one or several persons acting as the subject(s) of the activity. The focus may be on behavior or on different psychological dimensions of human behavior (i.e., affective, cognitive, motivational, or sensorimotor dimensions).
>
> The physical activity can take place in competitive, educational, recreational, preventative, and rehabilitation settings and includes health-related exercise. (p. 223)

This generic use of the term *sport psychology* includes all psychological topics related to exercise and sport. Sport psychology is such a huge area of study, however, that it can be separated into specific content areas.

The following systems for organizing the content within exercise and sport psychology are not mutually exclusive and are somewhat artificial. The three systems do, however, highlight a multitude of interest areas and facilitate awareness of the diverse content areas within exercise psychology. Delineation of various specializations within sport psychology include: the *exercise psychology* and *sport psychology* (System 1), as well as *health psychology*, *performance enhancement*, and *educational sport psychology* (System 2), and *clinical sport psychology* and *research sport psychology* (System 3).

System 1: Exercise and Sport Psychology

This organizational system emphasizes fundamental differences among the environments of exercise and sport that differ in competitiveness, training intensity, and types of participants. Exercise participants tend to focus on the process of becoming fit, friendly games of competition, personal meaning of physical activity, and enjoyment. Sport participants focus on high-intensity training, game outcome or winning, and maximal performance. The distinction between exercise and sport psychology in this system also is used by Division 47 of the American Psychological Association and throughout this book.

Exercise psychology. As previously emphasized, exercise psychology focuses on wellness, or the establishment of optimal mental health through physical activity. Researchers in exercise psychology often examine the relationship between exercise and psychological well-being. More specific topics of interest include exercise and changes in mood, stress management, mental health, flow, the exercise high, enhanced self-concept, improved self-efficacy, and exercise addiction. Personal meanings in exercise, individual characteristics related to exercise preferences, and sources of exercise enjoyment are additional areas of interest in exercise psychology. Exercise psychologists investigate the roles of fun and enjoyment in exercise adoption and adherence, and the underlying mechanisms that may mediate or cause various changes in mental health.

Exercise psychologists also investigate the types of exercise programs that can effectively elicit specific psychological benefits. Applied exercise psychologists develop, supervise, and test the effectiveness of exercise programs in meeting participants' exercise goals. These goals differ for specific populations: young children, teens, young adults, the elderly, male and female participants, psychotherapy clients, and psychiatric patients. Common exercise psychology topics examined throughout this textbook are outlined in Table 1.3.

Sport psychology. In contrast to exercise psychology, sport psychology includes psychological topics of interest to people associated with highly organized competitive sport, namely, athletes, coaches, sport administrators, and parents. Thus, specialists in sport psychology work with athletes and others associated with sport. Sport psychologists can emphasize the ultimate goal of winning by assisting athletes (and coaches) in reaching peak performance through mental training strategies, optimal levels of arousal, and goal setting. Sport psychologists employ various mental training techniques, such as stress management, self-talk, and imagery, to help participants improve sport performance.

Table 1.3
Areas of Interest Within Exercise Psychology

Design of specific exercise programs to maximize the psychological benefits

Exercise addiction and commitment to exercise regularly without injury

Exercise adoption, maintenance, and adherence to lifetime exercise

Exercise as a stress management technique: reducing psychological stress and seeking eustress

Flow and peak experiences in exercise as unique experiences

Fun and enjoyment in physical activity

Gender and sex-role influences on exercise choice and participation

Mental health benefits of exercise such as stress management, self-concept, and self-esteem

Mechanisms that mediate the various mental health benefits of exercise

Mindfulness or paying attention to the moment while exercising

Mood changes after exercising, both desirable and undesirable

Overuse injuries in exercise settings: psychological precursors, treatment, and prevention

Personal meaning of exercise or personal significance of specific physical activities

Personality and exercise preferences: sensation seeking, optimism, and trait anxiety

Psychological benefits of exercise for specific populations, such as clinical populations, the elderly, children, physically disabled populations, and populations with health problems

Psychotherapeutic benefits associated with exercise, especially for those with depression and anxiety

Quality of life and exercise: subjective well-being, happiness, and cultural influences

Running or exercise high: predisposing factors, general characteristics, and ways to facilitate it

Self-concept, self-esteem, self-confidence, and self-knowledge as influenced by specific types of exercise programs such as rock climbing and aerobic dance

CASE STUDY 1.1

Choosing to Pursue Graduate Study in Exercise Psychology

Julie Plans to Be a Coach

Julie was an undergraduate student majoring in exercise science at a Midwestern university. She had always wondered why it was that she loved competing on her university's varsity volleyball team so much. She decided that she wanted to earn a degree that would enable her to be a coach. A coaching career seemed logical because Julie was an enthusiastic volleyball player and wanted to enable others to find the same personal fulfillment in the sport as she did.

Julie Considers Graduate School

Something unexpected happened as Julie pursued her professional interests in coaching. During her junior year of undergraduate studies, Julie began to wonder whether she might want to attend graduate school. Julie was fortunate to have a professor in exercise and sport psychology who appreciated her interest in coaching and thought that she had great academic potential.

When Julie began her undergraduate studies, completing her undergraduate degree was her main goal. During her sophomore and junior years, Julie began to consider continuing her academic studies and attending graduate school. After completing her class in exercise and sport psychology, Julie became even more aware that there was a vast world of psychological knowledge related to coaching about which she knew relatively little. She was excited about connecting sport psychology to her interest in coaching. She also wondered why it was that some of her friends did not participate in any type of physical activity.

Julie Applies to Several Graduate Schools

After talking with her coach and the professor of her exercise and sport psychology class, Julie began the task of investigating graduate programs. Based on many individuals' input, a newsletter of a professional exercise and sport psychology organization, and correspondence with directors of various graduate programs, Julie successfully selected several graduate pro-

grams in exercise psychology and started the application process.

Julie was exceedingly pleased to learn that she had been awarded graduate assistantships at several different universities. Her grade point average was high, and her professors and coaches had written strong letters of support.

Julie had great difficulty choosing between two of the universities in particular. They were so different from one another. One offered a large graduate stipend and was in the Western U.S., a place where Julie always wanted to live. The other graduate program was less glamorous, but was known to be a stronger academic program at a more highly respected university. The second program also included exercise psychology as well as sport psychology.

Julie Selects a Graduate School

After considerable contemplation, Julie discussed her quandary with a variety of people including her parents, professors, and friends. Julie finally selected the graduate program and chose the program at the university that offered multiple specializations for study in exercise and sport psychology. Thus, Julie had the opportunity to decide the specific area in which she would specialize after she took some initial graduate courses and had more information about the broad areas of exercise psychology and sport psychology.

Conclusion: Identifying Graduate School Options

The possibility of further study can be a daunting concept for undergraduate as well as master's students who entertain the possibility of further graduate study. Although the prospect of additional years in school immediately may not be an attractive option, it is important to keep professional opportunities open. Try to avoid rejecting the possibility of further university study outright at this time. It is important to contemplate diverse professional options, because it is almost impossible to predict your professional goals three, five, and even ten years into the future.

Exercise and sport psychology offer attractive areas of investigation and application for students contemplating diverse career opportunities. Case Study 1.1 highlights the unexpected sequence of events and thoughts that often leads to graduate school and a specialization in exercise psychology.

The focus on elite athletes in the United States and throughout the world attracts many psychologists and sport scientists to sport psychology, especially to performance enhancement. It is exciting to be the sport psychologist for a professional football team or for an Olympic team! Because the number of professional sport psychology positions available with elite athletes is limited to a small number of teams, such positions are highly sought. To broaden their professional opportunities, sport psychologists are beginning to apply their professional expertise to a broader range of performers such as dancers, singers, actors, public speakers, and business executives as well as athletes.

System 2: Health Psychology, Performance Enhancement, and Social Psychology

This system highlights the broad content area of sport psychology that includes health, performance enhancement, and the social aspects of physical activity. The Association for the Advancement of Applied Sport Psychology (AAASP) emphasizes this tripartite organization of content and employs it as a base for organizing the program speakers at its annual conference, in determining the composition of its executive board, and in publishing research articles in its journal, the *Journal of Applied Sport Psychology*.

Health psychology. Health psychology is a specialization that includes psychological topics related to mental and physical health. There are many health psychology subareas, such as the personality profiles of cancer and heart disease patients and the effectiveness of psychological interventions in the prevention and treatment of disease. These subareas are of limited professional interest to exercise and sport psychologists. It is important to note, however, that health is much more than an absence of disease.

A holistic view of health emphasizes the interconnectedness of body, mind, environment, and spirit. Multiple determinants of an individual's health include exercise, genetic endowment, diet, socioeconomic and family background, social support, risk-taking behavior, spiritual beliefs, and the environment. These components constantly interact and affect people's present and future health. People are powerful creators of their own health as they make conscious choices about exercise, nutrition, social situations, careers, daily schedules, and priorities.

A sub-specialty within health psychology focuses on physical activity. In exercise-focused health psychology, an emphasis is placed on interrelationships of physical activity, health (physical and mental), and quality of life for participants. Health psychology with an emphasis on exercise and sport focuses on psychological factors in exercise and sport, particularly as they relate to health promotion, disease development and remediation, and coping with illness. Exercise-related health psychology issues include

- Exercise addiction,
- Exercise adoption and adherence in a variety of populations,
- Mood alteration,
- Management of daily stress levels,
- Psychological adjustment problems related to exercise injuries, and
- Eating disorders among exercisers.

Performance enhancement. Performance enhancement is the glamorous area within exercise psychology. Although the number of potential clients is small, performance psychologists hope to work with professional teams and world-class amateur athletes as well as with other well-known individuals such as movie stars. Performance-enhancement specialists also work with university, high school, and community teams as well as with exercisers and leaders in business and industry who are interested in applying "mental" skills to enhance their performance. Performance-enhancement techniques include visualization, stress management, and goal clarification to improve sport and other types of performance.

Social psychology. Social psychology focuses on social interactions and groups of people in physical activities. Social psychology topics of interest include group and team cohesion, team spirit, group goal-setting, sportsmanship and moral behavior, and gender and sex-role influences in exercise and sport. The dynamics of race in exercise and sport, aggression in sport, exercise psychology issues associated with youth sport participants, and interactions of players, coaches, and parents also are topics of interest in social psychology. Specialists in social psychology also have particular interests in the developmental effects of exercise participation (or lack of) on children and youth.

System 3: Educational, Clinical, and Research Psychology in Exercise and Sport

This system focuses attention on the professional expertise of exercise and sport psychologists and on the specific services that they provide, rather than on the clientele served. The U.S. Olympic Committee (1983) formalized this organizing system to emphasize that specialists in each of the three areas—educational, clinical, and research psychology—need different professional competencies and training.

Educational exercise/sport psychology. Educational exercise psychologists teach or conduct education sessions for exercisers who have no obvious psychological problems. Educational exercise psychologists teach other members of the general population how to enhance the psychological benefits of their exercise programs and how to use exercise to further develop their psychological well-being.

These specialists also teach psychological techniques to improve their performance quality. Doctoral-level specialists in this area tend to have strong academic expertise in the sport and exercise sciences and focus on members of the general population who do not have apparent psychological problems.

Clinical exercise/sport psychology. In contrast to educational exercise/sport psychologists, clinical psychologists treat individuals who have psychological problems. Clinical psychologists in exercise and sport are licensed as psychologists in the state in which they conduct individual and group practices. They have completed graduate programs that concentrate on developing counseling and therapeutic skills, and possess the clinical expertise necessary to treat athletes and exercisers who have specific psychological problems, many of which are related to exercise and sport.

Some of the more common issues in clinical exercise psychology include eating disorders, exercise addiction, substance abuse, fear of success and failure, and the therapeutic use of exercise to treat mental disorders. Clinical exercise and sport psychologists often have private practices and treat diverse clients who have exercise- and nonexercise-related personal problems.

Research exercise/sport psychology. Research is a critical component of all specializations—regardless of whether it is exercise psychology, sport psychology, health psychology, performance enhancement, social psychology, or educational or clinical exercise/sport psychology. The research category emphasizes that some exercise psychologists focus nearly exclusively on research: theory testing, data collection, and the generation and testing of new knowledge in exercise settings.

Research psychologists work on the clarification, refinement, and development of current psychological concepts and practices in exercise. By collecting data and publishing the results and conclusions of their studies, researchers test the effectiveness of the services provided by exercise psychologists. Researchers also provide exercise psychology practitioners and other movement specialists with new ideas and possible programs for their practices.

Conclusion

This text employs the first system that separates content into Exercise Psychology and into Sport Psychology and focuses nearly exclusively on exercise psychology. Although this text focuses on exercise psychology, it includes health psychology and social psychology in the second system, and the educational and research components in the third system. Understanding the three classification systems allows you to gain awareness of the diverse content areas, professional expertise, and professional opportunities within exercise psychology.

Foundations of Exercise Psychology

Exercise psychology has implications for nearly all segments of the American population. Exercise psychologists focus on the psychological benefits and problems associated with exercise for members of normal populations, psychiatric populations, and those who have movement- and other health-related disabilities. Exercise psychology is applicable to everyone regardless of their current level of physical ability, age, health, or activity. Exercise psychologists encourage people to be physically active by conveying the diverse benefits of exercise.

Hypokinetic Disease

Physical inactivity, or hypokinetic disease, is a serious health hazard comparable to smoking in its deleterious effects on health. Health care costs are skyrocketing at such a frightening rate that health insurance is a national concern. At the same time that health costs are spiraling upward, people are living longer. The average life expectancy for individuals increased from the age of 47 in 1900 to 73 years in 1980 (Fries, 1980). Life expectancy in the United States today is approximately 79 years for females, 73 years for males, and differs for individuals of different ages, genders, and ethnic backgrounds (Spirduso, Francis, & MacRae, 2005; U.S. National Center for Health Statistics, 1991). It is comforting to know that by living longer, each of us has more time to do the things that we each hold dear.

As the length of life increases, there is a nagging question: What about the *quality* of our lives, especially during our later years? In other words, will we enjoy the later stages of our lives and be able to do the things we want to do? Or does living longer simply mean that we will develop amore chronic diseases before we die and be restricted in the activities we can pursue? What benefits will these extra years provide?

The good news is that both the functional *quality* of health and the compression of morbidity, remaining healthy until one's death, depend on health behaviors. These behaviors include exercise, nutrition, tobacco abstinence, weight management, and medical care as well as important genetic and environmental considerations and medical progress (Spirduso et al., 2005; USDHHS, 1996). Major goals of exercise psychologists are to encourage, assist, and enable more people to be physically active and to establish lifelong exercise behaviors that enhance their quality of life.

Exercise and Quality of Life

There is little doubt that our quality of life is determined to a large extent by our own behavior. This book explores the role of exercise in enhancing people's lives. Quality of life depends on our psychological well-being, stress management, our ability to have fun, our freedom from disabling diseases, and the maintenance of physical abilities such as adequate strength, flexibility, and energy to participate in enjoyable activities (Berger & Motl, 2001; Spirduso et al., 2005). A program of frequent exercise can contribute to a variety of life-quality components:

- Enhancing psychological well-being;
- Increasing positive mood states and reducing negative ones;
- Managing stress—consciously raising or lowering ongoing stress levels;
- Enhancing self-concept, self-awareness, and body image;
- Creating opportunities for peak experiences;
- Establishing and maintaining high levels of mental as well as physical strength, endurance, and flexibility;
- Facilitating and maintaining weight loss;
- Enhancing health; and
- Possibly increasing longevity and slowing the aging process.

Exercise Adoption and Adherence

Despite the many benefits of exercise and their desirability, approximately 10% to 20% of the American adult population exercises sufficiently to maintain adequate levels of physical well-being. An additional 25% to 60% of Americans do not exercise at all in their leisure time. The remaining percentage of the population does exercise sporadically, but the health benefits are uncertain (Dishman & Buckworth, 1996). Some of the key questions explored throughout *Foundations of Exercise Psychology* include the following:

- Why do some people exercise?
- Do these reasons change as an individual moves from initially adopting an exercise program to becoming a habitual exerciser to establishing a lifelong exercise program?

- Do young and old exercisers have different exercise goals?

From questions such as these, other questions arise. For example, do some people enjoy exercise and others hate it? What factors make exercise enjoyable? Are some types and forms of physical activity more conducive to psychological well-being than others? *Foundations of Exercise Psychology* addresses these questions and many others.

Organization of the Book

Section A: Introduction and Key Concepts

The introductory section explores basic issues in exercise psychology. In Chapter 1, you have read about the content of exercise psychology and the definitions of *play*, *exercise*, and *sport* as three types of physical activity. In Chapter 2, "The Emerging Field of Exercise Psychology," you will examine the historical development of exercise psychology and learn about key exercise psychology organizations and journals that disseminate state-of-the-art information for professionals in the field.

Section B: Exercise and the Quality of Life

The eight chapters of section B represent a major focus of the book. In Chapter 3, you will find a survey of the factors that contribute to subjective appraisal of well-being. Chapter 4 highlights the relationship between exercise and various aspects of self, particularly *self-concept* and *self-esteem*. Chapter 5 explains key models and measures of mood and self-regulation of mood. Chapter 6 investigates multiple relationships between exercise and mood. The next two chapters in this section focus on the general topic of stress. Chapter 7, "Stress: Definitions and Management Strategies," defines key terms and explores models that explain the occurrence of stress and examine coping techniques. Chapter 8 focuses exclusively on the use and effectiveness of exercise as a stress management technique that interacts with physiological and psychological stress responses. Chapter 9 explores possible relationships between exercise participation and personality characteristics such as *sensation-seeking*, *self-motivation*, *anxiety*, and *locus of control*. Chapter 10, the final chapter in this section, considers psychological factors that are related to the occurrence of exercise-induced injuries and psychological techniques that facilitate the recovery process.

Section C: Motivation to Exercise

The six chapters in the motivation section highlight the importance of motivation and the multiple factors influencing the transformation of exercise goals into reality. In Chapter 11, you will investigate the basic models of exercise behavior such as the *health beliefs model*, *transtheoretical model*, and the *theory of reasoned action*. Then in Chapter 12, you will become acquainted with personal, environmental, programmatic, and situational factors related to exercise adoption and adherence. Chapter 13 focuses on a variety of approaches to enhance exercise adherence. The personal meanings of exercise explored in Chapter 14 present additional reasons for exercising throughout one's life span. Chapter 15 introduces the reader to peak moments in exercise that include *peak experience*, *peak performance*, and *flow experiences* as another facet of intrinsic motivation in exercise. The final chapter in this section, Chapter 16, highlights three situations in which the motivation to exercise has become too strong: *eating disorders*, *substance abuse*, and *exercise addiction* or *dependence*.

Section D: Exercise and Specific Populations

The three chapters in Section D focus on specific populations of exercisers: women, men, children, youth, and older individuals. Chapter 17, "Gender Issues in Exercise," explores social influences on the exercise participation of men and women, media images of female and male exercisers, and gender differences in the importance of weight control, body toning, and muscle development. Chapter 18 focuses on children and youth in sport. This chapter examines young people's motives for participation, the importance of enjoyment for exercise adherence, the relationship of coordination to perceived competence, and the need for a balanced perspective concerning the importance of exercise for young children. Chapter 19 considers issues directly related to older exercisers: misconceptions regarding the need for exercise, the undesirability of age-grading exercise activities, the psychological benefits of exercise for older populations, and exercise as the long-sought fountain of youth.

Section E: Exercise Guidelines to Maximize the Benefits

The two chapters in this section focus on practical guidelines to encourage desirable psychological changes associated with exercise throughout a lifetime of participation. Chapter 20 explores the types of exercise and their individual characteristics that are related to psychological well-being. Chapter 21 focuses on the practice or training guidelines of exercise *intensity*, *duration*, and *frequency* that are related to optimizing the psychological benefits of physical activity.

Summary

Exercise psychology includes all psychological issues and theories related to physical activity, especially to exercise. More specifically, exercise psychology focuses on wellness, or the optimal mental and physical health of exercisers. Specialists in exercise psychology investigate diverse topics in direct reference to exercise—for instance, *mood alteration*, *flow*, *improved self-efficacy* and *self-concept*, the *exercise high*, *stress management*, *exercise addiction*, and *exercise as treatment* for mental health disorders, as well as exercise for *fun*, *enjoyment*, and *personal fulfillment*.

These three forms of physical activity have differing characteristics, but are not mutually exclusive. Exercise, the focus of this text, involves planned and purposive physical activity. It generally has physical and psychological fitness emphases, and often has socially competitive elements as exemplified by a friendly game of tennis. Less competitive than exercise, play is spontaneous and self-directed. Play is not restricted to children and can be an integral component of exercise and sport. Sport occurs in a more structured environment, is highly competitive, and has an emphasis on physical skill and winning.

There are many useful ways to organize the diverse contents of exercise psychology. One system includes *health psychology*, *performance enhancement*, and *social psychology*, areas that focus on three key research and applied interests. The separation of exercise psychology into *educational*, *clinical*, and *research practice* emphasizes different services that specialists offer. A third system for partitioning the content into manageable pieces is the twofold division of exercise and sport psychology. This system, employed in this text, focuses on the types of physical activity in which individuals participate: exercise and sport.

Exercise psychology refers to psychological principles and concepts that are of value to exercisers. These recreational participants in physical activities concentrate on improving their *fitness*, *skill*, *health*, and *appearance*. Exercisers also participate for personal enjoyment and friendly levels of competition.

Separate chapters in the *Foundations of Exercise Psychology* focus on a broad range of exercise psychology topics. Specific topics include emergence of the field and those related to life quality, namely, exercise and *subjective well-being*, *enhanced self-concept* and *self-esteem*, *mood alteration*, *personality considerations in exercise choice*, exercise as a *stress management* technique, and psychological factors associated with exercise-induced injuries. Motivation-related topics include models of exercise behavior, factors and strategies related to exercise adoption and adherence, the search for personal meaning in exercise, the facilitation of peak experiences, and the exercise motivation concerns of eating disorders, substance abuse, and exercise addiction. Exercise population considerations include gender issues in exercise and issues directly related to young and old participants. The concluding chapters present practical guidelines for maximizing the psychological effectiveness of exercise to include mode and practice considerations.

Can You Define These Terms?

athlete
_____

exercise
_____

explicit rules
_____

humanistic model of exercise
_____

implicit rules
_____

medical model of exercise
_____

physical activity
_____

play
_____

sport
_____

System 1: Exercise psychology versus sport psychology
_____

System 2: Health psychology, performance enhancement, and social psychology
_____

System 3: Educational, clinical, and research exercise psychology
_____

triviality barrier
_____

Can You Answer These Questions?

1. What are the differences among play, exercise, and sport? Provide several examples of each.
2. Is play an important element in exercise and sport? Please explain your response.
3. Do you personally include play in your exercise or sport activities? Give an example.
4. What is an athlete? Do you consider yourself an athlete? Explain the basis of this decision.
5. Differentiate between the process and product of exercise.
6. Describe the content areas in exercise psychology.
7. Which system for organizing the content of sport psychology do you prefer? Explain the basis for your decision.
8. What is research, and why is research an important emphasis in exercise psychology?

CHAPTER 2

The Emerging Field of Exercise Psychology

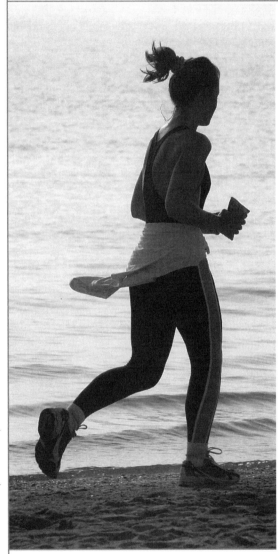

Photo courtesy of © iStockphoto.com

After reading this chapter, you should be able to

- Describe the emergence of exercise psychology as a field of study in the United States,

- Appraise the purpose and need for certifying exercise psychologists,

- Outline the requirements for Certified Consultant, Association for the Advancement of Applied Sport Psychology,

- Discuss the value of accrediting exercise psychology programs,

- Identify the interrelationship between research and application in exercise psychology,

- Describe the role of the International Society for Sport Psychology in the development of the field, and

- Distinguish between the interest areas and the general membership composition of key exercise psychology organizations:

  a. American College of Sports Medicine (ACSM)

  b. Association for the Advancement of Applied Sports Psychology (AAASP)

  c. Division 47 of the American Psychological Association (APA)

  d. International Society of Sport Psychology (ISSP)

  e. North American Society for the Psychology of Sport and Physical Activity (NASPSPA)

  f. Sport Psychology Academy (SPA)

Introduction

This chapter introduces you to the emerging specialization of exercise psychology. Specialists in exercise psychology have investigated a variety of factors influencing

- Exercise initiation, adoption, maintenance, and adherence;
- Psychological responses to exercise;
- Exercise addiction;
- Psychological precursors to exercise-related injuries; and
- Personal meanings in physical activity.

The birth and subsequent growth of exercise psychology have been fairly recent. For example, the North American Society for the Psychology of Sport and Physical Activity (NASPSPA), founded in 1967, was the first professional organization in the United States that included some emphasis on exercise psychology. The Association for the Advancement of Applied Sport Psychology (AAASP) has an even greater emphasis on exercise psychology, but was not founded until 1985. The subsequent formation of Division 47, Exercise and Sport Psychology, within the American Psychological Association (APA) in 1986 further established exercise psychology as a distinct field of inquiry.

Development of Exercise and Sport Psychology Throughout the World with Emphasis on the United States

The historical development of exercise psychology provides a broad perspective on the science and application of exercise psychology today. Exercise psychologists help people create exercise programs that encourage them to maximize enjoyment, facilitate exercise adoption and adherence, set and reach their exercise goals, and then reap the psychological benefits of exercise.

Exercise psychologists belong to some of the professional organizations described in this chapter to remain up-to-date in their profession, attending annual conferences to learn about new approaches and the latest research. The quality of service that exercise psychologists provide to their clients depends on both their familiarity with current scientific research and their ability to artfully select, apply, and research principles to meet clients' needs. If you are interested in exercise psychology, you should consider applying for a reduced-cost student membership in one of the exercise psychology organizations to learn more about key issues in the field.

The Early Years: 1898–1949

In the United States and throughout the world, the early research focused on sport rather than exercise psychology. Thus, development of exercise psychology is closely interwoven with sport psychology. Early investigators tended to focus on athletes. It was not until the mid-1960s that researchers of sport psychology branched out to include exercisers in all types of physical activity.

Norman Triplett (1863–1934), a psychologist who studied cycle racers (Triplett, 1898), is credited with being the first sport psychologist in the United States. However, Coleman Griffith (1893–1966) is considered the "father" of sport psychology in the United States because he established the first sport psychology laboratory in 1925 and carried out a systematic line of research in this laboratory at the University of Illinois (Browne & Mahoney, 1984). Griffith's books, *Psychology of Coaching* (1926) and *Psychology of Athletics* (1928), emphasize the early interest in sport rather than in exercise psychology. As World War II approached, the scientific community began to focus on combat-related research, and research in exercise (and sport) psychology temporarily ceased.

1950–1970: Increasing Professional Activity

Following World War II, John Lawther published a pioneering sport psychology text, *The Psychology of Coaching*, in 1951. Exercise psychology began to emerge as an active field of academic inquiry in the late 1960s. Even in the 1960s, though, the emphasis continued to be on sport.

Illustrating the burgeoning field of sport psychology, Bruce Ogilvie and Tom Tutko (1966), two psychologists from California, published a book, *Problem Athletes and How to Handle Them*, and a questionnaire entitled the *Athletic Motivation Inventory* (AMI). Both the book and inventory aroused considerable controversy. One obvious ethical question was "Who are *problem athletes*?" Are athletes "problems" simply because they do not follow the rules of autocratic coaches, or are they "problems" because they are not playing up to their capabilities and winning? Since scores on the AMI were used to cut athletes from team membership, many sport psychologists concluded that this was unethical use of the Inventory.

These philosophical questions and ethical issues still are discussed today. For example, what are a sport psychologist's professional responsibilities to individual athlete clients, coaches, and team organizations? Tom Tutko retired, but Bruce Ogilvie continued to be active as a sport psychologist until his death in 2003. Based on his multiple contributions to sport psychol-

Table 2.1

Establishment of Exercise and Sport Psychology Organizations

Year Founded	Organization	Organizational Components
1965	ISSP	*Exercise* and sport psychology Minor focus on motor learning, control, and development
1967	NASPSPA	*Exercise* and sport psychology Motor learning and control Motor development
1979	SPA	Sport psychology
1985	AAASP	*Health and exercise* psychology Social psychology Performance enhancement and intervention psychology
1986	Division 47 of APA	*Exercise* and sport psychology

ogy, Bruce Ogilvie is considered to be a founding father of *applied* sport psychology.

During the latter half of the 1960s, two landmark organizations emerged: the International Society of Sport Psychology and the North American Society for the Psychology of Sport and Physical Activity. See Table 2.1 for a listing of these and other key exercise and sport psychology organizations.

The International Society of Sport Psychology (ISSP) held its first meeting in Rome in 1965 and its second meeting four years later in Washington, DC. Numerous exercise psychology presentations were included in the 1968 meeting of ISSP and published in the proceedings. Some of these included "The Role of Play and Sport in Healthy Emotional Development" by Emma McCloy Layman, "Physical Activity Attitudes of Middle-Aged Males" by Dorothy Harris, "The Relationship between Physical Performance and Personality in Elementary School Children" by Roscoe C. Brown, Jr., "The Social Psychology of Play and Sport" by Gerald Kenyon, "Physical Fitness Correlates of Psychiatric Hospitalization" by William P. Morgan as well as a host of other exercise and sport psychology topics (Kenyon & Grogg, 1970).

The North American Society for the Psychology of Sport and Physical Activity (NASPSPA) was formed in 1967 and initially met in conjunction with the American Alliance for Health, Physical Education, Recreation, and Dance (AAHPERD). As the lengthy name of NASPSPA implies, the organization included the whole psychology of physical activity: exercise and sport psychology, motor learning and control, and motor development.

Formation of ISSP in 1965 and NASPSPA in 1967 was crucial in developing communication among exercise and sport psychologists throughout the world by providing annual conferences to facilitate research and the exchange of ideas. Although the names of these organizations include the term *sport psychology*, both organizations have examined exercise as well as sport psychology interests since their inception. Additional information about these organizations will be included later in the *Professional Organizations* section of this chapter.

The 1970s: Growth of Academic Information and a New Organization

During the 1970s, several early leaders in exercise and sport psychology wrote textbooks that have become landmarks in the field. These leaders include Bryant Cratty and Miroslav Vanek (1970), who wrote *Psychology and the Superior Athlete*; Jack Scott (1971), who attracted considerable attention with his book, *The Athletic Revolution*; and Robert Singer (1972), who authored *Coaching, Athletics, and Psychology*.

Dorothy Harris (1973) wrote a widely used text-

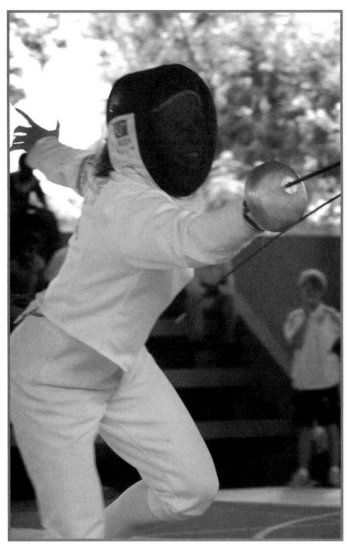

Photo courtesy of US Army

interest in exercise and sport psychology. Representing this growth of interest, a second U.S. organization, the Sport Psychology Academy (SPA), held its first meeting in 1979. This organization, still part of AAHPERD, attracts participants from the 25,000 AAHPERD members who primarily are teachers, coaches, and researchers. In 2005, there were 1,322 members of the SPA according to Alan L. Smith, who was Chair of the Sport Psychology Academy (personal communication, March 7, 2005).

The 1980s: New Organizations

The 1980s gave birth to two new exercise and sport psychology organizations in the United States. As highlighted in Table 2.1, AAASP began in 1985 with John Silva, an exercise and sport scientist, as its first president. Division 47, Exercise and Sport Psychology, within the APA began in 1986 with William P. Morgan, also an exercise and sport scientist, as its first president. Formation of AAASP and Division 47 of APA was particularly important to the development of exercise psychology within the United States.

Association for the Advancement of Applied Sport Psychology (AAASP). The original three programmatic and membership sections within AAASP were 1) Health and exercise psychology, 2) Social psychology, which often includes an exercise psychology component, and 3) Performance enhancement and intervention. As previously noted, performance enhancement is nearly synonymous with sport psychology to the layperson who is unfamiliar with exercise and sport psychology. The organizational structure of AAASP, however, emphasizes the need for "sport psychology" to encompass much more than performance enhancement—namely, health and exercise psychology, as well as the social psychology of exercise and sport.

American Psychological Association (APA), Division 47. The Division of Exercise and Sport Psychology in APA, which includes "exercise" in its name, clearly identifies psychologists' focus on exercise as well as sport psychology. As emphasized by both AAASP and Division 47 of APA, exercise psychology includes factors influencing the psychological benefits of exercise and exercise behaviors in diverse settings. Each of these organizations is described more fully later in this chapter.

The 1990s: Certification

AAASP. A milestone in exercise and sport psychology was the establishment of certification criteria by AAASP in 1991. The certification requirements describe the adequate and necessary coursework and practicum experience needed to serve as an educa-

book, *Involvement in Sport: A Somatopsychic Rationale for Physical Activity* that included numerous chapters that focused on exercise psychology. Some of the chapters in her text included exercise psychology chapters such as "Do Adults Play? The Meaning of Physical Activity," "Theories of Physical Activity Involvement," "Motivational Factors Influencing Physical Activity Involvement," "Does Inactivity Promote Obesity?", "Body Image: The Relationship to Movement," "Kinesthetic Satisfaction," and "Personality and Involvement in Physical Activity." These chapters are as relevant today as they were in 1973 and mark the beginning of the scientific study of exercise psychology (Mutrie, 2005). To commemorate Harris's many contributions, the Association for the Advancement of Applied Sport Psychology (AAASP) has honored, since 1992, an emerging scholar/practitioner in exercise or sport psychology who has made significant contributions to AAASP with a Dorothy V. Harris Memorial Award.

Since the mid-1970s, the increasing number of new textbooks and edited books illustrates the growing

tional exercise and sport psychology consultant. The specification of minimal preparation also provides colleges and universities with guidelines for courses and practicum experiences for students who aspire to be exercise and sport psychology consultants in the areas of exercise psychology and sport psychology. These certification requirements of AAASP also serve as a useful guide if you wish to select a university that offers a strong specialization in exercise or sport psychology. Consult the AAASP web site at *www.aasponline.org* for the most recent information about becoming a certified consultant of AAASP. Basic requirements for Certified Consultants include the following:

- Current membership in AAASP;
- *A doctoral degree* in a related area of study, or program equivalent to three full-time academic years of study at an accredited institute of higher education as evidenced by an official university transcript;
- *Completion of three-credit hour courses, primarily at the graduate level,* in the 12 specific areas identified in Table 2.2,;
- *400 hours of practical internship experience* that must be supervised by a certified consultant of AAASP or another qualified specialist in exercise or sport psychology (Note: In 2002, AAASP approved certification for exercise and sport psychologists with master's degrees as described later in this chapter); and
- *Attendance at three AAASP conferences* prior to applying for certification (Burke, Sachs, & Smisson, 2004).

In 1995, the United States Olympic Committee (USOC) and AAASP coordinated efforts in the recognition of well-qualified exercise and sport psychologists. Upon attaining certification by AAASP, individuals can apply to the USOC for inclusion in the USOC Sport Psychology Registry. The Registry was established in 1983 as a mechanism for identifying outstanding professionals in the field of sport psychology. The only requirement for inclusion in the USOC Registry, in addition to obtaining AAASP certification, is membership in the APA and completion of an application form.

Value of AAASP certification. The AAASP certification requirements are helpful in providing brief descriptions of what exercise or sport psychologists have studied, the extent of their practicum experiences, and what they are qualified to do. Overall, certification identifies professionals who are minimally qualified to work as exercise and sport psychologists. The courses required for certification are listed in Table 2.2 and need primarily to be graduate level courses. Requirements for certification by AAASP

were modified in 1994 and again in 2003. Most likely, they will change again in the future. The certification requirements are not etched in stone, but they do identify the types of courses that prospective undergraduate students, and especially graduate students, should complete if they are interested in becoming exercise or sport psychologists.

If you are planning to specialize in exercise psychology and these courses are not offered at your present university, you might consider attending a university where a specialization is available. Program strengths and the faculty's academic interests are important as you apply to graduate programs. For information about graduate programs in exercise and sport psychology, consult the most recent edition of the comprehensive *Directory of Graduate Programs in Applied Sport Psychology* (Burke et al., 2004). This *Directory of Graduate Programs* is a publication sponsored by AAASP and can be purchased from Fitness Information Technology at www.fitinfotech.com. The Directory includes in-depth descriptions of the more than 100 master's and doctoral degree programs in exercise and sport psychology in the United States, and also in a wide range of countries including Australia, Canada, Great Britain, and South Africa.

If you wish to obtain additional information about certification, contact the current secretary-treasurer of AAASP, whose name is listed as a member of the Executive Board and appears in each issue of the *Journal of Applied Sport Psychology*. The secretary-treasurer of AAASP will assist you in locating the name and address of the current chairperson of the Certification Review Committee, who can provide the most current certification requirements. The *Directory of Graduate Programs in Applied Sport Psychology* also provides additional information about becoming a Certified Consultant, AAASP (Burke et al., 2004).

2000 and Beyond: Issues in the Field

Current issues in exercise psychology tend to focus on the necessary qualifications of exercise psychologists, whether there is a need to create an accreditation system for rating university programs, and the employment opportunities for new professionals in exercise psychology. Additional issues include attracting new students to the study of exercise psychology, broadening the scope of exercise psychology to include more diverse populations of exercisers in a variety of settings, and clarifying the desirability of a primary background in exercise science or in psychology.

Professional qualifications of specialists in exercise psychology. The AAASP certification guidelines broadly define the necessary but minimal qualifications of both exercise and sport psychologists. Thus, certifi-

Table 2.2

Required Coursework for Becoming a Certified Consultant by the Association for the Advancement of Applied Sport Psychology

Courses[a]	Description and Details
Either Sport Science or Psychology Courses	
1. *Professional ethics and standards* _____	One course, or parts of several courses on professional ethics and standards
2. *Sport psychology subdisciplines* _____	Three courses: two must be at the graduate level. One course may be an independent study course. Courses in the subdisciplines of health/exercise psychology, social psychology of sport, and intervention/performance enhancement
3. *Research design, statistics, and* _____ *psychological assessment*[b]	One course in any of these three areas
4. *Biological bases of behavior:* _____ *neuropsychology, psychopharmacology*[c]	A course in biomechanics, kinesiology, comparative psychology, exercise physiology, sensation, physiological psychology, psychopharmacology
5. *Cognitive-Affective bases of behavior*[c] _____	A course in cognition, emotion, learning, memory, motivation, thinking, perception, motor development, or motor learning/control
6. *Social bases of behavior*[c] _____	A course in cultural/ethnic group processes, sociology of sport, social psychology, organizational and systems theory, or gender roles in sport
Primarily Sport Science Courses	
7. *Biomechanical and/or physiological bases* _____ *of sport*	One course in kinesiology, biomechanics, or exercise physiology
8. *Historical, philosophical, social, or motor* _____ *behavior bases of sport*	One course on the history of sport, philosophy of sport/physical activity, sociology of sport, motor learning/control, or motor development
9. *Skills, techniques, and analysis within* _____ *exercise or sport, and related experiences such as coaching*	A course that includes the teaching of sport skills and techniques, formal coaching experiences, or organized participation.
Primarily Psychology Courses	
10. *Psychopathology and its assessment* _____	One course in abnormal psychology or psychopathology
11. *Counseling skills*[b] _____	Course work designed to foster basic skills in counseling (e.g., course work in basic interventions in counseling, supervised practica in counseling, and clinical or industrial psychology)
12. *Individual behavior*[c] _____	A course in developmental psychology, personality theory, health psychology, individual differences, or exercise behavior

[a] A maximum of four courses can be completed at the undergraduate level.
[b] Graduate course work only.
[c] At least two of four courses (Content Areas: #4, 5, 6, and 12) must be met through psychology courses, rather than sport science scores.

cation is awarded to individuals, not to academic programs or institutions. Course requirements for certification focus on the movement sciences, psychology, and specifically on exercise and sport psychology.

An often-debated issue in exercise psychology is whether the primary preparation of the exercise psychologist comes from psychology or from movement sciences. This issue is complex because most states in the United States and provinces in Canada require psychologists of all types to be licensed by the state or province in which they reside. Thus, individuals with a primary background in movement or exercise science can be *specialists* in exercise psychology. They cannot identify themselves as *exercise psychologists* since use of the word *psychologist* requires licensure. In contrast, psychologists with little or no background in movement sciences or exercise psychology ethically cannot identify themselves as *exercise* psychologists even though they are psychologists.

Determination of the "best" training for exercise psychologists differs from person to person and often reflects the individual's own professional background. Because exercise psychology is truly a merger of exercise science and psychology, informed exercise psychologists recognize the credibility of individuals from both backgrounds with the caveat that they have different professional competencies if they are working with exercisers and athletes who are members of the general population and with exercisers and athletes who have psychological problems.

Certified Consultant, AAASP: For specialists with Master's Degrees. In 2002, AAASP extended the possibility of certification to specialists in exercise and sport psychology who have completed master's degree programs. Master's degree applicants need to complete the same requirements as applicants who have completed doctoral degrees. These include (1) the same coursework listed in Table 2.2, and (2) the 400 hours of supervised experience for obtaining *Provisional Certification*. With the completion of the requirement of an additional 300 hours of supervised practicum hours (i.e., a total of 700 hours), a master's degree individual can be a fully Certified Consultant, AAASP. Certified Consultant application forms are available on the AAASP web site, *www.aaasp online.org*. These application forms are useful when applying for certification and also when planning your sequence of courses at the undergraduate, master's, and doctoral levels of study.

APA Proficiency in sport psychology. Although the new APA Proficiency is in sport psychology, rather than in exercise psychology, it may be of interest to some specialists in exercise psychology. In 2003, the APA's Council of Representatives approved the Proficiency. Proficiency status indicates that sport psychology is recognized as a specific part of the practice of psychology. The useful purposes of the Proficiency in Sport Psychology are (1) to assist the public in recognizing the services and skills of sport psychologists, and (2) to assist psychologists in recognizing the knowledge and skills necessary for sport psychologists. As noted in *ESPNews*, the newsletter of APA Division 47,

> The APA Proficiency recognizes specialization in sport psychology as a post-graduate specialization after a doctoral degree in one of the primary areas of psychology. The Proficiency encompasses training in psychological skills of athletes, in the well being of athletes, in the systematic issues associated with sports organizations, and in the developmental and social aspects of sports participation. (American Psychological Association, Division 47, 2003, p. 13)

The APA Proficiency emphasizes specialized knowledge in sport psychology that includes many of the same areas of study required for AAASP Certification such as the social and historical foundations of sport, principles of applied sport psychology, developmental and social issues related to sport participation, and knowledge of the biobehavioral bases of sport. See *www.apadiv47.org* for additional details about the *Proficiency in Sport Psychology*.

The Proficiency focuses more on psychologists working with *athletes* at age-group, high school, collegiate, professional, and master's/senior levels of competition than on psychologists working with the use of exercise for psychological well-being and exercise adherence. Key procedures and practices identified in the APA Proficiency include psychological skills training for athletes, goal-setting and performance profiling for athletes, and visualization and performance planning for athletes (American Psychological Association, Division 47, 2003). Perhaps in future years, the scope of the Proficiency will be broadened to include exercisers and associated with recreational and health-related physical activities since Division 47 includes a strong exercise emphasis.

Accreditation of programs of study. Desirability of accrediting university programs in exercise psychology is closely related to the certification process. Certification focuses on the competencies and qualifications of the individual who is certified. In contrast, accreditation focuses on the quality of an entire program of study at a university. Accreditation of a program includes a large number of quality indicators: number of full-time faculty who have specializations in exercise psychology, number and breadth of courses offered, and opportunities for supervised practicum experiences. Accreditation provides students with assurance of program quality. However, determining the exact factors to be included in the accreditation

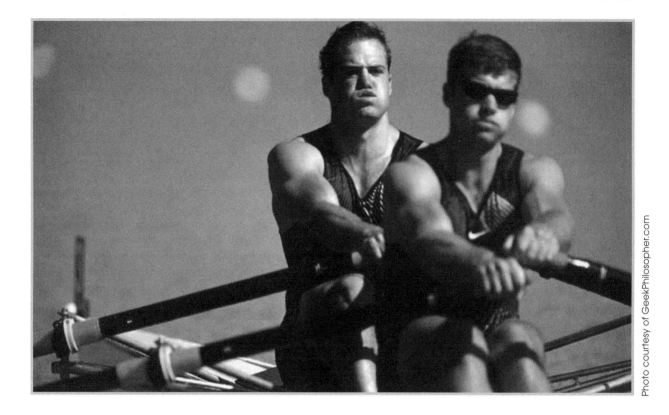

process and identifying an organization responsible for the accreditation require considerable planning and financial support. Thus, accreditation continues to be a widely discussed possibility in the newly burgeoning field of exercise psychology.

Employment opportunities. Potential employment opportunities for exercise psychologists are vast. However, in actuality, many exercise psychologists are employed in colleges and universities where they teach courses in exercise psychology. Exercise psychologists tend to be housed in exercise and sport science departments, such as departments of kinesiology, physical education, human movement, and exercise and sport science. Some exercise psychology faculty are also included in psychology departments, especially in departments with strong concentrations in educational, counseling, and health psychology.

In addition to teaching at universities, specialists in exercise psychology also work as

- Managers of corporate fitness programs,
- Personal trainers,
- Coaches,
- Physical education teachers,
- Counselors in physical rehabilitation programs with diverse clients, and
- Exercise specialists with older populations.

Many exercise psychologists have doctoral degrees in exercise and sport psychology and master's or undergraduate degrees in related areas that enhance their employment opportunities. For example, if you had a major in exercise physiology at the undergraduate level and a specialization in exercise psychology at the graduate level, you would have ideal qualifications to be a personal trainer or director of corporate fitness. Illustrating the employment versatility of a graduate degree in exercise psychology, completing a master's degree in exercise psychology would enable you as a teacher of physical education to employ your pedagogical skills and physical education background in a way that encourages a lifetime of participation, enjoyment of physical activity, and the use of exercise for stress management, mood alteration, enhanced self-concept, and flow.

Exercise Psychology and the Scientist-Practitioner Model

Specialists in exercise psychology focus on helping people reach their personal exercise goals. This includes assisting people in discovering and creating programs that fit their exercise goals; guiding the choice of exercise to encourage participants to maximize their personal enjoyment; and facilitating exercise adoption, maintenance, and adherence of their exercise program. At first glance, this seems different from the sport psychologist's emphasis on performance enhancement and winning. However, there is considerable overlap between exercise and sport psychology. *Exercise psychology* focuses on the psychological health and well-being of the participants. *Sport psychology* emphasizes psychological well-being in athletes to help them reach their maximal potential. Rather than fragment the content of exercise and sport psychology, it is important that researchers and practitioners in both areas work together, share ideas, and advance the field of exercise and sport psychology.

The Importance of Research Skills

Exercise psychologists—whether they consider themselves specialists in health psychology, social psychology, clinical psychology, or educational psychology—need to develop solid research skills. Essentially, research tests the effective-

ness of new ideas and techniques, problem solving, and theory development. Without well-designed research studies, there would be no objective information about the value of one approach or technique in comparison to another. Exercise psychologists use research methodology to test hypotheses and to eliminate personal bias in determining effective exercise psychology practices and procedures.

This research must be vitally linked to existing theory and knowledge as well as to daily practices in practical settings. If not based on research findings, services to clients are of unknown value and benefit. Figure 2.1 depicts the scientist-practitioner model. Connections are vital between theory development,

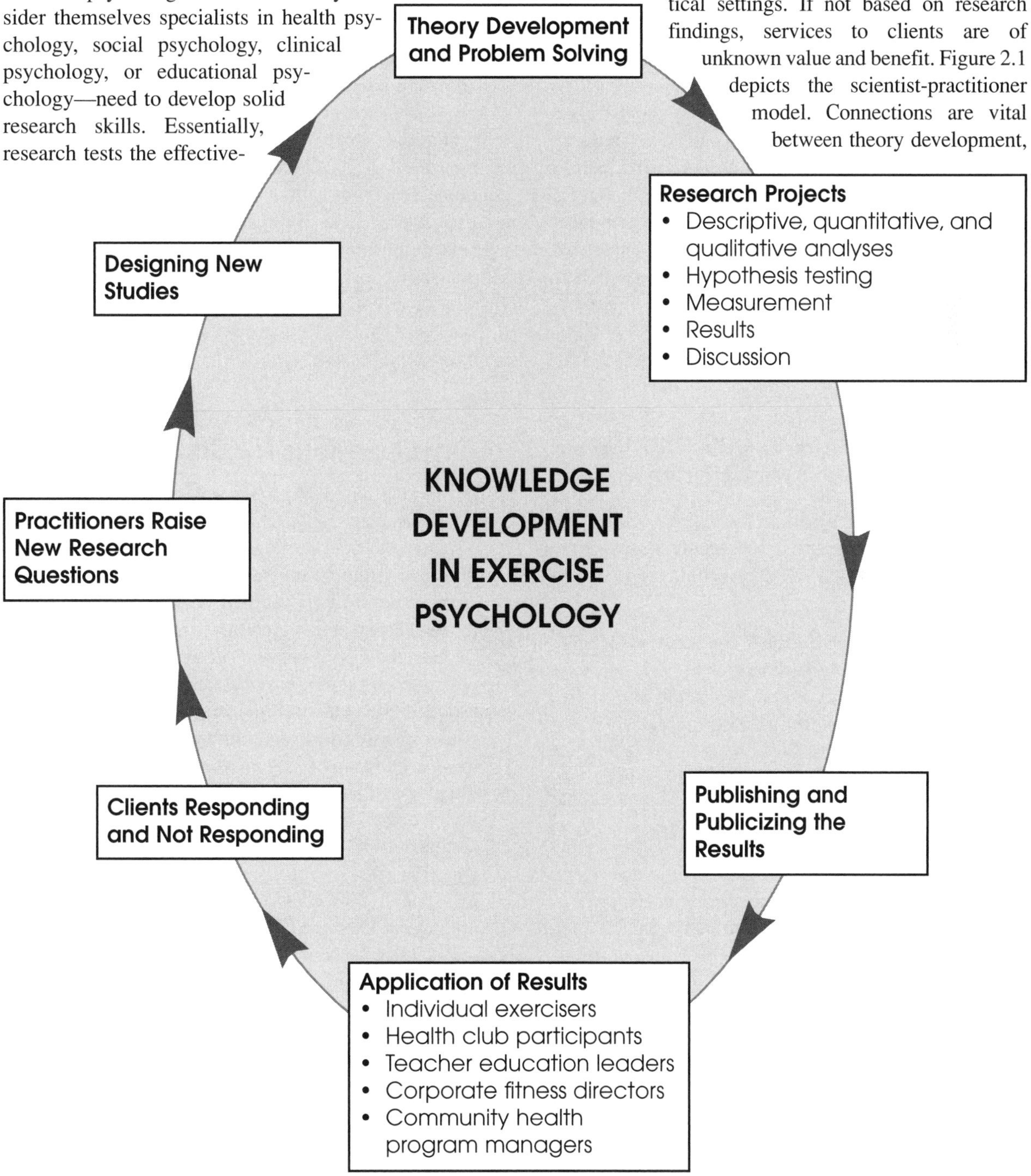

Theory Development and Problem Solving

Research Projects
• Descriptive, quantitative, and qualitative analyses
• Hypothesis testing
• Measurement
• Results
• Discussion

Designing New Studies

KNOWLEDGE DEVELOPMENT IN EXERCISE PSYCHOLOGY

Practitioners Raise New Research Questions

Clients Responding and Not Responding

Publishing and Publicizing the Results

Application of Results
• Individual exercisers
• Health club participants
• Teacher education leaders
• Corporate fitness directors
• Community health program managers

Figure 2.1. The scientist-practitioner model: Theory, research, application, and continuation of the cycle.

research, application of research findings, the raising of new research questions, additional studies, and the development or refinement of new theories.

Application of Research Results in Diverse Settings

Specialists in exercise psychology need a basic level of research skills to be able to read, interpret, and use information in research publications. In addition, physical therapists, coaches, personal trainers, and educators need to be able to appraise the current research and to incorporate new exercise psychology ideas and approaches into their respective specializations. (Figure 2.1 illustrates the need to apply research-based results by diverse professionals in exercise-related settings.) Individual exercisers, health club participants, teacher education leaders, corporate fitness directors, and leaders of community health programs observe the successes, failures, and inconsistencies of their new research-based applications in their programs and then can design new studies to further investigate their concerns. A major point stressed throughout this book is that theory and research form the basis of the applied practice of exercise psychology.

Unanswered Questions and Use of the Scientist-Practitioner Model

Here are some examples of the many unanswered questions in the newly emerging field of exercise psychology:

- Which types of exercise are most associated with desirable mood changes?
- How long (as indicated by the length of exercise session) does a person need to exercise to experience these benefits?
- Do these benefits occur right away, or does the exerciser need to establish some minimal fitness level prior to experiencing the benefits?

These questions and others can best be answered from a scientific approach based on theory development, application of the research information in the real world, and then formulation of new research questions based on the success of the application, which is illustrated in Figure 2.1.

According to the *scientist-practitioner model*, research and practice continually interact and strengthen one another. The knowledge base of exercise psychology needs continual development and refinement to establish information that is valuable to diverse movement specialists. State-of-the-art knowledge is in constant flux as the results of new research studies emerge

and practitioners incorporate the findings into their procedures. Theories, ideas, and hypotheses change as researchers provide new ideas and approaches that practitioners can apply.

For example, current research findings suggest that exercise programs at light and moderate intensities are more likely to provide positive mood changes than are high-intensity programs that deplete the participants' physical and psychological resources. Researchers can alert exercise practitioners to the likelihood that exercise intensity may be associated with differential changes in mood. Practitioners then can pass this information on to their clients, test the benefits of light and moderate exercise programs, and provide new insights—such as the role of an individual exerciser's preferences in the exercise intensity and mood relationship—to researchers for further investigation. Some exercisers truly may prefer high-intensity exercise. A preference for specific exercise intensity may have implications for mood alteration. The cycle of generating new information about exercise and mood alteration continues from researcher to practitioner and from the practitioner back to the researcher in the cycle depicted in Figure 2.1.

Benefits of Professional Organizations for Students

By joining an exercise psychology organization you will learn firsthand about the latest research and key issues in the field by receiving copies of the organization's newsletters and professional journals. Professional organizations continue to contribute greatly to the development and growth of exercise psychology.

Attending national and international conferences will enable you to meet individuals with diverse interests and competencies in exercise psychology as you gather in a single location for concentrated interaction. Program sessions focus on key issues and theories in exercise psychology. Conference participants meet and interact with other exercise psychologists who have similar interests. Attending conferences also provides participants with renewed professional energy, new ideas, new approaches, and sources of information that are invaluable when they return home to their individual exercise psychology practices and universities.

Receiving published newsletters and journals several times a year is another way that you benefit from joining professional organizations such as ISSP, NASPSPA, and AAASP. These publications keep members abreast of current issues, developments, controversies, and the latest research in exercise psychology. Professional organizations and the people in them can be considered the lifeblood of exercise psychology.

Professional organizations in exercise psychology

seek student members by offering reduced membership fees. If you are contemplating a possible career in exercise psychology, you should join at least one professional organization while still a student. Benefits include information about future conferences and necessary registration forms, familiarity with the "hot" topics within the field that might be of interest, and copies of the organization's journal.

By joining a professional organization, you also will gain information about faculty with whom you might want to study in the future, familiarity with the major graduate programs at other universities, availability of graduate assistantships, and current job opportunities. As a service to students, AAASP has held a Graduate Program Fair in recent years as part of the annual conference. The Fair acquaints you with graduate programs at specific universities. In conclusion, attending conferences enables you to meet the people whom you have read about, to interact with other students attending the conference, and to speak with directors of graduate programs at a variety of colleges and universities. The membership fee is money well spent.

The following section on professional organizations assists you in deciding whether any of the professional exercise/sport psychology organizations are allied with your future career directions. Each organization has a different focus based on its goals and member characteristics. See Table 2.3 for the Web addresses of organizations in exercise and sport psychology. After deciding to join a specific organization, you can locate a membership application either on the Web or in the journal published by the organization. If this information is unavailable, the officers of the organization are usually listed in the journal.

Table 2.3

Web Addresses for Exercise and Sport Psychology Organizations and Listserves

Organization	Web Address
American Academy of Kinesiology and Physical Education (AAKPE)	www.aakpe.org
American Alliance for Health, Physical Education, Recreation, and Dance (AAHPERD)	www.aahperd.org
American College of Sports Medicine (ACSM)	www.acsm.org
American Psychological Association, Division 47 (APA, Div 47)	www.psyc.unt.edu/apadiv47
American Psychological Association, Division 47: Listserve	div47@lists.apa.org
Association for the Advancement of Applied Sport Psychology (AAASP)	www.aaasponline.org
International Society of Sport Psychology (ISSP)	www.issponline.org
North American Society for the Psychology of Sport and Physical Activity (NASPSPA)	www.naspspa.org
Sport Psychology Academy (SPA)	www.aahperd.org/academy action/academies/ psych.html

CASE STUDY 2.1

What Graduate Program Should I Choose: Exercise Science or Psychology?

Chris was a master's student entering the second year of a 2-year master's program in exercise psychology. He had an undergraduate degree in psychology, soon would have a master's degree in exercise psychology from a department of exercise science, and was contemplating the continuation of his graduate studies. Chris knew that he needed to start applying for admission and for assistantships at universities sometime during the early fall, but had no idea whether he should pursue further work in exercise science or psychology.

Type of Department: Sport Science, or Psychology

As the result of conversations with his graduate advisor, Chris learned that the department in which his degree was located was an important consideration when choosing a doctoral program. The quality of the academic program and his determination of what he really wanted to do once he graduated also were important considerations when selecting a university. For example, if Chris wanted to be a psychologist in private practice, he needed to complete his doctorate in psychology. If, however, he wanted to teach at a university, his degree could be from departments in either exercise and sport science or psychology.

Membership in Professional Organizations

To gather the information needed in the decision-making process, Chris renewed his student membership in two professional organizations: Division 47 of APA and AAASP. He carefully read their newsletters and journals to become more familiar with issues in the field and with the active researchers in exercise psychology. Chris also had an opportunity to participate in the four-day annual meeting of AAASP, since it was within driving distance of his home university. This meeting, which occurred during the fall semester when he was enmeshed in the process of applying to doctoral programs, was invaluable. Chris met other master's program students who also were contemplating doctoral programs, and they shared their perceptions of programs. At the conference, he also met with many faculty members at universities offering doctoral programs, including those at the universities he was most interested in attending.

Chris subsequently became a member of the sport psychology listserv that is organized by Dr. Michael Sachs at Temple University.[a] At first, he was a passive observer of the online discussions, but later became an active participant himself and asked questions about graduate programs in clinical aspects of exercise psychology.

The Thinking Process: What Do I Really Want to Do Professionally?

After much contemplation, Chris decided he wanted to teach at a university, but that he also wanted to be able to work with exercisers who might also have clinical problems such as eating disorders, substance abuse, and exercise addiction. He then applied for doctoral programs in exercise psychology that were offered in psychology departments. That way, he could apply for licensure as a psychologist within his home state.

Maximizing the Information Available when Selecting a University Program

Chris looked through the most recent *Directory of Graduate Programs in Applied Sport Psychology* (Burke, Sachs, & Smisson, 2004), contacted the directors of potential programs that would enable him to earn a doctorate in psychology, and completed numerous application forms. Throughout the long process, Chris learned about the differences among the various programs he was applying to, had telephone conversations with the program directors, and clarified his own thinking about what it was that he really wanted to do. Although he hated to pay the application fees, Chris applied to five doctoral programs to see which ones might be interested in him and to learn about potential assistantships. He knew that the assistantships would provide much-needed financial assistance as well as work-related experiences that would allow him to enhance his exercise psychology skills and knowledge.

The Decision

After being accepted at four universities, Chris was awarded assistantships at two of them. He carefully considered the following: (1) whether the programs were in exercise science or psychology departments, (2) the content and quality of the programs, and (3) the financial assistance available. He chose a doctoral program that was offered by a department of exercise science and one that included numerous courses offered by the psychology department. The doctoral program also emphasized both the research and application aspects of exercise psychology. By planning for the doctoral programs early in the fall, Chris was able to gain admission to a university that fit his professional aspirations and his financial need.

---

[a] Contact Dr. Michael Sachs (V5289E@VM.TEMPLE.EDU) for information about joining the sport psychology listserve.

As noted in Case Study 2.1, student membership in professional organizations is of great value and can help you in choosing a specific master's or doctoral program. By contacting the organization's treasurer, you can obtain needed information about membership application. The following section

- Highlights specific organizations to help you choose one for joining that best suits your professional interests, and
- Describes the diverse research journals in the field that you will read as you become more active in the research-practitioner process.

International Organizations in Exercise Psychology

The International Society of Sport Psychology (ISSP) was founded during a meeting of interested individuals in Rome, Italy, in 1965. More than 400 individuals from 27 countries attended the Rome meeting of the ISSP. The second meeting was held 4 years later in Washington, DC, and the ISSP has been holding international conferences every 4 years since 1965. Meeting locations include Ottawa, Canada (1981), Copenhagen, Denmark (1985), Singapore (1989), Lisbon, Portugal (1993), Netanya, Israel (1997), Skiathos, Greece (2001), and Sydney, Australia (2005). It is anticipated that in 2009, the meeting will be in Morocco. At the ISSP World Congress in Sydney, participants from more than 50 different countries participated.

Ferruccio Antonelli was the first president of the ISSP. He also served as editor of the organization's *International Journal of Sport Psychology* from its first issue in 1970 until 1988. Between 1988 and 2000, Antonelli was honorary editor of the quarterly journal, which includes exercise as well as sport psychology research from all parts of the globe. Recently, the ISSP discontinued sponsorship of the *International Journal of Sport Psychology* and now sponsors another journal: the *International Journal of Sport and Exercise Psychology*, which first was published in 2003.

Reflecting the international interest in exercise psychology, national organizations have been formed throughout the world. The *Journal of Applied Sport Psychology* (AAASP, 1989), available in your college or university library, provides an in-depth account of the international development of exercise psychology. Examples of the many exercise and sport psychology organizations throughout the world include the following:

- College of Sport Psychologists within the Australian Psychological Society, founded in 1991,
- British Association of Sport and Exercise Sciences, launched in 1985,

- Canadian Psychomotor Learning and Sport Psychology Committee, begun in 1969,
- Chinese Society of Sport Psychology, founded in 1980,
- Italian Association of Sport Psychology, established in 1974,
- Sport Psychology Association of India, founded in 1986,
- Korean Society of Sport Psychology, founded in the late 1980s and currently enrolling 270 members (Chung, 1996), and
- Sport Psychology Association of Nigeria, begun in 1973.

U.S. Organizations in Exercise Psychology

The primary exercise and sport psychology organizations in the United States include the North American Society for the Psychology of Sport and Physical Activity (NASPSPA), the Sport Psychology Academy (SPA), the Association for the Advancement of Applied Sport Psychology (AAASP), and the Exercise and Sport Psychology Division of the American Psychological Association (APA). The American College of Sports Medicine (ACSM) focuses primarily on exercise physiology, but it also has an active exercise psychology section. Each of these organizations has a different emphasis within exercise psychology and has a distinctive membership base. Joining one or more of the following organizations provides students with valuable information for pursuing graduate study in exercise psychology.

The North American Society for the Psychology of Sport and Physical Activity (NASPSPSA)

Started in 1967, NASPSPA was the first sport psychology organization in the United States. The founders included Dr. Arthur Slater-Hammel (Indiana University), a researcher in motor learning; Dr. Roscoe Brown, Jr., a sport scientist at New York University who later became president of Bronx Community College; and Dr. Gerald Kenyon, a sport sociologist at the University of Wisconsin. In its early years, NASPSPA members gathered for a few days prior to the national convention of the American Alliance of Health, Physical Education, Recreation, and Dance (AAHPERD). Beginning with its annual conference in 1975, NASPSPA has held its annual meeting independent of any other organization.

Since its inception, NASPSPA has offered a broad interpretation of the content within sport psychology.

Its three program and membership areas include

- Exercise and sport psychology,
- Motor learning and control, and
- Motor development.

These membership areas emphasize the co-development of academic specializations that focus on the learning of motor skills, psychological considerations, and motor development. Because each of the three divisions receives equal program emphasis at the annual meeting, exercise psychology presentations constitute approximately a third of the program sessions held. In contrast to other exercise and sport psychology organizations, however, NASPSPA focuses primarily on research and has a strong membership interest in exercise as well as sport psychology. *The Journal of Sport and Exercise Psychology*, sponsored by NASPSPA, also focuses on research and is an outstanding source for diverse research topics in exercise and sport psychology. NASPSPA has a loyal group of exercise psychology members who value its research emphasis.

As in any organization, the number of members fluctuates from year to year. In the year 2005, according to its secretary and treasurer, A.L. Smith, the NASPSA had 508 members (personal communication, September 18, 2005; see Table 2.4). The exercise and sport psychology portion of the NASPSPA member-ship had 278 members in 2004. As shown in the table, the motor learning and control area had 261 members in this specialization. Motor development was the area with the fewest members. Combining the number of members interested in motor learning and in motor development, however, illustrates that less than half of the NASPSPA membership reports exercise and sport psychology as a primary interest. The strong student contingent within NASPSPA included 222 members, or 44% of the membership, in 2004. This large student membership argues well for the continued growth of NASPSPA as students become professional members and emphasizes widespread interest in the research emphasis in exercise and sport psychology.

The Sport Psychology Academy (SPA)

Founded in 1979, SPA had nearly 1,322 members in the year 2005 (A. L. Smith, personal communication, March 7, 2005). The reason for the huge membership in this organization is that SPA is part of AAHPERD, which had over 25,000 members in the year 2005 (D. Loy, personal communication, March 21, 2005). Because SPA members must join AAHPERD, most SPA members are primarily physical educators (in contrast to psychologists) who have practical and applied interests in exercise psychology. Of the four

Table 2.4
Membership Characteristics for NASPSPA, N = 508 (A.L. Smith; Secretary and Treasurer, North American Society for the Psychology of Sport and Physical Activity; personal communication, September 18, 2005)

Interest Areas [a]

Exercise and Sport Psychology	Motor Learning and Control	Motor Development
$n = 278$	$n = 261$	$n = 175$
39%	37%	25%

Types of Memberships

Professional	Student	Honorary/Retired
$n = 285$	$n = 222$	$n = 1$
56%	44%	0%

[a] Some of the 508 members have interests in more than one area. Thus, the number of members listing interests in specific areas totals 714.

exercise psychology organizations in the United States, SPA focuses the most on practical use of exercise and sport psychology information. As indicated by a former chairperson of SPA,

> The primary purpose of the . . . Sport Psychology Academy is to service the needs of the physical educators, coaches, and athletes. We are not in the business of clinical or counseling psychology, but rather we are a unique subdiscipline within physical education, which focuses on the mental aspects of performance. Our primary function is to teach and research performance enhancement strategies that can be used by *sport and recreation performers* [italics added]. (Cooke, 1993)

Annual meetings of SPA are held several days prior to and during the AAHPERD annual conference. Although SPA does not publish a journal, it publishes an electronic newsletter that contains information about the annual program. (See the SPA website listed in Table 2.3 to obtain a copy of the most recent Academy newsletter.) The primary focus of SPA is to interpret useful exercise and sport psychology research for physical education teachers and coaches. Each year since the early 1980s, the SPA has recognized outstanding dissertation research with a dissertation award. The 2005 recipient was Tiffanye Vargas-Tonsing, whose dissertation was entitled, "An Examination of Pre-Game Speeches and Their Effectiveness in Increasing Athletes' Levels of Self-Efficacy and Emotion."

The Association for the Advancement of Applied Sport Psychology (AAASP)

Dr. John Silva, a faculty member in the Department of Physical Education at the University of North Carolina, Chapel Hill, founded this organization in 1985. A unique aspect of AAASP is its emphasis on the integration of research and practice.

The scientist-practitioner model is a key consideration in AAASP program content at the annual conference and in the determination of which articles to publish in the *Journal of Applied Sport Psychology*. Journal articles include objective data as well as implications for professional use. As noted in Figure 2.1, exercise psychology techniques and approaches need continual testing to determine if they are effective, under what type of conditions they are effective, and for which exercisers. Researchers examine these types of questions for applied practitioners. Practitioners' use of various exercise psychology approaches and techniques gives rise to questions that point to a need for addtional research. Practitioners can conduct their own field research to answer these questions or work with other researchers to continually expand the knowledge base of exercise psychology.

Recognizing that exercise and sport psychology is a true cross-disciplinary field, AAASP has attracted nearly equal numbers of psychologists and sport scientists. In 1992, there were 370 psychologists, 327

Table 2.5

Membership Characteristics for AAASP, N = 1,125
(M. Fry, personal communication, March 29, 2005)

Professional Background of Members

Psychologists	Psychology and Sport Science	Exercise and Sport Science	Other and Not Reported
n = 247	*n* = 155	*n* = 219	*n* = 504
22%	14%	19%	45%

Types of Memberships

Professional	Student	Honorary/Retired	Not Reported
n = 534	*n* = 557	*n* = 11	*n* = 23
47%	50%	1%	2%

sport scientists, and 64 members from other disciplines. Since its formation in 1985, AAASP has attracted a large student membership. Of the 1,125 members of the organization in 2004, 557 or approximately 51% of the AAASP membership were students (M. Fry, personal communication, March 2, 2005). (Refer to Table 2.5 for additional membership information about the academic and professional backgrounds of AAASP members as you contemplate joining an exercise psychology organization.)

Members of AAASP are fairly evenly distributed between psychology and exercise/sport science. Students are integral members of the Association, and they organize conference sessions on topics reflecting student interests such as certification and job opportunities. A student member serves on the executive board; there is a student column in each issue of the newsletter; and students plan conference sessions and make presentations at the annual meeting. Each year, AAASP recognizes student members with awards for outstanding thesis and dissertation. In 2005, Emma Stodel was recognized for her dissertation, "Mental Skills Training for Enjoyment: Exploring Experiences, Processes, and Outcomes with Recreational Golfers." Jay Goldstein received the AAASP Master's Thesis Award for "An Empirical Test of a Motivational Model of 'Sideline Rage' and Aggression in the Parents of Youth Sport Soccer Players" (AAASP, 2005).

The tripartite organizational structure of AAASP focuses on three broad interest areas within exercise and sport psychology:

- Health psychology, which includes much of exercise psychology;
- Social psychology, which also includes exercise psychology; and
- Performance enhancement and intervention.

Health psychology, social psychology, and performance enhancement are equally represented by the presentations and keynote speakers at the annual fall conference, in the *AAASP Newsletter*, on the executive board, and in the editorial structure of the *Journal of Applied Sport Psychology*. As previously noted, AAASP is the only organization that certifies consultants in exercise and sport psychology.

American Psychological Association (APA), Division 47

The Division (47) for sport and exercise psychology of APA was established in 1986 and is the newest exercise psychology organization in the United States. A distinguishing aspect of Division 47 is the requirement that a doctoral degree in psychology (or equivalent training in sport science) is required for becoming a regular member of APA. Students are welcomed as affiliate members of APA. Due to the membership requirements, there are considerably more psychologists than physical educators in this organization.

The presidency of Division 47 tends to rotate naturally between specialists in sport science and psychology. The first two presidents—Dr. William P. Morgan from the University of Wisconsin and Dr. Dan Landers from Arizona State University—had exercise and sport science backgrounds. Recently, the presidency rotated from Dr. Robert Singer, Department of Exercise and Sport Science at the University of Florida, to Dr. Shane Murphy, a psychologist with Gold Medal Psychological Consultants, to Dr. Kate Hays, a psychologist in private practice. Further illustrating the sport science and psychology backgrounds of the leadership of Division 47, the 2005–2006 President was Frank M. Webbe, Florida Institute of Technology, who is a psychologist, and the President Elect is Penny McCullagh from California State University, Hayward, whose background is in sport science.

New divisions in APA are formed when sufficient members of the organizations indicate a willingness to join and pay divisional dues in a specific interest area. As indicated by the identification number of the Exercise and Sport Psychology Division, it was the 47th interest area established within APA. Establishment of Division 47 indicates that psychologists have become increasingly interested in the scientific, educational, and clinical foundations of exercise and sport psychology.

In 2005, Division 47 had 968 members, 109 of whom were student members (K. Cooke, personal communication, March 1, 2005). Division 47 publishes *The Exercise and Sport Psychology Newsletter*, which is sent to all members three times a year. The *Newsletter* provides a forum in which members communicate about pertinent issues related to the field of exercise and sport psychology. The Division has sponsored several texts published by the American Psychological Association. Examples of these include

- *Exploring Sport and Exercise Psychology* (Van Raalte & Brewer, 2002),
- *You're On! Consulting for Peak Performance* (Hays & Brown, Jr., 2004), and
- *Working It Out: Using Exercise in Psychotherapy* (Hays, 1999).

Division 47 also sponsors an annual dissertation award competition to recognize students' research that has potential for contributing to the theoretical and applied base of exercise and sport psychology. In 2005 the Dissertation Award recipient, Amy Latimer, examined "Bridging the Gap: Promoting Physical Activity Among Individuals with Spinal Cord Injury Within the Context of the Theory of Planned Behavior" (American Psychological Association, Division 47, 2005).

APA has approximately 150,000 members, and

more than 13,000 people from all divisions attended the 2004 annual conference in Hawaii (P. Miyamoto, personal communication, March 28, 2005). The size of membership can be overwhelming. A major advantage of attending an APA conference is the opportunity to hear presentations by a large number of world-famous psychologists from all areas of specializations within psychology, including exercise and sport psychology.

The American College of Sports Medicine (ACSM)

This organization focuses primarily on physiological adaptation to exercise and sport. Within the past few years, however, exercise psychologists have become actively involved in the organization by presenting papers and by organizing symposia at the annual meeting, which generally is held early in June. An increasing number of exercise psychologists are publishing their research in the organization's journal, *Medicine and Science in Sports and Exercise*.

The unique advantage of joining and participating in ACSM is an opportunity for a joint focus on the psychology and physiology of exercise. Mind and body are an integrated whole, and it is important to examine psychophysical changes associated with exercise and sport. Physiologists and psychologists are recognizing the need for interdisciplinary approaches to furthering our understanding of exercise and sport. ACSM is another large organization and has 18,483 members, of which 3,601 are student members (H. Lloyd, personal communication, March 1, 2005). Many of the members are physicians, and dues are fairly expensive. As with all of the organizations mentioned here, student members pay less than professional members.

Summary

The historical development of exercise psychology provides a broad perspective of exercise psychology as it is today. In the United States and throughout the world, early research focused on sport rather than on exercise psychology. Exercise psychology became an identifiable area of study in the late 1960s. Early topics included a focus on the psychological benefits of exercise and associated areas, such as setting and reaching exercise goals, creating exercise programs that encourage participants to maximize enjoyment, and encouraging adherence to exercise programs.

Between 1898 and the 1960s, exercise psychology was nearly inseparable from sport psychology. It was the second meeting of the International Society of Sport Psychology in 1968 that helped to identify exercise psychology as a separate area of investigation. Harris's (1973) book, *Involvement in Sport: A Somatopsychic Rationale for Physical Activity*, also

attracted scholarly focus on exercise psychology as a new field of specialization. Since the mid-1970s, new professional organizations and textbooks have appeared that included foci on exercise psychology. Some of these professional organizations included NASPSPA that was founded in 1967, AAASP in 1985, and Division 47 of APA, which were founded in 1986.

Requirements for professional certification of specialists with doctoral degrees were developed by AAASP in the 1990s, and certification of exercise psychology specialists with master's degrees was added in 2003. Current issues in exercise psychology include the determination of ideal professional qualifications, the desirability of accreditation for university programs of study, and the development of additional employment opportunities for new professionals.

It is important for professionals within exercise and sport psychology to recognize their commonalties. Exercise (and sport) psychologists need diverse combinations of academic strengths (educational, research, and clinical expertise) as they continue to create new professional opportunities in a variety of settings. These opportunities include university positions in diverse departments, corporate fitness centers, rehabilitation and medical settings, senior centers, and private practice.

Professional organizations—their foci, professional backgrounds of members, and publications and annual conferences—illustrate the diversity and commonality of interests among professionals within the growing field of exercise psychology. The International Society of Sport Psychology (ISSP), founded in Rome in 1965, facilitated the sharing of diverse research and applied international perspectives. The first U.S. organization, the North American Society for the Psychology of Sport and Physical Activity (NASPSPA), founded in 1967, is research based. NASPSPA provides members with interests in exercise and sport psychology, motor learning, and motor development many opportunities to examine broad issues of psychology in physical activity. These two organizations that emerged in the 1960s signaled a growing interest in exercise psychology. They provided the necessary channels for communication among professionals through meetings, newsletters, and journals.

The burgeoning field of exercise and sport psychology now includes the Sport Psychology Academy (SPA), which was founded in 1979, and professional organizations in many different countries. Some of these include Australia, Brazil, Canada, China, Great Britain, India, Italy, Nigeria, South Korea, and the United States.

The most recent exercise psychology organizations within the United States include the Association for the Advancement of Applied Sport Psychology (AAASP), which was founded in 1985; American Psychological

Association's (APA) Division 47, founded in 1986; and a growing contingent within the American College of Sports Medicine (ACSM).

As the name of AAASP implies with the inclusion of the word "applied," this dynamic organization emphasizes the scientist-practitioner model by stressing the interrelationships between research and practice. Division 47, Exercise and Sport Psychology, of APA primarily is composed of psychologists interested in all types of physical activity. ACSM members tend to be sport physicians and sport scientists who

concentrate on the psychophysical aspects of exercise psychology, the epidemiological benefits of physical activity, mood alteration in exercise and sport, and the mind-body and body-mind relationships.

In conclusion, exercise psychology could become a major research and applied field in the 21st century— as the American public realizes that exercise is a major influence on health, the quality of life, and personal satisfaction. The following chapters examine different ways that exercise contributes to psychological well-being and the quality of life.

Can You Define These Terms?

American Alliance for Health, Physical Education, Recreation, and Dance (AAHPERD)
___

American College of Sports Medicine (ACSM)
___

American Psychological Association, Division 47 (APA, Div 47)
___

Association for the Advancement of Applied Sport Psychology (AAASP)
___

International Society of Sport Psychology (ISSP)
___

North American Society for the Psychology of Sport and Physical Activity (NASPSPA)
___

Sport Psychology Academy (SPA)
___

Scientist-practitioner model
___

Can You Answer These Questions?

1. What is the scientist-practitioner model?

2. As an undergraduate student, which certification-required courses have you completed? Identify those that still remain for future study.

3. Do you anticipate being able to complete the course work requirements by the time you complete your master's degree? If not, what has hampered you in this process?

4. If you were completing your doctorate, would you anticipate completing all certification requirements by the time you complete your course work? If not, what are the impediments to your progress?

5. Do you think the requirements for being a Certified Consultant of AAASP are adequate to establish a minimum level of competency for sport psychologists? What is the basis for your decision?

6. If you were going to become a member of a professional organization in exercise psychology, which one would you choose? On what basis did you make this decision?

7. Would you choose a different professional organization if you were a regular professional member rather than a student member? Why might you change your choice of organizations?

CHAPTER 3

EXERCISE AND QUALITY OF LIFE

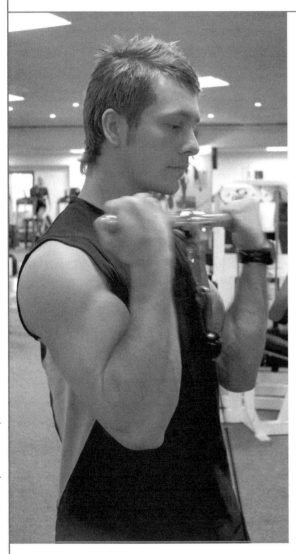

After reading this chapter, you should be able to

- Define *quality of life* and compare it to *subjective well-being* and *happiness*,

- Distinguish between the *health-enhancement* and the *disease-prevention models of exercise*,

- Identify and describe factors that influence quality of life,

- Identify and describe key measures of quality of life,

- Discuss the likelihood of acute and chronic mood changes after exercise in specific populations,

- Summarize the role of exercise as a stress management technique,

- Distinguish among distress, stress, and eustress,

- Explain how the following types of peak moments in exercise differ from one another: peak performance, peak experience, flow, and the exerciser's high,

- Define exercise enjoyment,

- Describe key sources of exercise enjoyment for young and older participants, and

- Review key roles of exercise in influencing life quality—in both desirable and undesirable directions.

Introduction

The diverse contributions of exercise to our lives can be captured by the phrase *quality of life*. Quality of life is an important issue for all individuals and is a multi-dimensional construct (e.g., Taillefer, Dupuis, Roberge, & LeMay, 2003; World Health Organization Group, 1995). This chapter focuses on the roles of exercise in establishing high levels of quality of life and the *health-enhancement model of exercise* (Berger & Motl, 2001; Berger & Tobar, in press). According to this model, health is a continuum that ranges from low or poor levels of health at one end, progresses through average or good levels of health at the midpoint, and continues to high or optimal levels of health at the other end of the continuum.

Quality of Life

Quality of life (QoL) reflects the harmonious satisfaction of personal goals and desires as defined in the current literature (Diener, 1994). On a practical base, QoL refers to behavioral functioning, or the ability to "do stuff," and to live long enough to do it (Kaplan, 1994, p. 451). "Doing Stuff" according to Kaplan's Ziggy theorem reflects the actual meaning of life, because the capability to perform activities is a central element in QoL.

Quality of life emphasizes subjective experiences, perceptions, and needs of the spirit, rather than objective conditions of life and affluence (Diener, 1994; Mroczek & Kolarz, 1998). Bradburn's (1969) classic description of psychological well-being, a major component of QoL, is an abundance of positive affect and an absence of negative affect. Quality of life also reflects the perceived degree to which individuals are able to satisfy their psychophysiological needs. Clearly, there are multiple factors that influence a person's assessment of QoL. The broad definition of QoL employed by the World Health Organization captures its many components:

> An individual's perception of their position in life in the context of the culture and value systems in which they live and in relation to their goals, expectations, standards and concerns. It is a broad construct incorporating in a complex way an individual's physical health, psychological state, level of independence, social relationships, personal beliefs and their relationships to salient features of the environment. (World Health Organization Group, 1995, p. 1405)

Depending on the type of exercise and its training parameters, exercise can be associated with a wide variety of benefits that are related to the quality of our lives. It is important to maintain a balanced perspective of exercise, however, by being aware that exercise can influence the QoL in both desirable and undesirable ways. In this chapter we discuss some of the desirable influences of exercise on the quality of our lives. These include

- Decreased negative affect,
- Increased positive affect,
- Optimal stress levels,
- Peak moments and flow, and
- Exercise enjoyment.

In addition to the factors listed above, exercise also enhances QoL by providing opportunities to enhance mood states and self-concepts, produce meaningful experiences, and slow the aging process. These later influences are briefly reviewed in this chapter and are the focus of subsequent chapters: Chapter 4 (Exercise and Enhanced Self-Concept and Self-Esteem), Chapter 5 (Mood and Exercise: Basic Mood Considerations), Chapter 6 (Mood Alteration, Self-Awareness, and Exercise: Multiple Relationships), Chapter 8 (Exercise as a Stress Management Technique), Chapter 14 (Personal Meaning in Physical Activity), and Chapter 19 (Exercise for Older Individuals).

Health-enhancement model of exercise. The health-enhancement model emphasizes that individuals who already are in good health can employ exercise activities to develop even higher levels of health. Through exercise, participants can improve their mood states, increase their vigor and vitality, decrease fatigue, and increase or decrease their stress levels as needed. Exercise also contributes to enhanced health and QoL by providing opportunities for peak moments and personal enjoyment. The health-enhancement model of exercise reminds us that positive health is directly related to our health behaviors and that exercise can facilitate our leading meaningful and purposeful lives.

Disease-prevention model of exercise. The health enhancement model is in direct contrast to the commonly employed *disease-prevention model of exercise*. As its name implies, the disease-prevention model focuses on the use of exercise to prevent and treat a variety of diseases such as coronary artery disease, osteoporosis, obesity, and cancer. Ideally, as a movement specialist with an understanding of exercise psychology, you will employ both models at appropriate times as you work with other health professionals to prevent and treat clients' diseases, and to enable healthy exercisers to enhance their QoL throughout all stages of life.

Definition of Terms

Subjective well-being and happiness. Subjective well-being is a key variable for measuring QoL (Andrews & Withey, 1976; Eid & Diener, 2004). Subjective well-being reflects the multidimensional evaluation of a person's life and includes cognitive judgments of life satisfaction and affective evaluations of moods and emotions. It can be conceptualized as a momentary state, or as a relatively stable trait. Whether subjective well-being is a state or trait characteristic depends on the timeframe of the assessment period (Eid & Diener, 2004). Theorized to be composed of at least three major components, subjective well-being includes the following:

- Appraisal of positive affect,
- Appraisal of negative affect, and
- Life satisfaction—which is more cognitive than affect-related (Pavot & Diener, 1993).

Happiness, a related term, is synonymous with subjective well-being (Seligman, 2002).

Positive, or hedonic, psychology. Terminology such as *quality of life*, *subjective well-being*, and *happiness* emphasizes a current focus in psychology on positive or hedonic psychology. Positive psychology emphasizes the phenomena of "elevation," health enhancement, "the good life," and personal strengths (Csikszentmihalyi, 1999; Seligman, 2002; Peterson & Seligman, 2004). Positive (or hedonic) psychology focuses on the positive aspects of life. With its root word of hedonism, hedonic psychology focuses on enjoyment, and other desirable psychological states. Hedonic or positive psychology focuses jointly on assisting people enhance their psychological strengths and on treating their weaknesses or psychological dysfunction such as anxiety, depression, and schizophrenia (Peterson & Seligman, 2004, p. 4).

Table 3.1

Positive Psychology: Virtues and Character Strengths (Peterson & Seligman, 2004)

Virtues	Character Strengths
Wisdom and knowledge	Creativity Curiosity Open-mindedness Love of learning **Perspective**
Courage	Bravery **Persistence** Integrity **Vitality**
Humanity	Love Kindness **Social intelligence**
Justice	Citizenship **Fairness** Leadership
Temperance	Forgiveness **Humility** Prudence **Self-regulation**
Transcendence	Appreciation of beauty and **excellence** Gratitude **Hope** Humor **Spirituality**

Note: Character strengths in bold print reflect strengths that may be developed through exercise and sport participation.

Examples of research issues within positive psychology, with its focus on life well-lived, include identifying and enhancing factors that contribute to psychological resilience, using turning points as opportunities for psychological growth, developing optimism, constructing meaning through engagement, and making the most of moments in our daily lives. See the edited book, *Flourishing: Positive Psychology and the Life Well-Lived* (Keyes & Haidt 2003), for reviews of each of these factors. In another book, *Authentic Happiness*, Martin Seligman (2002), a respected researcher, clinical psychologist, and former president of the American Psychological Association, identified the characteristics and strategies of people with positive outlooks as he examined ways to cultivate and experience positive emotional states such as happiness, glee, fun, contentment, meaning, and gratification.

To further positive psychology research, Seligman has developed the web site, *www.authentichappiness.com*. The Signature Strengths Survey at this web address enables Seligman to collect data to develop further his classification of virtues and character strengths. Seligman's basic premise is that strength of character makes the good life possible (Peterson & Seligman, 2004). The more often individuals use their strengths of character on a daily basis, the higher their perceived QoL. The Signature Strengths Survey also enables participants to test themselves on the virtues and character strengths identified in Table 3.1. The five strengths of curiosity, gratitude, hope, love, and vitality appear to be particularly strong predictors of life satisfaction, a major component of QoL (Peterson & Seligman, 2004).

Completing the Signature Strengths Survey provides an opportunity for self-reflection. It requires less than 30 minutes and helps test-takers to identify their personal psychological strengths. Consider completing the Survey to learn your signature strengths. Then, try to use them to analyze and enhance your own QoL, and the role of exercise within it.

Christopher Peterson and Martin Seligman (2004) continued to develop a classification system of character strengths and virtues in *Character Strengths and Virtues: A Handbook and Classification*. The book is designed to serve as a counterpart to the *Diagnostic and Statistical Manual of Mental Disorders* (DSM; American Psychiatric Association, 2000), the primary guide for diagnosing psychological disorders. Although Peterson and Seligman (2004, p. 9) cannot forecast the success of their classification system of character strengths and virtues, they indicate that they will be satisfied with the classification system if it provides ways of thinking about strengths, their naming, measurement approaches, and encourages development of the science of positive psychology. In support

of the health-enhancement model of health and exercise, Peterson and Seligman noted that they disavow the disease model in their approach to character and emphasized "that character strengths are the bedrock of the human condition and that strength-congruent activity represents an important route to the psychological good life" (p. 4).

The first Master's of Applied Positive Psychology Degree Program that began in 2005 at the University of Pennsylvania will further develop positive psychology as an area of scientific study. For information about the master's degree program, visit the web site at www.pennpositivepsych.org.

Throughout this chapter, the health-enhancement model of exercise is used to explore several key areas in which exercise may contribute to the good life and to flourishing. Other chapters in this text, such as those on exercise and self-concept, mood alteration, stress management, and personal meaning, also have implications for the QoL. Ultimately, however, both the perception of QoL and the role of exercise in enhancing it reside with the individual.

Factors Influencing Quality of Life

Quality of life reflects a person's assessment of his or her life as a whole. It refers to an overall sense of well-being and accompanying positive and negative feelings. It reflects only minimally specific life domains such as work, love, or even financial status. Quality of life refers to psychological and cognitive experiences and illustrates a paradox. Sociodemographic variables such as income, education, marital status, and age are important, but they explain only a small portion of the individual differences in our perceptions of life quality (Mroczek & Kolarz, 1998).

It seems that individual differences in quality of life, happiness, and subjective well-being are universally related to four broad sets of factors. These include

- *Contextual and situational factors* such as positive and negative affect (especially the frequency of their occurrence), emotion, stress, and physical health (Morris, 1999);
- *Personality factors* such as extroversion, neuroticism, optimism, and self-esteem (Diener & Lucas, 1999);
- *Sociodemographic factors* of age, education, marital status, gender, income, social class (Mroczek & Kolarz, 1998; Nolen-Hoeksema & Rusting, 1999); and
- *Subjective life satisfaction factors* (Oishi, Diener, Lucas, & Suh, 1999).

In addition, cross-cultural influences such as individualistic and collectivist values and the financial affluence of the country predict the global life satisfaction

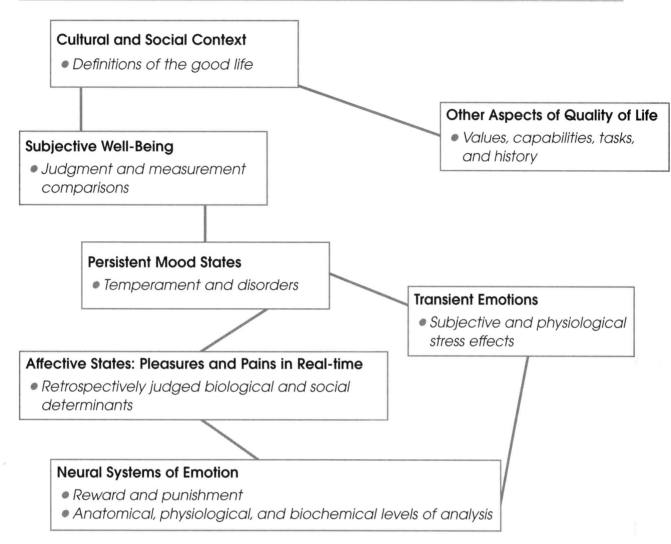

Figure 3.1. Factors of analysis in the quality of life. From *Well-Being: The Foundations of Hedonic Psychology*, p. x, by D. Kahneman, E. Diener, and N. Schwarz (Eds.). (1999). New York: Russell Sage Foundation. Copyright 1999 by Russell Sage Foundation. Adapted with permission.

of people living in different countries. In poorer nations, for example, financial satisfaction was strongly associated with life satisfaction (Oishi et al., 1999). In wealthy nations, home-life satisfaction was more strongly related to life satisfaction and subjective well-being than was financial satisfaction. As concluded by Oishi and colleagues, "universalist theories of SWB [subjective well-being] . . . need to be supplemented with theories that account for cross-cultural differences in values" (pp. 989–990).

Among nations that are equally wealthy, are individualistic, and emphasize personal autonomy rather than the common good, however, the factors of personality, sociodemographic variables, contextual variables, situational variables, and subjective experience are major influences on subjective well-being. Of the four primary factors that influence the quality of our lives, exercise contributes primarily to the

- Contextual and situational factors, especially to mood, emotion, stress levels, and physical health, and
- Subjective life-satisfaction factor that reflects how pleased we are with our lives.

A more complex version of the factors that influence the QoL is depicted in Figure 3.1. In the introduction to their book on well-being, Kahneman, Diener, and Schwarz (1999) describe QoL as including multiple factors and different levels of interaction. The factors emerged in response to the question, what makes for a *good life*? In other words, what is it that makes our lives pleasant or unpleasant and provides a subjective sense of well-being?

As illustrated in Figure 3.1, numerous factors contribute to the QoL. Macro *cultural and social context* are important for both the person who is responding to the question "What is a 'good life'?" and for the evaluator or researcher. Another influence on the "good life" is the *other aspects factor*, which includes objective characteristics such as crime rate, poverty, and pollution as well as values, capabilities, and tasks. The *subjective well-being factor* involves personal judgments and the comparisons of ourselves with other people, our past, our ideals, and aspirations. The *persistent mood states factor*, especially positive moods, and *transient emotions factor*, which include both subjective and physiological stress effects, are two additional contributors to our QoL. *Pleasures and pains factor* and the *neural systems of emotion factor* are based on subjective, biochemical, and physiological processes. These factors are integral components when determining QoL and illustrate the complexity of the concept. Despite the complexity, it is useful for movement specialists to know specific ways in which exercise can contribute in a desirable direction to clients' and their own QoL.

Approaches to Measuring the Quality of Life

To investigate the contributions of exercise to QoL, researchers need to measure participants' QoL before and after exercise programs to assess change. Measurement of QoL is so important that more than 300 scales have been developed to reflect various definitions of life quality (Spilker, Molinek, Johnston, Simpson, & Tilson, 1990).

Delighted-Terrible Scale

A typical paper-and-pencil measure of QoL is the Delighted-Terrible Scale, which asks this single question: "How do you feel about your life as a whole?" (Andrews & Whithey, 1976). As illustrated in Table 3.2, participants base their responses to this question according to the past year and expectations in the near future. As the name of the scale implies, the seven response options vary from *delighted* to *terrible*. Single-item quality-of-life measures include a "good/bad" dimension that has a natural zero point that is neither unpleasant nor pleasant (Kahneman et al., 1999).

Satisfaction with Life Scale (SWLS)

In contrast to single-item scales, other QoL measures reflect a global assessment of subjective well-being and include multiple items. For example, the Satisfac-

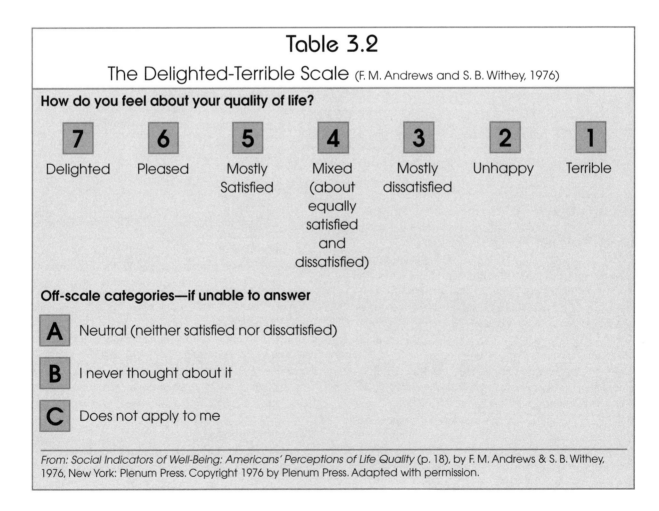

Table 3.2
The Delighted-Terrible Scale (F. M. Andrews and S. B. Withey, 1976)

How do you feel about your quality of life?

7	6	5	4	3	2	1
Delighted	Pleased	Mostly Satisfied	Mixed (about equally satisfied and dissatisfied)	Mostly dissatisfied	Unhappy	Terrible

Off-scale categories—if unable to answer

A Neutral (neither satisfied nor dissatisfied)

B I never thought about it

C Does not apply to me

From: Social Indicators of Well-Being: Americans' Perceptions of Life Quality (p. 18), by F. M. Andrews & S. B. Withey, 1976, New York: Plenum Press. Copyright 1976 by Plenum Press. Adapted with permission.

> # Table 3.3
> ## The Satisfaction With Life Scale (SWLS); Diener, Emmons, Larson, & Griffin, 1985)
>
> **Instructions:** Using the rating scale provided below, please indicate your agreement with each item. Place the appropriate number on the line preceding the item. Be open and honest in your response.
>
> **Rating scale**: **(1)** strongly disagree, **(2)** disagree, **(3)** slightly disagree, **(4)** neither agree nor disagree, **(5)** slightly agree, **(6)** agree, **(7)** strongly agree.
>
> _____ 1. In most ways my life is close to my ideal.
>
> _____ 2. The conditions of my life are excellent.
>
> _____ 3. I am satisfied with my life.
>
> _____ 4. So far I have gotten the important things I want in life.
>
> _____ 5. If I could live my life over, I would change almost nothing.

tion with Life Scale (SWLS) includes items shown in Table 3.3 (Diener et al., 1985; Pavot & Diener, 1993). Satisfaction with life can be assessed for a specific domain of life—such as school, work, and family—or globally. It is the global aspect of satisfaction with life that is most related to QoL.

The SWLS is a valid and reliable measure that is appropriate for a wide range of age-groups. Scores on SWLS are highly related to peer-reported subjective well-being (Pavot, Diener, Colvin, & Sandvik, 1991). In non-experimental survey settings, variability in global subjective well-being and personality (self-esteem, optimism, neuroticism, and extraversion) are independent as reflected by inconsistent and relatively small relationships. In contrast to experimental studies, both personality and occasion-specific mood states do not seem to affect reports of subjective well-being as measured by the SWLS (Eid & Diener, 2004).

SF-36 Health Survey (SF-36)

The SF-36 Health Survey (SF-36) is widely employed to measure health-related QoL and illustrates the importance of functional health and psychological well-being in QoL. This 36-item inventory includes eight subscales: four mental-health-related and four physical-health-related sub-subscales that quantify health-related QoL. It also includes a Health-Transition scale as noted in Table 3.4. The mental-health-related QoL sub-scales are Vitality, Social Functioning, Role-Emotional, and Mental Health. The physical-health-related QoL sub-scales are Physical Functioning, Bodily Pain, Role-Physical, and General Health (Ware, 2004). (See Table 3.4 for examples of test items in each of the SF-36 scales.) An advantage of using the SF-36 is that raw scores on the scales can be trans-

formed into normalized scores ranging from 0 to 100, with 100 representing the best possible score, to facilitate comparison of scores with national and international norms (Ware, Kosinski, & Gandek, 1993, 2000). Version 2 of the SF-36 Health Survey (SF-36v2) incorporates improved wording of items, instructions, and Survey format (Ware, Kosinski, & Dewey, 2000).

Conclusions

In a comparison of several different measurement strategies that included single-item measures, multiple-item scales, and memory search procedures, Pavot and Diener (1993) concluded that the various types of self-report measures demonstrated good reliability across a one-month period—despite fluctuations in transient mood states. Single-item inventories are valid measures of subjective well-being. Multi-item inventories, however, are less susceptible to item placement and contextual factors. The self-report measures of subjective well-being also correlate highly with reports by peers, family members, and friends (Pavot & Diener, 1993). For additional measurement considerations, such as comparisons of intensity and quality of subjective well-being across contexts, see Diener (1994) and Kahneman et al. (1999).

Importance of Quality of Life

The importance of life quality is illustrated by a quest for understanding the nature of "happiness" that goes back to the Golden Age of Greece. Aristotle and the Epicureans viewed happiness as the supreme good; all else in a person's life was viewed as a means to experiencing this highly desirable state. Once an individual attains happiness, nothing else is desired (Diener,

Table 3.4

The SF-36 Health Survey Version 2 (SF-36v2)—Your Health in General
(Ware, Kosinski, & Dewey, 2000)

Instructions: Please answer every question. Some questions may look like others, but each one is different. Please take the time to read and answer each question carefully, and mark an X in the one box that best describes your answer. *Thank you for completing this survey!*

Rating scale: The subscales differ from one another in the wording of the response choices. See Ware, et al., 2000, for specific response choices for various subscales.

Scale	No. of Items	Sample Items
Mental Health-Related Quality of Life		
Vitality	4	Did you feel full of life?
		Did you feel worn out?
Social Functioning	2	During the **past 4 weeks**, to what extent has your physical health or emotional problems interfered with your normal social activities with family, friends, neighbors, or groups?
		During the **past 4 weeks**, how much of the time has your **physical health or emotional problems** interfered with your social activities (**like visiting with friends, relatives, etc.)**?
Role-Emotional	3	Did work or other activities **less carefully than usual**
		Accomplished less than you would like
Mental Health	5	Have you felt so down in the dumps that nothing would cheer you up?
		Have you felt calm and peaceful?
Physical Health-Related Quality of Life		
Physical Functioning	10	**Vigorous activities**, such as running, lifting heavy objects, participating in strenuous sports
		Walking **more than a mile**
Bodily Pain	2	How much **bodily pain** have you had during the **past 4 weeks**?
		During the past **4 weeks**, how much did **pain** interfere with your normal work (including both work outside the home and housework)?
Role-Physical	4	Had **difficulty** performing the work or other activities (for example, it took extra effort)
		Were limited in the **kind** of work or other activities
General Health	5	I seem to get sick a little easier than other people
		I expect my health to get worse
Reported Health Transition	1	**Compared to one year ago,** how would you rate your health in general **now**?

1994). In addition to the longstanding interest in happiness, as human beings live longer, researchers are becoming even more concerned about the QoL. Quality of life becomes increasingly important as the human lifespan expands.

Quality of Life and Exercise

Exercise has much to contribute to the life quality of individuals throughout their lifespan (Berger & Tobar, in press). For example, a representative randomized controlled trial examined the effectiveness of a 24-week multi-modal program that included exercise and behavior modification (Atlantis, Chow, Kirby, & Singh, 2004). The program included aerobic exercise,

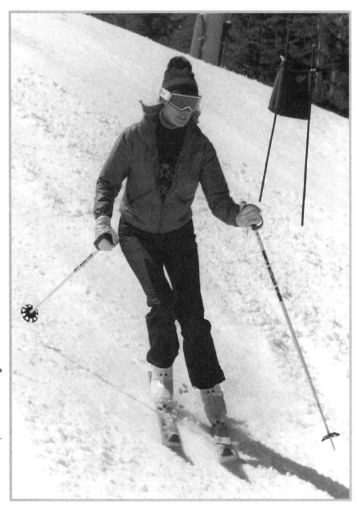

weight training, and behavior modification and was associated with significant benefits. These included increases in health-related QoL and decreases in depression and stress within a heterogeneous employee population. In this study, volunteer participants working in an Australian casino were stratified by gender and their combined depression, anxiety, and stress scores (i.e., mental health) prior to random assignment

to treatment: (1) exercise and behavior modification, or (2) a wait-list control. They performed aerobic exercise on a variety of equipment at an intensity of 75% age-adjusted maximal heart rate three days a week for a minimum of 20 minutes. Participants performed the weight-training portion of the program in multiple sets (sets of 10 and 3 sets) for 30 to 45 minutes, two days a week or more. After the 24-week program, exercisers in comparison to the wait-list controls reported impressive increases in health-related QoL as measured on the SF-36 Health Survey. These exercisers significantly improved their scores on Vitality, Mental Health, Physical Functioning, Bodily Pain, and General Health. Participants in the lowest and middle tertiles measured at baseline reported greater improvements in these QoL scales than those in the highest tertile on the Mental Health scale.

To better understand the relationship between exercise and QoL, this chapter explores selected aspects of the relationship as indicated by changes in mood states and stress levels in members of "normal" populations, the occurrence of peak moments in exercise, and the enjoyment of physical activity. (Refer to Case Study 3.1 for an illustration of the roles that exercise can play in the life quality of two individuals, Tass and Stephen.) Exercise is directly related to their QoL by providing opportunities for mood enhancement, stress management, peak moments, and personal enjoyment.

Specific Aspects of the Relationships between Exercise and Subjective Well-Being in the General, Nonclinical Population

The relationship between physical activity and subjective well-being is complex. One contributor to this complexity is that there are many types or modes of physical activity. For example, the term *exercise* may refer to

- Acute and chronic exercise,
- Aerobic or anaerobic activities,
- Competitive and noncompetitive recreational physical activities,
- Group or solitary activities, and
- Activities performed by individuals who differ greatly in fitness and skill levels.

The psychological benefits of exercise, much like the physical benefits, probably differ for the various types of exercise identified above.

Other contributors to the complexity are that even within a single exercise mode such as tennis, many factors vary. Such factors include the training characteristics of intensity, duration, and frequency; the exer-

CASE STUDY 3.1

Exercise and the Quality of Life: Tass and Stephen

Tass and Stephen, recent college graduates, had just married and had new, high-responsibility jobs. Stephen was managing a new business, and Tass was the manager of a local restaurant. Tass and Stephen knew that exercise could enhance the quality of their lives in multiple ways, and yet they had trouble exercising on a regular basis. They were aware that exercise definitely improved their subjective well-being by improving desirable mood states such as vigor and decreasing undesirable mood states such as depression and anxiety. Each of them felt better after exercising than before they started.

Stress Management and Mood Enhancement

In addition, exercise, depending on its type, helped Stephen and Tass either decrease or increase their stress levels as needed to reach optimal levels. Stephen truly appreciated the stress management benefits of exercise. Sometimes when he was stressed out, he went in-line skating and just focused on the repetitive, rhythmical movements of his arms and legs as they worked in synchrony. Stephen was a highly skilled skater; thus, he did not need to pay very much attention to the skill of in-line skating. He would just let his mind wander to whatever it was at the moment that popped into his awareness. Sometimes it was part of a conversation he had had with his new wife; other times, it was something that he wanted to fix up in his new house. Still other moments, his thoughts jumped to something needing attention at work. Occasionally, his mind was blank, and he thoroughly enjoyed moving mindfully and letting his body "take over" the skating. In-line skating was enjoyable, and Stephen often returned home feeling refreshed, tired but energetic and in a more upbeat mood than before he started.

Other times, though, when stressed, Stephen would just fall into a chair at the end of the day, watch TV, and experience considerable feelings of depression. Moving itself was difficult. He knew that he should exercise, but sometimes he felt it took too much effort.

Peak Experiences, Eustress, and Enjoyment

In the winter, Stephen thoroughly enjoyed the exercise activity of snowmobiling. Sometimes he and his buddies would hitch the snowmobiles on a trailer behind a truck and head out to one of the wilderness areas in his home state of Wyoming. They explored the backcountry and used nearly every muscle in their bodies as they held onto the handlebars while jumping over creek beds, climbing steep mountainous terrain, and traversing some of the mountains diagonally as necessary to prevent turning upside down.

The physical exertion while surrounded by the Wyoming wilderness was a peak experience. Sometimes it was associated with eustress, a euphoric, desirable form of stress, as Stephen tested his physical strength and endurance against the breathtakingly beautiful, but challenging terrain.

Snowmobiling definitely added to Stephen's quality of life, and often he and Tass went snowmobiling together. They both enjoyed the social interactions, the camaraderie of the other couples who were snowmobiling, the awesome beauty of nature, and, of course, the exercise. The cold weather, physical exertion, joint activity, and scenic beauty provided them separately and together a wonderful tiredness and feeling of being at peace with the world.

Exercise Commitment and Adherence

Recognizing the need for aerobic fitness, Tass and Stephen also exercised at their local health club. Their exercise sessions tended to be somewhat sporadic and depended on their work schedules.

Stephen recognized that he needed to exercise more, but just did not have the commitment to exercise that Tass had. He was envious of her dedication. Tass truly was committed to her exercise program and usually went out for a 45-minute jog each morning prior to going to work. Stephen knew it was a good idea, but just did not enjoy that type of activity. Thus, he decided to remain with his in-line skating on alternate days, weather permitting.

Flow and the Exercise High

Stephen and Tass both were exercising on a somewhat regular basis and learned to follow their own preferred types of activities. Each of them experienced peak moments. Stephen found peak experiences during the snowmobiling and flow during his in-line skating. Tass occasionally encountered the exercise high during her morning jog and, like Stephen, could get caught up in flow in-line skating when her skill matched that needed for the terrain. She found that she tended to experience flow when she was exercising alone rather than when she was with Stephen or a group of her friends. In conclusion, both Tass and Stephen were aware that their habitual exercise activities added to the quality of their lives.

cise environment; psychological characteristics and backgrounds of the participants; and the instructors' characteristics and approaches to exercise.

Further contributing to the complexity of the relationship is that the type and extent of the psychological benefits (and decrements) of exercise may differ for specific groups of people. These groups include participants who vary in age from preschoolers to the elderly, and those who are from normal and psychiatric populations. Individuals who have chronic diseases, as well as those who exhibit high levels of health also may report differing benefits of exercise.

A final contribution to the complex relationship between exercise and subjective well-being, the term *subjective well-being* itself includes multiple facets such as the absence of negative affect, the presence of positive affect, and high levels of life satisfaction (Diener, 1994; Mroczek & Kolarz, 1998). Despite such complexities, there is a strong consensus that many types of exercise are associated with enhanced subjective well-being, or a sense of "feeling better" (Berger, 1996; Berger & Motl, 2000; Craft & Landers, 1998; Hays, 1998, 1999; Morgan, 1997).

An Associative, Rather than a Causal Relationship

The relationship between physical activity and subjective well-being is one of *association*, rather than *causality*. An associative relationship means that when one event such as exercise occurs, another event such as *feeling better* also occurs. Measuring psychological well-being before and after an exercise session and finding changes supports an associative relationship. Many individuals feel better after exercising, and thus exercise and psychological well-being are associated with one another. The causes of these changes may not be the physical exercise itself, but a host of associated factors. The important conclusion is that the relationship between exercise and subjective well-being is robust and has been supported in a wide variety of studies.

Influences within the exercise experience and environment—such as having a "time-out" from daily hassles, being outside in nature, or interacting with friends—may cause the desirable changes in psychological well-being, and thus the exercise itself may not be *causing* the changes in well-being (Berger, 1996). An example of a study supporting a causal relationship between exercise and well-being would be one in which specific increases in physical fitness as a result of a training stimulus were differentially related to predictable increases in mood states, self-esteem, or other measures of psychological well-being in a dose-response relationship. Until such research evidence is available, we need to recognize that the relationship between exercise and subjective well-being is associa-tive, rather than causal. The consistency of the associative benefits, however, is impressive and lends support to a possible causal relationship.

Exercise and Acute Mood Changes

Acute changes in mood states are short-term changes measured immediately before and after a single exercise session. When exercisers report how they feel *right now at this very moment* both before and after a single exercise session, they tend to report desirable changes in mood after exercising. Exercisers often report acute decreases in anxiety, depression, anger, and fatigue, and increases in vigor (Berger, 1996; Berger & Motl, 2000; Morgan, 1997; Thayer, 1996). These measurable benefits reflect exercisers' perception that immediately after exercising, they "feel better" than they did before exercising.

Two to four hours of benefits. The acute changes in mood appear to last from 2 to 4 hours after exercising for members of nonclinical populations (Raglin & Morgan, 1987; Thayer, 1996). This may seem to be a short length of time. However, experiencing more positive moods for 2 to 4 hours can have a highly desirable influence on exercisers' QoL. During this period, desirable changes in mood can improve participants' social interactions with friends, influence their choice of study and work projects, and improve their work efficiency.

There also is a *ripple effect* for these benefits that occurs. The improvements in social interaction and productivity may affect your QoL for even longer periods of time than the 2 to 4 hours. For example, they can influence key people in your life who may change their reactions to you as a result of more positive interactions produced during the initial 2 to 4 hour period. The desirable changes in social interactions, mood states, stress levels, and productivity also may have a compounding effect—if they are experienced on a daily basis.

Undesirable as well as desirable changes. It is important to note that the mood changes can be in undesirable directions, especially when participants exercise at intensity levels and exercise durations that are close to their maximum capabilities. Longer exercise sessions and high intensity exercise sessions are not always "better" in regard to enhancing the psychological benefits. Thus, as an exercise psychology specialist, it is important for you to recognize that there are possible differences in the training stimuli required for the psychological and performance benefits of exercise.

Exercise mode and training parameters. As suggested in Chapter 6, which covers mood alteration and exercise, and in Chapter 20, which examines the types of exercise that are best for facilitating the psychological benefits, some types of physical activity are more likely to be associated with mood benefits than are others (Berger & Owen, 1988). Exercise that (1) is aerobic or that changes participants' breathing patterns, (2) has a relative absence of competition, (3) has predictable movement patterns, and (4) has repetitive and/or rhythmical movements seem particularly conducive to mood alteration. In addition to type of activity, practice or training factor—such as exercise intensity, frequency, and duration, as examined in Chapter 21—may be related to the direction and extent of the mood changes.

Exercise and Chronic Changes in Mood

There may be longer-lasting, or chronic, psychological benefits of exercise, especially for people who are clinically anxious or depressed. These long-lasting, chronic changes are reflected by mood scores that are measured at the beginning and end of an extended program of exercise. The exercise programs investigated in the studies may last for a few weeks, months, or even years. See Berger and colleagues (1988), Brown and colleagues (1995), and O'Connor and Puetz (2005) for studies of chronic mood changes associated with exercise.

The mood states of Energy and Fatigue as measured by the Profile of Mood States (POMS; McNair & Heuchert, 2003, 2005) and the Vitality scale of the SF-36 Health Survey (Ware & Sherbourne, 1992) have direct implications for QoL since energy and fatigue affect the ability and interest in "doing stuff." People who are high in energy and vitality can pursue both more difficult and a wider variety of activities in their daily lives than those who are low. Those who are high in fatigue have difficulty in pursuing the tasks of daily living and often are too tired to pursue their dreams. In addition to detracting from enhanced QoL, fatigue and low energy are associated with chronic illnesses such as cancer, chronic fatigue syndrome, congestive heart failure, chronic obstructive pulmonary disease, multiple sclerosis, and obesity.

Patrick O'Connor and Timothy Puetz (2005) reviewed the relationship between *chronic exercise* and the two mood states of energy and fatigue as reported in more than 100 studies. In their examination of experimental investigations and epidemiological evidence, O'Connor and Puetz (2005) reported that specific populations differed in their reports of exercise-related increases in energy and decreases in fatigue. More specifically, the results of this review of chronic physical activity, which ranged from 10 to 20 weeks in length, suggest the following.

- **Members of the general adult population report mixed changes in energy and fatigue after exercising.**

Approximately half of the 15 experimental studies reviewed showed chronic increases in energy with long-term exercise training. Other studies reported no meaningful changes in either energy or fatigue with long-term exercise programs. The lack of consistent findings is not surprising since exercise intensity and duration would seem to influence participants' feelings of energy and fatigue after exercising. Light and moderate exercise would seem to lead to increased energy and decreased fatigue. High intensity exercise may be related to decreased energy and increased fatigue.

- **Fatigued members of the population who have medical conditions such as cancer and heart failure tend to report chronic increases in the frequency and intensity of feelings of energy.**

- **Athletes (and exercisers) who overtrain report chronic increases in fatigue and vigor as measured by the POMS**.

  The effect of exercise training on the mood states of fatigue and vigor depends on the volume (duration and frequency) and intensity of the training stimulus and exhibits a dose-response relationship. Except for athletes who have become stale, the undesirable mood changes of overtraining are reversed when the training stimulus is reduced (Berger & Tobar, in press). This same relationship between exercise intensity, duration, and frequency probably would apply to exercisers, and would explain the mixed results reported for exercisers by O'Connor and Puetz (2005).

It is difficult to attribute chronic or long-term mood changes in nonclinical populations to the exercise program itself. When exercisers' mood states are measured prior to starting the exercise program and then again at the end of a lengthy exercise program, their changes may be due to the exercise program, or to a host of other seasonal and life-related influences. Thus, claims for mood benefits in members of nonclinical or the general population are most creditable when they are restricted to acute changes, or those reported immediately after exercise sessions during which investigators can control for extraneous factors that might influence participants' mood states.

In contrast to the general population, members of psychiatric populations have reported more lasting or chronic changes in mood after exercising as their depression and/or anxiety levels decrease (e.g., Hays, 1998, 1999; Dunn, Trivedi, Kampert, Clark, & Chambliss, 2005). For example, in a 3-day-a-week progressive resistance training intervention program conducted for 10 weeks, older adults who initially met the criteria for clinical depression reported significant decreases in depression, increased QoL, and increased strength as measured at the beginning and end of the program (Singh et al., 1997). Exercisers that are clinically anxious, depressed, or highly stressed have more opportunity for long-lasting improvements in mood. Consideration of the psychological benefits of exercise for clinical populations is presented in chapter 6, "Mood Alteration, Self-Awareness, and Exercise: Multiple Relationships."

A Need for Caution: Possible Mood Decrements

Exercise can have negative influences on the QoL (Berger & Tobar, in press). There is a dark side to exercise. Too much exercise as reflected by long duration and high intensity and frequency can have an undesirable influence on mood (O'Connor, 1997; O'Connor & Puetz, 2005). If overtraining (i.e., the long duration and high intensity exercise) continues for an extended period of time without sufficient recovery, staleness may occur (Tobar, in press). Exercise also can add to the stress of daily life. It can be one more thing to include in an already overloaded schedule. In addition, exercise dependency or compulsion, exercise-related injuries, exercise-related eating disorders, and even extreme competitiveness are not conducive to enhanced QoL as noted in Chapter 16, the examination of exercise concerns.

Mood decrements also can be related to feeling physically inept, noting little or no improvement in progress in development of physical skills, experiencing overtraining or burnout, and losing a competitive match (e.g., Berger, Butki, & Berwind, 1995; Hays, 1999; O'Conner & Puetz, 2005). Potential mood changes might include increased anxiety and anger, decreased energy and increased depression, fatigue, and disappointment. Even though exercise can decrease the QoL, sufficient data support the conclusion that habitual physical activity often is associated with desirable changes in subjective well-being.

Use of Exercise to Moderate Daily Stress Responses

Another way in which habitual exercise is related to QoL is by serving as a stress management technique. We do not think about it often, but too little stress (i.e., boredom), as well as too much stress, can have detrimental influences on QoL. Both result in "distress," which in everyday usage is shortened to the word "stress." As suggested in Chapter 7, distress detracts from our zest for living and our QoL.

Distress: A Definition

Distress or stress can be defined as "a relationship with the environment that the person appraises as significant for his or her well-being and in which the demands tax or exceed available coping resources" (Lazarus & Folkman, 1986, p. 63). Although individuals vary in their optimal or preferred levels of stress, a continual or chronic state of distress tends to be associated with physical symptoms: illness, high blood pressure, and rapid pulse rate (Seaward, 1997). Too much stress also is associated with psychological symptoms as reflected by increased anxiety, depression, hostility, and personal unhappiness. Various stress management techniques including exercise are useful in reducing the deleterious effects of stress.

The Spice of Life

Emphasizing the desirability of creating optimal levels of stress in our daily lives, stress has been referred to as the "spice of life" (Selye, 1975, p. 83). Stress provides each of us with zest, excitement, and memorable times, such as a strict work/school deadline pushing us to produce some our best work, and giving us a strong sense of accomplishment in meeting the deadline.

Because stress is integrally related to subjective well-being, it is important to learn to regulate stress levels along a continuum that progresses from "too little" at one extreme, to "optimal," to "too much" at the other extreme.

Eustress

In contrast to distress, the term *eustress* refers to a highly desirable type of stress—a specific type of stress that is exhilarating, exciting, and challenging (Berger, 1994). The thrill of eustress can be associated with participating in high-risk physical activities such as rock climbing and downhill skiing, and it also can occur in competitive types of exercise, especially when the competition is intense. Experiencing optimal levels of stress through exercise contributes directly to the quality of everyday life.

Effectiveness of Exercise as a Stress Management Technique

Exercise is one of the few stress management techniques that can assist in both raising and lowering participants' stress levels. Exercise is an ideal activity that enables participants to reestablish a personally optimal level of stress. For example, physical activity serves as a technique for increasing stress levels when participating in competitive physical activities and in high-risk physical activities such as rock climbing, downhill skiing, and scuba diving. Exercise also is a technique for reducing stress levels, particularly when it is non-competitive, rhythmical physical activity that promotes abdominal breathing. Activities such as jogging, swimming, weight training, and hatha yoga, for example, can be stress reducing. Exercisers in these types of activities have a time-out from a busy day, a time to think and to problem-solve while exercising, and an opportunity to experience their bodies in movement.

Exercise plays a key role in moderating both psychological and physical stress symptoms. The psychological and physical changes associated with exercise can interact to produce the "feeling better" sensation. Psychological changes associated with habitual exercise include decreases of state and trait anxiety, depression, and stress, and increases in positive mood states, self-esteem, and feelings of attractiveness (Berger, 1994). These changes provide exercisers with greater psychological resources for coping with stressful situations. As concluded by Rostad and Long (1996) in their comprehensive review of exercise as a stress management technique, the results of the 46 studies reviewed indicated "some improvement on psychological and physiological variables" (p. 216).

It seems that individuals who are fit or who exercise habitually have reduced stress symptoms. This is true in both normal and clinical populations who have exercised for 6 weeks or longer (Petruzzello et al., 1991; Rostad & Long, 1996). Additional research is needed to determine the role of expectancy, the effectiveness of particular types of exercise, and the effectiveness of exercise as a stress management technique for individuals who are not particularly stressed. Despite remaining questions, research supports the effectiveness of exercise in reducing stress levels (Long & van Stavel, 1995; Rostad & Long, 1996; Tomporowski et al., 2005).

Effectiveness of Exercise Compared to Other Approaches for Enhancing Quality of Life

Exercise seems to be as effective as more traditional mood alteration and stress management approaches such as reading, Benson's relaxation response, quiet rest, and eating a sugar snack in reducing anxiety, tension, depression, and anger (Berger et al., 1988; Long & van Stavel, 1995; Thayer, 1996). The effectiveness of exercise is particularly impressive, because the participants in some of the studies were randomly assigned to treatment. Thus, exercise can reduce stress and enhance mood even in individuals who are not self-selected exercisers.

The observation that the benefits of exercise are comparable, but are not superior, to other mood and stress management techniques emphasizes the need

for realistic claims regarding the benefits of exercise. Further investigation is needed to clarify whether the psychological benefits of exercise and other techniques differ from one another in regard to the patterns of change on mood profiles, duration of the benefits, and possible underlying mechanisms. A particularly appealing aspect of exercise is that it can enhance our subjective well-being while providing a wide variety of additional benefits, including health enhancement and improved physical appearance by increasing our muscle definition and reducing body fat percentage.

Peak Moments in Exercise Settings and the Quality of Life

Another way that exercise can add to the quality of our lives is by offering opportunities to experience peak moments. Peak moments include a broad spectrum of sporadic, but highly valued, states (Berger, 1996; Csikszentmihalyi, 1991, 1997; McInman & Grove, 1991; Privette & Bundrick, 1991, 1997). They provide a base for vivid, often reviewed memories that help define our lives and give depth of meaning, as suggested in later chapters that focus on peak moments and flow (Chapter 15), as well as personal meaning in exercise (Chapter 14). Peak moments share characteristics that are similar, but still are conceptually distinct from one another as reflected by the following.

- *Peak performance* is superior functioning and reflects a high standard of accomplishment.
- *Peak experience* reflects a psychological state that includes intense joy and enjoyment.
- *Flow* is a psychological state that is intrinsically enjoyable, and often is a matching of personal ability and task difficulty.
- The *exerciser's high* is a euphoric state often characterized by feelings of power, control, and ability to perform impossible feats such as leaping over oncoming cars when jogging.

These rewarding and memorable moments often occur in exercise and sport activities. They are unplanned, highly rewarding bonuses of exercise. When exercisers describe peak moments such as flow, peak performance, and peak experiences, they report many similarities in experiential, psychological, and performance states. The characteristics of flow described by Jackson and Eklund (2004) in *The Flow Scales Manual* can be expanded from being specific to flow to reflecting similarities across different types of peak moments. The following characteristics may occur in different combinations and strengths within peak moments:

- Autotelic, or intrinsically rewarding, experience,
- Balance between situational challenge and the participant's skills,

- Clear goals,
- Concentration on the task at hand,
- Loss of self-consciousness,
- Merging of action and awareness,
- Perception of control,
- Transformation of time, and
- Unambiguous feedback.

For more details, see Csikszentmihalyi (1991, 1997), Jackson and Eklund (2004), Jackson and Csikszentmihalyi (1999), Marsh and Jackson (1999).

Types of Peak Moments

Although peak moments are quite similar to one another, there are subtle differences between them. Peak performance, for example, typically is considered to be a peak moment, but not all peak moments are peak performances. Each type of peak moment is an important contributor to the QoL. See Table 3.5 for a summary of the characteristics of peak performances, peak experiences, flow, and the exerciser's high.

Peak performance. An outstanding physical performance reflects superior functioning and can occur in a wide variety of activities. Peak performance can include feats of physical strength or skill such as that displayed in an exquisite tennis match, creative expression, intellectual mastery of challenging material, and even work-related endeavors (Privette & Bundrick, 1987, 1989, 1997). Peak performance can be spontaneous, or in response to a placebo, biofeedback, or hyp-

nosis (Privette, 1983). A peak performance often occurs when the participant has a clear focus on the task at hand and a strong sense of intention. Examples of exercise-related peak performances include a hole in one in golf, a perfect serve in tennis, and an effortless 10-mile jog for a runner who usually is exhausted after jogging 5 miles. A peak performance increases our perceptions of competence, excellence, mastery, and self-efficacy that permeate many aspects of our lives. Such perceptions tend to promote feelings of satisfaction and well-being that are crucial to our QoL.

The major characteristics that describe peak performances are listed in Table 3.5. Additional characteristics of peak performance also may include awareness of power and an insufficiency of words to describe the moment. Some peak performances may trigger ecstasy, and thus are also peak experiences (Privette & Bundrick, 1997). Interestingly, participation with others as occurs in team games may hinder the likelihood of experiencing a peak performance. Being with others may disrupt the exerciser's concentration (Privette & Landsman, 1983).

Peak experience. A peak experience includes any experience that evokes strong, positive affective states such as peace, joy, illumination, or ecstasy (see Table 3.5). Such experiences often produce a loss of self and freedom from outer restrictions. They can be considered moments of highest happiness (Privette & Bundrick, 1987). Peak experiences are memorable, fulfilling, and personally meaningful moments that

Table 3.5
Major Characteristics of Peak Moments
(Jackson & Eklund, 2004; Privette, 1983; Sachs, 1984)

Peak Performance	Peak Experience	Flow	Exerciser's High
High Level of Performance	Joy and Happiness	Complete Concentration	Euphoric State
Clear Focus	Fulfilling and Meaningful	Enjoyment	Feelings of Unusual Strength or Power
Fulfillment	Loss of Self	Feeling of Control	Glimpses of Perfection
Intention	Passive	Freedom from Self-Consciousness	Gracefulness
Spontaneous	Spontaneous	Lost in Time and Space	Complete Concentration
Strong Sense of Self	Transpersonal	Play	Spirituality

affect the quality of our lives (Maslow, 1968). Maslow suggested that peak experiences are associated with fully functioning individuals (self-actualizers), who tend to report more numerous peak experiences than do less fully developed individuals.

Recently, exercisers who successfully swam the English Channel reported the completion of the swim as a peak experience. Reflecting on the personal meaning of finishing the swim, they reported increased self-confidence, awareness of unlimited potential, transcendence into daily life, and increased effectiveness at work (Hollander & Acevedo, 2000). Another example of a peak experience within the realm of exercise is running on a deserted beach during a beautiful sunset while hearing the seagulls calling to one another overhead. This peak experience could include the sound of waves lapping at the edge of the sand, and feeling the wonderful sensation of a body in motion.

Although peak experiences in exercise settings are important contributors to a high QoL, little is known about them. One problem with researching peak experiences is that they cannot be planned; thus, they are difficult to capture in laboratory settings. The percentage of people who report peak experiences in general, and specifically in exercise, also is not clear. In one study of university students, only 3 of the 214 students tested did not report having a peak experience (Allen, Haupt, & Jones, 1964). The results of this study suggest that peak experiences are rather common. In contrast, Keutzer (1978) reported that 61% of a national sample had *not* reported an experience that made them feel as though they "were very close to a powerful, spiritual force that seemed to lift them out of themselves" (p. 77).

Flow. Flow is another type of peak moment. We use the word "flow" in our everyday language as illustrated by the phrase "go with the flow." This phrase means that we should stay with the present moment and thus captures some of the term's meaning. Csikszentmihalyi (1975) initially proposed the concept of flow as a positive psychological state in which people are so caught up in the present moment and the activity that nothing else seems to matter. Flow is an optimal experiential state that occurs when a person's skills in an activity match the required challenges of the task (Csikszentmihalyi, 1991; Jackson & Marsh, 1996; Jackson, Thomas, Marsh, & Smethurst, 2001).

Enjoyment and freedom from self-consciousness also are central elements in the flow state as noted in Table 3.5. The experience of flow is so intrinsically enjoyable that exercisers seek it out (Csikszentmihalyi, 1993, 1997). Flow often results in feelings of control, complete concentration, and being totally in tune with the activity, and is likely to promote feelings of happiness and well-being (Csikszentmihalyi, 1997; Jackson & Csikszentmihalyi, 1999; Jackson & Marsh, 1996).

The nine subscales within the Flow-State Scale reflect key dimensions of flow (Jackson & Eklund, 2004; Jackson & Marsh, 1996). These include the same dimensions as those listed earlier in this chapter for peak moments. Flow subscales are as follows: (1) Challenge-skill balance, (2) Action-awareness energy, (3) Clear goals, (4) Unambiguous feedback, (5) Concentration on task, (6) Sense of control, (7) Loss of self-consciousness, (8) Transformation of time, and (9) Autotelic experience.

Not all activities are equally conducive to flow. When interviewing university students ($N = 123$) between 20 and 50 years of age, Privette and Bundrick (1987, 1989) reported that sport was a major source of flow experiences. In contrast, no university student mentioned having a flow experience at school or work, in relationships or sickness, or in connection with religious events.

The type of exercise and sport activities may facilitate or detract from the occurrence of the flow experience and have implications for promoting its occurrence. In fact, both within-individual factors and exercise/sport environmental factors may affect the flow experience (Jackson et al., 2001). Exercise activities that are structured and continuous or endurance-based (rather than start-stop) in nature may facilitate flow. In contrast, competition may either facilitate it or decrease the likelihood of its occurrence (Jackson et al., 2001). Although these results in the study by Jackson and colleagues (2001) may reflect the particular study sample of university students, Csikszentmihalyi (1991) and Jackson and Csikszentmihalyi (1999) have reinforced the possibility of experiencing flow more often when participating in specific types of exercise and sport activities.

The exerciser's, or runner's, high. Runners, in particular, tend to report occasionally experiencing peak moments and a euphoric state while exercising. Thus, the terminology *runner's high* has developed. This experience, however, would seem to extend to other activities. As a result, the term, *runner's high,* has been broadened to *exerciser's high* in this text.

The exerciser's high is a particularly strong peak moment that contributes to our QoL. The diversity of descriptions expressed by runners and other exercise participants is remarkable, but troublesome (e.g., Masters, 1992). Examination of personal descriptions of the exerciser's high has suggested widely different experiences ranging from an enhanced sense of well-being to euphoric states. Common descriptions of the exerciser's high include euphoria, imaginary feats of unusual strength and power, gracefulness, spirituality, sudden realization of your potential, glimpses of perfection, movement without effort, and the experience of spinning out and letting your mind just flow from one set of thoughts to another (Berger, 1996; Masters, 1992; Sachs, 1980, 1984; see Table 3.5).

Despite the many descriptions of the exerciser's high, it is not easy to define. Sachs (1984) proposed that the exerciser's or runner's high is "a euphoric sensation experienced during running, usually unexpected, in which the runner feels a heightened sense of well-being, enhanced appreciation of nature, and transcendence of barriers of time and space" (p. 274). Subsequently, Berger (1996) defined the exerciser's high as a specific type of peak experience characterized by euphoria, a heightened sense of well-being, feelings of psychological/physical strength and power, a glimpse of perfection, and even spirituality (p. 346).

The percentages of runners in various studies who report experiencing an exercise high vary greatly. Sachs (1984) estimated that somewhere between 9% and 78% of runners have experienced a runner's high. Among runners who have experienced an exercise high, the frequency of such an experience varies from rarely (i.e., only several times during their running careers) to an average of 29.4% of daily runs (Sachs, 1980). The exerciser's high is a personally important occurrence for exercisers who experience it. Because of its ability to enhance QoL, we need research that further explains the exerciser's high as well as provides information about related factors that trigger the exerciser's high.

Models of Peak Moments

Theories and models that account for various types of peak moments in a wide variety of activities illustrate their richness and depth.

Feeling and performance model. The "feeling and performance model" classifies peak moments on the two orthogonal dimensions, feeling and performance (Privette & Bundrick, 1987, 1991, 1997). As depicted in Figure 3.2, the *feeling dimension* on the vertical axis ranges from one extreme of misery, to worry and boredom, through neutrality, to enjoyment and joy, and then to the extreme of ecstasy. The *performance dimension* on the horizontal axis ranges from an extreme of total failure to inadequacy and inefficiency to mediocrity to effectiveness, high performance, and

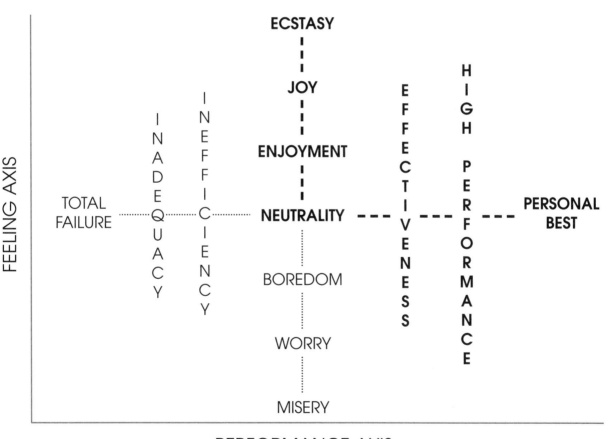

Figure 3.2. Feeling and performance model. From "Measurement of Experience: Construct and Content Validity of the Experience Questionnaire," by G. Privette and C. M. Bundrick (1987). *Perceptual and Motor Skills, 65,* p.318. Copyright 1987 by C. H. Ammons and R. B. Ammons. Adapted with permission.

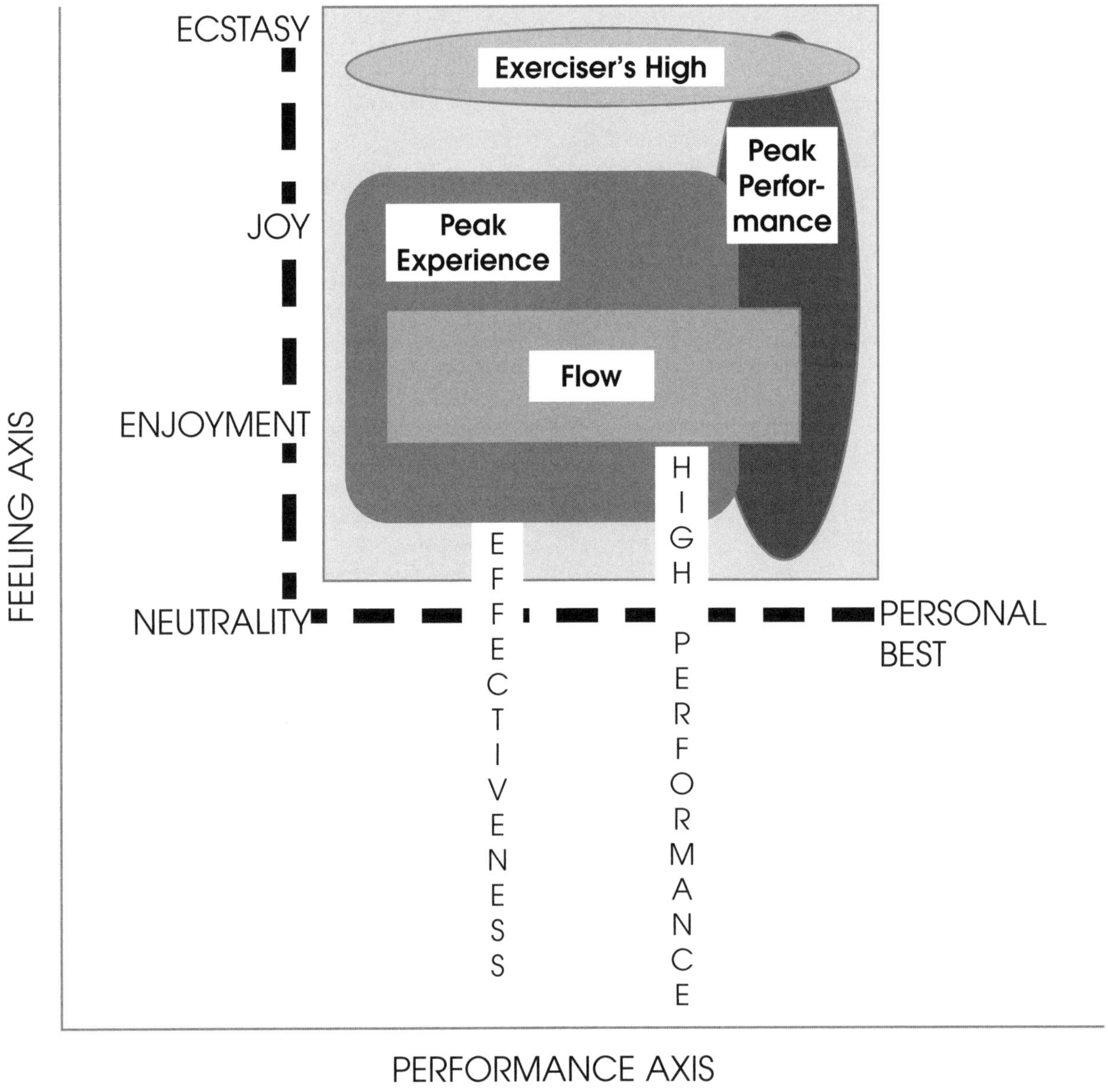

Figure 3.3. Peak moments quadrant of the feeling and performance model.

personal best. The feeling and performance dimensions have been validated by Privette and Bundrick (1991, 1997).

Employing the feeling and performance model, any experience can be classified according to the two dimensions of feeling and performance (see the two axes in Figure 3.3). For example, the state in the bottom left corner of the figure is characterized by total failure and misery, which would describe an experience of an extremely poor or embarrassing performance and the accompanying negative feelings. The center of the figure is neutral and typifies many everyday experiences consisting of average performance and neutral feelings. Such everyday experiences generally are somewhere between enjoyment and bore-

dom and between inefficiency and effectiveness.

The entire top-right quadrant of the feeling and performance model depicted in Figure 3.3 contains the diverse, yet somewhat similar peak moments. When behavior is in the top-right quadrant of the feeling and performance model highlighted in the Figure, we perform well and experience positive feelings of enjoyment, joy, and occasional ecstasy.

Although placement of specific types of peak moments within the feeling and performance model is inexact, *peak moments* are highlighted here for your consideration and contemplation. *Peak performance* is located at the extreme right end of the performance axis and may be at any place along the feeling axis. Peak performance reflects an unusually high standard of accomplishment and can be associated with the feeling states of enjoyment, joy, and ecstasy. An exercise performance that is the participant's *personal best* is the highest form of peak performance and reflects optimal physical functioning. In contrast, *flow* is a psychological state and is represented in the middle section of Figure 3.3 since a personal best is not required. Flow extends to the right-hand side of the figure since flow often is associated with a relatively high level of performance quality (Jackson, Thomas, Marsh, & Smethurst, 2001). Flow is associated with enjoyment and joy, rather than ecstasy. Flow has fairly equal components of feeling and performance states. A large portion of the top right quadrant area toward joy represents *peak experiences*, which may or may not be accompanied by peak performance. The *exerciser's high* is located near ecstasy on the feeling dimension and may occur in performances that range anywhere from the neutrality position along the horizontal axis in Figure 3.3 to the personal best position in the figure.

Flow model. Csikszentmihalyi (e.g., 1991, 1993, 1997) has proposed a model for the one specific peak movement of flow as a delicate balance between per-

sonal skill level and task demands. The flow model describes the occurrence of flow experiences in everyday life, which includes those in physical activity. As represented in Figure 3.4, this model describes exercise ability that exceeds the demands of the task, the task is too easy, and you may experience *boredom*. If your exercise ability is inadequate for the task, the task is too difficult and you probably will experience *anxiety*. An example of an anxiety-producing situation is playing golf with a friend who is a professional golfer when your golf skills are at a beginning level. In contrast, if both the perceived challenge of the task and your skill level are low, you may experience *apathy*. The enjoyable, pleasurable, and rewarding experience of *flow* results when the demands of the task require intense concentration and when there is a match between the participant's personal ability and the demands of the task.

To better understand the elusive flow experience, Kimiecik and Stein (1992) have suggested a need to examine the *person-by-situation* framework. The *person-based factors* can be separated further into dispositional and state components. Dispositional components include personal characteristics that are fairly

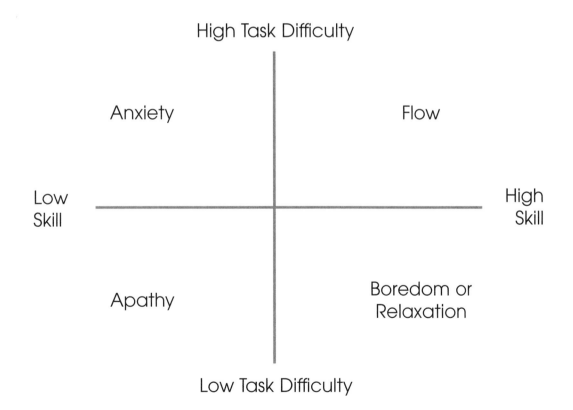

Figure 3.4. Model of the flow state: Task difficulty and personal skill. From *The Flow Scales Manual*, p. 4, by S. A. Jackson and R. C. Ekland (2004). Morgantown, WV, Fitness Information Technology. Copyright 2004 by R. C. Eklund and S. A. Jackson.

permanent, such as goal orientation (i.e., task and ego orientations), attentional style, trait anxiety, trait confidence, and perceived exercise competence. State components are more changeable and include game goals, concentration, state anxiety, self-efficacy, and perceived game ability.

The *situational-based factors* include type of exercise (e.g., self-paced vs. other dependent), the importance of the competition, opponent's ability, teammates' interactions and behaviors, and competitive flow structure. This person-by-situation framework highlights some of the factors that may interact to promote flow experiences, and perhaps other peak moments.

Conclusions: Peak Moments

The peak moments of peak performance, flow, exercise high, and peak experiences are likely to affect the physical activity experience and our lives. In general, peak moments are profound, rewarding, memorable, and moving experiences that can greatly enhance the QoL. It seems that researchers have accurately characterized peak moments, with the possible exception of the exercise high. Examining how and why peak moments occur in physical activity settings is a challenging area for future research and one that you may choose to pursue. With the recent advances in measurement (Jackson & Ekland, 2004; Marsh & Jackson, 1999), researchers may be able to better understand factors that foster peak moments. Understanding and facilitating peak moments in diverse groups of exercisers may unlock the gate to the pursuit and promotion of exercise as an attractive and rewarding form of recreation. Exercise activities that become intrinsically meaningful are pursued for their own sake, rather than avoided.

Enjoyment of Exercise and Our Quality of Life

Opportunities for enjoyment are another important contribution of exercise to QoL. As emphasized by the burgeoning focus on positive psychology, enjoyable activities enhance our QoL by providing hedonic, interesting, rewarding, and truly memorable experiences (Kahneman et al., 1999). As Mihaly Csikszentmihalyi (1991) suggested,

> When people ponder further about what makes their lives rewarding, they tend to move beyond pleasant memories and begin to remember other events, other experiences that overlap with pleasurable ones but fall into a category that deserves a separate name: *enjoyment* [italics added]. (p. 46)

Enjoyment adds zest and feelings of contentment and appreciation to our lives. It also may produce feelings of accomplishment, euphoria, and happiness (Kendzierski & DeCarlo, 1991), which, in turn, may add meaning and "zip" to our daily routines.

Definitions of Enjoyment

We know what enjoyment means, but like many words in daily use, enjoyment has been a difficult construct to define. In *The Oxford American Dictionary and Thesaurus* (2003), enjoyment is "pleasure, delight, joy, gratification, satisfaction, relish, zest . . . " (pp. 477–478). This definition highlights the importance of enjoyment for improving life quality; experiences of enjoyment result in positive feelings and perceptions of satisfaction.

Enjoyment, a positive affective state. Some researchers suggest that enjoyment is related to positive affective states. For example, Scanlan and Simons (1992) defined sport enjoyment as "a positive affective response to the sport experience that reflects generalized feelings such as pleasure, liking, and fun" (pp. 202–203). Wankel (1993) also described exercise enjoyment as "a positive emotion, a positive affective state" (p. 153). He further speculated that positive feeling states are a common element of exercise enjoyment (Wankel, 1997).

Enjoyment and flow. Enjoyment may be similar to flow-type experiences, and positive affect may be a byproduct of an enjoyable experience. According to Csikszentmihalyi (1991), enjoyment is an optimal experience, one of high quality, and it serves as an end in itself. Enjoyment often occurs in autotelic or intrinsically rewarding activities and seems to result in desirable affective states such as happiness, vigor, pleasure, and relaxation (Motl, Berger, & Leuschen, 2000). Reflecting these descriptions, enjoyment is "an optimal psychological state (i.e., flow) that leads to performing an activity for its own sake and is associated with positive feeling states" (Kimiecik & Harris, 1996, p. 256).

This definition of enjoyment by Kimiecik and Harris (1996) sparked a debate with Wankel (1997) and perhaps other researchers. Wankel (1997) suggested that Kimiecik and Harris misinterpreted or inaccurately reported aspects of previous research (e.g., Wankel & Kreisel, 1985; Wankel & Sefton, 1989), and utilized inconsistent logic in building a definition of enjoyment based on flow. The commentary between Wankel (1997) and Kimiecik and Harris (1996) illustrates the lack of agreement and difficulty in defining enjoyment.

Enjoyment, a positive emotion. Like all emotions, enjoyment has affective, behavioral, and physiological components. Enjoyment is a positive emotion that includes appetitive or approach tendencies, rather than aversion or avoidance tendencies. Enjoyment consists of distinct facial expressions associated with the contraction of eye muscles. There also are specific physiological responses in the central (CNS) and peripheral nervous systems associated with enjoyment, which include cerebral asymmetry in EEG activity reflecting more left-hemisphere activity, especially in the anterior temporal region and autonomic nervous system (ANS) activation (Frank et al., 1997). These characteristics of enjoyment indicate that enjoyment is more than a simple positive affective state that is measurable by self-report. Enjoyment also includes distinct facial expressions and physiological reactions in the CNS and autonomic nervous system (ANS), and has neuroanatomical and neurobiological bases (LeDoux & Armony, 1999).

Benefits of Exercise Enjoyment

Enjoying exercise as an activity or process has many benefits. A few of these include the participation in exercise on a regular basis and thus the adherence to exercise. Enjoyment also is related to mood enhancement and the "feel better" sensation after exercise sessions. Finally, exercise enjoyment can simply add to the number of our overall positive experiences in a day.

Exercise adherence. As Bob Singer (1996) observed, "There's got to be a way to associate regular involvement in vigorous physical activity as something we look forward to and are dedicated to—something we miss when we don't do it" (p. 249). One way to make physical activity enticing and desirable is to increase exercisers' enjoyment. In fact, enjoyment is a commonly cited reason for participating in exercise (Carpenter & Coleman, 1998; Wankel, 1993). Anticipation of enjoyment may be important for initial attraction to physical activity. Experiencing enjoyment during or following exercise and sport may be related to sustained commitment and participation in physical activity. Very simply, if we enjoy an activity, we are likely to participate in it on a regular basis.

Researchers have begun to examine enjoyment as a predictor of exercise behavior. Using cross-sectional research designs, they have investigated enjoyment in relation to physical activity, physical education classes, and sport commitment in youth and adults (e.g., Paxton, Browning, & O'Connell, 1997; Sallis, Prochaska, Taylor, Hill, & Geraci, 1999). Sallis, Prochaska, and colleagues (1999) reported that enjoyment of physical education was significantly related to physical activity levels in five of six subgroups of participants separated according to gender and grade (grades 4–6, grades 7–9, and grades 10–12). Since enjoyment of physical education classes was related to physical activity levels, it was concluded that enhancing young people's enjoyment of physical education classes should be considered a health-related goal by society and particularly by physical education teachers. Enjoyment and commitment to involvement in physical activity in adults and youth also have been examined in longitudinal or in intervention research designs (Dilorenzo et al., 1998; Sallis et al., 1999). For example, Sallis, Calfas, and colleagues (1999) reported that enjoyment of physical activity predicted physical activity levels across a 16-week course in college-aged male students who were randomly assigned to an intervention.

Enhancement of mood changes. Enjoyment may be linked to the psychological benefits associated with physical activity, especially mood changes. Berger and Owen (1986) and Koltyn, Shake, and Morgan (1993) provide indirect evidence of a relationship between enjoyment and acute changes in mood. When Berger and Owen examined the relationship between acute bouts of swimming and mood changes, college students enrolled in swimming classes reported short-term improvements on a variety of subscales on the Profile of Mood States (POMS) during the fall semester (Berger & Owen, 1986). In the summer session, however, there was no evidence that swimming was related to mood alteration. Berger and Owen speculated (1986) that the lack of mood changes during the summer could be attributed to extremely warm water and air temperatures, which may have affected perceptions of enjoyment. Koltyn et al. (1993) found a similar effect of unpleasant exercise conditions when analyzing the impact of cold water temperature on acute mood states. Thus, it seems that unpleasant environmental conditions may affect perceptions of enjoyment, which affect the mood changes associated with physical activity.

Recently, enjoyment of physical activity has been linked more directly to desirable short-term mood changes. The possible relationship between an activity, its enjoyment, and acute mood change was examined in rock climbers and students participating in a health education class who listened to a lecture and watched a video on rock climbing (Motl et al., 2000). Climbers and students in the health education class completed the POMS before and after their respective activities. They also completed a measure of activity enjoyment after the activity. Analyses indicated that both exercise enjoyment and participation in the activity were related to acute changes in mood as measured by the POMS. A subsequent path analysis and a series of simple and multiple regression analyses suggested that enjoyment mediated the acute mood changes reported by rock climbers and students in a health education class. In other words, participating in an enjoyable activity promoted mood change, rather than a particular mood state influencing perceptions of enjoyment.

Exercise enjoyment may help to balance the psychological stress associated with everyday activities. Berger (1994, 1996) and Wankel (1993) also have dis-

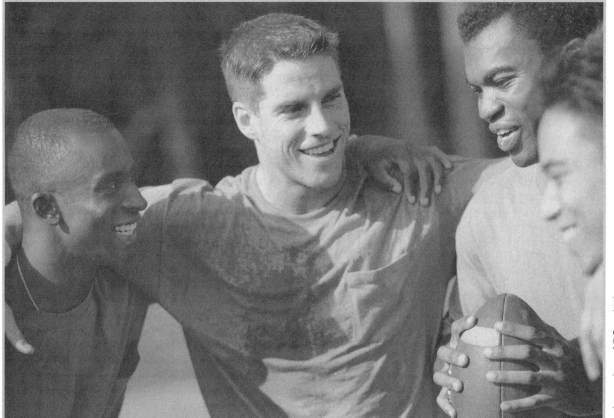

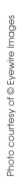

cussed the importance of enjoyment during exercise in counterbalancing the mood disturbances resulting from stress and hassles of everyday life. Enjoyment clearly plays a role in the diverse mental health benefits associated with exercise.

Sources of Enjoyment

Understanding common sources of enjoyment in exercise may assist you as a teacher, coach, personal trainer, or other type of movement specialist in facilitating the occurrence of this desirable and rewarding experience. In this section, you will focus separately on potential sources of enjoyment for adult exercisers and for youth sport participants because sources of enjoyment within these two groups may differ.

Youth sport participants. Three sources of enjoyment—intrinsic, social, and extrinsic factors—consistently have been identified in youth sport participants. *Intrinsic factors* related to enjoyment include accomplishment, challenge, excitement, fun, and skill improvement (Wankel & Kriesel, 1985; Wankel & Pabich, 1982, Wankel & Sefton, 1989). *Social factors* that are sources of enjoyment consist of being with friends and being on a team. *Extrinsic factors* include receiving awards, winning, and parental approval. For youth participants, intrinsic sources of enjoyment are rated as the most important, and these are followed in

order of importance by social and then by extrinsic sources (Wankel & Pabich, 1982).

Specific sources of enjoyment reported by elite figure skaters fit into four major themes (Scanlan et al., 1989):

- *Perceived competence.* Perceived competence is intrinsic to exercise and is characterized by factors such skill mastery, performance accomplishment, and competitive achievement.
- *Physical activity of skating itself.* The physical act of skating itself also is intrinsic to the exercise experience and is characterized by factors such as movement sensations, self-expressiveness, flow/peak experiences, and athleticism.
- *Social and life opportunities.* Social and life opportunities include both extrinsic and social benefits and facilitate developing and maintaining a broad base of friends and acquaintances, as well as interacting with coaches, parents, and athletes, traveling, and other life opportunities associated with high personal visibility.
- *Social recognition of competence.* Social recognition of competence is extrinsic to exercise participation and includes performance acknowledgment and social recognition.

These sources of enjoyment for skaters seem appropriate for exercisers in many types of activities.

Other factors probably contribute to exercise enjoyment in youth sport participants. Some of these focus on participants' characteristics and include their task orientation, perceived competence, and learned helplessness (Boyd & Yin, 1996; Oman & McAuley, 1993). We seem to enjoy participating in activities in which we are skilled and in which we feel competent. Perceived parental involvement, pressure, and satisfaction (Babkes & Weiss, 1999) and perceptions of success (Briggs, 1994) also are sources of enjoyment for youth sport participants.

In conclusion, the sources of enjoyment for youth sport participants include intrinsic, social, and extrinsic factors. Intrinsic sources are the most important sources of enjoyment and range from developing and improving physical skills to experiencing our bodies in motion, expressing ourselves, and simply having fun. Social sources also are important and include membership on a team and new friendships, desirable parental involvement, and positive interactions with coaches. Extrinsic sources are least important for sport enjoyment and include receiving trophies and social recognition of competence. Whether the sources of enjoyment for youth sport participants are applicable to young and adult exercisers is not yet established, but many of them seem to be appropriate.

Adult exercisers. Numerous factors contribute to adult exercisers' enjoyment of physical activity. Some of these factors include the broad categories of

- Personal factors,
- Situational factors,
- Exercise leaders and the environments they create, and
- Size of an exercise group.

For example, the size of an exercise group may be one influence on adult exercisers' perceptions of enjoyment (Widmeyer, Carron, & Brawley, 1990). As group size increases, enjoyment may decrease. In this particular study, smaller groups composed of 3 players reported more enjoyment than did larger groups of 12 players. Obtaining physical exercise and the positive feelings of fatigue associated with competition also were related to enjoyment scores for members of the small and moderate-size (6 players) exercise groups. In the larger group, strongest predictors of enjoyment were perceptions of reduced influence and responsibility.

Leadership behavior may influence participants' enjoyment as well as their exercise-related mood states and perceptions of self-efficacy (Turner, Rejeski, & Brawley, 1997). College-aged women ($N = 46$) in a ballet class indicated that a socially enriched environment that included frequent technical instruction, technical support, and positive feedback was more enjoyable than a bland exercise condition. Their enjoyment of ballet also was related to acute changes in mood, but it is uncertain whether enjoyment caused the mood changes, or vice versa.

When adult males were interviewed to determine factors that affected their exercise enjoyment and continued exercise involvement, the exercise "maintainers" reported that enhancing their physical sport skills, developing social relationships and going out with friends, achieving mental and physical outcomes, releasing competitive drives, and satisfying curiosity were important qualities within the exercise experience (Wankel, 1985). These elements, along with exercise intensity, exercise variability, and consistent leadership, may influence enjoyment. In a related study of exercise enjoyment, Heck and Kimiecik (1993) interviewed male and female adult exercisers to define exercise enjoyment. Analysis of the interviews identified two key components of enjoyment: social interaction and competition. Other sources of enjoyment included the exercise environment, flow experiences, emotional and physical outcomes, and distraction from daily hassles and demands.

Potential interactions among personality, exercise mode, and exercise environments. A variety of interactions may help to explain why some people find specific types of exercise to be enjoyable, other people prefer other types of exercise, and still others do not find any type of exercise to be enjoyable. It is clear that not all types of exercise are enjoyable to all individuals, and that exercisers differ in their personal preferences for specific types of physical activity.

There may be an identifiable personality profile that enables an exerciser to enjoy swimming numerous repetitive laps in a pool, rather than participating in the thrilling activity of rock climbing. In a study of enjoyment and personality, lap swimmers reported high scores on trait anxiety and low scores on sensation seeking; rock climbers reported the opposite personality profile (Motl & Berger, 1997). These differences in personality may have influenced the adult exercisers' enjoyment of swimming and rock climbing.

The interrelationships between exercisers' personality characteristics and the actual exercise environment may influence perceptions of enjoyment. For example, exercisers who have high levels of concern about the appearance of their bodies, or social-physique anxiety, may not enjoy exercising in gyms or aerobics classes. These exercise environments often present a strong physique-evaluative component that could produce anxiety rather than enjoyment (Focht & Hausenblas, 2004). In order to enjoy their exercise sessions, exercisers who have a high level of social-physique anxiety may need to participate in physical activity environments that contain less of an evaluative component. Such environments may include specifically designed exercise classes and may be conducted in their homes, local neighborhoods, or parks.

Conclusions: The Benefits of Exercise Enjoyment

Enjoyment is linked to QoL (Kahneman et al., 1999), and physical activity may be one way of experiencing enjoyment and thus improving QoL. Numerous factors within the exercise experience contribute to enjoyment. Some of these include mood enhancement or feeling better, opportunity for thrills and excitement, the occasional peak moment, mind-body-spirit unity, communing with nature, escape from the cares of the day, and opportunities for a sense of playfulness and frivolousness. You will explore some of these factors later in Chapter 14, which focuses on personal meaning in exercise. The depth and breadth of factors contributing to enjoyment are as diverse as the array of personal meanings associated with physical activity.

Summary

Quality of life emphasizes a state of excellence and an enhanced sense of well-being. Quality of life is a more comprehensive concept than either subjective well-being or happiness. Although the study of exercise and the QoL of life still is in its infancy, accumulating research evidence supports the likelihood that habitual physical activity, and especially exercise, influences our QoL in many different ways. Multiple interacting factors challenge researchers who are investigating somatopsychic and psychosomatic relationships that are related to QoL.

Exercise is associated with subjective well-being, especially desirable mood states. The mood benefits most clearly related to exercise tend to be acute or short-term in non-psychiatric populations, rather than chronic and long-term. Chronic mood changes tend to occur in populations with clinical diagnoses of anxiety and depression. The mood benefits of exercise will be described in greater depth in Chapter 6, which focuses on mood alteration and self-awareness. The importance of exercise enjoyment, exercise type, and practice considerations in the relationship between exercise and mood alteration are the topics of Chapters 20 and 21.

Another way in which exercise contributes to our QoL is by serving as a stress management technique. Different types of exercise enable participants to either decrease or increase their stress levels and thus move toward their optimal levels of stress for personal functioning and enjoyment.

Some types of exercise, especially noncompetitive, repetitive, and predictable types of exercise, are associated with decreases in ongoing levels of stress. Other types of exercise, especially those that are performed in competitive settings or at high exercise intensities, are stress producing. In addition, high-risk physical activity provides opportunities for a special form of stress

known as eustress, an exhilarating form of stress. Although exercise is only one of many available stress management techniques, exercise is particularly appealing because it simultaneously provides a variety of health benefits and desirable changes in appearance.

Examining the relationship between exercise and the QoL, it is important to recognize that exercise can have negative influences if participants habitually overtrain, become dependent on exercise, or use exercise in conjunction with disordered eating behaviors. Some of these exercise-related concerns will be explored in Chapter 16. Examples of undesirable consequences of exercise include overuse injuries, exercise compulsion, increased fatigue and decreased energy and other undesirable mood states, and feelings of stress. Further information about stress and the use of exercise as a stress management technique is provided in Chapter 7 on stress and in Chapter 8 on exercise as a stress management technique.

Providing opportunities for peak moments and flow is another way that exercise can add to the quality and meaning of life. Peak performance, peak experience, flow, and the exerciser's or runner's high are examples of different types of peak moments that exercise participants report. Although our understanding of peak moments is limited by the difficult nature of defining these elusive and fleeting moments, the current research emphasizes a critical need to move beyond describing the experiences. Understanding the experience of peak moments may be one piece of the puzzle for encouraging more people to be physically active. In addition, experiencing peak moments in exercise settings also affects our QoL.

Finally, exercise influences our life quality by providing opportunities for personal enjoyment. Enjoyment is "an optimal psychological state (i.e., flow) that leads to performing an activity for its own sake and is associated with positive feeling states" (Kimiecik & Harris, 1996, p. 257). Enjoyment is linked to QoL by providing rewarding, interesting, and truly memorable hedonic experiences.

Daily "doses" of enjoyment may counterbalance the stress and hassles of everyday life, reduce the likelihood of developing depression, and contribute to positive mood states. Enjoyment of exercise appears to result from factors such as body-mind integration, close interactions with the beauty of nature, peak moments, physical achievement, increased self-awareness, skill mastery, and social interactions. Some of the personal factors are examined in more depth in Chapter 14, "Meaning in Exercise."

In conclusion, this chapter focuses on some of the many ways in which exercise can influence the quality of our lives. Exercise influences QoL by providing a source of enjoyment and opportunities for peak moments, as well as desirable, short-term mood changes and a stress management technique. These influences on the QoL and others, such as enhancing positive self-concept and self-esteem, opportunities for heightened personal meaning, and the delaying of the aging process, will be explored throughout the remaining chapters of *Foundations of Exercise Psychology.*

Can You Define These Terms?

acute changes in mood

character strengths

chronic changes in mood

desirable mood changes associated with exercise

disease prevention model of exercise

exercise enjoyment

exerciser's high

eustress

feeling and performance model

flow states

flow model

happiness

health enhancement model of exercise

hedonic psychology

mood decrements

peak experiences

peak moments

peak performance

person-by-situation framework

quality of life

ripple effect

runner's high

self-report measures

stress

stress management

subjective well-being

virtues

Can You Answer These Questions?

1. What are the three major constructs that influence subjective well-being? Do you think that one construct is more important than the others?

2. How is the quality of life a broader concept than subjective well-being?

3. Based on the diverse influences on life quality, what is your current quality of life? Be sure to explain the basis for your conclusions.

4. According to Seligman's virtues and character strengths, what are your personal psychological strengths, as measured at the web site www.authentichappiness.com?

5. Does exercise influence your quality of life? Please provide a detailed reply.

6. How do the mood benefits of exercise differ for members of clinical and nonclinical populations?

7. How long do the acute mood benefits of exercise tend to last?

8. What are the differences between eustress, stress, and distress?

9. What are possible undesirable influences of exercise on participants?

10. Why are peak performances, peak experiences, flow, and the exercise high all considered to be peak moments in exercise?

11. How do you differentiate between peak performance, peak experience, flow, and the exercise high?

12. What characteristics are common to nearly all types of peak moments?

13. Which theory or model of peak moments do you prefer? How did you select your preference?

14. What are the basic sources of exercise enjoyment?

15. As a movement specialist, why is it important for you to assist your students and clients in enjoying exercise?

CHAPTER 4

Exercise and Enhanced Self-Concept and Self-Esteem

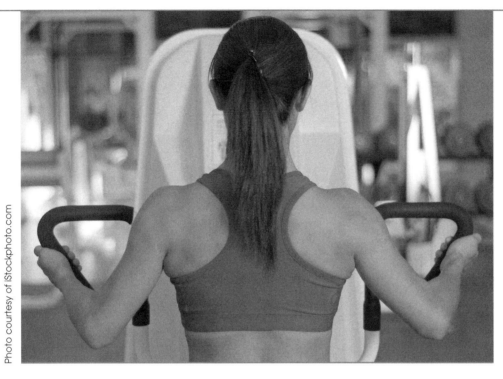

Photo courtesy of iStockphoto.com

After reading this chapter, you should be able to

- Describe the relationship between exercise and perceptions about the physical self,

- Define the term *self-concept* and distinguish it from terms such as *self-esteem*, *self-efficacy*, and *self-identity*,

- Discuss the multidimensionality of self-concept, and

- Identify available measures of self-concept and self-esteem.

Introduction

Our personal view of self may not be the same or even compatible with the way others see us. Life's lessons help us to develop perceptions of our own strengths, vulnerabilities, personality, and ways of relating to others. Many of us invest a lot of effort in striving to know who we are, and sometimes what we conclude pleases us and sometimes it does not.

The views you have of the various parts of your self, or your *self-concept*, represent the very core of your personality. Self-concept is the epicenter around which other traits develop and exist, and it is integral to psychological well-being. Perceptions of the self may take various forms, for there are numerous parts of the self and many ways in which to view them. Unfortunately, those who have contributed to the ever-increasing body of literature in this area tend to use a variety of related terms—sometimes synonymously and appropriately, sometimes improperly. It is therefore necessary to carefully differentiate among them. In the preface to his book, *The Physical Self: From Motivation to Well-Being*, Fox (1997) addresses this problem. Table 4.1 presents a number of terms used and defined in his book (pp. xii–xiii). They are included here in an effort to establish a basis for understanding the relationship between exercise and perceptions of the self.

Table 4.1
Looking at the Self: Different Perspectives

body esteem: The value or worth an individual attaches to his or her body. Similar to self-esteem, it represents an overall judgment based on body criteria that the individual feels are important.

body image: The mental representation an individual has of his or her body.

identity: The integration of beliefs, values, self-perceptions, and behaviors into a consistent, coherent, and recognizable self-package. It is more than a self-description—more akin to a self-theory. This term is used more frequently in the sociology literature, with some writers maintaining that an individual can have separate identities in different domains of life.

perceived ability: A more specific statement of competence restricted to a limited set of behaviors such as playing soccer, doing mathematics, or conducting relationships with similar-sex peers.

perceived competence: A statement of personal ability that generalizes across a domain such as sport, scholarship, or work.

self-concept: The individual as known to the individual. This is a self-description profile based on the multitude of roles and attributes that we consider make up our self. Examples might be "I am a father," "I am a friend," "I am a golfer." Some theorists include within the self-concept evaluative statements such as "I am a really talented golfer," whereas others exclude them.

self-confidence: A general term reflecting the degree to which an individual feels he or she is able to successfully meet the demands of a social context.

self-efficacy: A statement of expectancy about one's ability to accomplish a specific task.

self-esteem: The awareness of good possessed by the self (Campbell, 1984, p. 9). This is a global construct that provides an overall statement of the degree to which an individual perceives himself or herself to be an "OK" person, dependent on whatever criteria that individual uses to determine "OK."

self-perceptions: An umbrella term that denotes all types of self-referent statements about the self, from those that are global to those that are specific in content.

self-worth: Essentially the same meaning as self-esteem.

From: *The Physical Self: From Motivation to Well-Being* (pp. xii–xiii), by K. R. Fox, 1997, Champaign, IL: Human Kinetics. Copyright 1997. Reprinted with permission. *Note*: Reference inside reprint: Campbell, R. N. (1984). *The new science: Self-esteem psychology.* Lanham, MD: University Press of America.

In their book, Baron and Byrne (1991) use the terms *self-identity* and *self-concept* interchangeably. They note that our self-concept influences the manner in which we process social information and experience motivation and feelings (affective states). To the contrary, other scholars draw a firm line of distinction between the two psychological constructs. Among these are Brettschneider and Heim (1997), who maintain that self-identity refers to an individual's descriptions of the self as a unique and distinctive entity. However, in expressing their self-identity, individuals must initially describe themselves adequately so the establishment of self-concept is antecedent to an expression of self-identity. Who am I? What's special about me? How am I different from others? When responding to these questions, we construct a self-identity and provide building blocks necessary for the establishment of the self-concept. Self-identity is more comprehensive and inclusive in that it comprises a clear statement of goals, values, and beliefs to which a person is devoted (Waterman, 1985).

Self-concept itself consists of numerous role identities, each of which may be characterized as a *dimension* or part of the self-concept. All of us fulfill a number of different roles, each with its own responsibilities and obligations. We could be—at the same time—student, child or grandchild, boyfriend or girlfriend, church choir member, dog owner, part-time employee at the local pizza shop, and member of a university's intramural basketball team. Some of us might also experience the equally important roles of parent, professor, consultant, author, homeowner, or jogger. Taken together, these identities contribute to the perceptions we hold about ourselves. In addition, our performance of these roles and the evaluation of our performance in the social environment are just as important as our self-perception. Somehow, we learn that we excel as student and choir member, but are off the mark as contributor to the intramural team. Perhaps the manager at the pizza shop lets you know, in no uncertain terms, that he considers you to be an undependable employee. But, on Valentine's Day, you read a carefully worded message from a girlfriend or boyfriend indicating that you are lovable, considerate, and wonderful. Our overall concept of self helps us integrate these various judgments about how effectively we are handling our different roles. Conversely, our interpretation of how well we carry them out influences the overall concept we hold of the self.

Self-Concept

In referring to self-concept, Marsh (1997) suggests that "everybody knows what it is" (p. 28). However, despite its widespread use in parlance and our general familiarity with the term, there are also a number of different definitions of self-concept. In most cases, the differences are due to alternative research emphases. Some scholars seem to be essentially interested in relationships *between* self-concept and a variety of other hypothetical constructs, whereas other researchers explore the essentially internal structure (*within*) of self-concept (Marsh, 1997). The former approach attempts to demonstrate a correlation between numerous aspects of self-concept (for example, physical, social, intellectual) and behavioral tendencies or observable performance. The latter approach emphasizes variables within self-concept and focuses on the construct's multidimensionality; that is, the interrelationships among the various parts of self-concept.

Multidimensionality Aspect of Self-Concept

As mentioned previously, most researchers in the field consider self-concept to be multidimensional, with each dimension having several facets (Byrne, 1984). However, there seems to be disagreement about the degree to which the facets are correlated. Some experts consider the facets to be independent of one another, whereas others believe them to be somewhat correlated. Again, today, the multidimensionality of self-concept (meaning that it consists of various kinds of self-perceptions) is by and large undisputed. We do not simply ask individuals about the way they see themselves; rather, we question them about particular aspects of themselves. The relationship of the many dimensions may be complex, and it is difficult for some persons to make distinctions among them. The more dimensions, or the more roles a person has, the more challenging it is to separate and evaluate them. Persons said to have high levels of self-complexity (Linville, 1987; Rothermund & Meninger, 2004) may be better suited to coping with the effects of stress. If one dimension of the self is viewed as doing poorly (e.g., role as parent), one or more other dimensions of the self may provide positive feedback that will take the sharp edge off the negative perception of parenthood. Many exercisers are thus able to enhance their overall concept of self by perceiving themselves to be "strong" in exercise (although weak in another dimension). Some evidence exists that we may also exhibit behaviors that strengthen our identity as exercisers. We may thus reinforce our perception of a strong exercise-self by continuing to exercise as well as by embracing symbols that represent exercise such as using rituals, wearing t-shirts and gym shoes, or carrying gym bags (Anderson & Cychosz, 1994).

According to Linville (1987), the greater the self-complexity, the greater the buffering effect against stress. This suggests that the less complex a person's concept of self, the more likely stress reactions will

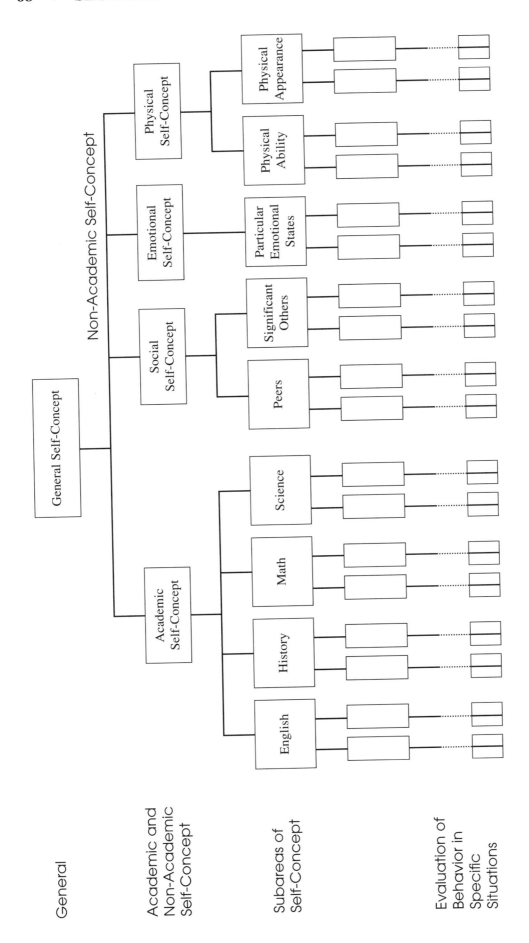

Figure 4.1. An example of the Hierarchical Structure of Self-Concept. From "Self-Concept: Validation of Construct Interpretations," by R .J. Shavelson, J. J. Hubner, and G. C. Stanton, 1976, *Review of Educational Research.*

spill over to one or two areas of the individual's life. With more aspects or roles in life, stress effects may be diffused. Perhaps this explains the alleged role of exercise as a stress-coping technique.

Hierarchical Organization of Self-Concept

It is helpful to think of the various dimensions of self-concept as being vertically aligned (Harter, 1990; Marsh & Redmayne, 1994; Shavelson, Hubner, & Stanton, 1976). If a hierarchical arrangement is assumed, then a person may hold a view of herself as a physically functioning entity who moves well or uses her body efficiently. This view is considered broad, general, or global and is located at the top of the self-concept hierarchy or taxonomy (see Figure 4.1). At a lower level might be her perception that she does not jump high but is graceful, or that she cannot run fast but is able to run far. At an even lower hierarchical level might be the view that she is a poor basketball player but quite a decent swimmer or ice skater.

Role Conflict

The perspective of the physical self is thus one of numerous dimensions, each of which has parts and subfacets. Further, all of the perceptions about parts and subparts of the self are based on standards that are *comparative,* or related to other people. That is, we tend to think of and evaluate ourselves in terms of others. Our concept of self is based substantially upon the similarities and dissimilarities we note among our physical, emotional, and intellectual attributes, and those of others.

On occasion, the different aspects of self-concept may be in conflict with one another. Along these lines is an interesting question posed in research hypotheses format by Miller and Levy (1996). Might females, for example, who participate in collegiate sport possess stronger perceptions (being more masculine) about their personal gender than non-athletes? That is, do female collegiate athletes (undoubtedly frequent and inveterate exercisers) see themselves as being more masculine than non-athletes? The answer generated by their research protocol is "no." They found no differences in a number of self-views, including gender identity.

Stability of Self-Concept

Each of the self's parts can change over time. In addition, parts of the self-concept are situation specific, although the overall view of the physical self (at the hierarchy's apex) remains fairly constant. Some research findings have suggested that self-concept is stable and we therefore tend to embrace or pay more attention to evaluations that support a broad view of self

and its parts. Individuals with negative self-concepts would accordingly be inclined to seek unfavorable evaluations more frequently than would those with more positive self-concepts (Swann, 1985; Swann & Hill, 1982; Swann, Hixon, et al., 1990). In keeping with such findings are results from other studies that actually show a tendency to reject information that does not support the self-concept (Greenwald & Pratkanis, 1984; Tesser & Campbell, 1983). Incoming information that bears upon who we are and what we represent is thus filtered. Information that is not consonant with our prevailing view of self is likely to be discarded, repressed, or ignored. If this is so, then this hypothesized screening process helps clarify the stable nature of self-concept.

Another tern, *self-presentation*, is used to refer to the processes by which people attempt to control and monitor how they are perceived and evaluated by others (Leary, Tchividjian, & Kraxberger, 1999). Since most people want others to view them in a favorable light, they attempt to regulate how others evaluate them. They attempt to do this by restructuring information about themselves that they themselves provide. They manipulate information they disseminate in order to achieve the impression that they covet and hide information that may depict them in negative ways (Leary et al., 1999). Participation in exercise may be linked to self-presentational concerns (Hausenblas, Brewer, & Van Raalte, 2004). Exercise may be pursued by people who desire to present themselves as fit and "in shape." They have confidence in their body image and are eager to share this view with others.

Not only do such findings support the speculation that self-concept is not easily modified, but they also bring the matter of attentional focus into play. If an individual attends more to information that supports his or her self view, then issues of information processing arise. That is, we are attracted to and inclined to absorb and deal with stimuli that are relevant to our particular world. We hear and see what we want to hear and see.

On the other hand, a larger and more convincing body of findings seems to encourage a situation-specific emphasis (McInman & Berger, 1993), wherein self-concept is responsive to such variables as other persons, evaluative feedback, and outcome of competitive experiences (Demo, 1985; Pedic, 1989; Tesser, 1988; Wells, 1988). This contrasts significantly with the above speculation that places a premium upon selective attention and processing of information. When a person receives flattering commentary (particularly from a significant other), vanquishes an opponent on the athletic field or in an important election, or wins an award, that person's self-concept may fluctuate in a positive direction. Alternatively, in negative situations, the self-concept may suffer. An interesting treatment of both sides of the "stability versus variability" issue is provided by Kernis and Goldman (2003).

Exercise is an experience (situation) with the potential for such fluctuations. It permits "feel good/bad" responses, positive or negative feedback from others (peers, leaders, etc.), and resulting alterations in mood, all of which can influence self-concept. As Markus and Wurf (1987) suggest, self-concept is a collection of general notions about the self that derive from past experiences. In other words, we should think of self-concept as describing something that "is best viewed as a continually active, shifting array of accessible self-knowledge" (Markus & Wurf, 1987, p. 306). Exercise can be an important causal element in this change in knowledge about the self.

Exercise and Self-Concept

Participation in an ongoing exercise program, in contrast to a single bout of exercise, is associated with change in self-concept (Ford, Puckett, et al., 1989; Nagy & Frazier, 1988; Plummer & Koh, 1987; Sorenson, Anderssen, et al., 1997; Taylor & Fox, 2005). For the most part, this change is positive; that is, exercise significantly enhances self-concept (e.g., Alfermann & Stoll, 2000; Hayden, Allen, & Camaione, 1986; Asci, 2003; Taylor & Fox, 2005). Moreover, persons who are high in measures of physical fitness tend to have higher self-concepts than do those with low fitness levels (Berger & McInman, 1993; DiLorenzo, Bargman, et al., 1999).

Both aerobic dance and aerobic exercise, in particular, have generated such positive change under certain conditions (Daley & Buchanan, 1999). One reason for this may be that these activities have been incorporated as independent variables in research designs so often. Groups of aerobic dance and aerobic exercisers (e.g., swimmers, joggers, and cyclists) are conveniently available to researchers. Another reason may be that certain characteristics of aerobic activities, rather than the activities as a whole, make them especially effective at changing self-concept.

To date, these characteristics have not been clearly identified, but they are likely to be a combination of neuropsychological, biochemical, and social-cognitive factors (Berger, 1996; Thayer, 1996). In other words, something inherent in or resulting from exercise (aerobic exercise in particular) influences the self-view. Perhaps it is the pleasure that some of us derive from exercise; perhaps it is complimentary remarks from others; or perhaps physiological effects of exercise somehow interact with our cognitive processes to alter self-concept. At the moment, we are not sure. Bolstering this speculation are the findings of Knapen, van de vliet, VanCoppenolle, David, Peuskens,

Knapen, and Pieters (2003), who reported improvement in self-concept after eight weeks of physical fitness training in nonpsychotic psychiatric patients, despite absence of changes in dynamic strength, muscular endurance, and physical work capacity. Butki (1998) reported a positive correlation between level of physical activity and various dimensions of self-concept in adolescent males and females located in public school psychological treatment centers.

In particular, the following three additional variables may be related to self-concept:

- percent of stored body fat (the lower the amount of body fat, the more positive the concept of self—particularly body image),
- frequency and type of exercise, and
- muscular strength (Balogun, 1987).

Reasons for participating in regular exercise as well as the amount of exercise accomplished may also influence body satisfaction and self-esteem. Exercisers whose motives were centered on health and fitness were observed to realize an increase in self-esteem; those who participated for reasons of weight control and muscle tone improvement were associated with lower self-esteem (Tiggeman & Willamson, 2000).

One kind of physical activity, namely Outward Bound survival courses, is consistently associated with positive changes in self-efficacy. Moreover, the longer the participation in the program, the greater the increase in self-concept (Marsh, Richards, & Barnes, 1986a). Outward Bound courses typically involve challenging and rugged outdoor activities such as rope climbing and rappelling, canoeing, hiking, swimming, and boating. It may be that mastery of the environment and overcoming its physical obstacles are contributors to the observed changes in self-concept.

Weight lifting has also been shown to enhance self-concept (Brone & Reznikoff, 1989). Perhaps this is so because weight-training programs are often conducted over comparatively longer periods of time, thus enabling strong changes in self-concept.

Motivation to exercise and self-concept. The link between motivation for exercise and perception of self appears to exist in two directions. The self is an essential determinant of exercise (Sallis et al., 1986; Sonstroem, 1988). People with strong feelings about the self—although not necessarily perceiving themselves as having high physical ability—are more likely to adhere to an exercise program (Valois, Shephard, & Godin, 1986) than are people with low self-worth (Duncan, McAuley, et al., 1993; Theodorakis, 1994). Thinking highly of oneself means liking oneself, and people who like themselves are inclined to be concerned about their physical appearance. Accordingly, they may wish that others view them in a positive way because these others are likely to respond favorably to individuals with attractive physical attributes. Hence, persons with high self-worth are willing to exercise regularly in order to bolster their physical image. Conversely, individuals with low self-concept are not inclined to participate in regular physical activity (Vanden Auweele, Rzewnicki, & Van Mele, 1997). Many factors interact in complex ways to determine our self-concept. As Marsh (1994) suggests, "Self-concept cannot be adequately understood if its multi-dimensionality is ignored" (p. 307).

In a series of studies, Kendzierski (1988, 1990, 1994) demonstrated that an individual's exercise self-schemas, or cognitive generalizations about important parts of the self (what he or she thinks about him or herself), are derived from past experiences and related to exercise intention. These schemas about the self are good predictors of exercise behavior. Those who think of themselves as exercisers are more likely to report that they have adopted an exercise program than are individuals who have no such self-schema.

The Physical Self

An important theme in this chapter is that the overall concept of self is strongly influenced by the individual's view of the *physical self*. Self-evaluation of the physical self, in particular, exerts a meaningful impact upon the development of general (overall) self-concept (Davis, Claridge, & Brewer, 1996). Our view of the physical self is so important to us that when we perceive our physiques being evaluated by others, we tend to experience heightened anxiety (Hart, Leary, & Rejeski, 1989; Crawford & Eklund, 1994). This phenomenon is referred to as *social physique anxiety* and is apparently more prevalent among women than men (Eklund, Kelley, & Wilson, 1997). Social physique anxiety is heightened when persons believe that their body will create an undesirable impression upon others in the immediate environment. It is believed that SPA is a personality trait which influences choice of exercise environment (e.g., gender of other exercis-

CASE STUDY 4.1 — *Struggling With the Physical Self-Concept: The Story of Ricardo*

Ricardo is a shy, thin, 10th grader of average height. Preferring his own company, he is not inclined to spend much time in the company of classmates or peers. During a conference with his homeroom teacher, who requested a meeting, his parents verify Ricardo's tendency to avoid being with others. Mr. Lowry had noticed Ricardo's tendency over a period of a few months and concluded that it would be in the boy's best interest for him to be better integrated with other students in his grade level. Mr. Lowry is also convinced of Ricardo's low concept of his physical self. He reached this conclusion after hearing Ricardo express displeasure with his thinness on a few occasions. One, in particular, occurred while Mr. Lowry was inquiring about Ricardo's high frequency of absences from physical education class. During conversation, the boy confessed to feeling embarrassed when obliged to "dress out" for gym. He felt that the other boys looked at him disparagingly and with ridicule because of his ungainly physique. Because Mr. Lowry feared that Ricardo's weak body image would negatively affect his general view of self and undermine his self-confidence, the teacher recommended to Ricardo's parents that they enroll him in a local fitness center where he could participate in an organized program of weight training under the direction of a personal trainer. The parents accepted the suggestion and acted accordingly. With some strategic manipulations suggested by the competent trainer, in combination with an appropriately designed heavy resistance program in which Ricardo participated 4 days a week, favorable results were soon apparent. At the conclusion of approximately 4 months, Ricardo's body weight had increased by 15%. Muscle mass underwent appreciable and obvious increase. Ricardo began to demonstrate increased confidence in his appearance. He became more interested in the clothes he wore. He began to show interest in cultivating social relationships. He became more outgoing and attended after-school functions that he previously had made efforts to avoid. His self-confidence and self-concept appeared to be positively changed. As his body shape changed due to a likely combination of exercise (weight training), enhanced nutrition, and physical maturation, Ricardo's body image improved. He sought social contact with schoolmates, and, as his teacher, Mr. Lowry, put it, "Ricky is now a really happy guy."

ers), as well as feelings about the environment and the exercise experience itself (Leary, 1992). Our perceptions of ourselves as physical entities are essential to the formation of our understanding about who and what we are, in a broader sense. Another way of expressing this is to say that the body, or the physical self, is the medium through which most of us experience reality, which is the basis for building concepts of self (see Case Study 4.1 for a story about Ricardo, a young man struggling with the concept of his physical self). Piaget, the eminent child development psychologist, believed this process occurred in what he described as the *sensorimotor stage*, or the very first stage of cognitive development. Here, children from birth to about 2 years of age cultivate reasoning, thinking, and problem-solving abilities by interacting with the environment through sensory and physical means (by using their bodies to acquire understanding of their world [Piaget, 1954]). Several studies have shown that children as young as 7 and 8 years of age have reported dissatisfaction with their bodies and concern about becoming overweight. A comprehensive literature overview by Ricciardelli and McCabe (2001) indicates that many of these children are engaged in weight-loss behaviors, such as eating less and exercising to lose weight. Negative views of the body in children are considered major risk factors for body image problems, exercise dependence, and eating disorders in adulthood (Smolak, Levine, & Schermer, 1999; Birch & Fisher, 1998).

Exercise and the Physical Self

Because body shape and function are basic elements of the physical self, they are affected by regular participation in vigorous physical activity, namely, exercise. In this way, self-perceptions and exercise are integrally related. Physical activity, when experienced in appropriately designed programs over extended periods, can enhance the body's form (mechanical) and function (physiological). These enhancements in turn may conceivably affect the personal view of self. Thus, the more we exercise or train (properly), the more we are likely to improve our self-esteem (Sonstroem, Harlow, & Josephs, 1994). This was demonstrated in dramatic fashion in a study conducted with persons with spinal-cord injury paraplegia who participated in an electrical-stimulation walking program. They, too, experienced changes in measures of physical self-concept (Guest, Klose, Needhamshropshire, & Jacobs, 1997). Interestingly, their depression scores also decreased, thus suggesting a strong influence of even artificially stimulated exercise upon psychological factors.

Exercise may enhance our perceptions of our physical abilities, our self-competence, and our self-acceptance. Improvement in function or performance

is what Bandura (1986) refers to, in his *social cognitive* viewpoint, as successful mastery experiences, or successful outcomes. These new and improved perceptions may also have a positive impact upon *self-efficacy* (expectations about future performance on specific tasks), which in turn influences effort, persistence, and achievement (i.e., motivation). Results from a study by Lox, McAuley, and Tucker (1995) also support this model. In their study of subjects at various stages of HIV-1 infection, the authors concluded that exercise should be considered as a therapeutic intervention for enhancing aspects of self-perceived well-being. Subjects in this study participating in aerobic and weight-training interventions demonstrated enhanced physical self-efficacy, positive and negative mood, and satisfaction with life. As McAuley (1994) and Sonstroem (1984) have suggested, exercise behavior, particularly adherence and compliance, can have a positive effect on self-perceptions. Thus, there is some evidence that when we exercise regularly, we tend to view the physical part of ourselves more positively. In a more recent study using diabetic adults, it was found that those actively involved in regular exercise had higher efficacy levels (for ability to deal with their disease) as well as higher self-concept scores than did individuals who were thinking about, but not yet involved in, a program of exercise (Plotnikoff, Brez, & Hotz, 2000).

Measures of Self-Concept Dimensions

Because there is more than a single approach to self-concept research, there are different theoretical understandings of its multidimensionality. This has led to a variety of measurement strategies. If self-concept is multidimensional, with each dimension having subparts that are arranged hierarchically, then instruments designed to assess self-concept would include items that explore perceptions of each dimension as well as its subparts. Given the overarching importance of self-concept and self-esteem, and their particular relevance to physical activity and exercise, it is imperative that they be assessed validly and reliably. What instruments and approaches are therefore available? We now turn to issues related to the measurement of self-concept and its various components.

Physical Self-Perception Profile

Fox and Corbin (1989) have developed the Physical Self-Perception Profile (PSPP), which is intended to examine perceptions of the physical self from a multidimensional perspective. The instrument, presented in five 6-item subscales, includes perceived sports competence, perceived bodily attractiveness, perceived physical strength and muscular development, perceived level of physical conditioning and exercise, and physical self-worth. The profile, emphasizing various independent facets of the physical self, represents a comprehensive approach that permits individuals to express perceptions about various aspects of their physical selves. The PSPP is available in forms for children as well as adults. This instrument is particularly applicable when teachers or exercise leaders wish to gather information about their student's or client's views about various aspects of their physicality.

Self-Description Questionnaire

Shavelson et al. (1976) developed a series of Self-Description Questionnaire (SDQ) instruments that were later revised (Marsh, 1990; Marsh & Shavelson, 1985). The various dimensions of self-concept as measured by these tests, refined for different developmental levels (preadolescent, adolescent, and young adults), are clearly distinct. The instruments have psychometric properties that indicate high construct validity (predicated upon a strong theoretical foundation)

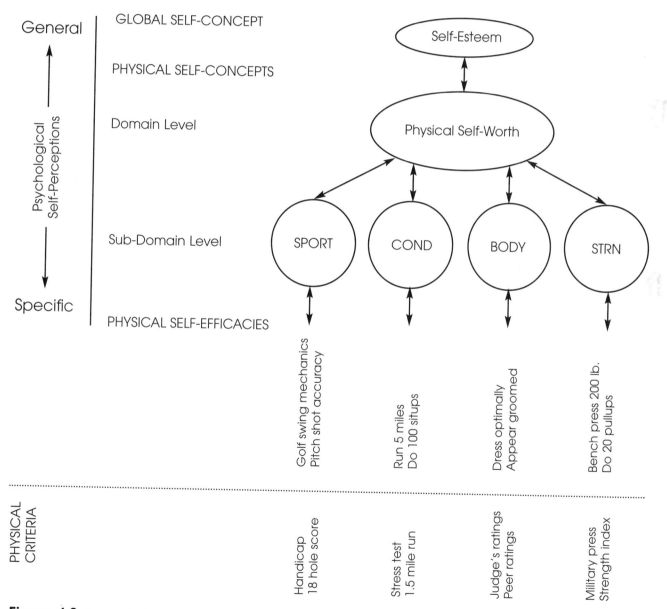

Figure 4.2. Expanded Exercise and Self-Esteem Model (EXSEM). From "Exercise and Self-Esteem: Validity of Model Expansion and Exercise Associations," by R. J. Sonstroem, L. L. Harlow, and L. Josephs, 1994, *Journal of Sport and Exercise Psychology, 16,* p. 38. Reprinted with permission.

and high internal consistency (reliability). The SDQ instruments measure a number of dimensions of self, but some of the scales are specifically directed towards physical self-perceptions. For instance, one scale relates to physical ability self-concept, whereas another relates to physical appearance self-concept. Women who participated in high school athletics scored differently on the physical ability self-concept than did non-athletes (Jackson & Marsh, 1986). In a study done by Marsh and Peart (1988), physical fitness was found to be related to physical ability self-concept, but only modestly related to physical appearance self-concept. Interestingly, those women who were participants in a cooperative aerobics program changed their physical ability self-concept scores in a positive direction (pre-post comparison) in contrast to those involved in competitive aerobics, who evinced a decline. Participants in an Outward Bound intervention enhanced their physical ability self-concept scores on the SDQ (Marsh, Richards, & Barnes, 1986a, 1986b). This suggests the changeability of physical self-perception scores (measured by the SDQ) and indicates a need for wholesome and effective interventions under the auspices of competent exercise leadership.

Exercise Identity Scale

There are numerous assessment instruments that provide an array of inventories and scales designed to assess self-perceptions about movement competence and physical fitness. Some, such as the Exercise Identity Scale, purport to determine the extent to which exercise describes one's concept of self (Anderson & Cychosz, 1994); that is, how importantly do number of weeks exercising, frequency of exercise per week, and duration and intensity of exercise bear upon the concept of self? Bracken (1992) has produced a multi-dimensional Self-Concept Scale that not only includes perspectives about various parts of the self, but also has performance related questions.

Expanded Exercise and Self-Esteem Model

A multidimensional approach to assessing physical self-concept, the Expanded Exercise and Self-Esteem Model (EXSEM), is currently in vogue. Moreover, as Sonstroem (1998) suggests, most of these assessment models are hierarchical in that there is an ordered array in which tertiary constructs determine secondary constructs, which, in turn, determine perceptions about the primary ones. General constructs are at the top of the hierarchy whereas lower-order components represent more specific ones. Lower-level constructs influence change in more general ones (see Figure 4.2).

Self-Concept Scale

Bracken (1992) has produced a multidimensional self-concept scale that not only includes perspectives about various parts of the self, but also has performance-related questions.

Social Physique Anxiety Scale

The Social Physique Anxiety Scale (SPAS) was developed in 1989 by Hart et al. as a trait measure of anxiety related to the physique. It is a 12-item scale that reliably and validly assesses anxiety experienced when one's physique is perceived to be evaluated by others (Petrie, Diehl, Rogers, & Johnson, 1996). Social physique anxiety, a concept that was introduced earlier in this chapter, represents a fear of negative evaluation about the physique (Martin, Rejeski, Leary, McAuley, & Bane, 1997).

The above instruments are offered here as examples of the large number of assessment tools that may be used to assess various perceptions about the physical self. A helpful source for an annotated list of instruments is the *Directory of Psychological Tests in the Sport and Exercise Sciences*, edited by Andrew C. Ostrow (1996).

Summary

The perceptions we hold about ourselves shape our behavior. Exercise exerts a strong influence upon these perceptions because it provides us with information about who we are from the standpoint of our physicality. Motivation to exercise is associated with self-perceptions and people with stronger and more positive self-views tend to be more highly motivated to exercise. As a cognitive process that involves thinking and describing ourselves to ourselves, *self-concept* is complex, multidimensional, and has a number of parts. Contemporary thinking suggests that in order to measure self-concept properly (i.e., Who am I?), an assessment of all of its aspects must be made.

Self-esteem, on the other hand, is more of an emotional or affective reaction because it reflects an evaluation of who we are (e.g., good, bad, positive, negative); self-esteem is a person's sense of self-worth or self-importance relative to each of the components of self-concept.

Self-identity refers to the roles we fulfill and is subsumed under the more overarching notion of self-concept. This means that when we attempt to determine who we are, we must consider the various roles (not merely parts, as referred to above) or identities we claim (e.g., husband, plumber, grandson, nurse). For many individuals, exercise or regular physical activity is included in this list of roles so that, among all the identities, there might also be aerobic dancer, martial artist, or tennis player.

Although some research findings suggest that self-concept is stable and not easily modified, a convincing number of recent studies point to situation specificity, which implies that self-concept is responsive to events, feedback from others, and the results of competitive experiences. For this reason, it may make more sense to view self-concept as an ongoing, modifiable cognitive operation. In this perspective, exercise would be among the experiences (and outcomes) with considerable potential to alter self-concept.

Can You Define These Terms?

body esteem
_____

body image
_____

identity
_____

perceived ability
_____

perceived competence
_____

physical self
_____

self-concept
_____

self-confidence
_____

self-efficacy
_____

self-esteem
_____

self-perceptions
_____

self-worth
_____

Can You Answer These Questions?

1. What are the components of self-concept?
2. Why does exercise exert a strong influence upon perceptions of the self?
3. Are the various components of self-concept meaningfully correlated among themselves? What is the nature of the correlation(s)?
4. Explain the following statement: "Self-concept is active, shifting, and unstable."
5. What is the social-cognitive viewpoint? Explain how this notion relates to expectations about future exercise performance.
6. What is the link between motivation to exercise and self-concept?
7. What instrument would you use if you wished to examine perceptions of the physical self from a multidimensional perspective in adults?
8. What is social physique anxiety?

CHAPTER 5

Mood and Exercise: Basic Mood Considerations

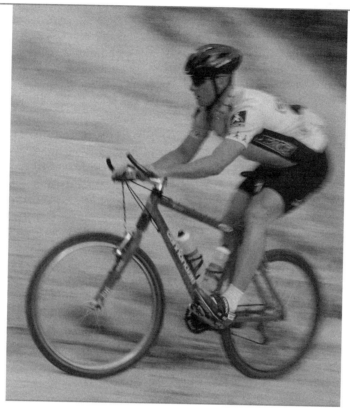

Photo courtesy of © Media Focus LLC

After reading this chapter, you should be able to

- Discuss the dilemma of a hedonic unipolar continuum versus a bipolar, independent dimensions model of mood,

- Explain the high-low arousal/negative-positive valence model of mood,

- Explain the energy-tiredness/tension-calmness model of mood,

- Define the meaning of mood, emotion, and affect,

- Discuss the relationship between mood and health behaviors,

- Identify some of the main mood states and describe each,

- Clarify state and trait measures of mood,

- Discuss the importance of mood and the role it plays in our daily lives, and

- Describe the "iceberg profile" of mood states commonly reported by exercisers.

Introduction

Regular exercisers often report that they "feel better" or are in a better mood after participating in physical activity. Anecdotal or personal reports of why a person exercises include observations such as having more energy, having a clearer mind, and feeling more "up." Examples of such anecdotal reports about the mood benefits of exercise include the following quotations. The first quotation is from Arnold Mandell, a psychiatrist who runs with his patients. The second quotation is from George Sheehan, now deceased, who was a running philosopher and cardiologist.

> . . . Colors are bright and beautiful, water sparkles, clouds breathe, and my body, swimming, detaches from the earth. A *loving contentment* [italics added] invades the basement of my mind, and thoughts bubble up without trails. *I find the place I need to live if I am going to live* [italics added]. (Mandell, 1979, p. 57)

> Exercise has the effect of defusing *anger and rage, fear and anxiety* [italics added]. Like music, it soothes the savage in us that lies so close to the surface. It is the ultimate tranquilizer. (Sheehan, 1992, p. 64)

Personal reports such as these have prompted exercise psychologists to explore the relationship between mood alteration and physical activity. Exactly what are people talking about when they say they "feel better" after exercising? "Feeling better" is vague because it includes a broad range of characteristics: enhanced mood, feelings of competency and self-efficacy, lower stress levels, decreased anxiety and depression, a sense of calmness or peace, and even feelings of personal power and strength.

This chapter focuses directly on one set of benefits associated with exercise, namely, mood: ways of describing and measuring mood, its importance in daily life, and the role of exercise in the self-regulation of mood (e.g., Berger, 1996; Berger & Owen, 1998; Gauvin, Rejeski, & Reboussin, 2000; Thayer, 2001). The following chapter focuses on types of mood changes that often occur after exercising and on some of the possible mechanisms that underlie the exercise-mood relationship. But, first, let us examine the definition of mood.

Differentiation Among Terms

Mood: A Definition

A typical definition of mood is a host of "transient, fluctuating affective states," both positive ones and negative ones, as noted in the test manual of an often employed mood inventory, the Profile of Mood States (POMS; McNair, Lorr, & Droppleman, 1971, 1992).

Moods usually are in our conscious awareness, which allows us to talk about them in conversations or rate them on questionnaires. Moods are composed of subjective feelings, and they have cognitive, behavioral, neurochemical, and psychophysiological manifestations (e.g., Izard & Ackerman, 1998; Matthews, Jones, & Chamberlain, 1990). Our moods remind us of the unity or integration of mind and body. As emphasized in the above definition of mood from the POMS Manual, shifts in mood states occur routinely and easily. Despite the variability in mood states, mood has very pronounced effects on our thoughts and judgments, behavior, feelings, and thus our overall quality of life.

Because moods are transient, they usually are *state measures* that reflect how an individual feels *at a particular moment in time*. The moment in time might refer to the present moment (i.e., "right now") or for a slightly longer period of time, such as "the past week, including today." It is important to note, however, that mood also can be a *trait measure*—if the inventory asks people to indicate how they have been feeling during a fairly long period of time such as the past year.

Some theorists suggest that mood ranges along a hedonic or happiness continuum that is exceedingly desirable or positive at one end and undesirable or negative at the other end. Despite this generalization, it is important to note that no specific mood *always* is desirable or undesirable. A particular mood needs to be appropriate to its context. Vigor, for example, often is a desirable mood, but if it occurs at bedtime, vigor may be detrimental to falling asleep. Fear can be immobilizing and detrimental to trying new activities; however, fear also can serve the adaptive function of warning us to seek a safe haven when harm is near (Izard & Ackerman, 1998). With this warning regarding the need for caution when assigning positive and negative values to mood, specific moods tend to occupy positions along a positive and negative continuum. Elation, energy, satisfaction, and vigor generally are examples of positive or desirable mood states that differ from one another in their degree of "positiveness." Moods that often are negative, or undesirable, include feelings of anger, depression, disappointment, and tension.

Exercise sessions are conducive to experiencing a variety of such mood states in a relatively brief amount of time. In a case study of a woman jogger, the exerciser reported feelings ranging from agony to ecstasy (Berger & Mackenzie, 1980). Some of the key moods associated with her exercise were feelings of aliveness, anger, competency, guilt, and power. Take a moment to reflect on your own exercise sessions and the multitude of moods that you experience. You might feel pleased that you scheduled time to exercise, proud of your exercise progress, worried about an overuse injury, happy to win an event, as well as a host of additional moods. Mood alteration, especially short-term

		Table 5.1	
		General Characteristics of Affect, Mood States, and Emotion	
Characteristic	**Affect**	**Mood**	**Emotion**
Cognitive	Non-cognitive, automatic response; Evolutionarily more primitive	Cognitive origin of subjective states	Cognitive origin of subjective states
Cause(s)	Non-specific causes Often unidentifiable causes	Non-specific causes Often unidentifiable causes Composite of multiple external & internal events	Response to specific events Antecedent-eliciting situations Usually directed at someone, or an event
Intensity	Composite of moods and emotions	Less intense than emotion Occasionally of high intensity	Higher in intensity than mood
Duration	Persists for longer periods than emotion	Persists for longer periods of time than emotion (e.g., day to day and throughout a day) Follows events over a longer period of time than do emotions	Brief duration (e.g., hour to hour; moment to moment) Rapid onset
Scales	Two broad categories Global indication of feeling states: Positive Affect and Negative Affect	Subscales vary from inventory to inventory Specific moods: Tension, Depression, Anger, Vigor, Fatigue, etc.	Subscales vary from inventory to inventory Anxiety, Depression, Disgust, Fear, Happiness, Surprise
Other	— — — — — — — —	Modulates thinking patterns by providing background color for daily behavior	Distinctive physiological manifestations (facial expression, etc.)

change, is an integral accompaniment to many exercise sessions.

Distinguishing Among the Terms: Affect, Mood, and Emotion

To understand the complex relationship between mood and exercise, it is important to identify factors that differentiate the terms *affect*, *mood*, and *emotion* (Berger & Tobar, 2006). These terms are similar and denote the broad categories of positive and negative feelings that are changeable. Although similar, there are some subtle differences between the terms (Schimmack, Oishi, Diener, & Suh, 2000; see Table 5.1).

Affect. Affect is a term denoting broad psychological states of positive and negative feelings (Isen,

2004). In a landmark study, Watson and Tellegen (1985) combined the results of numerous key studies of mood in a factor analysis and concluded that one-half to three-quarters of mood variations can be explained by two separate dimensions: positive affect and negative affect.

- *Positive affect* denotes a zest for life, or an individual's favorable engagement with the environment. It includes the mood states of elation, energy, enthusiasm, relaxation, and vigor.
- *Negative affect* indicates subjective feelings of distress and being upset. These feelings include anger, depression, fatigue, hostility, jitteriness, and tension.

Positive affect, which can be influenced by exercise, has many desirable results (Isen, 2004). It facilitates creativity, problem solving, and flexible, systematic thinking. Positive affect also can serve as a retrieval cue for positive memories.

In conclusion, affect includes both positive and negative dimensions, as well as emotions and mood states (Gohm & Clore, 2000). Thus, affect is a global indication of how we are feeling. Multiple mood states are included in these two broad dimensions of affect. Since affect has cognitive, neurological, physiological, motivational, and behavioral components, it needs multiple and integrated levels of analyses (Isen, 2004). As noted by Thayer (1996, p. 6), "Affect has a certain surface quality or immediacy associated with it."

Mood. In contrast to affect, both mood and emotion refer to more specific feelings. Mood tends to be undirected and has a variety of internal and external causes. Moods often do not have distinct or specific causes, whereas emotions do (Schimmack et al., 2000; Morris, 1989). Thus, the cause-and-effect relationship between specific events and moods is not as readily identifiable as it is for emotions.

Moods tend to follow events that occur over a longer period more than those that cause various emotions. For example, a sunny, warm day may evoke positive *mood states* relatively slowly. In contrast, the experience of someone crashing into your car while running a red light suddenly evokes pronounced autonomic changes and the *emotions* of fear and anger. Intentionality is one of the primary criteria for the scientific distinction between emotions and moods (Schimmack et al., 2000). Feeling relaxed is a mood state; feeling ashamed is an emotional state.

A primary function of mood is to modulate our thinking patterns and to provide background color to all that we do (Davidson, 1994). Mood states persist longer than do emotions. Mood states also tend to be less intense than emotions (Davidson, 1994). However, it is important to note that occasionally moods can be intense and overwhelm us (Thayer, 1996).

Emotion. Emotions are directed at someone or something. Emotions such as pride, joy, and fear often are higher in intensity than moods and usually are in immediate response to specific events or stimuli. Emotion-laden stimuli include the joy of movement, elation over finishing a marathon, pride in executing a perfect dive, and the anxiety over being invited to make a speech.

In contrast to moods, emotions also are accompanied by distinctive facial expressions (Davidson, 1994). Basic or core emotions include happiness, sadness, anger, fear, disgust, and surprise (Cacioppo, Berntson, Klein, & Poehlmann, 1998). Emotion is composed of subjective feeling states. Emotions also have broad cognitive, behavioral, neuropsychological, and psychophysiological manifestations (Schaie & Lawton, 1998). In addition to the qualities listed in Table 5.1, emotions have been proposed to have six primary features:

- *Physiological arousal* that is a departure from the physiological baseline,
- *Physiological expressions* that may influence the behavior of other individuals,
- *Valence* that indicates the pain and pleasure that accompany emotions,
- *Cognitive antecedent* that may be rational or irrational,
- *Intentional object* since they are about something or directed toward someone, and
- *Action tendency* that results in specific behavior or if not behavior, wishes for specific results (Elster, 2004).

Concluding caveat. Despite the carefully delineated differences between affect, mood, and emotion, it is important to note that many of these distinctions "can be found wanting when carefully scrutinized" (Davidson, 1994, p. 51). Discussions of these distinctions were continued at the recent Amsterdam Symposium and are summarized in the edited text, *Feelings and Emotions* (Manstead, Frijda, & Fischer, 2004). As reflected in the Symposium proceedings, the distinctions between mood, affect, and emotion can be regarded as correct for much of the time, but not all of the time.

Trait and State Characteristics of Mood

As previously noted, mood is more often a state, rather than a trait, characteristic. As a state characteristic, it is subject to change and can be influenced by exercise (Berger & Tobar, 2006). You might say to a friend, "I am in a great mood." This statement probably means that you are in a better mood *at this moment* than you are most of the time, and thus the statement refers to your present mood state. Mood states tend to change and thus are related to a single, specific exercise ses-

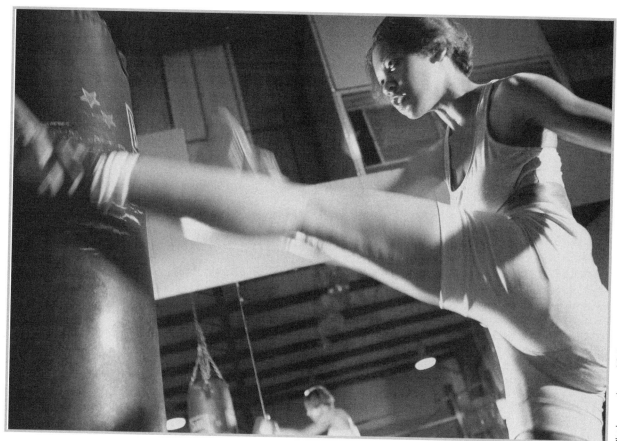

Photo courtesy of © Eyewire Images

sion. In comparison to their mood states prior to exercising, participants tend to feel elated, energetic, and less fatigued, depressed, anxious, and confused after exercising (e.g., Berger, 2004; Giacobbi, Hausenblas, & Frye, 2005; Gauvin, Rejeski, & Reboussin, 2000).

Mood on occasion also can be a trait characteristic. There also are general levels of mood that characterize the way that you feel *most of the time*, and these moods are considered to be *traits*. Some individuals simply are more energetic, less fatigued, higher in arousal, and more positive most of the time than are others. These general, more permanent moods are traits that reflect personal baseline levels.

Mood states and traits are measured by the same inventory. However, to measure mood traits, the instructions to mood inventories would ask respondents to indicate how they have been feeling for the *"past six months"* or even the *"past year"* to reflect a more stable, trait characteristic. To measure the state aspects of mood, the instructions would ask respondents to indicate how they feel *"right now, at this moment"* they are taking the test, or *"during the past week, including today."*

Mood states fluctuate around general baseline or *trait levels of mood* and include moment-to-moment fluctuations or changes. These temporary fluctuations are generalized changes in feelings. As previously

noted, mood states are reactions to a broad base of events and usually are not directly related to specific events, such as finding money lying on the sidewalk, or having an argument.

Models of Mood

Bipolar and Unipolar Continuum Models

Bipolar model. According to the bipolar model, mood is a continuum that differs from one extreme of positiveness (e.g., happiness) to the opposite extreme of negativeness (e.g., sadness). The two extremes of a bipolar dimension of mood as represented on a continuum are mutually exclusive, and cannot coexist. As the word "bipolar" implies, a person's mood state on a particular dimension is someplace along a continuum ranging from exceedingly positive or desirable at one end of a continuum, to negative or undesirable at the other end (Russell & Carroll, 1999). According to the bipolar model represented in Figure 5.1, we cannot be both happy and sad at the same time. In other words, the presence of happiness would reflect the absence of sadness. Further illustrating bipolar mood dimensions, we cannot be both elated and depressed at the same time, or calm and tense.

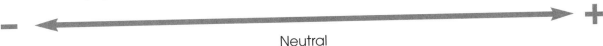

Figure 5.1. Illustration of the bipolar model of mood.

Unipolar model. In contrast to the bipolar model, the unipolar model of mood suggests that positive and negative mood states are distinct and independent of each other (Russell & Carroll, 1999; Watson and Tellegen, 1985). If the mood states are independent, we can experience positive mood states (e.g., happiness) and negative mood states (e.g., sadness) at the same time, rather than only one or the other. According to the unipolar model, happiness is an independent mood state that can be measured on a scale ranging from an absence of happiness to extremely high levels of happiness. Sadness also can be considered an independent mood state, and moods can range from not at all sad to extremely sad. According to the unipolar model, the fact that you are not happy does not automatically mean that you are sad (see Figure 5.2 for an illustration of this model). Happiness and sadness are two independent mood states.

Although mood states tend not to be preceded by recognizable antecedent events, the following examples serve as illustrations of why we might experience diverse mood states simultaneously. We *simultaneously* may be *happy* about graduating from college, *sad* about relocating and moving away from friends, and *anxious* about the progress in our job search. Another example of conflicting positive and negative mood states attached to a situation is feeling *sad* when a close family member dies. We may feel *happy* that the person no longer has to suffer the pains of illness,

and feel *lonely* as we contemplate the shortness of the human life span. As a result of these simultaneous, sometimes conflicting mood states, some researchers have suggested that positive and negative moods are not at opposite ends of a continuum, but are independent and uncorrelated dimensions of mood (Diener & Suh, 1998; Russell & Carroll, 1999).

Combined bipolar and unipolar models. A relatively new model combines the unipolar and the bipolar models into a single, integrative model that accounts for some of the contradictory findings in the research literature. In this model, mood is context related, with specific situations determining the amount of separation between the positive and negative valence (Zautra, Potter, & Reich, 1998). Positive and negative mood states are two separate dimensions during normal or nonstressful periods of time. The relationship between the two dimensions changes, however, during periods of unusually high amounts of negative life events. During stress, the dimensions become inversely correlated. Thus, in times of stress, positive and negative mood states are at the opposite ends of a single continuum and are bipolar, or opposite, one another.

The theory underlying this combined bipolar/unipolar model is that positive and negative mood states are unrelated to one another during normal times. They become opposites of one another during times of stress in order to conserve information-processing resources. Obviously the interrelationships among

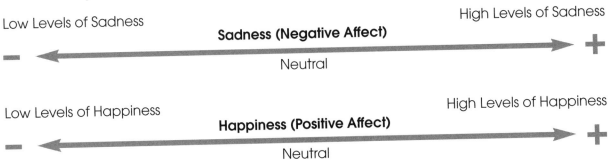

Figure 5.2. Illustration of the unipolar model of mood.

various mood states are complex, and future research will augment our present conceptualizations (Zautra et al., 1998).

Conclusions. Both the unipolar and bipolar models are widely accepted; however, some theorists suggest that the bipolar model is becoming the predominant theory (e.g., Russell & Carroll, 1999). There also is a lack of consensus concerning the actual number of separate, independent dimensions of mood in each of the models (e.g., Matthews et al., 1990; Thayer, 1996). Supporting the existence of independent dimensions of mood, desirable (positive) and undesirable (negative) mood states may be processed by different portions of the brain. They also may be associated with different neural structures (Folkman & Moskowitz, 2000). Desirable mood states may be processed by the left hemisphere, and undesirable mood states, by the right hemisphere. Each of the mood inventories reviewed later in the chapter reflect different models of mood but still capture diverse mood benefits often associated with exercise.

Two-Dimensional Models of Mood

Several continuums or dimensions of mood help clarify interrelationships between various mood states. Mood states seem to fall along two independent dimensions, and they can be organized in a circular, two-dimensional space (Remington, Fabrigar, & Visser, 2000). Each of the following models is a useful depiction of mood, even though they are quite similar to one another.

Circumplex model. This model includes arousal as one dimension and positive/negative valence as another dimension. The two dimensions are independent (orthogonal) of one another but do intersect as represented in Figure 5.3. The *arousal dimension* would seem to be highly related to physical activity. Most types of physical activity increase physical arousal in diverse physiological systems. In fact, sleep experts suggest that exercise should be avoided several hours prior to sleeping—if falling asleep is a problem. The

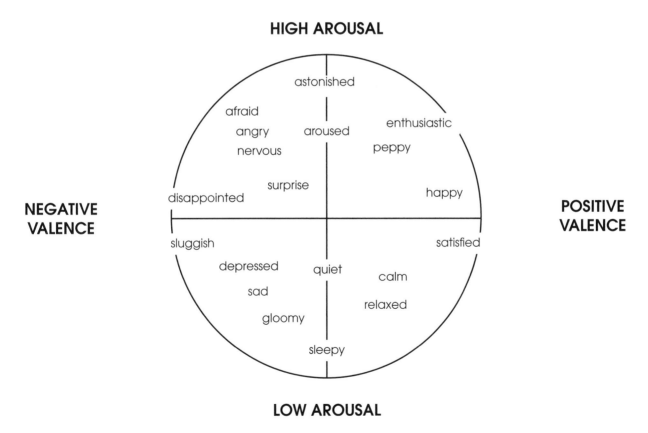

Figure 5.3. A two-dimensional, circumplex model of mood: High-low arousal and positive-negative valence. *Note:* From "Variations in the Circumplex Structure of Mood," by L. A. Feldman, *Personality and Social Psychology Bulletin, 21,* pp. 807, 811. Copyright 1995 by the Society for Personality and Social Psychology, Inc. Adapted with permission.

arousal dimension ranges between the two extremes of high and low and can be positive or negative as depicted in Figure 5.3 (Feldman, 1995).

When the negative-to-positive valence dimension and the arousal dimension intersect as diagramed in Figure 5.3, four distinct quadrants are formed within a circle. These include

- High arousal-positive valence (pleasant),
- Low arousal-positive valence (pleasant),
- High arousal-negative valence (unpleasant), and
- Low arousal-negative valence (unpleasant).

Because specific mood states can be situated within a circle that is formed to enclose each of the four quadrants, the model is described as the *circumplex model* of mood (Feldman, 1995; Remington et al., 2000). Specific mood states represent different positions within the quadrants depicted in Figure 5.3. Moods representing high levels of arousal and a positive valence include states such as enthusiasm and pep. Feeling calm and feeling relaxed are positive mood states, but are characterized by considerably lower levels of arousal as depicted in the figure. Being aston-

ished or sleepy are neutral states in regard to positive and negative valence but are exact opposites of one another in their respective levels of arousal. Negative moods in the high-arousal quadrant include fear and anger. Negative moods that are low in arousal include depression and gloom.

The exact placement of moods within the circle or circumplex seems to depend on how mood is measured: by self-report inventories or by semantic concepts that people use to describe their subjective mood experiences. In addition, the positive-negative valence seems to be a more important component than is arousal when people self-report their mood states (Feldman, 1995).

Energy-tiredness and tension-calmness model. Another separate but somewhat similar model of mood is one in which mood differs in accordance with two other independent dimensions. The *energy-tiredness* dimension is similar to the arousal dimension in the previous model. The *tension-calmness* dimension is the second continuum (Thayer, 1996). Refer to Figure 5.4 for a representation of these unipolar dimensions, which vary from more to less on energy and calmness.

Both the energy-tiredness and tension-calmness

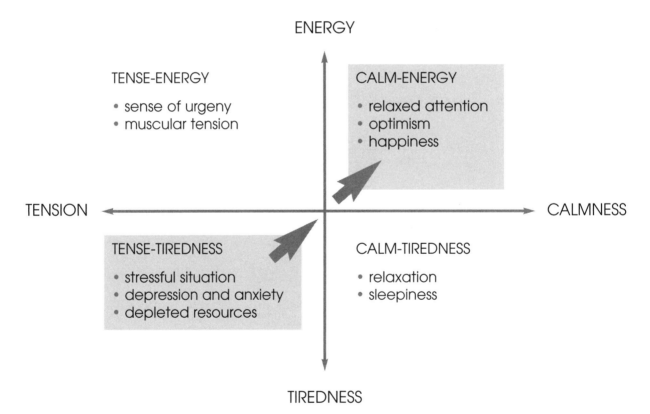

Figure 5.4. A two-dimensional model of mood: Energy-tiredness and tension-calmness. *Note*: From *The Origin of Everyday Moods: Managing, Energy, Tension, and Stress* (p. 150) by R. E. Thayer, New York: Oxford University Press, 1996. Copyright 1996 by Oxford University Press. Adapted with permission. Reprinted from "Subjective well-being in obese individuals: The multiple roles of exercise," by B. G. Berger, *Quest, 56*, p. 59. Copyright 2004 by National Association for Physical Education in Higher Education. Reprinted with permission.

dimensions seem to be affected by physical activity. For example, light and moderate levels of physical activity often are associated with increased energy (Thayer, 2001). In contrast, high-intensity training is associated with feelings of tiredness. In fact, habitual feelings of tiredness are symptomatic of overtraining (Tobar, in press). Various types of exercise may serve to decrease feelings of tension and to move toward the calmness end of the second continuum.

As illustrated by the quadrants created by the two dimensions or continuums, moods can be characterized as fluctuating along a tension-calmness dimension and an energy-tiredness dimension. The quadrants of tense-energy, tense-tiredness, calm-energy, and calm-tiredness are pictured in Figure 5.4. Specific mood states within each of the quadrants represent differences in the feelings of calmness and energy. Mood states in the tense-energy and tense-tiredness quadrants often reflect feelings of time urgency. In contrast, mood states in the calm-energy and calm-tiredness quadrants reflect relaxation.

The arrows in Figure 5.4 highlight Thayer's theory that people try to self-regulate their mood states and specifically decrease feelings of tense tiredness and increase feelings of calm-energy (e.g., Thayer, 2001). Exercise, eating/snacking, drinking alcoholic beverages and coffee, and social interaction often are employed as self-regulating/mood-enhancing activities (Berger, 2004; Thayer, 2001, p. 4; Thayer, Peters, Takahashi, & Birkhead-Flight, 1993). Although there are desirable as well as undesirable mood states within most of the quadrants, people try to change mood states within the tense tiredness quadrant. Managing mood, especially increasing energy, is a particularly important key to reducing overeating. Exercise has been proposed as a particularly effective approach to enhance mood (the focus of the next chapter) and to reduce the tendency to snack and add extra pounds (Berger, 2004; Thayer, 2001). The quadrants within the energy-tiredness and tension-calmness model of mood are theorized to facilitate different types of activities (Thayer, 2001).

The *tense-energy* quadrant facilitates completion of mundane tasks that might otherwise be left undone and the meeting of deadlines. Some individuals, especially those who are characterized as having Type A personalities and habitually create time-pressured situations, may prefer maintaining higher levels of tense-energy than do others (Thayer, Newman, & McClain, 1994). Although mood states reflecting tense-energy can be productive, they take their toll. Tense-energy denotes a sense of time urgency and stress, which often are characterized by muscular tension, particularly in the jaws, neck, shoulders, and back. Maintaining a constant state of tense-energy results in feelings of fatigue and movement into the tense-tiredness continuum.

Tense-tiredness is related to stressful situations, but also reflects a depletion of resources and energy. The tense-tiredness quadrant includes moods such as depression, anxiety, tension, and other generally undesirable mood states. Tense-tiredness is so unpleasant that it motivates self-regulation in the form of overeating to avoid this state and to move toward mood states in the calm-energy quadrant. Tense-tiredness also detracts from the quality of sleep, and even from falling asleep, as you reflect on the day's activities and urgent things left undone. In general, frequent mood states in the tense-tiredness quadrant detract from the overall quality of life.

The calm-energy and *calm-tiredness* quadrants are more desirable than those of tense-energy and tense-tiredness. High levels of *calm-energy* provide for relaxed attention, feelings of pep, and optimal functioning. Mood states related to calm-energy are ideal for work productivity, especially on creative or problem-solving types of tasks. The mood states of optimism and happiness are associated with high energy and low tension. The calm-energy quadrant is associated with "feeling good" and reflects the mood states that most of us would like to maintain.

Feelings of *calm-tiredness* reflect the mood states of relaxation and ideally occur just before bedtime, as well as at other times of the day. In this quadrant, thoughts generally are not focused on work or problems—even minor ones. Although the calm-tiredness quadrant includes desirable mood states, most people would not rate them as desirable as those in the calm-energy quadrant. As its name implies, mood states of tiredness and sleepiness characterize this quadrant (Thayer, 1996, 2001).

Conclusions

Individuals differ in their personal predispositions to be in positive or negative moods, in their levels of arousal, and in the relative concentrations of energy-tiredness and tense-calm moods. These personal predispositions can be considered relatively permanent or trait aspects of mood (Morris, 1989). Daily events, both internal and external, often influence mood fluctuations around an individual's baseline or trait levels of mood.

The Importance of Mood in Our Daily Lives

Mood states fluctuate throughout the day. Thus, they seem to be trivial and rather unimportant at first glance. Upon closer inspection, however, it becomes clear that mood is an integral component of daily life. Mood is a prism that sheds colors and light on much of what we do. Mood influences our feelings of happiness, appreciation of the moment, the likelihood that we will provide assistance to others, appraisal of stressful situations, and the quality and meaning of our lives in general. As observed by Thayer (1996), a noted psychologist who wrote *The Origin of Everyday Moods: Managing Energy, Tension, and Stress*, moods influence the quality of our days:

> Even an unpleasant social interaction can be tolerable if our mood is positive. On the other hand, if we are in a bad mood, an activity that usually is very pleasant, one that otherwise gives us great enjoyment, can be boring and uninteresting. When our mood is low, even the most positive events become meaningless. (p. 3)

Psychosomatic, or Mind-Body, Relationship

Mood is closely intertwined with physical health in ways that are just beginning to be understood. Mood states are key elements in both somatopsychic and the psychosomatic relationships. Illustrating the psychosomatic relationship, mood states such as distress may influence a person's immune system, health habits, and even the onset and time-course of specific diseases (Melamed, 1995). Heart disease, stroke, and flare-ups of chronic autoimmune diseases such as rheumatoid arthritis and asthmatic attacks may be associated with the activating mood states of fear and anger through both direct and indirect paths (Leventhal, Patrick-Miller, Leventhal, & Burns, 1998). Long-term phlegmatic moods of hopelessness and fatigue may be associated with the development of cancer and the reoccurrence of myocardial infarction (Leventhal et al., 1998).

Both direct and secondary pathways for interactions between mood states and the immune system support the mind-body relationship. Direct pathways include mood states affecting both the number and activity of B and T lymphocytes, macrophages, antibodies, leukocytes, reactivity to pathogens, and shift in energy balance (Maier, Watkins, & Fleshner, 1994). An illustration of these interactions is the observation that the positive moods created by laughter and by social support or interactions are thought to influence the course of a disease and be "good medicine."

Secondary pathways by which mood may interact with illness include lifestyle factors that are deleterious to health. For example, undesirable mood states may influence eating patterns that result in dietary deficiencies, obesity, and eating disorders. Undesirable mood states also may be related to smoking, illicit drug use, and sedentary behavior or lack of physical activity (Cohen & Rodriguez, 1995; Thayer, 1989, 1996; Thayer et al., 1994).

Somatopsychic, or Body-Mind, Relationship

In addition to the mind influencing the body as implied by the term psychosomatic, the reverse also may occur. Our bodies or state of health influences our moods and reflects the somatopsychic or body-mind relationship. A person who is ill often lacks energy, has low-quality sleep, and may feel tense or depressed. In their review of stress-related mood states and illness, Leventhal and colleagues (1998) indicate that the relationships between illness, a lack of energy, and feelings of depression are fairly typical. This multi-pronged response to illness represents a conservation of resources, which are needed for the destruction of invading pathogens. These physiological changes are experienced as both an illness and as emotional distress.

Additional evidence of the somatopsychic relationship is that even when a person is not physically ill, but simply tired, the person may experience a variety of undesirable mood states such as depression, tension, and even anger. To reduce physical feeling of tiredness, some individuals exercise at the end of a day and report more positive mood states—even feelings of energy and revitalization after exercising. By expending physical energy, they may experience more energy. Further evidence of the somatopsychic relationship is that reducing muscular tension by stretching or participating in a hatha yoga session often results in mood elevation (Berger & Owen, 1988, 1992; Thayer, 1996). As observed by Thayer (1996), moods are described as the windows to both our mental and physical states and truly reflect the unity of mind and body.

Self-Regulation of Mood

Because of the importance of mood, its self-regulation is an essential component of a well-lived life. Consciously altering our moods can assist in establishing healthy habits and lifestyles, boost our immune systems, and enhance our general zest for living. With or without conscious awareness, most individuals attempt to maintain desirable moods and mitigate negative ones. For example, we try to change our moods that are in the tense-tiredness and tense-energy quadrants to those in the calm-energy quadrant depicted in Figure 5.3. When we are experiencing calm-energy, we also self-regulate our moods to maintain our desirable mood states.

As suggested by various techniques listed in Table 5.2, each person tries to establish and/or maintain desirable mood states, to reduce tense arousal, and/or to raise energetic arousal with a variety of approaches. Mood-altering activities include having a cup of coffee, going for a walk, talking to a friend, or exercising.

Table 5.2

Procedures for Changing Negative Moods into Positive Ones and for Maintaining Positive Moods

Procedures	References
Active mood management	
Exercise	Berger & Motl, 2001, 1996; Gallup & Castelli, 1989; Giacobbi, Hausenblas, & Frye, 2005; Thayer, 1996; Thayer et al., 1994
Light therapy	Golden et al., 2005; Thayer, 1996
Music & guided imagery therapy	Campbell, 1997; McKinney, Antoni, Kumar, Tims, & McCabe, 1997
Prayer	Gallup & Castelli, 1989
Walking	Berger & Owen, 1998; Osei-Tutu & Campagna, 2005; Thayer et al., 1994
Yoga	Berger & Owen, 1988, 1992a; Thayer, 1996
Distraction & seeking pleasurable activities	
Keeping busy, avoidance	Thayer et al., 1994
Listening to music	Clark & Teasdale, 1985; Fried & Berkowitz, 1979; Rippere, 1977; Thayer et al., 1994
Social support and ventilation	
Social interaction	Thayer, 1996; Thayer et al., 1994
Passive mood management	
Alcohol & recreational drug use	Thayer et al., 1994
Coffee	Brice & Smith, 2002; Thayer, 1996; Thayer et al., 1994
Food, especially good tasting	Thayer, 1996; Thayer et al., 1994

To change a negative mood into a positive one, we need to modulate our states of arousal and tension to optimal levels. Optimal arousal and tension differ for specific activities such as studying for an exam, engaging in social interaction, and falling asleep.

Changing a negative mood to a more positive one necessitates avoiding some of the automatic effects of mood, such as the production of mood-congruent thoughts and behaviors (Morris, 1989). For example, when we are depressed, we tend to dwell on depressive memories and thoughts. When we are angry, we tend to think about other times and places where we also have been angry. This vicious cycling begets additionally depressive or angry mood states.

Procedures for changing negative moods into positive ones include active mood management, distraction and pleasure-seeking activities, social support and ventilation, and passive mood management as illustrated in Table 5.2. In fact, moderate exercise has been rated among the most successful approaches to mood alteration in diverse studies (Thayer et al., 1994). This may be due to its primary mood effect of enhancing energy

and secondary mood effects of reducing tension (Thayer et al., 1994). In fact, the results of four studies focusing on the self-regulation of mood led to the conclusion that exercise is effective in changing bad mood, raising energy, and reducing tension as reported by Thayer:

Of all the behavioral categories described to self-regulate mood, a case can be made that *exercise is the most effective* [italics added]. This behavior was self-rated as the *most successful at changing a bad mood, fourth most successful at raising energy*, and *third or fourth most successful at tension reduction* [italics added]. Furthermore, even though all subjects did not rank exercise first in regulating energy and tension, its value is apparent by its primary use by some knowledgeable individuals. (Thayer et al., 1994, p. 921)

The Measurement of Mood

Because of the pervasiveness of mood and its implications for the quality of our daily lives, it is important to be able to measure it with valid and reliable measures.

As might be expected from the numerous theoretical conceptualizations of mood, there are a variety of mood inventories that reflect the structure of mood experiences. Inventories of mood commonly employed in exercise and sport settings include the Profile of Mood States (McNair et al., 1971, 1992; McNair & Heuchert, 2003, 2005), the Positive Affect-Negative Affect Scale (Watson, Clark, & Tellegen, 1988), the revised form of the Multiple Affect Adjective Check List (Lubin & Zuckerman, 1999), and the Activation-Deactivation Adjective Check List (Thayer, 1986). In addition, several inventories have been designed specifically to measure mood states associated with how people feel after exercising. These include the Exercise-Induced Feeling Inventory (Gauvin & Rejeski, 1993) and the Subjective Exercise Experiences Scale (McAuley & Courneya, 1994). Prior to examining the characteristics of specific mood inventories, it is necessary to identify key issues in the measurement of mood. These include the difference between state and trait measures, diurnal variations, and types of scores derived from the inventories.

State and Trait Measures of Mood

Instructions for the inventories differ according to the researcher's interest in measuring immediate mood states, or the more general mood traits. Depending on the issues under investigation, instructions for completing mood inventories range from the state instructions of "How are you feeling right now?" to the trait instructions of "How have you generally been feeling for the past six months (or for an even longer period of time)?" Responses to the inventory employing the state set of instructions reflect an individual's mood at a particular moment and change according to recent activities or an experimental treatment. Responses to the same inventory employing the trait instructions capture more general, or typical, mood states.

Diurnal Variations in Mood States

Mood states may vary as a result of the time of day and thus are described as "diurnal" (Thayer, 1989). Although diurnal mood variations may not be large, they have implications for testing procedures in studies of mood and exercise. *Desirable mood states* such as energetic arousal, vigor, or energy tend to be strongest in the middle of the day around noon and to be lower in the early morning, the afternoon, and evening (Thayer, 1989, 1996). In contrast to the expected noontime peaking of desirable moods, other researchers have observed the most positive mood scores of the day at 9 A.M. on the four subscales of Positive Engagement,

Revitalization, Tranquility, and Physical Exhaustion (Gauvin et al., 2000). After 9 A.M., these specific mood-state scores tended to change in less desirable directions throughout the remainder of the day. Each of the four mood states, however, followed patterns of change that were dissimilar from one another throughout the day, especially after noon. In contrast, *undesirable mood states* did not seem to be as influenced as much by the time of day as by specific undesirable events or interactions (Gauvin et al., 2000).

Some investigators have found no diurnal variations in the mood benefits associated with exercise (Trine & Morgan, 1997). Trine and Morgan recruited male and female runners, who habitually had been morning, noontime, or evening runners for the preceding month, for the study. These runners reported significant reductions in anxiety after running. This reduction was present regardless of the time of day they ran—whether they were running at a time of day that was merely convenient for their schedules, or running at their preferred time of day. Clearly more research about the diurnal effects of exercise on mood is needed to reconcile these conflicting results, some of which may reflect the specific mood inventories employed.

Based on the possibility that time of day may influence positive, but not negative, mood states, test administrators should make an effort to compare exercisers' mood states in various activities at approximately the same time of day until more definitive research is available. If investigators are primarily comparing a person's mood states before and after a *single* exercise session, however, time of testing is less important. When testing individuals after only a single exercise session, the research question would be whether the person reports more positive moods and less negative mood states after exercising, regardless of the person's initial mood states at that particular time of day. Despite possible diurnal variations in mood states and the participant's initial mood scores, exercise tends to be associated with desirable changes in both positive and negative mood states.

Types of Scores: Raw Scores, *T* Scores, *z* Scores, and Percentile Scores

An individual's set of subscale scores on a mood inventory can be reported as raw scores that reflect a summation of actual answers to the questions. Depending on the normative data available for a specific inventory, however, raw scores can be converted to standardized T scores, standardized z scores, or percentile scores. Raw scores, z scores, and T scores (but not percentile scores) can be used in any kind of mathematical operation.

Various types of standardized scores, such as T scores and z scores that are based on a normal curve, are useful for comparing an individual's score to that of a larger, comparable population and scores on diverse measures with one another. A raw score of 14 on a scale measuring tension is not very informative, because it provides no information about either the average score or the range score that people tend to report. However, knowledge that a score of 14 is equivalent to a T score of 51 means that the individual scored near the mean (a T score of 50) of a comparable sample of individuals. The T scores have a standard deviation of 10. Thus, T scores between 40 and 60 on the POMS represent scores that approximately 68%, or two-thirds, of the population would have—if the scores within a sample of individuals are normally distributed (e.g., follow the normal curve). The advantages of both T and z scores are that they facilitate comparison of various groups of people and the comparison of one subscale score to another. In contrast, percentile scores are useful for reporting test information to individuals, because people tend to have more personal experience with scores reported as percentiles than with T scores.

Comparing scores across subscales. In addition to providing comparisons to other populations, use of standardized T scores facilitates the comparison of an individual's scores with a variety of subscales differing in the overall number of items by employing a common scale. Regardless of whether there are 5 or 50 items in a scale, a T score of 40 on one scale is comparable to a T score of 40 on another scale. Thus with the use of T scores, scores on a variety of scales can be compared with one another.

The mood profile composed of the six mood states on the POMS illustrated in Figure 5.5 exemplifies the use of T scores for comparing scores on one subscale to another. Both groups of exercisers completed the POMS before and immediately after exercising on three different occasions. Because their mood scores were averaged across three exercise sessions, their scores did not represent one potentially unique exercise experience, but how they generally felt before and after an exercise session. The swimmers and yoga participants reported mood benefits after physical activity even though their pre-exercise scores (except for Vigor) were at or below the mean for college students. In this particular study, male participants in hatha yoga reported significantly greater mood benefits than did male swimmers on the scales of Tension, Anger, and Fatigue (Berger & Owen, 1992).

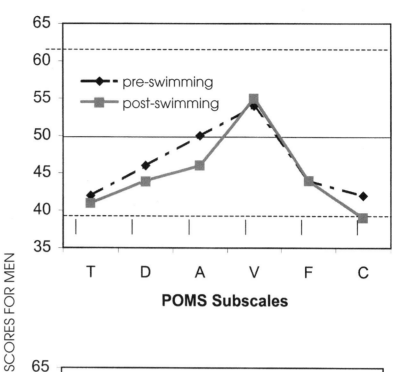

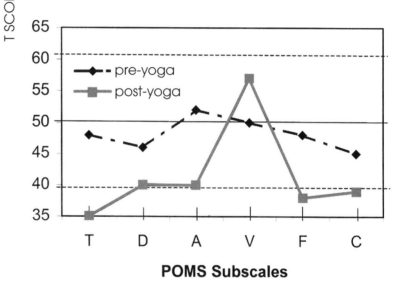

Figure 5.5. POMS scores of men before and after exercise sessions of hatha yoga and swimming (Berger & Owen, 1992a).

Interpreting percentile scores. Percentile scores indicate the proportion of all the test takers who scored lower than the specified raw score. Intuitively easy to understand, percentile scores are useful for reporting results on a single scale to the individual test taker. For example, if the score of 14 reflects the 66th percentile, you would interpret the percentile score of 66 as indicating that 66% of a comparable sample scored lower on Tension. Percentile scores *cannot* be used in mathematical operations. Percentile scores exaggerate differences in the middle scores and dramatically underemphasize differences in extreme high and low scores. Thus, T scores and z scores are superior for the comparing a person's scores on various scales.

Mood and Affect Questionnaires Commonly Employed in Exercise Settings

The Profile of Mood States, the Positive Affect-Negative Affect Schedule, Activation-Deactivation Adjective Check List, Multiple Affect Adjective Check List, Exercise-Induced Feeling Inventory, and Subjective Exercise Experiences Scale are presented in the following section as examples of typical mood inventories employed in studies of exercise and mood alteration. The samples of inventory items in the various tables provide initial information that is helpful for selecting a mood inventory for a study that you might be planning to conduct. The inventories also provide a more in-depth understanding of specific mood states.

On each of the inventories, participants rate how they feel according to a set of instructions indicating a particular timeframe. For shorter timeframes, mood state scores are more changeable. Mood states may fluctuate throughout a day and from one day to the next. However, when using the longer timeframes of trait measures, mood tends to be more stable. Specific subscales included within questionnaires and the items in each subscale differ from one questionnaire to another. Selecting the "best" questionnaire depends on the specific hypotheses under investigation, the ability of the questionnaire to capture the items of interest, as well as the questionnaire's validity and reliability.

Profile of Mood States (POMS)

The Standard Form of the POMS is a mood inventory that includes 65 adjectives that describe how people feel. Although initially developed for use with psychiatric outpatients, the POMS has been used extensively with college students and with the general adult populations (McNair, Lorr, & Droppleman, 1971, 2003). Normative data is available for these populations as reported in the *Technical Update* (McNair & Heuchert, 2003, 2005). The POMS has been employed in diverse exercise settings as reviewed by Berger and Motl (2000). Because of its length, completing the POMS requires approximately 10 minutes. This is time consuming, especially when mood is measured multiple times in a single exercise session.

Several abbreviated versions of the POMS are available. The POMS Brief Form (POMS-B; McNair, Lorr, & Droppleman, 1989, 2003) contains 30 items and has 5 items in each of the six subscales (McNair & Heuchert, 2003, 2005). It requires approximately five minutes to complete. Another abbreviated version of the POMS by Bob Grove and Harry Prapavessis (1992) includes 40 items. This version includes the same six subscales of the Standard Version of the POMS and an additional subscale for Esteem-Related Affect.

Subscale characteristics. There are six subscales in the 65-item Standard Form of the POMS (McNair et al., 1971, 1992), and each contains 7 to 15 items as described in the *Profile of Mood States Technical*

Table 5.3

Examples of the Profile of Mood States (POMS) Items

Instructions: Below is a list of terms that describe feelings people have. Please read each one carefully. Then fill in ONE circle to the right which best describes **how you feel right now at this moment.** [a].

Rating Scale:

| 0 = Not at all | 1 = A little | 2 = Moderately | 3 = Quite a bit | 4 = Extremely |

Subscales	Sample Item	Answers	Subscales	Sample Item	Answers
Tension	Anxious	⓪①②③④	Anger	Grouchy	⓪①②③④
Depression	Sad	⓪①②③④	Vigor	Energetic	⓪①②③④
Fatigue	Exhausted	⓪①②③④	Confusion	Uncertain about things	⓪①②③④

Note: From *Profile of Mood States Technical Update* (pp. 5-7), by D. M. McNair and J. W. P Heuchert, 2005, North Tonawanda, NY: Multi-Health Systems (MHS). Reprinted with permission.

[a] The POMS can be employed with any of the following instructions depending on whether state or trait characteristics of mood are of interest: (1) "How you feel right now at this moment," (2) "How you have been feeling during the past week including today," or (3) some other specified rating period indicating by filling in a blank on the new style of inventories.

Update (McNair & Heuchert, 2003, 2005). Specific POMS subscales include

- *Tension-Anxiety,*
- *Depression-Dejection,*
- *Anger-Hostility,*
- *Vigor-Activity,*
- *Fatigue-Inertia, and*
- *Confusion-Bewilderment.*

As suggested in the POMS *Technical Update*, *Tension* refers to heightened musculoskeletal tension as defined by the terms *tense*, *on edge*, and *restless*. *Depression* reflects feelings of personal inadequacy and personal worthlessness, and a sense of emotional isolation from others. *Anger* is defined by the terms *furious* and *ready to fight*. *Vigor* suggests moods of ebullience and high energy. *Fatigue* represents feelings of inertia, low energy, and weariness. *Confusion* refers to cognitive inefficiency and muddle-headedness (McNair & Heuchert, 2003, 2005). After converting raw scores to *T* scores to adjust for the differing number of items in the subscales, scores on the six subscales can be connected with one another to form a POMS profile that is depicted in Figure 5.5.

See Table 5.3 for representative items in the various subscales. Respondents rate how accurately the 65 adjectives describe their feelings along a five-point scale. Although five of the six subscales reflect undesirable mood states, POMS scores still can reflect desirable changes in mood. For example, exercisers who report post-exercise decreases in their initially low pre-exercise levels of Tension and Depression would appear to "feel better" after physical activity.

Total mood disturbance score. Scores on the POMS six subscales also can be combined into a single *Total Mood Disturbance (TMD)* score. Total Mood Disturbance reflects a person's overall state of well-being. It is formed by summing the five "negative" raw scores on the subscales of Tension, Depression, Anger, Vigor, Fatigue, and Confusion, and then subtracting the "positive" score on Vigor from the score of the other five subscales (McNair & Heuchert, 2003, 2005). The single TMD score does not provide as much information about mood as do scores on the six subscales. However, TMD has value in providing global information briefly to test takers. The *TMD* score also is of value in statistical analyses when the number of participants is small and the small number precludes tests of significance for each of the subscales.

Bipolar version of the POMS. A Bipolar Version of the POMS (POMS-Bi) that includes 77 adjectives representing desirable and undesirable mood states is also available (Lorr, McNair, & Heuchert, 1980, 2003). Each subscale in the POMS-Bi includes two mutually exclusive moods as reflected in the following listing. The subscales are bipolar because an exerciser cannot

be both composed and anxious at the same time. The POMS-Bi includes revised versions of four of the six subscales contained in the Standard Form, and another subscale that is a combination of two subscales, namely, the Vigor and Fatigue subscales. In addition in the POMS-Bi, there is a new bipolar subscale: Confident-Unsure.

Although the POMS-Bi has not been employed extensively in exercise settings, it would appear to be of value in measuring exercise-related mood states as reflected by the following subscales.

- *Composed-Anxious.* Adjectives in this subscale range from composed, relaxed, and serene to anxious, tense, and uneasy.
- *Elated-Depressed.* Adjectives in this subscale range from cheerful, lighthearted, and joyful to dejected, discouraged, and lonely.
- *Agreeable-Hostile.* Adjectives represent feelings ranging from friendly, kindly, and sympathetic at one pole and angry, annoyed, and grouchy at the other.
- *Energetic-Tired.* This subscale includes the desirable feelings of alertness, liveliness, and pep, and the often undesirable feelings of drowsiness, exhaustion, and sluggishness.
- *Confident-Unsure.* This subscale measures feelings of being bold and forceful and the undesirable feelings of being unsure and timid.
- *Clearheaded-Confused.* Adjectives in this subscale reflect feelings of being attentive and efficient and their opposite of being confused, dazed, and mixed-up (Lorr, McNair, & Heuchert, 1980, 2003).

Positive Affect-Negative Affect Schedule (PANAS)

The PANAS is a 20-item self-report inventory that also is widely employed in exercise psychology studies. As the name implies, the Positive Affect-Negative Affect Schedule includes two orthogonal, or independent and uncorrelated, dimensions (Watson et al., 1988):

- *Positive Affect,* and
- *Negative Affect.*

Subscale characteristics. The Positive Affect (PA) dimension is considered to be a single construct as measured by the PANAS. High scores on PA are characterized by a zest for life and include positive mood states such as arousal, enthusiasm, excitement, happiness, high energy, and pleasurable engagement. In contrast, low scores on PA are characterized by an absence of these feelings.

The Negative Affect (NA) dimension concerns subjective distress and feelings of being upset or unpleasantly aroused, and is usually characterized by feelings of anxiety, hostility, and nervousness (Crawford & Henry, 2004; Watson et al., 1988). Low scores on NA are characterized by an absence of these feelings. Research findings indicate that the specific negative mood states of Depression (characterized by feelings of personal hopelessness, deficiency, and worthlessness), Fatigue (characterized by feelings of mental and physical tiredness), Confusion (characterized by feelings of bewilderment and uncertainty), Anger (feelings that vary from mild annoyance or aggravation to

---

Table 5.4

Positive Affect—Negative Affect Scale (PANAS); Watson, Clark, & Tellegen, 1988)

Instructions: The illustrative items in this scale consist of words that describe different feelings and emotions. Read each item and them mark the appropriate answer in the space provided next to that word. Indicate to what extent (INSERT APPROPRIATE TIME-RELATED INSTRUCTIONS HERE[a]).

Rating Scale:

1	2	3	4	5
Very slightly or not at all	A little	Moderately	Quite a bit	Extremely

_____ 1. Interested[b]	_____ 11. Irritable
_____ 2. Distressed	_____ 12. Alert[b]
_____ 3. Excited[b]	_____ 13. Ashamed
_____ 4. Upset	_____ 14. Inspired[b]
_____ 5. Strong[b]	_____ 15. Nervous
_____ 6. Guilty	_____ 16. Determined[b]
_____ 7. Scared	_____ 17. Attentive[b]
_____ 8. Hostile	_____ 18. Jittery
_____ 9. Enthusiastic[b]	_____ 19. Active[b]
_____ 10. Proud[b]	_____ 20. Afraid

Note: Scores are achieved by summing the raw scores of each of the items for both subscales.

[a] The PANAS can be employed with any of the following seven-time instructions depending on the desire to measure state or trait characteristics:

Moment . . . . you feel this way right now, that is, at the present moment
Today . . . . you have felt this way today
Past few days . . . . you have felt this way during the past few days
Week . . . . you have felt this way during the past week
Past few weeks . . . . you have felt this way during the past few weeks
Year . . . . you have felt this way during the past year
General . . . . you generally feel this way, that is, how you feel on the average

[b] Denotes items in the Positive Affect subscale; unmarked items are from the Negative Affect subscale.

fury and rage), and Tension (characterized by feelings of nervousness, apprehension, worry, and anxiety) are typically highly intercorrelated (Watson & Clark, 1997; Watson & Tellegen, 1985). See Table 5.4 for the 10 adjectives in each of the two subscales.

The PANAS subscales provide reliable, valid, and largely independent measures of Positive and Negative Affect regardless of the participant population, or specific timeframe of the response set (Watson et al., 1988; refer to Table 5.4 for a compilation of the 10 items in each subscale). Test takers rate themselves on

a 5-point scale ranging from 1 (*very slightly*) to 5 (*extremely*) as illustrated in Table 5.4. Each of 20 mood items can be rated for any of the seven time-frames listed in the Table. Test administrators employ the instructional set of how a person feels "right now" or "today" to measure the highly fluctuating PA and NA mood states. The instructional set of how someone felt "during the past year" or "generally feels" measures more permanent or trait PA and NA.

The PANAS is a well-constructed questionnaire that measures the two dimensions of positive and negative

---

Table 5.5
Activation-Deactivation Adjective Check List, Short Form(AD ACL);
Thayer, 1986, 1996

Instructions: Each of the words below describes feelings or moods. Please use the rating scale next to each word that describes your feelings *at this moment*.

Rating Scale:

1=definitely do not feel   3=slightly feel   2=cannot decide   4=definitely feel

Dimensions	Descriptors	Items
Energetic Arousal	General Activation: Calm-Energy	____ Full of pep
		____ Active
		____ Vigorous
		____ Energetic
		____ Lively
	General Deactivation: Calm-Tiredness	____ Placid
		____ At rest
		____ Calm
		____ Still
		____ Quiet
Tense Arousal	High Activation: Tense-Energy	____ Tense
		____ Jittery
		____ Clutched-up
		____ Intense
		____ Fearful
	Deactivation: Tense-Tiredness	____ Drowsy
		____ Sleepy
		____ Tired
		____ Wide awake[a]
		____ Wakeful[a]

Note: Scoring for each of the quadrant descriptors is achieved by summing the scores for individual items.

[a] Scoring reversed

affect. Depending on the purpose of the testing and information desired, however, there may be a need for information about more specific mood states such as anger and tension rather than global Positive Affect and Negative Affect. To accommodate this need, Watson and Clark (1994) have created the PANAS Expanded Form (PANAS-X), which measures 11 specific affects: Attentativeness, Fatigue, Fear, Guilt, Hostility, Joviality, Sadness, Self-Assurance, Serenity, Shyness, and Surprise. (See David Watson's University of Iowa faculty website, www.psychology.uiowa.edu/Faculty/Watson, for information about the PANAS-X.)

Since the scales are independent, exercisers can score high in both PA and NA, low in both, or they can score high in PA and low in NA, or visa versa. To examine the statistical properties of the PANAS, the inventory was administered to 1,003 members of the general adult population (females = 537; males = 466) from a variety of organizations, community centers, and recreational clubs in the United Kingdom (Crawford & Henry, 2004). Results of this investigation of UK adults from a non-clinical sample indicated that the PANAS is a reliable and valid measure of PA and NA. In addition, scores are relatively independent of the demographic variables of gender, age, education, and occupation. Although the two dimensions of mood are relatively independent as initially determined, they are *not completely* independent of one another as reflected by 5.8% of shared variance between the two subscales (Crawford & Henry, 2004). Negative Affect and Positive Affect are distinct dimensions, but they may be modestly, negatively correlated with one another. As Positive Affect increases, Negative Affect tends to decrease.

Activation-Deactivation Adjective Check List (AD ACL)

The Activation-Deactivation Adjective Check List (AD ACL) is based on Thayer's (1986) multidimensional model of mood presented earlier in this chapter. The AD ACL seems to capture mood states intuitively related to exercise settings. As the name implies, this multidimensional inventory measures a person's immediate state of arousal and provides a rapid assessment. The two core dimensions depicted in Figure 5.3 are

- *Energy*, which includes *tiredness* as its opposite, and
- *Tension*, which includes *calmness* as its opposite.

Energy and Tension, two dimensions of arousal, are NOT totally independent of one another. At moderate levels, they are positively correlated with one another. Thayer (1986) suggests that moderate tension enhances energy. At higher levels of intensity, these dimensions are negatively correlated. High levels of tension decrease energy. The reverse also is true. Heightened energy decreases feelings of tension.

Energetic arousal. This dimension reflects general activation/deactivation and includes (1) calm-energy and (2) calm-tiredness, an ideal pre-sleep state. Energetic Arousal is theorized to be affected by exercise activities, the sleep-wake cycle or a circadian rhythm, and nutrition (see Table 5.5).

Tense arousal. The Tense Arousal dimension includes both (1) tense-energy and (2) tense-tiredness. Tense Arousal reflects the preparatory emergency responses of stress and may decrease after some types of physical activity. Because exercise serves as a major influence on activation—on both Energetic Arousal and on Tense Arousal—it is not surprising that Thayer (1996) has conducted several studies of brisk walking. These studies will be described in the next chapter, which focuses specifically on exercise and mood alteration.

AD ACL Check List properties. A major advantage of this inventory is that it requires only 10 to 60 seconds to complete, depending on the version employed (Thayer, 1986). There is a standard 50-item form and also two shortened forms that include 20 and 25 activation-related adjectives. Test takers rate each adjective on a four-point scale. Refer to Table 5.5 for examples of some of the adjectives.

Multiple Affect Adjective Check List (MAACL-R)

The revised version of the Multiple Affect Adjective Check List is another measure of mood states that is employed in exercise settings (Lubin & Zuckerman, 1999; see Table 5.6 for subscales and sample test items in each). The MAACL-R includes 132 adjectives and the following five subscales:

- *Anxiety,*
- *Depression,*
- *Hostility,*
- *Positive Affect, and*
- *Sensation Seeking.*

Test takers simply check which of 132 adjectives on the MAACL-R best describe their mood states. Some individuals may check as few as 15 adjectives; others might check all 132 items. By indicating how they generally feel, the score would be a trait measure of mood. By indicating how they feel right now, the score is a state measure. Two of the five MAACL-R subscales measure desirable mood states. The positive affect subscale reflects a global aspect of mood. The Sensation Seeking Scale would appear to be especially appropriate for participants in high-risk exercise activities such as rock climbing, scuba diving, and skydiving.

Table 5.6

Multiple Affect Adjective Check List (MAACL-R)

Instructions: On this sheet you will find words which describe different kinds of moods and feelings. Fill in the circles ○ beside the words which describe **how you feel now—today.**[a] Some of the words may sound alike, but we want you to **check all the words** that describe your feelings. Work rapidly.

Negative Scales	Sample Item	Positive Scales	Sample Item
Anxiety	○ frightened	Positive Affect	○ good-natured
Depression	○ discouraged	Sensation Seeking	○ adventurous
Hostility	○ annoyed		

Note: From the MAACL-R: *Manual for the multiple affect adjective check list—revised* (p. 2), by B. Lubin and M. Zuckerman, 1999, San Diego: Educational and Industrial Testing Service (EdITS). Reprinted with permission.

[a] Trait instructions substitute the phrase "describe how *you generally feel*" in place of state instructions of "describe how you *feel now—today.*"

Subscale characteristics. Key terms reflecting the five mood scales within the MAACS-R include the following. *Anxiety* represents feelings of nervousness, tension, and fear. *Depression* reflects feelings of being sad and being lost. *Hostility* includes feelings of being disagreeable, cross, and disgusted. *Positive Affect* suggests being glad, happy, and pleased. *Sensation Seeking* includes feelings of enthusiasm, adventurousness, and energy. The subscales of Anxiety, Depression, and Hostility can be combined into a higher-order affect of *dysphoria*. The Positive Affect and Sensation Seeking scales can be combined into a Well-Being scale.

Alternate versions of the MAACL-R. Alternate versions of the Multiple Affect Adjective Check List include a shortened version that includes 66 adjectives for the five subscales and requires only one and a half to two minutes to complete. The Short Form of the MAACL-R has reliability and validity coefficients that are almost identical to those for the Standard Form of the MAACL-R (Lubin, Van Whitlock, Reddy, & Petren, 2001). In addition, there is a version of the MAACL-R that is available for use with young children and with adults who have a sixth-grade education (MAACL-R6; Lubin, Van Whitlock, & Rea, 1995). There also is a version for those who have a fourth-grade reading level (Lubin & Van Whitlock, 1998).

Exercise-Induced Feeling Inventory (EFI)

The Exercise-Induced Feeling Inventory (EFI) is the first inventory reviewed in this chapter that is designed specifically for exercise settings to capture the unique and distinct mood-related influences of exercise (Gauvin & Rejeski, 1993). The EFI is a brief inventory that includes only 12 adjectives. These adjectives capture four distinct feeling states hypothesized to be specifically related to the stimulus properties of acute bouts of physical activity (Gauvin & Rejeski, 1993). The EFI items include biological, psychological, and social influences commonly included in physical activity. In contrast to many of the mood inventories that are not designed specifically for measuring changes in mood associated with physical activity, the EFI includes a preponderance of positive mood states.

As illustrated in Table 5.7, the four independent subscales in the EFI are Revitalization, Tranquility, Positive Engagement, and Physical Exhaustion.

- *Revitalization* refers to feeling energetic, revived, and refreshed.
- *Tranquility* refers to feeling calm, peaceful, and relaxed.
- *Positive Engagement* is characterized by enthusiasm and happiness and is very similar to Positive Affect within the PANAS.
- *Physical Exhaustion* is similar to the Fatigue subscale in the POMS and includes being tired and worn out.

Based on the face validity of the inventory's 12 items contained in Table 5.7, the subscales seem to be associated with exercise.

Subscale properties. The psychometric properties of the EFI are reported to be sound. The factor structure, which is the four subscales, has been supported by confirmatory factor analysis with the comparative

Table 5.7
Exercise-Induced Feeling Inventory (EFI)

Instructions: Please use the following scale to indicate the extent to which each word below describes **how you feel at this moment in time**. Record your responses by filling-in the appropriate circle next to each word.

Response choices:

1=Do not feel (DNF)   2=Feel slightly   3=Feel moderately   4=Feel strongly
5=Feel very strongly (FVS)

1. Refreshed	1 2 3 4 5	7. Happy	1 2 3 4 5
2. Calm	1 2 3 4 5	8. Tired	1 2 3 4 5
3. Fatigued	1 2 3 4 5	9. Revived	1 2 3 4 5
4. Enthusiastic	1 2 3 4 5	10. Peaceful	1 2 3 4 5
5. Relaxed	1 2 3 4 5	11. Worn-out	1 2 3 4 5
6. Energetic	1 2 3 4 5	12. Upbeat	1 2 3 4 5

Note: Subscale scores are obtained by summing or averaging the numerical values of items in each of the four subscales. Positive Engagement items are 4, 7, and 12; Revitalization items are 1, 6, and 9; Tranquillity items are 2, 5, and 10; and Physical Exhaustion items are 3, 8, and 11.

From: "The Exercise-Induced Feeling Inventory: Development and Initial Validation," by L. Gauvin and W. J. Rejeski, 1993, *Journal of Sport & Exercise Psychology, 15,* p. 409. Copyright 1993 by Human Kinetics Publishers. Adapted with permission.

fit index greater than .90. The subscales also have been reported to have good internal consistency, with each subscale usually having a reliability coefficient greater than .80. The subscales also share expected variance with related constructs, are sensitive to exercise interventions, and appear responsive to the different social contexts in which exercise may occur (Gauvin & Rejeski, 1993).

Subjective Exercise Experiences Scale (SEES)

The final mood inventory included in this chapter is the Subjective Exercise Experiences Scale, another 12-item mood inventory designed specifically for exercise settings (McAuley & Courneya, 1994). The three subscales in this inventory are more general than those in the preceding EFI and focus on mood states in response to exercise. The three subscales include

- *Positive Well-Being,* which is characterized by feeling positive and terrific,
- *Psychological Distress,* characterized by feelings of being miserable and discouraged, and
- *Fatigue,* which is characterized by feeling tired and drained.

The SEES subscales. The first two subscales would seem to make the SEES quite similar to the PANAS. Fatigue, the third subscale, could be either a negative or a positive mood state—depending on the exerciser's experience with physical activity, fitness level, and even enjoyment of being physically tired. However, extreme fatigue probably is a negative mood state for most individuals, especially when there is absolutely "nothing left." Fatigue clearly is part of the exercise experience and is influenced by factors such as exercise intensity, duration, frequency, and training states or fitness levels.

Middle-aged exercisers completing a submaximal cycle ergometer graded exercise test tended to report larger decreases on the Psychological Distress (22% change) subscale than increases on the Positive Well-Being (6% increase) subscale (McAuley & Courneya, 1994). Of course, the direction as well as size of the mood changes on the subscales may vary according to the type of exercise, age, exercise experience, and fitness levels. These and other influencing factors will be examined in the following chapter. Because Fatigue scores tend to increase after exercising, it is interesting to note that participants in physical activity can experience enhanced Positive Well-Being, as well as increased Fatigue.

Table 5.8

Subjective Exercise Experiences Scale (SEES)

Instructions: By circling a number on the scale below for each of the following items, please indicate the degree to which you are experiencing each feeling *now*, at this point in time, *after exercising*.

I FEEL:

		(Not at all)			(Moderately)		(Very much so)	
1.	Great	1	2	3	4	5	6	7
2.	Awful	1	2	3	4	5	6	7
3.	Drained	1	2	3	4	5	6	7
4.	Positive	1	2	3	4	5	6	7
5.	Crummy	1	2	3	4	5	6	7
6.	Exhausted	1	2	3	4	5	6	7
7.	Strong	1	2	3	4	5	6	7
8.	Discouraged	1	2	3	4	5	6	7
9.	Fatigued	1	2	3	4	5	6	7
10.	Terrific	1	2	3	4	5	6	7
11.	Miserable	1	2	3	4	5	6	7
12.	Tired	1	2	3	4	5	6	7

Note: Subscale scores are obtained by summing or averaging the numerical values of items in each subscale. The Positive Well-Being subscale includes items 1, 4, 7, & 10. The Psychological Distress subscale items 2, 5, 8, & 11. The Fatigue subscale includes items 3, 6, 9, & 12.

From: "The Subjective Exercise Experience Scale (SEES): Development and Preliminary Validation," by E. McAuley and K. S. Courneya, 1994, *Journal of Sport & Exercise Psychology, 16,* pp.176–177. Copyright 1994 by Human Kinetics Publishers. Adapted with permission.

Psychometric properties. See Table 5.8 for the 12 adjectives in the SEES. Each subscale has four items that are rated on a 7-point Likert scale. The three subscales of Positive Well-Being, Psychological Distress, and Fatigue have acceptable internal consistency when employed for both children and adults (Markland, Emberton, & Tallon, 1997; McAuley & Courneya, 1994). Reliability coefficients of the various subscales have ranged between .73 and .92.

Selection of a Mood Inventory

When selecting one of the mood inventories reviewed for measuring mood states before and after an exercise session, or for inclusion in a study that you are planning, you will discover that choosing the "best" inventory is very challenging. Each inventory has advantages and disadvantages. No single inventory can be described as better than the others, which makes selection difficult. Some of the difficulties in selecting a mood measure are illustrated in Case Study 5.1 with

Angela, who faces the difficulty of choosing an inventory for a study that she is planning. Key considerations in inventory selection include the following: identification of potential measures, determination of statistical properties and usefulness, and selection of an inventory that best measures mood states of interest.

Summary

Exercisers often report that they "feel better" after exercising. Both the anecdotal reports and the results of research studies suggest that there is a decrease in negative affect and an increase in positive affect after exercising. In order to understand what is meant by the reports of "feeling good," it is important to distinguish between affect, emotion, and mood.

Affect is a global indication of how a person is feeling and includes separate positive and negative affective states. Thus, affect is all-inclusive. In contrast to affect, moods and emotions capture more specific feelings both desirable and undesirable. Moods and emotions

CASE STUDY 5.1 — *Choosing a Mood Inventory*

Angela Contemplates a Topic for Her Master's Thesis

Angela is very excited to have completed much of the coursework for her master's degree and finally to have time to focus on her thesis project: examining the changes in mood states in different types of physical activities. Angela has been an avid exerciser all of her life and notices that she feels "better" after exercising and that the nature of this "feeling better" experience seems to differ from one activity to another.

Starting the Process

The specific activities of interest to Angela were common recreational activities in her home state of Montana. After considerable thought, Angela decided to investigate the comparable mood changes associated with three activities that differed according to degree of activation: rock climbing (which was high activation), jogging (which was moderate activation), and hatha yoga (which was low activation). Angela is an avid rock climber and found this activity to be thrilling, personally challenging, and energizing due to its involvement with nature and the accompanying physical risk of the activity. Jogging certainly was not as exciting as rock climbing, but after jogging, Angela felt supercharged and psychologically and physically strong. In contrast, after hatha yoga, Angela found that she was calm rather than supercharged, very alert, and relaxed. In addition, after yoga, Angela was aware that her muscles were less tense than the muscular tightness or firmness she experienced after jogging and rock climbing. These physical activities seemed to represent the different quadrants in Thayer's (1996) two-dimensional model of mood depicted in Figure 5.2.

Checking the Research Literature

Angela sought answers in the research literature, but was unable to locate many studies that contrasted state changes in mood for the specific exercise activities that interested her. Thus, after discussing her interests and the literature with her advisor, Angela decided to investigate this phenomenon to examine the scientific bases for her personal exercise experiences.

Angela Considers Various Mood Inventories

Based on the research literature for mood and exercise, Angela discovered that many different inventories were employed. She had no idea which inventory would be an ideal measure for use in her study. Thus, Angela began the important process of inventory selection.

Identifying Possible Inventories

First, Angela created a list of possible inventories, their statistical properties, and their subscales. Most of the inventories were reasonably valid and reliable, and had normative data available for interpreting the scores. Thus, the statistical properties were necessary considerations, but were not of great help in differentiating inventories for inventory selection. Angela certainly wanted to choose the best available inventory because she wanted to find "answers" to her questions. However, she was unsure which mood inventory to select.

Determining Inventory Usefulness

Angela then began to consider the usefulness of specific subscales in the inventories in helping her answer questions about how people in the different exercise activities, characterized by differing levels of activation, feel after exercising. Specific inventories considered included the following.

The **Positive Affect-Negative Affect Scale (PANAS)** included the two subscales of Positive Affect and Negative Affect. Limiting mood to these two subscales just did not seem to yield quite enough information about the variety of potential mood changes that participants in the different activities of rock climbing, jogging, and hatha yoga might experience.

The standard form of the **Profile of Mood States (POMS)**, with the six subscales of Tension, Depression, Anger, Vigor, Fatigue, and Confusion, seemed to only capture primarily negative mood states. As a result, Angela was hesitant to employ the inventory, since she wanted to also measure positive mood states. Angela did note, however, that the widespread use of the inventory in the exercise psychology literature was an appealing aspect of the POMS, and she considered employing this inventory in her study.

CASE STUDY 5.1 (cont.)

The **Activation-Deactivation Adjective Check List (AD ACL)**, with the inclusion of Calm-Energy, Calm-Tiredness, Tense-Energy, and Tense-Tiredness subscales, seemed directly related to Angela's interest in the mood differences associated with the three types of exercise. Because Angela was uncertain that the AD ACL was her preferred inventory, she continued to examine potential measures of mood.

Angela was pleasantly surprised to discover that the **Multiple Affect Adjective Check List (MAACL-R)** included a measure of Sensation Seeking that seemed to be particularly related to her project, especially to differentiating between the mood changes associated with rock climbing, jogging, and hatha yoga. However, the other subscales of Anxiety, Depression, Hostility, and Positive Affect did not seem to be of as much interest as those in the AD ACL.

One of the two commonly employed mood inventories designed specifically for exercise and sport seemed especially relevant to Angela's basic research question concerning activation levels and mood alteration. The **Exercise-Induced Feeling Inventory (EFI)** included the measures of Revitalization, Tranquility, Positive Engagement, and Physical Exhaustion. The more that Angela analyzed the EFI, the more the subscales appeared to have an important relationship to her general topic.

As Angela completed her examination of mood inventories, she reviewed a second inventory that was specifically designed to be employed in exercise environments. The **Subjective Exercise Experiences Scale (SEES)**, with its three subscales of Positive Well-Being, Psychological Distress, and Fatigue, had strong psychometric properties, but would not provide the specific mood-related information she sought.

Angela Makes Her Inventory Selections

After reflecting even more on the inventories, gauging her initial reactions to them, and revisiting her thesis advisor's suggestions, Angela made her test selections. She decided to employ the EFI, because the subscales appeared related to the different level of physical activation in rock climbers, joggers, and hatha yoga participants. In addition, Angela decided to select the POMS as a second inventory to provide a broader view of participants' mood responses to exercise and to enable her to compare her results to those widely disseminated in the research literature.

By selecting two mood inventories, Angela could compare the effectiveness of the inventories with one another for distinguishing between her groups of rock climbers, joggers, and hatha yoga participants. With the EFI, Angela was able to measure Revitalization, Tranquility, Positive Engagement, and Physical Exhaustion. With the POMS, she was able to measure six additional mood states of Tension, Depression, Anger, Vigor, Fatigue, and Confusion. Angela was pleased that she spent sufficient time to examine numerous inventories and chose two of them that included subscales related to her research hypothesis.

---

are general underlying feeling states that permeate our lives. Intentionality is the best criterion for distinguishing between emotions and moods. Moods are undirected and have no specific causes. Emotions are feeling states that are directed at someone, such as when we feel angry with someone or have feelings of jealousy. More subtle differences between mood and emotions are that moods persist for longer periods, and are less intense than emotions.

Mood can be conceptualized as including a variety of dimensions. Examples of these include positive and negative dimensions and dimensions of high and low arousal. These dimensions can be combined in a variety of ways in various models of mood and capture a wide variety of mood states. Regardless of how mood is conceptualized, moods can influence our social interactions, health-related behaviors, and immune systems.

The ability of physical activity to moderate mood states has important implications for the quality of life. Exercise can be an effective approach to the self-regulation of mood and will be explored in depth in the next chapter. It seems that exercise can be associated with both desirable and undesirable changes in mood. Acute changes reflect mood states measured before and after an exercise session. Measures of mood commonly employed in exercise settings include the Profile of Mood States (POMS), the Positive Affect-Negative Affect Scale (PANAS), the Activation-Deactivation Adjective

Check List (AD ACL), and Multiple Affect Adjective Check List (MAACL-R). Two inventories, the Exercise-Induced Feeling Inventory (EFI) and the Subjective Exercise Experiences Scale (SEES), have been designed to measure mood states directly related to the exercise experience. Most of the inventories reviewed in this chapter provide a variety of scores that facilitate analysis of the relationship between exercise and mood alteration: raw scores, percentile scores, z scores, and T scores.

Can You Define These Terms?

Activation-Deactivation Adjective Check List (AD ACL)

affect

bipolar model of mood

chronic mood change

circumplex model of mood

diurnal variations in mood

emotion

Exercise-Induced Feeling Inventory (EFI)

hedonic

iceberg profile

Multiple Affect Adjective Check List (MAACL-R)

mental health model

mood states

mood traits

Positive Affect-Negative Affect Scale (PANAS)

percentile scores

psychosomatic relationships

Profile of Mood States (POMS)

raw scores

Subjective Exercise Experiences Scale (SEES)

self-regulation of mood

somatopsychic relationships

T scores

two-dimensional model

unipolar model of mood

z scores

Can You Answer These Questions?

1. What is mood?

2. How does mood differ from emotion and affect?

3. Which model of mood seems to best capture your own mood states most accurately? Explain the basis for your decision.

4. Which inventory seems to best capture your own exercise mood states? Please explain your decision and considerations.

5. What are the respective uses of raw scores, T scores, z scores, and percentile scores?

6. How can the same inventory be used to measure both mood states and mood traits?

7. What techniques do you use to regulate your moods? Which ones do you find to be most successful? Are these the techniques that you employ most often?

8. Is mood alteration one of the reasons that you exercise? Please explain your responses.

9. How do you measure the acute and the chronic mood changes associated with exercise programs?

CHAPTER 6

Mood Alteration, Self-Awareness, and Exercise: Multiple Relationships

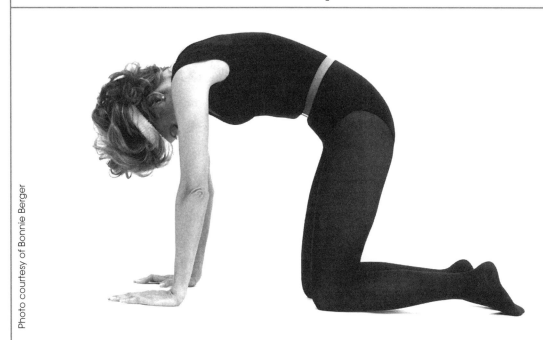

Photo courtesy of Bonnie Berger

After reading this chapter, you should be able to

- Elaborate on the effectiveness of exercise in the self-regulation of mood,

- Describe the "iceberg profile" of mood states commonly reported by exercisers,

- Discuss the role of enjoyment in the exercise-mood relationship,

- Clarify the types of exercise that might be most conducive to mood alteration,

- Specify training factors that might influence desirable and undesirable mood changes associated with exercise,

- Identify the *mental health model* of mood as it applies to exercisers,

- Describe the mood changes associated with exercise in nonclinical populations,

- Identify the mood changes associated with exercise in psychiatric populations,

- Discuss opportunities for developing self-awareness present in the exercise experience,

- Elaborate on the length of time during which the mood changes associated with exercise tend to persist, and

- Present possible solutions to the quandary: *so many benefits, so few participants.*

Introduction

In this chapter, you will explore the general mood changes associated with exercise—desirable as well as undesirable ones. You also will examine the possibility that the mood changes associated with exercise differ in clinical and nonclinical populations. Other important aspects of the relationship between exercise and mood alteration identified in this chapter include the time-course of the mood changes, specific aspects of the exercise experience that might influence the mood changes as outlined in a proposed exercise taxonomy, and possible mechanisms that might explain the relationship. Finally, you will become familiar with the opportunities that exercise presents to participants for increasing their awareness of their exercise responses and the role of exercise in their lives.

Analyzing Your Own Exercise Experience

As an initial step in understanding the relationship between exercise, mood alteration, and self-awareness, please take a moment to complete the project in Case Study 6.1. In this brief self-study, you have an opportunity to reflect on your own exercise sessions.

As you analyze your responses to the questions in the case study, it would be informative to determine whether the mood changes and their directions of change are similar to those reported in the experimental studies reviewed in this chapter. Some of the important questions about your mood states as visualized in the case study are as follows:

1. Did your mood states change *after* exercising in comparison with your mood states *before* exercising?
2. Were the mood changes in desirable or in undesirable directions, or a combination of both?
3. What exercise or environmental factors may have contributed to these changes?

Your replies to these questions and the additional ones posed in the case study might change as you reflect on participation in different types of physical activities, different exercise settings, and activities that differ in your enjoyment. Keep these personal mood responses to exercise in mind as you read this chapter in order to compare your personal mood responses to those of larger segments of the general population.

Exercise and Mood Alteration

The term *mood alteration* includes all changes—both desirable and undesirable mood changes. The term *mood enhancement* denotes changes in desirable directions. As emphasized in the chapter on quality of

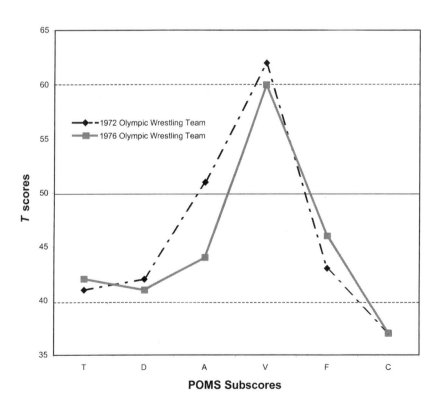

Figure 6.1. POMS scores of Olympic wrestlers. *Note:* From "The Trait Psychology Controversy," by W. P. Morgan (1980), *Research Quarterly for Exercise and Sport, 51,* p. 64. Copyright 1980 by the American Alliance for Health, Physical Education, Recreation, and Dance. Adapted with permission.

CASE STUDY 6.1

A Case Study Focusing on Your Own Exercise Experience

Take a moment to reflect on your own exercise sessions and some of the diverse moods that you may experience. It is quite likely that before, during, and after your exercise sessions you might feel a variety of mood states. For example, you may be feeling

- *Angry* about losing an event or match;
- *Energized* and *rejuvenated*, or *exhausted*—depending on the intensity and duration of your exercise session;
- *Excited* about your skill accomplishments;
- *Pleased* that you managed to find some exercise time for yourself in an overloaded day;
- *Proud* of your fitness progress;
- *Motivated* to exercise more, either more frequently or more intensely;
- *Relaxed* after the expenditure of energy; or
- *Worried* that your body may be showing signs of an overuse injury, as well as a host of other mood states.

How do you feel before, during, and after an exercise session? Use yourself as a case study to examine the mood changes associated with exercise. You will need to first collect the data and then analyze it.

Collecting the Data

Instructions: Focus specifically on your *favorite type of exercise*. For example, it might be tennis, golf, hatha yoga, or swimming laps. Visualize yourself participating in the activity for a full five minutes. For example, visualize how it feels when you are moving and the typical sequence of events from beginning to end of a session. In addition, visualize how you feel immediately before and after exercising. Use a full five minutes to develop these images and reflections. Then, answer the following items.

1. Identify your favorite activity:

2. My mood states **before** exercising:

3. My mood states **immediately after** exercising:

4. My mood states **one hour after** exercising:

5. My mood states **3 or more hours after** exercising:

Analyzing the Data

Clarifying your exercise-related mood states will enable you to compare your personal exercise responses with some of the general trends reported throughout this chapter. To continue with this self-analysis, answer the following questions.

1. Did your general mood state change from before to immediately after exercising?

   Yes _____ No _____

2. If your mood did change, in which directions were the changes for specific mood states when compared from before to after exercising?

3. What particular mood states changed the most?

4. For how long a period did a specific mood state remain changed?

5. Did some mood states remain changed for longer periods of time than did others?

In conclusion, it seems that mood alternation is an integral component of many exercise sessions. As you read about the mood and exercise relationship throughout this chapter, compare your introspective experiences recorded here with those reported in the literature. You may respond to exercise in many of the same directions and with the same specific mood changes as most individuals. You also may experience some unique changes in mood since the literature reflects the general tendencies of large groups of exercise participants.

Awareness of specific factors that influence the mood changes enables diverse specialists in the movement sciences to design exercise programs that are conducive to desirable changes in mood—if that is a high priority of the participant. Desirable mood changes also seem likely to enhance exercise adherence, because many individuals engage in activities that enable them to regulate their mood states.

life, mood enhancement is a primary component of an active lifestyle. Many exercisers report the desirable mood constellation of mood states referred to as the *iceberg profile,* which William P. Morgan (1980) identified more than 25 years ago. Morgan was investigating the mood states of athletes who hoped to qualify for Olympic teams. Among this elite group, he noticed that Olympic as well as intercollegiate wrestlers and oarsmen who were most successful were high in Vigor, but relatively low in Tension, Depression, Anger, Fatigue, and Confusion (i.e., the iceberg profile; see Figure 6.1 for the Profile of Mood States [POMS] scores of these athletes). In contrast, the Olympic-level "runner-ups" tended to have higher Anxiety and lower Vigor scores than those of the Olympic qualifiers.

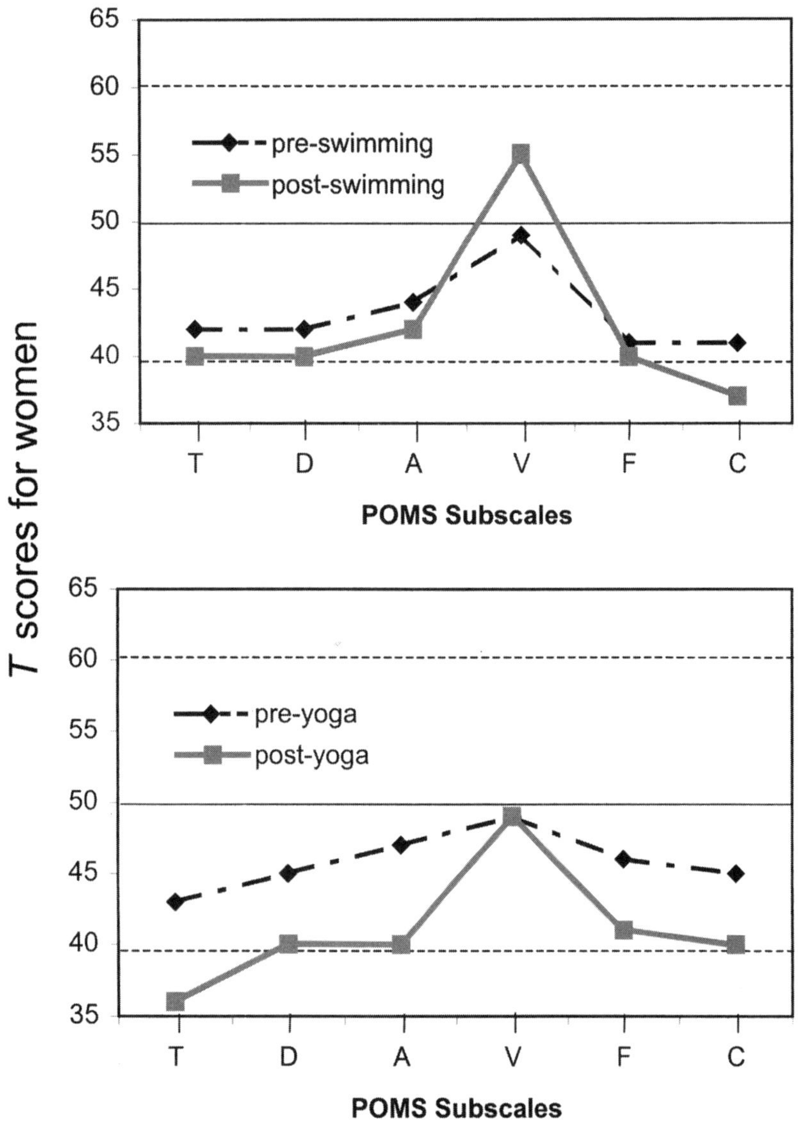

Figure 6.2. POMS scores of women before and after hatha yoga and swimming sessions (Berger & Owen, 1992a).

Iceberg Profile

The *iceberg profile* was aptly named, because the line connecting the mood scores is in the shape of an iceberg with only a tip (Vigor) rising up above the mean, or *T* score of 50. See the before- and after-exercise mood scores of recreational exercisers in swimming and hatha yoga in Figure 6.2. The swimmers' post-exercise mood states clearly represent the iceberg profile. After swimming, the one positive POMS subscale of Vigor is elevated and is above the mean of 50. The remaining POMS scores are submerged beneath the surface, or the mean of the general population. Yoga participants also exhibited a prominent iceberg profile after exercising, even though their Vigor scores were at the mean. Such desirable changes in mood may be one of many factors that contribute to exercisers' commonly reported "feeling better" phenomenon.

As illustrated in Figure 6.2, exercise participants often report the same iceberg profile commonly observed for elite athletes. Athletes tested by Morgan tended to have *T* scores for Vigor that were above the mean (ranging between 60 and 63) and *T* scores on Tension, Depression, and Confusion below the mean (in the low 40s). The *T* scores of the exercisers in Figure 6.2 were similar to those of the athletes in Figure 6.1 on all of the POMS subscales except Vigor. Exercisers' *T* scores for Vigor were between 48 and 57 and thus were slightly lower than those of the athletes. It is unlikely that these small differences in Vigor are meaningful in day-to-day living. However, it is the general relationship between exercisers' before- and after-exercise mood states, with the reporting of desirable changes after exercising, that is important.

Many exercisers have personally experienced the mood benefits of physical activity as reflected in Figure 6.2 and as described in the following observation of Breathnach (1998), a popular author who has written a best-selling book, *Something More: Excavating Your Authentic Self:*

> *A half hour of walking every other day increases your vitality and energy level and you find yourself less depressed. Suddenly you become more relaxed and fun to be around. You smile, maybe even laugh* [italics added]. You catch a reflection of yourself in a mirror and you're pleasantly surprised. (p. 86)

In contrast, exercisers and athletes who habitually overtrain, or participate in high-intensity/long duration exercise sessions that are physically exhaustive, may report a reverse iceberg profile. These exercisers and athletes who push the envelope of training tend to have low scores on the Vigor and high scores on the Fatigue subscales of the POMS. They also may report elevations in Tension, Depression, Anger, and Confusion (e.g., Hooper, Mackinnon, & Hanrahan, 1997; O'Connor, 1997; Tobar, in press). Not all exercise is conducive to desirable changes in mood states as reviewed in the following sections. Thus, exercise specialists need to be familiar with factors that influence the exercise-mood relationship as they design exercise programs that facilitate their clients' mood enhancement and perhaps their program adherence.

Mood Benefits

Positive exercise experiences of increased vitality and energy and decreased depression, as described by Breathnach (1998), have prompted exercise scientists to investigate diverse facets of the relationship between participating in physical activity and mood alteration. A fairly consistent finding is that desirable mood changes occur after exercising (e.g., Gauvin, Rejeski, & Reboussin, 2000; Long & van Stavel, 1995; North, McCullaugh, & Tran, 1990).

Meta-analyses have been conducted to examine exercise-related changes in anxiety (e.g., Calfas & Taylor, 1994; Long & Stavel, 1995; Petruzzello, Landers, Hatfield, Kubitz, & Salazar, 1991) and depression (e.g., Calfas & Taylor, 1994; Craft & Landers, 1998; North et al., 1990). In meta-analyses, the data from many studies on the same topic are *combined* and *statistically analyzed* as a group to determine the strengths of aggregate relationships. Results from meta-analyses are informative, because they include statistical analyses from many studies on the same topic. Meta-analyses generally have supported the mood benefits of exercise.

Many of the benefits of exercise are identified in a position statement that summarized the state-of-the-art knowledge field and was published by the International Society of Sport Psychology (ISSP, 1992). Although the ISSP position statement was published approximately 15 years ago, it still represents conclusions from the research of today.

> Individual psychological benefits of physical activity include: positive changes in *self-perceptions* and *well-being*, improvement in self-confidence and awareness, positive *changes in mood, relief of tension,* relief of feelings such as *depression* and *anxiety* [italics added], influence on pre-menstrual

Photo courtesy of Bowling Green State University

tension, increased mental well-being, increased alertness and clear thinking, increased *energy and ability to cope with daily activity,* increased *enjoyment of exercise* [italics added], and social contacts, and development of positive coping strategies. (p. 95)

Implications of Mood for Quality of Life

As reviewed in Chapter 3, the desirable mood changes commonly associated with physical activity have important implications for psychological well-being.

If a person "feels better" for several hours after exercising, then that person interacts with people, events, and a variety of projects in a more positive manner. By interacting more positively with others during this time, other people are more inclined to react favorably to the exerciser at other times.

Personal Interactions

Mood enhancement with exercise can affect a person's social interactions. For example, if a person is highly stressed and feeling hostile, the person may respond brusquely to coworkers who ask for assistance. As a result of that person's abruptness, coworkers might have hurt feelings, say something negative about that person to other coworkers, and/or might not provide needed assistance to the brusque and hostile person in the future.

Social interactions can affect our lives both positively and negatively. If the stressed, hostile person had exercised that day, she or he might have been in a more positive mood. As a result, she or he may have responded more positively, either verbally or behaviorally, to the initial request for assistance. Supporting the role of mood in personal interactions, people in positive mood states created by experimental manipulations have responded more positively to requests for assistance than have people who have been exposed to experimental manipulations designed to produce negative mood states.

Enhanced Psychological Well-Being

Improved mood states after an exercise session simply make a person's day more enjoyable. Often after exercising, we are in a positive mood in comparison to our own personal baseline level. Our more positive mood states may reflect (1) lower-than-normal levels of undesirable moods (such as anxiety, depression and sadness, anger and hostility, fatigue, and confusion) or (2) higher levels of desirable mood states such as vigor. When we are in positive moods, we might catch ourselves whistling as we walk down a hallway, smiling when we meet acquaintances walking across campus, and having a clear mental focus as we complete daily projects.

With desirable changes in mood—whether they be an increase in positive moods or a decrease in negative moods—life is more enjoyable even though the actual life events we encounter remain the same. In more desirable mood states, we tend to enjoy our activities, friends, and lives even more than usual. If habitually participating in physical activity can enhance our moods, mood enhancement would seem to provide us with a good reason for returning the next day for additional physical activity (Carels, Berger, & Darby, in press).

Flourishing

The desirable mood states associated with exercise can be directly related to the positive psychology concept of flourishing. As described by Keyes and colleagues (Keyes & Haidt, 2003; Keyes, 2005), *flourishing* denotes individuals who have positive feelings about their emotional, psychological, and social well-being and about their lives in general. Flourishing individuals (N = 3,032) between the ages of 25 and 74 years experienced fewer physical health problems, tended to miss fewer days at work, and were more productive (Keyes, 2005; Tracey, 2005). Approximately 18% of the adults tested fit Keyes' criteria for *flourishing*. Most adults (65.1%) fall into the category *moderately mentally healthy*. While these individuals are not flourishing, they are free of mental illness. The remaining 16.9% are *languishing* (i.e., mentally unhealthy; Keyes, 2005). Nearly as many Americans were languishing (mentally unhealthy) as were flourishing (mentally health). Exercising for mood alteration may be one of several approaches that could enable a larger portion of the population to flourish. Exercise psychologists and other movement specialists can design exercise experiences that promote desirable mood states, enhanced vitality, decreased fatigue, mental health, and ultimately flourishing.

A Taxonomy to Maximize the Benefits

To better understand the relationship between exercise and mood alteration, Berger and her colleagues (Berger, 1983, 1984, 2004; Berger & Motl, 2000; Berger & Owen, 1988, 1992a, 1998; Berger & Tobar, 2006) developed a taxonomy to help participants maximize the likelihood of mood benefits being associated with their exercise sessions (see Figure 6.3 for key elements in the taxonomy). Based on the research literature as well as anecdotal reports, Berger and colleagues suggest that exercise sessions that include a greater number of the taxonomy guidelines are more conducive to mood alteration than are sessions that include fewer of the guidelines.

As noted in Figure 6.3, the taxonomy contains three primary requirements. These include exercise enjoyment, specific mode or type of exercise guidelines, and key training guidelines. Both exercise mode and training considerations have subcategories that seem to be related to mood alteration. The taxonomy is introduced only briefly in this chapter. It is described in more depth in Chapters 20 and 21, where you will explore specific research studies that support and disagree with the proposed exercise guidelines that appear to maximize psychological benefits. The taxonomy is presented as a working model, designed to

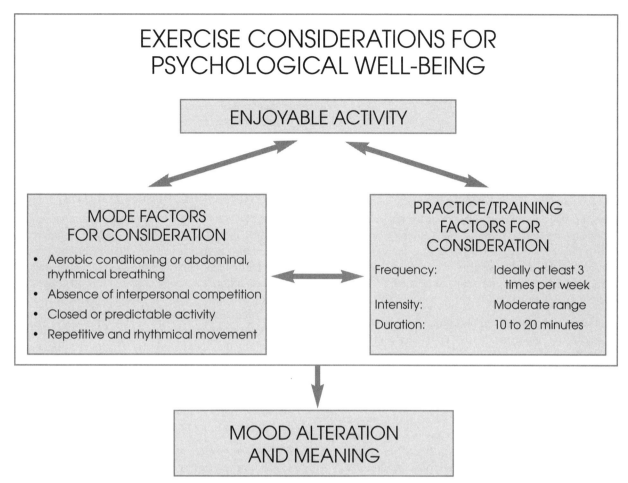

Figure 6.3. Taxonomy for enhancing mood benefits of exercise. From "Subjective Well-Being in Obese Individuals: The Multiple Roles of Exercise," by Bonnie G. Berger (2004), *Quest, 56*, p. 50. Copyright 2004 by the National Association for Physical Education in Higher Education. Used with permission.

clarify some of the components of exercise mode and practice/training considerations that may be related to mood alteration associated with exercise.

Need for Exercise Enjoyment

The enjoyment factor encourages you as an exercise specialist to consider individual differences and preferences when designing a specific exercise program that is conductive to mood enhancement. As specified in Chapter 3, enjoyment is "pleasure, delight, joy, gratification, satisfaction, relish, and zest . . . " (The Oxford American Dictionary and Thesaurus, 2003, pp. 477–478). Activities that are enjoyable to the participant are more likely to be associated with desirable changes in mood than are activities that are not (Motl, Berger, & Leuschen, 2000). Participating in an enjoyable exercise session may help individuals cope with everyday demands and hassles by adding to the overall positive experiences in a day. Exercise enjoyment also may serve to increase exercise adherence as the individual returns to the activity for another enjoyable session and to have "time for oneself" within a hectic day.

Enjoyment emphasizes the differences between various exercise modes and training factors. Some individuals tend to enjoy specific exercise activities such as rock climbing, tennis, jogging, and swimming more than they enjoy the others. In addition, the enjoyment factor suggests a need to consider exercise training factors as they relate to preferred exercise intensity, duration, and frequency (e.g., Ekkekakis & Lind, 2005). Both mode and training parameters are related to exercise enjoyment and mood alteration as illustrated by the bi-directional arrows in Figure 6.3.

Individual differences in enjoyment, as reflected in exercise preferences, need to be taken into account when designing exercise programs that facilitate mood alteration (Berger, 2004; Berger & Tobar, 2006). Emphasizing the importance of the exercise enjoyment for exercise practitioners when designing exercise programs, Ekkekakis and Lind (2005, p. 8) concluded that "it seems clear that exercise recommendations for overweight adults should take into account not only what is safe and effective from a physiological standpoint but also what is tolerable and enjoyable from a psychological perspective." Although their study of self-selected and imposed exercise intensity on mood and perceived exertion focused on overweight women, their recommendation to consider exercise enjoyment and perceived exertion preferences probably can be generalized to broad populations (e.g., Berger & Tobar, 2006).

Mode or Type of Physical Activity

Some types or modes of physical activity are more likely to be associated with mood alteration than others for most participants. Although there are a multitude of factors that distinguish among exercise modes, the basic mode guidelines in the taxonomy include four primary characteristics. These characteristics are presented here as a working model to clarify exercise mode considerations that may be related to mood alteration (Berger, 2004; Berger & Tobar, 2006).

- *Abdominal, rhythmical breathing* is the first exercise mode guideline in the taxonomy and is an important component in many stress management techniques. Abdominal, rhythmical breathing is likely to be associated with desirable changes in mood states. It occurs almost automatically when participating in aerobic exercise activities such as swimming and jogging. Thus there is substantial literature supporting the relationship between aerobic exercise and mood alteration. Abdominal, rhythmical breathing also occurs in lower intensity exercise activities such as hatha yoga, and in weight training, as participants coordinate inhalation and exhalation with specific components of their movements. Participating in yoga and weight training also are associated with mood benefits.
- *Absence of interpersonal competition*, or its *relative* absence, is another exercise mode guideline. A relative absence of interpersonal competition helps exercisers avoid comparisons with others and the often-accompanying mood states of anxiety, envy, or discouragement. Absence of interpersonal competition also enables exercisers to avoid the stress of competition and a variety of undesirable mood states often associated with losing an event or match, overtraining, or exhaustive exercise sessions.
- A *closed and predictable environment* is a third guideline. In closed environments, there are few unanticipated events, and the sequence of movements is predictable. In closed, predictable environments such as swimming and jogging, participants do *not* need to attend closely to their exercise environments. As a result, exercisers have the opportunity to let their attention and thoughts wander. They also can engage in self-reflection and stream-of-consciousness thinking, and/or have an absence of thought and enjoy a sense of solitude.

- *Repetitive and rhythmical movement* is a final exercise mode guideline in the taxonomy. Repetitive and rhythmical movements are closely associated with predictable environments and again occur in activities such as jogging, swimming, aerobic dance, and sometimes in downhill skiing, tennis, and weight training. Repetitive and rhythmical movements seem to enhance opportunities for thinking in general, for self-reflection, and at other times for a complete absence of thought.

Practice, or Training, Factors

In addition to specific types of exercise, a variety of training factors such as exercise frequency, intensity, and duration as well as various personal characteristics of the participants such as fitness levels may be related to the direction and scope of mood changes. Specific practice or training guidelines that may be related to mood alteration include the usual physical fitness guidelines of frequency, intensity, and time (FIT) considerations that can be adjusted for psychological as well as for physical benefits (Berger, 2004; Berger & Motl, 2000; Berger & Tobar, 2006). Note that in the commonly employed acronym "FITT," the second "T" includes *Type* of exercise, which is included earlier in the taxonomy.

- *Frequency: How often to exercise?* Recommended training guidelines often include a minimal exercise frequency of two to three times a week in order to establish a basic level of fitness. A minimal fitness base reduces the physical discomfort that can occur while exercising. A minimal fitness level may be necessary for the activity to be enjoyable, and this level may change from one individual to another. Despite the recommended exercise frequency that would seem to enhance exercise enjoyment, the mood benefits of exercise seem to occur even on the first day of exercise (e.g., Carels et al., in press; Berger, 2004; Thayer, 1996). However, to facilitate exercise comfort, adherence, and—ultimately—enjoyment, a minimum frequency seems to be a conservative recommendation.
- *Intensity: How hard to exercise?* Exercise intensity is a second training factor and generally is indicated by the participant's heart rate, or VO_2 max, as measured in a graded exercise test conducted according to carefully prescribed guidelines (American College of Sports Medicine, 2006). Exercise intensity should be "moderate" or approximately 60 to 80% of heart rate max (HR_{max}) to avoid the undesirable mood changes that have been associated with high-intensity exercise (80 to 100% HR_{max}). Moderate-intensity exercise also helps the participant avoid the physical discomfort, pain, and lack of desirable mood changes that often are asso-

ciated with high-intensity exercise (e.g., Ekkekakis & Lind, 2005). Considerably more is known about mood changes associated with moderate- and high-intensity exercise, than with low-intensity exercise.

● **Duration: How long to exercise?** Recommended length, or duration, of an exercise session for mood alteration is approximately 20 to 30 minutes—or less (Berger, 1996, 2004). Desirable mood changes tend to occur during this length of time, and this duration of exercise is less conducive than longer duration to overuse injuries. Recent studies suggest that as little as 10 to 15 minutes of walking may be conducive to calmness and relaxation (Carels et al., in press; Ekkekakis, Hall, VanLanduyt, & Petruzzello, 2000).

Possible Mood Decrements

The mood benefits after exercising are not automatic. Sometimes, there may be no mood changes, or even changes in an undesirable direction. Thus, it is important to be aware that there are many types of exercise modes and training parameters of exercise. Jogging is very different from rock climbing, and both can be performed in a variety of ways (at differing intensities, durations, and frequencies) and environments. It seems to make intuitive sense that not ALL exercise is conducive to enhancing mood states (Ekkekakis & Lind, 2005; O'Connor, 1997; Tobar, in press). When examining the mood benefits of exercise, it is important to consider its multiple influences on quality of life, and especially to recognize that exercise can have undesirable influences on life quality, and on mood in particular.

Exercise-related injuries, eating disorders, exercise dependence or addiction, and even extreme competitiveness are not conducive to psychological well-being and mood enhancement as highlighted in Chapters 10 and 16. For example, becoming upset after losing a competitive event, noting physical ineptness, prolonged overtraining to physical exhaustion, and making slower-than-expected progress with performance enhancement can lead to undesirable changes in mood. These mood decrements might include increased tension, anxiety, disappointment, depression, anger, fatigue, and decreased energy. In support of such undesirable changes, participants in high-intensity or long-duration exercise who are at recreational and elite levels have reported undesirable state changes in mood (Tobar, in press). Various combinations of high intensity and/or long duration exercise can result in overtraining, staleness, and burnout (O'Connor, 1997; Tobar, in press).

In a study of overweight women that focused on affect and exercise intensity, Ekkekakis and Lind (2005) indicated that participants reported no changes in the mood state of pleasure-displeasure as measured by the Feeling Scale (Hardy & Rejeski, 1989) after an

exercise session performed at a self-selected intensity. Exercise intensity was relatively high during the last 10-minutes of the 20-minute session and averaged 85–87% of their peak heart rate. The same overweight women reported a decline in desirable feeling states after exercising at an imposed intensity that was 10% higher than the self-selected intensity. For the final portions of the 20-minute imposed-intensity treadmill session, the even higher level of exercise intensity was approximately 93–94% of the women's peak heart rate (Ekkekakis & Lind, 2005). This study supports the need for moderate rather than high-intensity exercise for mood alteration.

Adding to the complexity of the exercise-mood relationship, individual psychological characteristics and environmental factors also seem to influence participants' responses to an exercise stimulus. For example, inactive women who scored high on social physique anxiety (concern about the physical appearance of their bodies) have reported increased state anxiety after exercising in a naturalistic setting. The naturalistic setting in this study was designed to elicit perceptions of evaluative threat (Focht & Hausenblas, 2003). In support of the negative influence of concern about one's appearance, another group of inactive women reported undesirable changes in mood or feeling states after exercising in front of a mirror—regardless of their predisposition towards body image concerns (Martin-Ginnis, Jung, & Gauvin, 2003). It seems that personal psychological characteristics such as social physique anxiety and concerns about body image are important moderators of mood responses to exercise (Focht & Hausenblas, 2004). Individual differences in social physique anxiety and potential evaluative exercise climates need consideration when designing exercise programs for mood enhancement. Consideration of these factors would decrease the possibility that a participant's physique is a barrier to the potential mood benefits and to exercise participation itself.

In conclusion, it is important to acknowledge the possibility of mood decrements and the factors that cause them. Despite such undesirable changes, however, evidence is accumulating that habitual physical activity *can be* associated with desirable implications for quality of life as indicated in the following sections.

Exercise and Mood Alteration in Non-Clinical Populations

A non-clinical or "normal" population is the terminology often employed to refer to individuals who have no major psychological problems. This distinction is important when examining the relationship between exercise and mood alteration. It seems that non-clinical and psychiatric populations report different mood benefits that accompany their exercise (North et al., 1990).

As noted earlier, non-clinical populations report exercise-related changes in mood that last for the relative brief duration of two to four hours. In contrast, clinical populations tend to report both larger decreases in depression and more lasting changes that range from several months to years than do non-clinical populations.

Although the following sections focus on the observance of mood changes with exercise interventions (i.e., changes in depression measured before and after exercising), there is a supporting body of evidence in the epidemiological literature indicating that depression and exercise levels are related. Epidemiological studies examine population trends, but include no interventions. This epidemiological body of evidence indicates that individuals who have higher levels of daily physical activity, in contrast to those with lower levels of daily physical activity, have lower levels of depression (e.g., Brown & Blanton, 2002; Cairney, Faught, Hay, Wade, & Corna, 2005). For example, in one study researchers examined the relationships among depression and the physical activities of a Canadian sample of 2,736 older adults above the age of 65 (Cairney et al, 2005). These included (1) activities of daily living such as gardening and house cleaning and (2) recreational exercise activities such as baseball, golfing, and jogging during the past three months. Results indicated that as much as 30% of the variation in depression in this older population was explained by the stress process model that included physical activity. Results of another epidemiological study indicated that physical activity and sport participation also may be associated with a major indication of depression and/or suicidal behavior among college students (Brown & Blanton, 2002).

Epidemiological studies such as these indicate that there is a demonstrable relationship between physical activity and mood in non-clinical populations. Within these correlational studies, however, it is not clear (1) whether people who are more physically active have more positive mood states as a result of the activity, or (2) whether people who have more positive mood states simply are more physically active. The following studies that include exercise intervention programs offer more substantial support for the mood changes associated with exercise.

Acute or Short-Term Mood Changes: Non-Clinical Populations

Mood changes associated with exercise tend to be acute or short-term in members of non-clinical populations (Berger, 1996; Morgan, 1997b; Sachs & Buffone, 1997). For example, before exercising, some individuals might be experiencing a variety of negative mood states. After exercising, they would tend to report lower levels of Tension, Depression, Anger,

Confusion, and possibly Fatigue if the POMS was the inventory administered. Other exercisers who are experiencing relatively positive mood states prior to an exercise session may feel even better than they did before the physical activity.

The changes from below-average scores to scores that are even farther below average on such mood scales as Tension and Depression are illustrated by the female swimmers and hatha yoga participants represented in Figure 6.2. Both sets of exercisers were in fairly positive moods prior to exercising as indicated by their pre-exercise scores' proximity to a mean T score of 50, which represents average mood scores. Their mood scores were even more positive after exercising. Because the women swimmers reported increased Vigor after exercising, their mood profiles more closely resembled the iceberg profile that seems to represent a high level of psychological well-being.

Members of a non-clinical population who report desirable changes in mood indicate that the acute benefits usually tend to last for two to four hours (Raglin & Morgan, 1987; Thayer, 1996). This may seem like a short length of time, and hardly worth our interest; however, upon reflection, it seems that experiencing more positive mood states for two to four hours and the accompanying "ripple effect" can have highly desirable influences on our lives. The more positive moods may influence exercisers' choice of work projects, social interactions with friends, colleagues, and family; work efficiency; and psychological well-being. Thus the short-term elevation in mood can provide important changes to an exerciser's overall quality of life when it is experienced on a daily basis.

Short-term mood alteration highlights the need for habitual exercise participation in order to reestablish the elevations in mood. Consciously or unconsciously experiencing such mood changes may serve as reinforcement for adhering to exercise programs. Individuals may return to exercise the next day in search of enhanced mood states: feelings of Vigor, Energy, and Clear-headedness as well as reductions in Tension, Depression, Anger, and Fatigue.

Chronic or Long-Term Mood Changes: Non-Clinical Populations

There also may be chronic or longer-lasting benefits as evidenced by stable changes in mood if they are monitored prior to exercising and then during a period of a few weeks, months, or even as long as a year (Brown et al., 1995; DiLorenzo et al., 1999; O'Neal, Dunn, & Martinsen, 2000). The meaning of long-term changes in mood—such as decreases in depression, tension, and anxiety, as well as increases in vigor—is difficult to interpret. For example, lasting or chronic mood changes associated with a long-term exercise program may be influenced by a variety of life events and factors, including exercise (Berger, Friedman, & Eaton, 1988).

When chronic mood changes are evident, the exercise program of several months actually may have produced the changes, or other seasonal, environmental, and life influences may have affected participants' mood states. People who feel depressed during the bleak winter months have automatic mood changes in the spring as the amount of sunshine increases, temperatures rise, and spring flowers appear. The desirable mood changes may last throughout the summer, but it would be erroneous to conclude that the daily exercise sessions were solely responsible for the changes. As encouraging as it is for the occurrence of chronic mood changes to last as long as a year, such changes are difficult to interpret. Attributing the mood changes to an exercise program is questionable.

In conclusion, members of non-psychiatric populations report acute, or short-term, rather than chronic mood changes with exercise (Berger et al., 1988; Brown et al., 1995). Until more knowledge is available about chronic changes in mood for members of a normal population, it is prudent to restrict claims for benefits to those reported immediately after exercise sessions. Clinical populations, as described in the next section, tend to report more lasting changes in mood as their anxiety or depression levels, or both, decrease (Martinsen, 1993; Martinsen & Morgan, 1997).

Exercise and Mood Alteration in Clinical Populations

Generalizations from exercise-related research with diverse psychiatric sub-populations are difficult, and research in the area is plagued by a variety of methodological difficulties unique to clinical populations. One methodological concern is the differing types (and measures) of depression and anxiety exhibited in clinical populations. Depression, for example, includes "mood disorder," "bipolar disorder," "cyclothymia," "major depression," and "dysthymia" which are considerably different from the mood state labeled "depression." Likewise, the mood state of anxiety or tension also is considerably more pronounced in psychiatric populations and can include personality disorders such as panic disorder, agoraphobia without panic disorder, simple phobia, and generalized anxiety disorder, as well as cognitive and somatic anxiety as reviewed by Berger, Owen, and Man (1993).

Mood Disorders

Mood disorders, including depression and anxiety disorders, are the focus of separate chapters in the major handbook for diagnosing psychiatric disorders, the *Diagnostic and Statistical Manual of Mental Disorders*

(DSM-IV-TM; American Psychiatric Association, 2000). The small number of participants in specific psychiatric diagnostic categories is another commonly encountered problem when designing exercise programs for psychiatric patients. The confounding effects of a variety of psychotropic medications further complicate assessing a possible relationship between exercise and decreases in anxiety and depression (Martinsen & Stranghelle, 1997). As noted in the review by Martinsen and Stranghelle, some of the medications also may detract from a patient's ability to exercise. Despite these difficulties, exercise may serve as a therapeutic modality for treating mood disorders and also may enhance the quality of life of psychiatric patients.

The Role of Exercise in Clinical Populations

Although physical activity has promise as a treatment modality for psychiatric patients, exercise therapy is not a highly established therapeutic approach. Egil Martinsen, a psychiatrist who served as a director of a psychiatric hospital in Norway, is a respected practitioner who has employed movement therapy and has conducted experimental studies to investigate its effectiveness. For more than 18 years, approximately 300 patients have been included in systematic studies of physical rehabilitation under Martinsen's supervision as part of their psychiatric treatment at various hospitals.

Martinsen's patients exhibited a wide range of psychiatric disorders and received a whole spectrum of psychotropic drugs while participating in exercise therapy. Psychiatric patients in both the walking/running treatment and the weight-training treatment reported decreased scores on depression and anxiety (Martinsen, 1993; Martinsen, Hoffart, & Solberg, 1989; Martinsen & Morgan, 1997). Recently, Martinsen and his colleagues (O'Neal et al., 2000) have provided basic "Recommendations for Supervising Exercise Training" for psychiatric patients, particularly patients with depressive disorders.

Depression in Clinical Populations

Within clinical populations, depression is characterized by a loss of interest or pleasure in many activities. It also may include changes in appetite, weight, and sleep; feelings of worthlessness or guilt; decreased energy; difficulty thinking or concentrating; and even thoughts of death or suicide (American Psychiatric Association, 2000). Thus, clinical depression involving mood episodes and mood disorders as categorized within the DSM-IV-TM is very different from the transitory mood state of depression experienced by non-clinical populations.

Defining depression. Depression is considered a "major depressive episode" if it lasts two weeks or longer, is characterized by the loss of pleasure in nearly all activities, and includes at least four of the additional symptoms listed in the DSM-IV-TM (American Psychiatric Association, 2000). Depending on how depression is measured and the population surveyed, somewhere between 10% and 25% of women and 5% and 12% of men in the general population have a lifetime risk of a major depressive disorder (Martinsen & Morgan, 1997). Standard treatment for depression includes medication, psychotherapy, and, in severe cases, electroconvulsive shock. These treatments are expensive, painful, and often have unpleasant side effects. Thus, a few therapists have begun to examine the effectiveness of exercise as a treatment modality in improving mood states (Martinsen, 1993; Martinsen & Morgan 1997). Exercise as a therapeutic approach is appealing because it has desirable side effects, and individuals who otherwise may not be treated with standard approaches for depression can employ it.

Studies of exercise and depression. A variety of studies support the possibility that exercise can have therapeutic benefits for people diagnosed with minor and major depression with the largest benefits for the more severely depressed exercisers (e.g., Craft & Landers, 1998). In a classic study of 28 outpatients classified with minor depression, Griest and colleagues (1979) compared running therapy with two types of individual psychotherapy. All three groups reported decreases in depression scores after 12 weeks of treatment. There were no differences in the amount of change in depression among the groups. Thus, the antidepressant benefits of running therapy were comparable to those for traditional psychotherapy.

Subsequent investigations have supported the effectiveness of exercise in reducing depression in psychiatric populations. In a representative study of four women classified with major depressive disorder, there was a significant reduction in depression (Doyne, Chambless, & Beutler, 1983). These results were observed after only six weeks of physical activity, and the changes in depression were larger than those in a pre-exercise screening phase. In another study of depressed women ($n = 6$), mood was measured immediately before and after exercising at 40%, 60%, and 80% VO_2 max. Results indicated that women who were depressed reported decreases in Depression and Total Mood Disturbance on the POMS (Nelson & Morgan, 1994). No mood changes were noted for the nondepressed females ($n = 5$) who completed exercise sessions at the same intensity levels.

There is some question as to whether the exercise activity for clinical populations needs to be aerobic. In some studies, the extent of improvement in aerobic fitness as a result of jogging and brisk walking has been related to the antidepressive benefits (Martinsen & Morgan, 1997; O'Neal et al., 2000). In other studies, participants randomly assigned to aerobic training of walking or jogging and those assigned to weight training (an activity that does not produce many aerobic benefits) reported significant reductions in depression (Doyne et al., 1987). Thus, it is uncertain whether the activity truly needs to result in aerobic conditioning for mood alteration. This questioning of the need for aerobic exercise in a clinically depressed population also has occurred in studies of normal populations (Berger & Owen, 1992a). As Berger and Owen (1992a) have suggested, it may be the change in breathing patterns rather than the aerobic component of exercise that is conducive to mood alteration.

These studies and others support the likelihood that physical activity has a therapeutic benefit for people with a variety of depressive disorders. There is a need, however, for continued research with depressed populations given the often small sample sizes, the tendency of depression to be confounded with other psychological disorders such as anxiety, and the potential confounding of results by various medications.

Anxiety in Clinical Populations

Anxiety includes a host of disorders such as panic attacks, agoraphobia or avoidance of places from which escape might be difficult, phobias, obsessive-compulsive disorder, posttraumatic stress disorder, and generalized anxiety disorder.

Diagnosing anxiety. Individuals diagnosed with a generalized anxiety disorder have had at least six months of worry and anxiety that are persistent as well as excessive (American Psychiatric Association, 2000). In addition, anxious individuals find it difficult to control their worry. The anxiety also must be accompanied by at least three of the following additional symptoms: fatigue, difficulty concentrating, restlessness, irritability, disturbed sleep, and muscle tension (American Psychiatric Association, 2000).

Studies of exercise and anxiety. In his review of the anxiolytic, or anxiety-reducing, effects of physical activity, Raglin (1997) noted that mental illness is a major problem in our society and that anxiety disorders are a prevalent form of mental illness that affects approximately 7.3% of the adult population. Thus, it is impressive that numerous reviews of the literature regarding the use of exercise for anxiety reduction indicate that exercise has resulted in significant reductions in state anxiety (a mood state), trait anxiety (a relatively permanent personality characteristic), and physiological correlates such as reduced blood pressure in clinical populations (e.g., Martinsen et al., 1989; O'Connor, Raglin, & Martinsen, 2000; Petruzzello et al., 1991).

The intensity of exercise appears to be related to changes in anxiety in clinical populations. Exercise performed at low intensities may be as effective as more vigorous physical activity in reducing anxiety disorders in patients hospitalized with anxiety disorders (e.g., Martinsen et al., 1989). The apparent mood benefits of low-intensity exercise are important, because low-intensity exercise seems more appealing than higher intensity exercise to a wide cross section of people, including clinical populations, who may be successful in initiating and maintaining such exercise programs. As Raglin (1997) notes, many studies of the anxiety-reducing benefits of exercise suffer from methodological problems such as not employing random assignment to treatment conditions, not considering the fitness levels of participants, and not controlling for the intensity of physical activity.

Despite such methodological problems, it seems that exercise is related to decreases in anxiety for members of clinical populations who have anxiety disorders as summarized in a recent review (O'Connor et al., 2000). These anxiety-reducing benefits also generalize to members of non-clinical populations who have high levels of anxiety. For example, one study investigated the anxiety-reducing benefits of cycling for a group of college women who studied more than their peers, a sign of high levels of anxiety (Breus & O'Connor, 1998). These women thought that academic requirements were the primary stressor in their lives, and had higher than average trait-anxiety scores as determined by test norms. They also had higher pre-exercise scores on state anxiety than did their peers. Results of this study indicated that a 20-minute cycling session at a fairly low exercise intensity (40% of the women's maximal aerobic capacity) was associated with significant reductions in state anxiety. In fact, this high-anxiety group of college students reported double the usual size of reduction in state anxiety following their cycling session than what usually is reported by nonanxious individuals (Breus & O'Connor, 1998). It seems that highly anxious individuals particularly benefit from the anxiety-reducing benefits of exercise.

Use of Exercise as Therapy in Private Clinical Practice

Psychotherapists who treat individual private clients or patients realize that exercise has a role in helping clients improve their psychological health (e.g., Hays, 1999; Johnsgard, 1989, 2004; Sachs & Buffone, 1997; Sacks & Sachs, 1981). In his recent book, Keith Johnsgard (2004), a psychology professor and psychotherapist, explored the relationships among exercise and mood alteration, self-esteem, anxiety and anxiety disorders, depression, and substance use, as well as

physical health and weight loss. To illustrate the importance of exercise in "conquering depression and anxiety," Johnsgard (2004, p. 269) provides a quotation from Friedrich Nietzsche, who wrote, "A man's stride betrays whether he has found his way . . . I love to run swiftly, and though there are swamps and thick melancholy on earth, whoever has light feet runs even over mud and dances as on swept ice."

In the introduction to her book, *Working It Out: Using Exercise in Psychotherapy*, Kate Hays (1999), a clinical psychologist in private practice and a previous President of Division 47 (Exercise & Sport Psychology) of the American Psychological Association, observes that psychotherapists are keepers of hope as they honor clients' pain and appreciate their potential. Based on this orientation, Hays provides experience- and research-based analyses of the use of exercise in

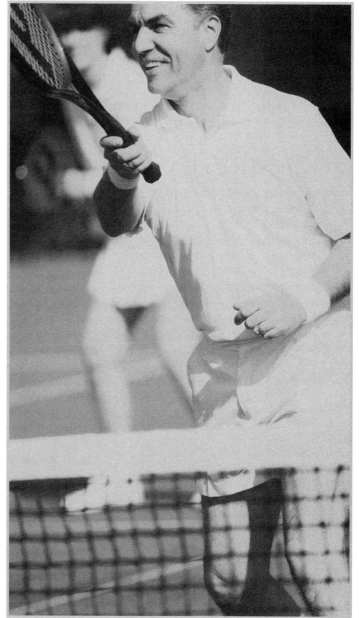

psychotherapy. These analyses include the basic theories underlying the body-mind connection and necessary considerations for choosing exercise as a therapeutic tool. Hays emphasizes the need to design exercise programs that reflect the client's stage of exercise readiness according to the transtheoretical model of behavior change or stage theory as developed by Prochaska, Norcross, and DiClemente (1994). Illustrating the complexity of exercise as a therapeutic technique, Hays devotes separate chapters to treating specific clients who are depressed, anxious, and stressed. Other chapters focus on treating clients who have eating disorders, substance abuse problems, and chronic mental illnesses. Additional chapters explore the role of exercise in treating trauma survivors and individuals of all ages. The major theme throughout this text for practicing therapists is as follows:

> Moving our bodies is one way to help move our minds—just as, in turn, our thoughts and feelings can alter our use of our bodies. In the broadest sense of the term, working out allows us to stretch not only our physical but also our mental muscles. The persistence of physical activity strengthens intrapsychic endurance, rhythmic routine soothes and smoothes our thoughts. The shared camaraderie of physical activity connects us with others. The unification of mind and body connects us with ourselves. *Exercise allows us to resolve, that is, work out, concerns, crises, and conflicts* [italics added]. (Hays, 1999, p. xi)

Effectiveness of Exercise in Comparison to Other Mood-Alteration Approaches

Physical activity often is associated with desirable changes in mood. However, there is no evidence that the relationship is causal. "Causal" means that it is the

---

Table 6.1
Factors That Can Influence the Relationship Between Exercise and Mood Alteration

Factors	Characteristics
Exercise Factors	
Mode, or type of exercise	Aerobic or rhythmical breathing, Non-competitive
	Closed
	Rhythmical and repetitive
Training parameters	Intensity
	Duration
	Frequency
Personal Factors	
Exercise enjoyment	Individual differences in exercise preferences
Clinical and non-clinical population	Classification according to DSM-IV
Initially high anxiety and depression	Mood state scores above/below 60th –40th percentile
Social physique anxiety	Concerns about physical appearance
Environmental Factors	
Evaluative environment	Mirrors, evaluative participants
Nature	Outdoors, woodlands, snow
Mood Measures Employed	
Acute, or short-term changes	Specific mood inventories
Chronic, or long-term changes	

physical activity itself that causes or precipitates the changes in mood. The lack of evidence for a causal relationship emphasizes that people who exercise may be in more positive mood states after exercising, but the cause or causes of these changes are unclear. The cause(s) may be the actual exercise itself, and thus the relationship would be causal. Or, the cause(s) may be a variety of situations *associated* with the exercise. Factors *associated* with the exercise experience that might influence mood include

- Being outside in nature,
- Interacting with friends,
- Becoming more physically skilled and fit,
- Simply leaving our cares behind,
- Having time to think,
- Or a host of other influences.

Obviously there also is a possibility that only people who initially are in relatively good moods have the necessary energy and motivation to exercise.

There are many ways to enhance our moods. Exercise is only one of many such approaches. An appealing aspect of the use of exercise for mood enhancement, however, is that exercise simultaneously provides a variety of health benefits (Blair, LaMonte, & Nichaman, 2004; U.S. Department of Health and Human Services, 1996, 2000). These include cardiorespiratory fitness, improving appearance by increasing muscle definition and reducing fat, and providing opportunities for social interaction. Other mood-enhancement techniques such as eating a sugar snack and talking with friends do not provide these health benefits. Many of the alternative mood enhancement techniques do, however, have the advantage of not requiring any planning or expenditure of energy and are thus "easier" and more enticing than exercise.

Questioning the effectiveness of exercise in comparison to other mood-enhancement techniques, researchers have investigated its benefits in comparison to those of quiet rest (Jin, 1992; Raglin & Morgan, 1987), Benson's relaxation response (Berger et al., 1988), and eating a sugar snack (Thayer, 1996). Comparing a broad selection of techniques for mood alteration helps to maintain perspective on the effectiveness of specific techniques for self-regulation. Illustrating the relative effectiveness of exercise in participants who were randomly assigned to treatment, Berger and her colleagues (Berger et al., 1988) reported that exercise and the highly established relaxation response were associated with similar short-term reductions on several POMS subscales, namely Tension, Depression, and Anger in non-clinical populations. Further illustrating the comparable effects of exercise, Jin (1992) found that following a mental/emotional stressor, the mood-alteration techniques of brisk walking, tai chi, reading, and meditation were associated with similar acute mood benefits on each of the six POMS subscales.

A conservative conclusion is that exercise is as effective as other techniques for mood enhancement, but not more so. More specifically, exercise appears to be a better antidepressant than relaxation techniques and quiet rest, equally effective to psychotherapy, and less effective than exercise and psychotherapy combined (North et al., 1990; Raglin & Morgan, 1987). A meta-analysis of 19 studies of clinically depressed patients that were published after the North et al. study, however, found no significant support for the superior effectiveness of exercise treatments in comparison to other treatment interventions (Craft & Landers, 1998). It seems that exercise has mood benefits that are comparable but not necessarily superior to other depression-management techniques. As previously noted, however, exercise has the advantage of providing concomitant psychological, physiological, social, and even spiritual benefits. Further investigation is needed to clarify whether the mood benefits of exercise and other strategies are associated with possibly different (1) duration of benefits, (2) patterns of change on mood profiles based on specific mood states, and (3) underlying mechanisms in non-clinical and clinical populations. See Table 6.1 for a summary of factors influencing the relationship between exercise and mood alteration.

Theoretical Mechanisms Underlying the Relationship Between Exercise and Mood Alteration

What mechanisms, or groups of interacting mechanisms, might explain the relationship between exercise and mood alteration? This important but still unanswered question captures the interest of many researchers. The relationships are not readily decipherable, and thus this section includes proposed mechanisms that are highlighted in Table 6.2. Essentially, the proposed mechanisms can be separated into the following categories:

- *Proposed physiological/biological mechanisms,*
- *Proposed psychological mechanisms,*
- *Potential social mechanisms,* and
- A *combination* of interconnected mechanisms: psychological, social, and physical processes.

Proposed Physiological Mechanisms

Potential physiological mechanisms underlying the exercise-mood relationship include, but are not limited to, the following: physical health, cardiorespiratory, beta-endorphin, cortisol, monoamine, and thermogenic (temperature elevation) hypotheses. Interested

Table 6.2
Theoretical Mechanisms Underlying the Relationship Between Exercise and Mood Alteration

Categories	Hypothesized Mechanisms
Physiological Mechanisms	Physical health Cardiorespiratory fitness Beta-Endorphin Monoamine Others
Psychological Mechanisms	Enjoyment Cognitve-behavioral Time-out Mastery Expectancy Others
Social Mechanisms	Being with friends Social interaction Others
Combination of Mechanisms	

students should refer to *Physical Activity and Mental Health*, edited by Morgan (1997b), and also see articles by North et al. (1990), O'Neal et al. (2000), and Petruzzello et al. (1991) for more detailed discussions of some of these proposed mechanisms.

Physical health hypothesis. Definitions of physical health include an absence of chronic diseases such as diabetes, heart disease, rheumatoid arthritis, obesity, cancer, and related limitations in daily activities (e.g., Cairney et al., 2005). Thus physical health often indicates a relative absence of disease, rather than optimal health characterized by high levels of vitality, strength, endurance, and energy. Despite this narrow conceptualization, physical health status can be a mechanism influencing the exercise-mood alteration relationship (Berger & Tobar, 2006; Cairney et al., 2005).

Physical health, as indicated by the prevention and progression of illnesses and their associated limitations, is influenced by exercise (Blair et al., 2004). In addition, physically active individuals may have fewer illnesses and more strength, endurance, and energy. As a result of these increases in physical health, exercisers may experience more positive mood states. The strongest relationship between physical health and positive mood states may be evident in the elderly (e.g., Cairney et al., 2005), whose health status may restrict the frequency of desirable activities: visiting

with friends, driving the car, and even exercise itself. People in poor physical health may exercise less and as a result be depressed, anxious, and fatigued.

Cardiorespiratory fitness hypothesis. Cardiorespiratory fitness is another commonly proposed physiological mechanism that may contribute to the relationship between exercise and feelings of psychological well-being. The rationale for the relationship is that some types of exercise are almost synonymous with respiratory fitness. Thus, exercise programs that produce greater cardiorespiratory fitness should be associated with greater psychological benefits than should programs that do not produce as large a change. This does not seem to be a totally accurate portrayal of the exercise-mood relationship as summarized by North and colleagues (1990) in their meta-analysis of the exercise and depression research. For example, decreases in depression occurred early in exercise programs prior to the development of cardiorespiratory fitness (Carels et al., in press; North et al., 1990). Participants in activities such as weight training and hatha yoga which produce little improvement in cardiorespiratory fitness also have reported decreases in depression and other undesirable mood states (Berger & Owen, 1988, 1992; North et al., 1990).

Beta-Endorphin hypothesis. The endorphin hypothesis has received considerable visibility in the popular press. Endorphins are produced in the brain, pituitary gland, and other tissues of the body and have "morphine-like" qualities in their reduction of pain and production of a euphoric state—similar to a runner's or exerciser's high. According to the endorphin hypothesis, elevations in beta-endorphins, which occur during an exercise session, produce the improvement in mood states. Researchers have provided some support for the endorphin hypothesis when administering the opiate receptor antagonist Naltrexone, which blocks the production of endorphins (Daniel, Martin, & Carter, 1992). When Naltrexone was administered to participants prior to exercising, the exercisers did not evidence an increase in endorphins or mood enhancement. Other studies, however, have not supported the endorphin hypothesis as reported in a review article by O'Neal et al. (2000).

Beta-endorphin levels in the bloodstream have not been related to mood changes in several studies employing the POMS to measure mood (Farrell et al., 1986; Farrell, Gustafson, Morgan, & Pert, 1987). These same studies also suggested that peripheral levels of corticotrophin, dopamine, epinephrine, norepinephrine, and growth hormone were unrelated to mood changes. Further lack of support for the beta-endorphin hypothesis is the observation that endorphin levels have been related to changes in Depression and Confusion scores reported by exercisers in a direction opposite to that anticipated (Kraemer, Dzewaltowski, Blair, Rinehardt, & Castracane, 1990). A problem in testing the relationship between endorphin production in the brain and its relationship to mood elevation is that the endorphin levels in the brain cannot be measured directly. Some of the equivocal relationship between beta-endorphins and mood change with exercise appears to be related to the blood-brain barrier (i.e., endothelial cell layer surrounding the capillaries in the brain). This barrier is relatively impermeable to peptides and other large molecules circulating in the bloodstream. As a result, changes in peripheral levels of endorphins circulating in the bloodstream would not be expected to modify opioid activity in the central nervous system as necessary for altered mood states.

Monoamine hypothesis. The monoamine hypothesis identifies another plausible mechanism underlying the relationship between exercise and mood alteration, especially depression (O'Connor et al., 2000; O'Neal et al., 2000). Neurotransmitter systems, especially the noradrenergic and serotonergic systems, form the underlying bases for much of the pharmacological treatment of depression and for anxiety. According to the monoamine hypothesis, if exercise produces chemical changes similar to those associated with drug therapy, it would explain the mechanism underlying the exercise-mood alteration relationship. Measuring these

physiological changes in the brain, however, is nearly impossible in human beings due to its invasive nature. Thus, current research evidence supporting the monoamine hypothesis has been restricted primarily to rodents and awaits further testing on human beings for more conclusive support (Dunn, Reigle, Youngstedt, Armstrong, & Dishman, 1996; O'Neal et al., 2000).

Conclusions. Other appealing physiological mechanisms that might account for the exercise-mood relationship include the brain-blood flow hypothesis and the hypothalamic-pituitary-adrenal (HPA) hypothesis. However, these hypotheses, like all hypotheses, required considerable testing. As exemplified by this brief analysis of proposed physiological mechanisms, no single mechanism consistently explains the relationship. Continued examination of physiological mechanisms that may influence the relationship between exercise and mood alteration is important for future research.

Proposed Psychological Mechanisms

Psychological mechanisms also may influence the relationship between exercise and mood alteration. Potential psychological mechanisms include exercise enjoyment, time-out from a busy day, distraction from one's daily routine, achievement of self-care, opportunity for self-talk, expectancy of benefits or a placebo effect, and psychological resources such as increased perception of control over one's life, improved self-concept, increased psychological energy, perceived mastery, self-efficacy, and self-esteem (e.g., Berger, 1996; Cairney et al., 2005; North et al., 1990; Petruzzello et al., 1991; Thayer, 1996). Although little current evidence identifies any single psychological variable or group of psychological variables that consistently mediates the exercise-mood relationship, this section identifies some of the proposed mechanisms that await further testing.

Enjoyment hypothesis. Enjoyment is one of the psychological mechanisms that may produce the psychological benefits of physical activity (e.g., Berger & Motl, 2001; Berger & Owen, 1988; Kimiecik & Harris, 1996). Participating in enjoyable types of exercise may help individuals counterbalance psychological stress associated with everyday demands and hassles. A study of seasoned rock climbers who had an average of 54 months of experience examined the role of enjoyment on the relationship between exercise and mood alteration. The rock climbers' enjoyment of the activity was associated with the extent of acute mood benefits on the POMS subscales of Tension, Depression, and Vigor when measured before and after a climb (Motl et al., 2000). Individuals who reported high levels of enjoyment had greater mood changes in desirable directions than did those who had comparably lower enjoyment scores. Enjoyment appeared to mediate the acute mood changes associated with rock climbing, rather than the mood changes influencing level of enjoyment. Thus, exercise enjoyment may be a factor contributing to mood alteration (see Chapters 3 and 21 for more information about exercise enjoyment).

Cognitive-behavioral hypothesis. A proposed cognitive-behavioral hypothesis for the link between exercise and decreases in depression (e.g., North et al., 1990) also might apply to a variety of mood states and other indices of psychological well-being such as feelings of self-efficacy and competency. According to this hypothesis, exercise might change the presence of

- Automatic, negative self-talk and thoughts,
- Systematic errors in logic, and
- Depressive/anxious/stressed and other undesirable schemata that underlie depression and other undesirable psychological states (North et al., 1990).

With changes such as the above in cognitive patterns, exercisers might "feel better" after participating in physical activity.

Time-out hypothesis. Another plausible psychological mechanism for mediating the relationship between exercise and psychological well-being is having some time out (Bahrke & Morgan, 1978). Distraction and escaping from our daily hassles and current concerns while exercising may provide a more balanced perspective as participants have an opportunity to reframe their thinking; gain new perspectives on daily activities, goals, and social interactions; and simply have an opportunity to relax. This possibility has been tested in several studies. It seems, however, that exercise is associated with greater and longer lasting mood benefits compared to other time-out activities such as reading and quiet rest (North et al., 1990; Raglin & Morgan, 1987). Although still untested, the time to think and to be with one's thoughts may provide the greater benefit.

Mastery hypothesis. The mastery hypothesis reflects the possibility that developing physical competencies, both the development of complex motor skills as well as increased physical fitness, may increase exercise-related feelings of accomplishment, self-mastery, self-efficacy, self-competence, and control (Petruzzello et al., 1991). These feelings of mastery also may generalize from exercise settings into other areas of life. Thus, mastery and success experiences in exercise settings subsequently may enhance psychological well-being. Bandura's (1997) theory of self-efficacy suggests that when mastering a difficult and effortful task such as exercise, we tend to have increased self-confidence and self-efficacy as well as the ability to cope with personal problems.

Expectancy hypothesis. Expectancy of benefits might be another factor mediating the relationship between exercise and acute mood alteration. Participants' beliefs about how they expect to feel after exercising can be based on actual reactions to an exercise session, previous reactions to similar sessions, and knowledge of how others have reacted to exercise. With all the media attention to the mood alteration and stress reduction benefits of exercise and to endorphin "highs," it is not surprising that some exercisers expect psychological benefits.

The expectancy hypothesis suggests that if we expect to feel better after exercising, we may do so because of expectancy, or this placebo-like effect. Despite this possibility, the mood changes associated with exercise do not seem to be related to our expectancy of feeling better (Berger, Owen, Motl, & Parks, 1998; King, Taylor, & Haskell, 1993). For example, in one examination of expectancy effects, joggers in two studies consistently reported significant mood benefits after exercising (Berger et al., 1998). However, the same joggers' expectation of benefits as measured by an open-ended question "Does exercise affect how you feel?" in one study and by an objective expectancy questionnaire in a subsequent study was not conclusively related to their mood changes. Of course, depending on specific exercise environments and exercise leaders, expectancy of psychological benefits may be either a strong or weak moderating influence.

Proposed Social Mechanisms

Social mechanisms that might underlie the relationship between exercise and mood alteration are the opportunity to be with friends while exercising and the accompanying discussion of ideas, problems, and life events. Many exercisers cite social interactions and friendships as reasons for participation in physical activity. In addition to serving as exercise motives and support for habitual exercise, the social interaction may provide opportunities to rebalance our perspectives on daily events, needed companionship, and just plain fun.

Despite the apparent logic for social mechanisms, North and colleagues (1990) did not find support for social interaction in their meta-analysis of the exercise-depression relationship. Surprised at this lack of support, they suggested that social support and interaction may be more important for beginning exercisers than for accomplished exercisers, who already have discovered the inherent rewards and appeal of exercise. Thus, there is a need to examine beginning, somewhat established, and long-term exercisers when testing the vole of social interaction as a mediator in the exercise-mood alteration process.

Additional Possibilities: A Combination of Mechanisms, the Changing of Mechanisms in Different Activities, and Individual Differences

There is little research evidence to support any single factor underlying the exercise-mood relationship. Identifying mechanisms underlying the relationships between exercise participation, mood alteration, and other psychological benefits seems to reflect the complexity of exercise settings and individual differences. Specific mechanisms, and even combinations of several mechanisms, may occur more readily in some types of exercise and specific training conditions than others. For example, a range of specific exercise intensities may be necessary to elevate endorphin levels; beyond that range, endorphin levels may fall. The same might be the case for the relationship of other physiological, psychological, and social mechanisms.

There also may be individual differences from one participant to another. As a result, a *person × exercise mode × training parameters × exercise environment* interaction may explain the complexity in elucidating underlying mechanisms. Continued research is needed to help unravel the elusive psychological, social, physiological and combined mechanisms that offer viable explanations for the mood alterations that occur after exercising. Like the simple aspirin, the exercise treatment is effective, but the causal mechanisms are unclear.

Mood and Exercise: Opportunities for Self-Awareness

In addition to providing an opportunity to enhance mood states, exercise provides occasions for participants to learn about themselves as they experience diverse moods connected to the movement process itself. Exercise provides multiple opportunities to look within ourselves and to ask questions such as

- "Why am I exercising?"
- "What's the purpose of all of this?" and even
- "Who am I?" as participants experience a broad range of mood states while exercising.

Asking such questions and experiencing and acknowledging some of the mood changes associated with exercise are initial steps toward enhanced self-awareness. The following poem by Price (1983) in her book *The Wonder of Motion: A Sense of Life for Woman* captures a few of the mood states such as joy, sadness, struggles, triumph, and peace that can occur in exercise and in sport.

Sport (and exercise) holds a mirror to a woman's life
all that she can know
of joy
or sadness

finds its counterpart in sport

she learns not only how she moves
but how she feels
and thinks
and struggles

how she *is tormented*
triumphs
and then finds *peace*

as she absorbs the
mood
drama
and *emotion*

which are the essences of her sport
so she *discovers*
all the *inward stresses*
that move *her being*.
(italics added) (p. 13)

To examine the role of exercise in enhancing mood alteration and self-awareness, Berger and MacKenzie (1980) analyzed the mood states and emotions of a woman jogger who maintained personal, dated diary entries of her thoughts that occurred during 32 different running sessions. The project was conducted during a four-month period in which the runner averaged three running sessions per week. On three additional occasions, the woman ran in a different location so that she might be interviewed immediately after her run. A trained clinician conducted psychiatric interviews, which were approximately 50 minutes in length. These three sessions were audio-recorded during weekly meetings near the end of the study and later were transcribed for data analysis.

The study was in search of an answer to the question "Why is sport (or exercise) meaningful to so many people?" Mood states and emotions were the focus of the study because they might accurately depict the authentic phenomenological experience of jogging. Three interviews were designed to go beyond the culturally acceptable answers to the question of "why." Results of the study indicated that there were four primary reasons for this woman—and presumably for other women and men—to participate in jogging. Three of the four propositions support the value of self-analyzing moods and emotions that emerge from exercise in the human quest for self-knowledge and increased self-awareness.

- *Proposition 1.* **Participating in physical activity is conducive to experiencing a wide spectrum of moods and emotions.** Over 30 different kinds of feelings and emotions ranging from agony to ecstasy were included: hostility, loneliness, pleasure, power, hopelessness, aliveness, competency, and control.
- *Proposition 2.* **Individual activities such as jogging are conducive to thinking in general and to introspection.** One example of the introspection included the following journal entry:

  > Jogging is a real gift to oneself. It's a form of self-affirmation to say that one is important enough to devote an entire hour to oneself. Too often we are doing things that we "must." . . . Time to get out of that trap . . . I have had enough of that shit . . . of blaming self, self-criticism. (Berger & Mackenzie, 1980, p. 8)

- *Proposition 3.* **Inner psychological needs were satisfied by the physical activity.** These psychodynamic needs included a near obsessive-compulsive constellation of behaviors with a focus on accomplishment, checklists, and schedules and overreliance on intellectuality with a shrinking of affective capacity. Another psychodynamic consideration was her relationships with her father and brother, who also were runners.
- *Proposition 4.* **This final proposition was that self-understanding can be enhanced by an awareness of the phenomenological experiences associated with exercise.** Mood-related issues of self-understanding included feelings of competitiveness with other joggers, and family influences on the drive to accomplish. For example, the woman reported,

  > There was one other jogger out today—a male who had a lot more speed than I . . . I was wondering how much stamina he had—felt a little insecure since he was going faster than I. What a competitor! Is it good or bad? Interesting. Will have to test my reactions another time. (Berger & Mackenzie, 1980, p. 14)

Supporting the value of exercise for enhancing self-awareness, George Sheehan (1992a), the noted running philosopher, describes the value of habitual physical activity as an avenue for increasing self-knowledge. Sheehan was a master at the self-knowledge process as he used his running experiences as raw material for personal insights that he described to the world at large. Asked in a public forum what he thought about when he exercised, Sheehan (1992a, p. 173) reported that his thinking was rather mundane and included two broad categories of thought, as well as a near absence of thought. One category was *free association*; his mind could wander anywhere it chose.

The other category of thought was to focus *on a single, specific problem* that he would have liked to solve before the end of the exercise session. On other occasions, there was a *total absence of thought*. During these runs, the physical motion became a mantra, and all external and internal stimuli were removed from his consciousness. As Sheehan observed,

> Motion becomes my mantra. Through it I gradually divest myself of *worry and anger, of fear and depression* [italics added]—and the reasons for them. I can reach a state when time is this never-ending moment and where this place is the entire world. This is the passive meditation of the East. (p. 174)

Many exercisers do the same types of thinking and introspection as Sheehan did, but in a less public forum. Exercisers, particularly those in solitary activities, can tune into their thought processes and feelings while running, swimming, skiing, or skating. If exercising alone, they might ask themselves where and for how long they might want to exercise, at what intensity, and for what purposes as well as observe their moods throughout their exercise session. In addition, they can note their moods as they experience personal improvement, reflect on daily hassles and uplifts, and/or examine past events, personal relationships in their lives, and former times.

The importance of self-awareness, its complexities, development, and centrality to human nature itself are explored in the book, *Self-Awareness: Its Nature and Development* (Ferrari & Sternberg, 1998). Social scientists are just beginning to become aware of how we human beings come to understand who we are in relation to others, the broader world, and ourselves. Physical activity presents wonderful opportunities to increase self-awareness and/or to have no thoughts or awareness of mood states, which can result in a true time-out experience. The exercise experience can present an opportunity to quiet our often-chattering minds, especially if the exercise is a relatively non-competitive, predictable, and rhythmical activity.

A Quandary: So Many Benefits, So Few Participants

People who reap the desirable mood states and elevated self-awareness associated with exercise would seem to have an important, immediate reason to return for more. Most people are familiar with the physical benefits of exercise such as lowering their blood pressure, lowering their resting heart rate, decreasing their body fat, and increasing their bone density (Blair et al., 2004; U.S. Department of Health and Human Services [USDHHS], 1996, 2000). These health benefits are highly desirable, yet they require lengthy participation in order for exercisers to begin to see these physiological changes.

Due to the effort required to exercise, the pace of modern society, and the tendency for the physiological benefits of exercise to require a long-term commitment, it is not surprising that estimates of the percentage of people who exercise sufficiently in the United States and other developed countries vary between 12% and 30% (Dishman & Buckworth, 1997; USDHHS, 1996, 2000). The percentages change according to the populations sampled, but the conclusions remain the same: A relatively small portion of the population is physically active.

The gulf between knowledge and behavior is huge. This is illustrated by the common suggestion: "Do as I say (knowledge), and not as I do (behavior)." Identifying factors that facilitate translating knowledge of what we "should do" into behavior that leads to high levels of health is an important need in exercise psychology (see Chapter 13 for determinants of exercise adherence).

A way to encourage a larger proportion of the population to be physically active is to provide nonexercisers with information about *immediate* psychological benefits of exercise and with positive exercise experiences, rather than with information about the *long-term* physiological benefits. As the running philosopher Sheehan (1992a) aptly captured,

> I will be fit because I must. I will find my sport because without it I will be incomplete. If I am fortunate I will find an area where movement of body joins movement of the mind and movement of the spirit—and discover that activity in which the subsequent repose coincides with heightened states of being, and affirmation of myself and all creation. (pp. 33–34)

Opportunities to experience enjoyment, enhanced mood states, and increased self-awareness when exercising may encourage more people to be habitual participants. As observed by Sheehan (1992a), "Once you find something that is playful and addictive and filled with satisfaction, your daily budget takes care of itself. New priorities are set. A new perspective, a new sense of proportion takes over" (p. 29).

In contrast to the physical benefits such as weight loss and increased bone density, which may take weeks and even months to effect—even though we are exercising every day—the mood changes associated with exercise seem to occur quickly after initiation of an exercise program. Illustrating the relatively rapid ability to experience the mood changes of exercise, beginning swimmers and joggers who completed the POMS before and after exercise sessions (at the beginning, middle, and end of a semester), reported mood benefits on each of the occasions (Berger et al., 1988; Berger et al., 1993). Similar mood changes have been reported by yoga participants at the beginning, middle, and end of a 14-week program (Berger & Owen, 1988, 1992a). These encouraging results would seem to have implications for becoming a habitual exerciser. Although the exact mechanisms are not known, many exercisers report feeling better after exercising. Regardless of whether the experience of feeling better is at a conscious or unconscious level, it would seem to be a powerful motivator to continue participating in physical activity.

The mood benefits of physical activity have implications for our social interactions, psychological well-being, and continued participation in exercise. It is important to identify influences on the complex relationship between physical activity and mood alteration. These include a focus on acute or short-term changes in mood, the chronic or long-term mood changes, the type of populations the participants represent, and the characteristics of the exercise activity itself.

Summary

Although physical activity can be associated with desirable as well as undesirable mood changes, many participants in physical activity report desirable changes in mood such as decreases in Tension, Depression, Anger, Fatigue, and Confusion and increases in Vigor. The mood changes associated with exercise often result in the iceberg profile.

Mood changes tend to be short-term or acute and tend to last two to four hours in members of the general population. Physical activity also has promise as a treatment modality for psychiatric patients. However, exercise therapy is not yet a widely accepted therapeutic approach by practicing clinicians. Based on diverse studies of psychiatric populations, hospitalized patients tend to report more stable or chronic changes associated with exercise therapy than do members of nonclinical populations. Patients have reported chronic decreases primarily in depression and anxiety.

Exercise enjoyment and type of physical activity and training parameters seem to influence the direction and extent of the mood changes. For example, there is some question as to whether the activity needs to be aerobic. Additional research is needed to investigate the relationship between various types of activities and mood alteration. A change in breathing patterns, rather than the aerobic component of exercise, may be conducive to mood alteration. In conclusion, exercise seems to be as effective as other mood-alteration approaches even though the underlying mechanisms are unclear at this time. Proposed underlying mechanisms include those that are physiological, psychological, social, and a combination of two or more categories.

In addition to being conducive to mood alteration, physical activity also provides participants with an opportunity for personal awareness and growth—learning about themselves as they experience diverse moods connected to the movement process. Increased self-awareness and awareness of one's reasons for exercising, inner mental life, and experiencing a wide spectrum of moods and emotions while exercising, seem to be recognized by exercisers as mental health benefits of physical activity. Despite mood and self-awareness benefits, a relatively small portion of the adult population is physically active. Perhaps the highly desirable mood benefits, opportunities for enjoyment, and opportunities for self-reflection might serve as inducements for greater participation in physical activity.

Can You Define These Terms?

acute mood change

anxiety

bipolar personality disorder

blood-brain barrier

chronic mood change

clinical population

closed environment

depression

endorphins

exercise duration

exercise enjoyment

exercise frequency

exercise intensity

iceberg profile of mental health

mechanisms for mood alteration

mode of exercise

mood decrements

nonclinical population

practice or training factors

ripple effect of mood

self-awareness

Can You Answer These Questions?

1. Do all exercisers experience mood benefits after physical activity? If not, what factors influence less desirable outcomes?

2. How can you facilitate the desirable mood changes associated with exercise?

3. Can you avoid mood detriments when you exercise? If so, how do you do this?

4.. How long after the cessation of exercise do positive changes in mood last within normal populations?

5. For what types of populations do acute and chronic mood changes tend to occur? Speculate on the possible reasons for these occurrences.

6. What roles might exercise play in the lives of psychiatric patients?

7. How effective is exercise in comparison to other approaches to mood alteration?

8. Why is the relationship between exercise and mood alteration described as an associative relationship rather than a causal one?

9. What are some of the hypothesized mechanisms possibly underlying the relationship between exercise and mood alteration?

10. Explain why a specific mechanism underlying the exercise-mood relationship makes the strongest appeal to you.

11. How would you design an exercise program to promote self-awareness?

12. Do you personally think that it is worthwhile to use exercise for mood alteration? Please provide a rationale for your response.

CHAPTER 7

STRESS: WHAT IS IT?

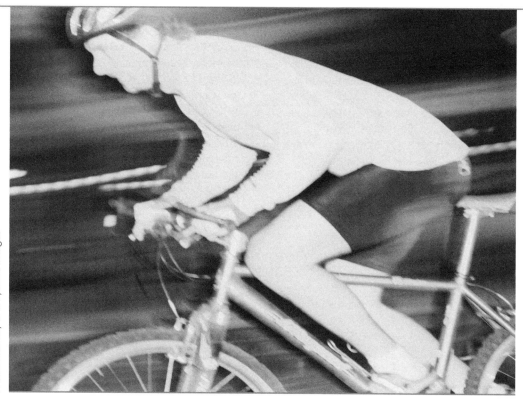

Photo courtesy of © Eyewire Images

After reading this chapter, you should be able to

- Define the terms *stress, stressor, distress,* and *eustress,*

- Discuss the relationship between life events and illness,

- Analyze the key models of stress:
  —Selye's general adaptation syndrome,
  —The identity disruption model,
  —The disparity model,
  —Conservation of resources model, and
  —Physiological toughness model,

- Distinguish between intra-individual and inter-individual differences in the stress response,

- Describe the interactional stress process, and

- Identify and analyze several coping and stress management techniques.

Introduction

Stress is integrally related to the quality of everyday life. We do not think about it, but both *too much* and *too little* stress can detract from our enjoyment of daily activities and overall quality of life. Sheehan (1992b), the running philosopher and cardiologist, has captured the dual-edged sword of stress: "Stress makes us fit, ready of mind, people of virtue and courage. Stress is what makes us complete. Through it we advance, grow, stay alive—but not without danger. Stress is a struggle that can also destroy" (p. 71).

Too much stress has undesirable health consequences, adds pressure to our daily lives, disrupts our thoughts, and even leads to panic. As a college student, you might be living in a high-stress environment. Stress could result from class assignments, financial needs, social interactions, deadlines, outside jobs, parental expectations, and other factors. These situations influence your ability to concentrate on studies, increase your worries, and decrease your resistance to colds, flus, and more serious diseases.

For exercise and sport psychologists, coaches, athletic trainers, physical therapists, and other types of movement specialists, it is important to realize that not all stress is "bad" or undesirable. Individuals who habitually encounter stress from having "too much to do" often are unaware that having "too little to do" also is stressful. In fact, we need a certain level of stress to add zest to our lives, to meet challenges, and to make us feel as if we are using our capabilities fully. Too few responsibilities, not enough challenges, and inadequate social interactions are boring situations that can produce stress. Each of us needs to maintain an optimal level of stress in our life to function at a high level. Optimal levels of stress provide us with many benefits. They provide us with energy and excitement, and help us to enjoy our daily activities, and to live life to the fullest.

The pervasiveness of stress in modern society and the seriousness of its diverse health effects were illustrated by a cover story in *Time Magazine* that appeared

Table 7.1

Stress: Definitions, Descriptions, and Theories

- Stress is a neutral term that denotes neither desirable nor undesirable states of being
- Stress is a broad concept adapted from the fields of physics and engineering where stress is something that produces strain
- "Stress is the spice of life" (Selye, 1975, p. 83)
- *Distress* refers to the negative aspects of stress; stress and distress are often employed as though they are synonymous
- *Eustress* is a thrilling, highly desirable form of stress that often is associated with risk taking
- Stress results in the fight-or-flight response and mobilizes the body for muscular activity in response to a perceived threat
- Stress is an undifferentiated state of heightened arousal and hormonal activity that results in the general adaptation syndrome (GAS; Selye, 1956)
- Stress is "a multihued blanket of complex design and fabric, woven from all the interrelated and variegated colored threads that enter into mind-body relationships" (Rosch, 1986, pp. x–xi)
- Stress "refers to a relationship with the environment that the person appraises as significant for his or her well-being and in which the demands tax or exceed available coping resources" (Lazarus & Folkman, 1986, p. 6)
- Stress results from situations and forces that challenge and test a person's capabilities
- Stress is a process, a series of events and reactions that highlights the unity of mind and body
- The identity disruption model's two-step stress-illness process is "(a) life events create alterations in identity and (b) identity disruption has negative effects on health" (Brown & McGill, 1989, p. 1103)
- The disparity model of stress suggests that stress is a process that results from a "call to action" and a subsequent response that one's personal capabilities or resources are insufficient (Lazarus, DeLongis, Folkman, & Gruen, 1985)
- According to the conservation of resources model, stress is a reaction to the environment in which there is a loss or potential loss of resources (Hobfoll, 1989)
- "Toughened" individuals respond to stressors effectively and view stressful situations as challenges rather than as threats (Dienstbier, 1989, 1991)

more than 20 years ago in 1983 (Wallis, Galvin, & Thompson, 1983). Today stress continues to be a major health hazard. In a recent examination of stress, culture, and community, Hobfoll (1998), a noted psychologist, observed

> No concept in the modern psychological, sociological, or psychiatric literature is more extensively studied than stress. The *sheer amount of scientific literature is so extensive that it is no longer possible to conduct a comprehensive review.* But the amount of research is only one facet of the attention given to stress. I submit that *stress is also the social-psychological concept of greatest interest to Western* society [italics added]. (p. 1)

With the recognition that no single chapter in an exercise psychology text can present a comprehensive view of the stress literature, we focus this chapter on important concepts and issues in the stress literature that are of particular interest to you as a movement specialist and as an exercise and sport psychologist. To help you understand the stress process and the role of exercise in reducing stress, this chapter focuses on the concept of stress, various components in the stress process, and important models of stress. This chapter also examines key coping strategies and identifies effective stress management techniques. In the next chapter, you will examine the role of exercise in the stress management process.

Important Concepts

Despite the immediacy and reality of stress symptoms, the concept of stress is vague and overly inclusive. The openness of stress to a myriad of definitions gives it much of its intuitive appeal but also makes stress exceedingly difficult to define. To preview the multiple definitions of stress employed throughout in this chapter, see Table 7.1.

Stress and *Distress:* Is There a Difference?

In actuality, *stress* is a neutral term that denotes neither desirable nor undesirable states of being. Some stress actually is desirable. Stress adds excitement, stimulation, and color to our lives. Our lives would be drab without some stress. On the other hand, too much stress damages our bodies. Selye (1975) aptly observed, "Stress is the spice of life" (p. 83). Similar to the spices in our food, too little or too much is undesirable, but the "right" amount is most enjoyable. As illustrated by Figure 7.1, too little as well as too much stress detracts from our performance of daily tasks as well as from our psychological well-being. In contrast, optimal levels of stress contribute to our psychological well-being.

Of course, we differ from one another in the optimal levels of stress that are conducive to our own personal psychological well-being. See Figure 7.2 for the

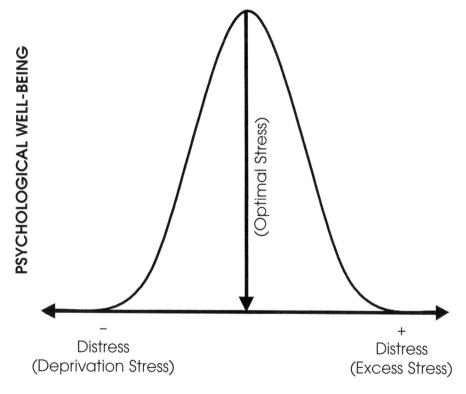

Figure 7.1. Stress continuum.

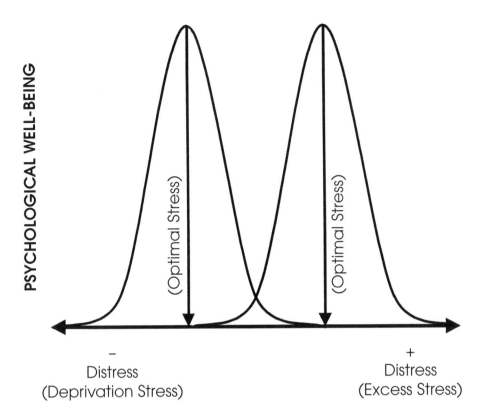

Figure 7.2. Individual differences in stress.

need to consider individual differences in optimal stress levels. The preferred stress levels of the two individuals represented in Figure 7.2 differ considerably with one another. Recognizing our optimal levels of stress and then regulating the stress in our daily lives and controlling our stress responses improve our quality of life.

After working in the area of stress for many years, Selye (1975) at the age of 68 poetically captured the important role of stress in our lives. The following quotation emphasizes the importance of regulating our daily stress levels as needed to maintain optimal functioning:

> It seems to me that man's ultimate aim in life is to express himself as fully as possible, according to his own lights, and to achieve a sense of security. To accomplish this, you must first find your *optimal stress level* [italics added], and then use your adaptation energy at a rate and in a direction adjusted to your innate qualifications and preferences. (p. 110)

Emphasizing the neutrality of stress, the word *distress* refers to the negative aspects of stress. In common usage, however, *distress* is shortened to the more common term, *stress*. Because stress and distress often are synonymous, these terms will be used interchangeably throughout this book. Stress "refers to a relationship with the environment that the person appraises as significant for his or her well-being and in which the demands tax or exceed available coping resources" (Lazarus & Folkman, 1986, p. 63). Lazarus (1999) still conceptualizes stress as resulting from personal appraisal.

Stress is *a process, a series of events and reactions, that highlights the unity of mind and body*. Stress begins as a cognitive or mental response to a stressor and results in physiological changes that are distributed throughout the entire body. For example, some of the immediate changes that reflect short-term or acute stress responses include

- A rapid heart rate;
- A rapid, shallow, thoracic breathing pattern;
- Increased blood flow to the muscles;
- Increased perspiration; and
- Inhibition of the digestive system.

Changes in the functioning of the immune system take more time. Many of these physical manifestations of psychological stress also result from exercise. In fact, physical exercise is a stressor.

Acute and Chronic Stress

Acute or short-term stress refers to time-limited stress that can occur when taking final exams, driving a car in a blinding snowstorm, and competing in a tennis tournament. *Chronic* stress is prolonged stress that extends for an indeterminate time period. Chronic stress "arises from harmful or threatening, but stable

Table 7.2
Stress: Symptoms and Illnesses

Symptoms	Illnesses
Anger	Cancer
Anxiety	Chronic fatigue syndrome
Chronic pain	
Forgetfulness	Clinical anxiety
High blood pressure	Clinical depression
Irritability	Colitis
Muscle tension	Epstein-Barr virus
Nervousness	Heart disease
Poor concentration	Phobias
Sleeplessness	Sleep disorders
Tiredness	Ulcers
	Upper respiratory infections

conditions of life, and from the stressful roles people continually fulfill at work and in the family" (Lazarus, 1999, p. 144). Both chronic and acute stress is associated with the same unpleasant symptoms, but chronic stress may influence the onset and development of serious physical and psychological illness. See Table 7.2 for some of the common symptoms and illnesses that may be related to stress.

Eustress, An Unusual, Exciting, Thrilling Form of Stress

The term *eustress* is derived from the Greek prefix *eu*, which means "good," and is a highly desirable, exciting form of stress. Eustress describes the stress that occasionally is associated with *competitive exercise activities* like tennis and squash when game outcome is uncertain. Activities *high in physical risk* such as rock climbing, scuba diving, bungee jumping, downhill skiing, whitewater rafting, and wilderness challenges also are potential sources of eustress. Some people find these activities exhilarating and eustress-producing; other people find them activities to be avoided at all costs due to fear and/or lack of enjoyment.

The term *eustress* that denotes this positive form of stress (Selye, 1975) further supports the view of *stress* as a neutral term. *Dis*tress is the negative, destructive form that includes both too little and too much stress. The positive excitement and challenges of eustress are in the eye of the beholder and vary from one person to

another. What is exciting and fun for one person, such as rock climbing, may frighten another person and be something to avoid. Despite individual differences, many people experience eustress in a variety of activities. Additional examples of activities in which people may report feelings of eustress include carnival rides, sexual activity, and simply testing how much we can accomplish in a day. Regardless of an individual's preferred level of excitement, risk, and challenge, a personally optimal level of eustress is thrilling and exhilarating. Eustress adds zest and a sense of contrast to our sometimes mundane lives.

Some eustress is desirable, but too much can have negative effects. The determining factors as to whether any stress is pleasant or unpleasant are the *intensity* and *frequency* of the demand upon an individual's adaptive capacities. Although little research has been conducted in regard to eustress, it remains an appealing concept. Research is needed to identify various activities that promote eustress and to explore its possible health-promoting benefits.

Stress and Stressors

As indicated in the preceding analysis of eustress, stress is a complex process. It occurs within an individual in response to events (stressors) that demand change and/or a response. *Stressors* are stimuli. These stimuli can be either desirable or undesirable events and can be either acute (time-limited) events or chronic (long-lasting) events. In addition, stressors can be external, objective situations that include major life events, more minor hassles, and uplifts. Internal stressors include thoughts, interpretations of life events and hassles, and imaginings. Regardless of whether the stressors are desirable or undesirable, acute or chronic, external or internal, they require energy for adaptation by the individual. As described in the next section, even positive life events can be debilitating—if too many occur within a short period.

Life Events

Life events are one type of stressor and include major life occurrences such as being fired, starting a new job, flunking out of school, getting cut from a sports team, taking final exams, receiving unanticipated money in the mail from your parents, and getting married. Undesirable life events are obvious stressors that require readjustment to the situation. However, a long-accepted view of stressors is that they can be either desirable (e.g., vacation, new job) or undesirable (e.g., failing a course, being fired). Both desirable and undesirable life events require adaptation by the individual. Such events can excite, irritate, endanger, and confuse. Refer to Table 7.3 for examples of common life events for college students and for adults. As indicated by the Life-Change Units (LCUs) listed for each life event, the events are weighted according to the severity of their stressfulness, which has been averaged across a large and diverse sample of people. For details, see R. H. Rahe, "Life Change, Stress Responsivity, and Captivity Research." In general, the higher the LCU, the more disrupting the life event is and the more readjustment it requires (Seaward, 1997a). Getting married has 76 LCUs and generally is more stressful than taking a vacation, which has 33 LCUs and thus a lower stress potential. Of course, there are always individual exceptions when the LCUs are based on group averages.

Refer again to Table 7.3, and take a moment to assess your own life events within the past 12 months. This will provide you with an objective measure of your current stress level. First, determine the life events that you have experienced within the past year. Then, add the total life-change units. The original Social Readjustment Rating Scale for adults by Holmes and Rahe (1967) had a listing of 43 events. A high score on this scale could result from having several highly rated events or from numerous events that require only moderate adjustment efforts. Life-event inventories represent a stimulus approach to stress. A stressor occurs as a stimulus, then you respond to it with elevated stress.

On the Social Readjustment Rating Scale, an LCU score below 150 is considered within an average range for stress. A score between 150 and 200 is elevated, and when you reach a score between 200 and 299, there is a moderate possibility of future illness. A score above 300 indicates a high possibility of illness within the next 6 to 12 months. It is important to note that a high LCU score does not predict illness for *all* people. However, a high score does seem to indicate a higher likelihood that you will have a major illness due to stress in the next year than if your score is low (Lazarus, 1999; Rahe, 1990). Some individuals, by nature of their genetic endowment, experiences, or personality, appear to be immune to the deleterious effects of stress.

Although Holmes and Rahe (1967) considered change to be stressful regardless of whether the effects were desirable or undesirable, opinions in the research community differ. It seems that negative events tend to

Table 7.3
The Abbreviated Social Readjustment Rating Scale

Instructions: Place an **X** beside each event that you have experienced in the past 12 months.

Life Events for College Students [a]	LCU [b]	Life Events for Adult Population [c]	LCU [b]
___ Death of a spouse	87	___ Death of a spouse	100
___ Marriage	77	___ Divorce	73
___ Divorce	76	___ Marital separation	65
___ Pregnant or fathered a pregnancy	68	___ Personal injury/illness	53
___ Sexual difficulties	58	___ Fired from job	47
___ Major change in recreation patterns	37	___ Pregnancy	40
___ A trip or vacation	33	___ Sexual difficulties	39
___ Change in eating habits	30	___ Gain a family member	39
___ Change in number of family gettogethers	26	___ Outstanding personal achievement	28
		___ Change in recreation	19
		___ Vacation	13
		___ Christmas	12

[a] Items are from *College Schedule of Recent Experiences*, by G. E. Anderson, 1972, M.A. thesis, North Dakota State University (as cited in McGuigan, 1992).
[b] Life change units
[c] Items are from "The Social Readjustment Rating Scale," by T. H. Holmes and R. H. Rahe, 1967, *Journal of Psychosomatic Research, 11*, pp. 213–218.

Table 7.4
Hassles and Uplifts: Commonly Reported Items

Hassles	% [a]	Uplifts	% [a]
Concerns about weight	52.4	Relating well with your spouse/lover	76.3
Health of a family member	48.1	Relating well with your friends	74.4
Rising prices of common goods	43.7	Completing a task	73.3
Home maintenance	42.8	Feeling healthy	72.7
Too many things to do	38.6	Getting enough sleep	69.7
Misplacing or losing things	38.1	Eating out	68.4
Yard work or outside home maintenance	38.1	Meeting responsibilities	68.1
Property, investment, or taxes	37.6	Visiting, phoning, or writing someone	67.7
Crime	37.1	Spending time with your family	66.7
Physical appearance	35.9	Home (inside) pleasing to you	65.5

[a] Figures represent the mean percentage of people checking the item each month averaged over 9 monthly administrations.
Note: From "Comparisons of Two Modes of Stress Measurement: Daily Hassles and Uplifts Versus Major Life Events," by A. D. Kanner, J. C. Coyne, C. Schaefer, and R. S. Lazarus, 1981, *Journal of Behavioral Medicine, 4,* pp. 1–39. Copyright 1981 by Plenum Publishers. Adapted with permission.

be *more highly* related to psychological and physical dysfunction than do positive ones (e.g., Barrett & Campos, 1991; Lazarus, 1999). In conclusion, both the positive and negative events in our lives require energy and personal adjustment. More substantial relationships between life events and illness are found if we rate the emotional importance of the life events to ourselves. For example, losing a job might indicate financial disaster for most people, but it may be a desirable situation for us if we have too many job possibilities. Obviously, there are many gradations of meaning and personal reactions to life events. Determining your own stress level and the stress levels of your exercise clients is a complex and difficult, but important task.

Daily Hassles and Uplifts

Hassles and uplifts are another type of stressor and include everyday events. Hassles are events such as getting a flat tire, time pressure, misplacing car keys, and fights with family and friends. Uplifts include having a rewarding exercise session, earning an A on an exam, and hearing from an old friend. In contrast to major life events, hassles and uplifts are minor stressors. They are less life-changing than life events, but do occur repeatedly and on a daily basis. Thus, they are important stressors. Hassles and uplifts generally are highly related to your appraisal of situations as influencing your goals and abilities to cope.

Hassles range from irritants, frequent annoyances, and low-intensity stressors to major difficulties, problems, and pressures. For a detailed examination of these hassles, see *Comparisons of Two Modes of Stress Measurement: Daily Hassles and Uplifts Versus Major Life Events* by Kanner, Coyne, Schaefer, and Lazarus. Basically, hassles are the irritating demands that characterize our *everyday* lives. Common hassles include being stopped in traffic, losing things, standing in a long line to register for courses, not getting enough sleep, a surprise quiz, and low grades on an exam. Hassles such as those listed in Table 7.4 often are based on unmet expectations that trigger frustration or an anger response. These microstressors are cumulative and can be potent sources of stress—especially in the relative absence of compensatory uplifts. Hassle scales usually measure both the frequency and intensity of occurrence (e.g., Rowlinson & Felner, 1988).

Uplifts are the opposite of hassles. They are pleasant surprises, treats, and events that make people feel good. Uplifts can be sources of joy, peace, and satisfaction. Typical uplifts include personal compliments, a great exercise session, hugging or kissing, a day off from classes, and a telephone call from a friend. Hopefully, uplifts occur more often throughout your day than do hassles. Table 7.4 includes some of the most frequent hassles and uplifts reported by a sample of 100 middle-aged adults. For a personal analysis of hassles and the importance of measuring the strength of their impact, assess the number of hassles and uplifts that you recently have experienced as outlined in Case Study 7.1.

Scores on the Hassles Scale (Kanner et al., 1981) have predicted present and future psychological symptoms and somatic illness—sometimes more strongly than life events (e.g., DeLongis, Coyne, Dakof, Fortman, & Lazarus, 1982; Kanner et al., 1981; Langens & Stucke, 2005; Rowlinson & Felner, 1988). In contrast to hassles, the relationship between uplifts and stress is not as clear. Apparently, an absence of hassles is more important for psychological well-being than are pleasant events—at least for men. Additional research is needed in this area to further explain the interrelationships between hassles, uplifts, life events, and health for men and women.

At the present time, both hassles and undesirable life events seem to contribute independently to distress levels, impaired emotional well-being, overall functioning, and physical health (Langens & Stucke, 2005; Rowlinson & Felner, 1988). Many life events such as the death of a parent are difficult, if not impossible to control.

Therefore, lowering the number of daily hassles holds considerably greater potential for reducing stress and enhancing the quality of life than does a focus on reducing life events. It also seems that *negative* stressors and hassles affect health more strongly than do positive life events and uplifts. Thus, avoiding vexing situations when possible or interpreting them more positively is conducive to enhanced levels of health—both on psychological and physiological bases.

Moderators of the Stress, Emotional Well-Being, and Illness Relationships

Although hassles and life-events have undesirable influences on psychological well-being and on illness, some individuals may be more vulnerable to stress than others (Langens & Stucke, 2005; von Känel, Mills, Fainman, & Dimsdale, 2001). Identifying possible psychological characteristics and coping behaviors such as exercise is important to help understand why some individuals cope well with stress, and others experience significant impairment.

CASE STUDY 7.1 — *Comparing Daily Hassles and Uplifts*

Take a moment to assess the number of hassles and uplifts you personally have experienced recently. See Table 7.4 for a listing of the most commonly reported microstressors of hassles and compensatory uplifts.

Self-Assessment

Rate how strongly you experienced each hassle and uplift during the past week on a five-point scale. The rating scale is as follows:

1 (not at all experienced as a source of stress),
2 (slightly experienced as a source of stress),
3 (moderately experienced),
4 (strongly experienced), and
5 (very strongly experienced).

Scoring Instructions

Indicate your rating (1 to 5) for each of the 10 hassles listed in the table, and then for each of the 10 uplifts listed. Add your ratings to form separate composite scores for hassles and for uplifts that you experienced in the past week.

Interpretation of Scores

To interpret your scores, examine how your assessment of recent hassles compares to your appraisal of weekly uplifts. If your hassle score is higher than your uplift score, analyze how you might change the relationship of the two. Common hassles for college students tend to fall into four primary categories: (1) assorted annoyances, such as money troubles, and health problems, such as colds; (2) changes in living conditions, such as decreased leisure time and inadequate sleep; (3) study stress; and (4) interpersonal stresss, such as arguments with family or friends (Langens, 2002). These need particular attention for remediation.

Absolute hassle and uplift scores also are important. Since a rating of 3 indicates that a hassle or uplift is of moderate importance, hassle and uplift scores between 20 and 40 are the norm for most people. If your scores are lower than 20 for uplifts, and higher than 40 for hassles, your stress levels need your attention. Employing some of the stress management techniques and coping strategies listed later in the chapter would be of potential benefit to your health and psychological well-being.

Evidence from a broad base of studies indicates that people who have the following personality and psychological characteristics tend to experience less stress and stress-related illnesses:

- High dispositional optimism (e.g., Matthews, Räikkönen, Sutton-Tyrrell, & Kuller, 2004; Segerstrom, Taylor, Kemeny, & Fahey, 1998),
- High internal locus of control (e.g., Hahn, 2000), and
- Low in trait anxiety and depression (e.g., Jones, Bromberger, Sutton-Tyrell, & Matthews, 2003; van Eck, Nicolson, & Berkhof, 1998; von Känel, Mills, Fainman, & Dimsdale, 2001),
- Do not to intensely experience their emotions (e.g., Ciarrochi, Deane, & Anderson, 2002), and
- Do not inhibit their emotional and motivational impulses (e.g., Langens & Stucke, 2005).

In contrast, people who are less optimistic, have external locus of control, high levels of trait anxiety, intensely experience their emotions and inhibit their emotional and motivational impulses are more affected by daily hassles and life events. For example, people who are highly optimistic are not as likely to experience negative mood states and immune changes as a result of daily hassles than those who are lower in optimism (Segerstrom et al., 1998). In addition, people who are high in emotional and motivational inhibition reported higher negative mood states and even more numerous daily hassles than people who are low in inhibition (Langens & Stucke, 2005).

These results indicate that stressful life events and daily hassles do not affect all people equally. Clearly there are psychological characteristics that moderate the relationship between stress, psychological well-being, and physical illness (Matthews, 2005; Suls & Bunde, 2005). Stress management techniques such as exercise, yoga, and meditation would seem to be particularly helpful to people who are strong reactors to life events and daily hassles.

Measuring Stress: Key Considerations

There are numerous ways to measure stress as illustrated in Table 7.3 through Table 7.5. As summarized in Table 7.5, multiple aspects of the stress process and response stress can be measured. The categories or broad types of stress measures in Table 7.5 illustrate the breadth of the stress response. Stress measures include biochemical markers, measurement of cardiovascular responses, measurement of immune responses, electromyographic recording devices, checklists of stressful life events, measures of affective responses, interview measurement of stressful life events, and hassle and uplift inventories (see an edited book enti-

Table 7.5
Common Stress Measures and Indices

Type of Measure	Specific Indices
Biochemical	• Sympathetic nervous system-adrenal-medullary arousal: adrenaline, nor-adrenaline • Pituitary-adrenal-cortical arousal: cortisol • Other: cholesterol, endorphins, immune system functioning, and uric acid
Physiological	• Blood pressure • Electromyographic (EMG) measures • Galvanic skin response • Heart rate
Psychological	• Anger • Anxiety • Depression • Impatience • Irritability • Lack of concentration • Intolerance • Mood • Neuroticism • Perceived control
Behavioral	• Facial expressions • Rate of speech • Restlessness • Sleep disturbances • Trembling • Task performance: memory, attention, and learning • Other specific behaviors: nail biting, eating problems
Self-Report	• Hassles and uplifts • Life events • Marital satisfaction • Mood inventories • Psychological questionnaires including anger, anxiety, and depression
Cognitive	• Attitudes • Autonomic nervous system activity • Beliefs • Forgetfulness • Perceived control

tled *Measuring Stress* [Cohen, Kessler, & Gordon, 1995] for a more detailed examination of stress measurement issues). As emphasized in the next chapter on exercise and stress management, it is difficult to decide which measures to use because of individualized reactions to stress.

The "best" stress measures in any particular situation depend on (a) the specific factors under investigation, (b) the orientation and interests of the stress therapist or researcher, and (c) the availability and limitations of the measure or equipment. The following sections familiarize you with specific considerations for choosing stress measures and in analyzing your own personal stress levels.

Inter-Individual Differences

As previously indicated, individuals differ from one another in their appraisal (a) of the personal importance of the stressor demands and (b) of their personal resources for responding. Both the importance of a stressor and individual resources influence our overall stress responses. These inter-individualized tendencies to exhibit stress also include a variety of responses. Some of these responses include the contraction of skeletal muscles, distractibility, irritability, and increases in blood pressure. These interindividual stress responses compound the difficulties of accurately measuring stress levels.

No single general activation pattern is common to all individuals (Barrett & Campos, 1991; Lazarus, 1999). Each individual's stress profile across many modalities is person specific. This is especially true when researchers examine both physiological modalities and psychological characteristics in a single study. One person may have a rapid heart rate, headaches, and forgetfulness when stressed. Another person in the same situation may be nauseated, fatigued, impatient, and short-tempered. Due to these interindividual differences, it is important to obtain pre-stressor measures of several different stress modalities and to observe baseline changes after a particular stressor for that individual.

Intra-Individual Differences

Further complicating the study and measurement of stress is the fact that the same individual can respond to various types of stressors with different symptoms. Intra-individual variations in stress responses emphasize that the stress profile of an individual may differ from one situation to another (Barrett & Campos, 1991). For example, the profile of a rapid heart rate and sweaty palms is one person's response to dental treatment. Forgetfulness and an upset stomach may be the same person's profile in response to taking an exam or to speaking in public (Barrett & Campos, 1991).

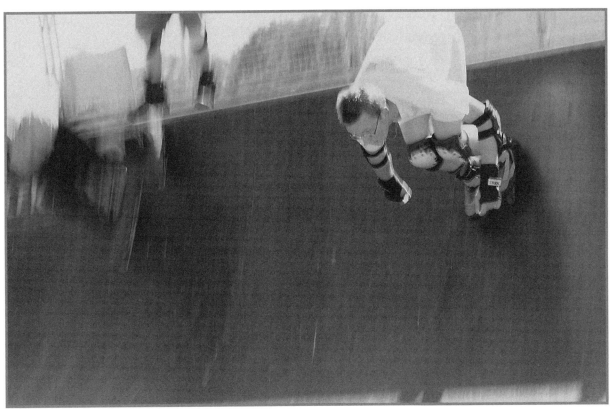

The Time Course of the Stress Response: Before, During, and Following a Stressor

Adding even more complexity to the measurement of stress, circulating stress hormones such as catecholamines and corticoids have a time course of production and excretion. Stress hormones can be secreted in anticipation of a stressor, during a stressful situation, and following a stressful event when reflecting on it afterward. Such variability in inter- and intra-individual stress responses and the time courses make it very difficult not only to measure stress responses, but also to conduct and interpret studies of stress.

Psychological Characteristics Mediating the Stress Response

As previously noted, psychological factors also influence an individual's vulnerability to stress. Some of these include self-efficacy, self-esteem, feelings of competency and control, self-confidence, social support, hardiness, and anticipation of an event to determine how a person appraises his or her personal resources (Lazarus, 1999). In addition, the focus of thought patterns—whether a person is employing task-oriented or self-focused coping responses—influences the likelihood of responding to a particular stressor successfully. The appropriate or effective thought pattern changes from one stressor to another and from one stage of the stress process to another (Lazarus, 1999). *Task-oriented* thoughts such as "I am going to study for my physiology exam for at least two hours" or "I will exercise today" can be more productive or successful ways to handle a stressor than can *self-preoccupying* thoughts such as "I am going to fail this course and be expelled from college" or "I hate exercise, and thus, I am not going to exercise, I will get fat, and no one will like me." With task-oriented thinking, individuals provide themselves with a plan of action that results in behavior directly addressing a specific life event, and this eventually reduces ongoing stress levels.

Paper-and-Pencil Stress Inventories

Life-event and hassle inventories are common paper-and-pencil measures of stress. The original life-event inventory was the Social Readjustment Rating Questionnaire (SRRQ), which later became the Social Readjustment Rating Scale (SRRS). Refer again to Table 7.3 for abbreviated versions of the adult and student forms of the SRRS. The SRRS measures a person's stress level. Scores on the SRRS have been linked to future illness. Measuring stress as the number of life events is appealing because of its apparent

---

Table 7.6
Stress Overload Inventory
(Girdano, Everly, & Dusek, 1997)

Instructions:
Choose the most appropriate answer for each of the following statements, and write the number of your response to the left of the question. Choose your response from the following:

(1)=almost never; **(2)**=seldom; **(3)**=often; and **(4)**=almost always.

How often do you...

___ 1. find yourself with insufficient time to do things you really enjoy?

___ 2. wish you had more support/assistance?

___ 3. lack sufficient time to complete your work most effectively?

___ 4. have difficulty falling asleep because you have too much on your mind?

___ 5. feel people simply expect too much from you?

___ 6. feel overwhelmed?

___ 7. find yourself becoming forgetful or indecisive because you have too much on your mind?

___ 8. consider yourself to be in a high-pressure situation?

___ 9. feel you have too much responsibility for one person?

___ 10. feel exhausted at the end of the day?

---

objectivity and simplicity. To increase accuracy of measurement, some life-event inventories have been modified to include the individual's report as to:

- Whether the event was desirable or undesirable, and
- The importance or impact of the stressor.

Rating event desirability and importance will result in separate positive and negative change scores. Marriage, for example, may be either a positive or a negative event depending on the perception of the respondent. In addition, the changes and meanings attached to getting married may be far more stressful for one individual than for another. When completing the Life Experiences Survey (LES), respondents rank

Table 7.7
Stress Deprivation Inventory
(Girdano, Everly, & Dusek, 1997)

Instructions:

Choose the most appropriate answer for each of the following statements, and write the number of your response to the left of the question. Choose your response from the following:

(1)=almost never; (2)=seldom; (3)=often; and (4)=almost always.

How often do you. . .

____ 1. feel that your work is not stimulating enough?

____ 2. lose interest in your daily activities?

____ 3. find yourself becoming restless during your daily routine?

____ 4. feel "insulted" by the simplicity of your work?

____ 5. wish your life were more exciting?

____ 6. find yourself becoming anxious from a lack of stimulation?

____ 7. find yourself becoming bored?

____ 8. feel that your usual activities are not challenging enough?

____ 9. find yourself daydreaming during work?

____ 10. feel lonely?

each life event on a scale of minus 3 (extremely negative) to plus 3 (extremely positive) to indicate the impact of the particular event on their life at the time of occurrence (Sarason et al., 1978). Adjustment is defined as a combination of the *intensity* of one's reactions and the amount of *time* necessary for coping with the event (Rhodewalt & Zone, 1989). Some researchers report that the frequency of life events alone is a better predictor of stress than are the personal impact scores (Rowlinson & Felner, 1988).

In addition to life-event, hassle, and uplift measures, numerous other paper-and-pencil inventories measure various aspects of the stress experience. In *Controlling Stress and Tension*, Girdano, Everley, and Dusek (1997) include more than 10 different stress inventories. Each inventory focuses on different stress dimensions such as overload, deprivation, adaptation, frustration, personal habits, self-perception, behavior patterns, personality, need for control, and occupa-

CASE STUDY 7.2

Measuring Your Own Stress Overload and Stress Deprivation

Complete the stress overload and stress deprivation inventories in Tables 7.6 and 7.7. Compute your total score for each inventory following the instructions provided in the tables. The higher your score, the greater your stress overload and your stress deprivation. Scores between 25 and 40 on each of the inventories are considered high (Girdano et al., 1997).

Overload

Items on the Stress Overload Inventory emphasize that stress often results from the perception that you have too much to do. A high overload score indicates that you perceive that you have too many responsibilities and that you should reduce your obligations in order to feel less stressed. If you are overloaded, trying to fit an exercise session into an already overwhelming day may be even more of an overload for you. Thus, for exercise to be a stress-reducing activity as described in the next chapter, you may need to reduce your daily list of "things to do."

Deprivation

In contrast, a high score on the Stress Deprivation Inventory indicates that your life is not optimally challenging or stimulating. The Stress Deprivation Inventory emphasizes that having too few challenges is stressful. If you score high on stress deprivation, you need to include more challenging and meaningful activities in your life. One of these challenges could be adding to or enhancing your own exercise program, especially by adding an exciting type of activity.

Optimal stress

Reflect on your optimal levels of stress overload and deprivation. How do they compare to your present levels? This awareness is an important step in maintaining your optimal levels of stress. As reflected in Figures 7.1 and 7.2, optimal stress levels are highly related to psychological well-being.

tional stress. Two of three paper-and-pencil inventories are the Stress Overload and Stress Deprivation inventories in Tables 7.6 and 7.7. Take a moment to analyze your current stress levels as suggested in Case Study 7.2.

Despite the difficulties in measuring stress, the measures are useful in increasing personal awareness of stress. Stress inventories provide important external validation of our often-unrecognized responses to general life events and day-to-day hassles and uplifts. High scores are a direct indication that changes may be needed. Each of us needs to actively manage our daily stress levels to make certain that they fluctuate as closely as possible around our optimal level to enhance our quality of life.

Models of Stress

This section on models of stress is helpful in explaining some of the components in the stress process. Each model has strong and weak points. Familiarity with some of the more common models provides you with an understanding of the complexities within the stress process and the multiple roles that exercise can play in interrupting the stress process.

General Adaptation Syndrome: A Reactive Model

Selye, considered the "father of stress," introduced the engineering term *stress* to the allied health fields in 1926 (Selye, 1975). Selye (1956) used the term *stress* to describe an undifferentiated state of heightened arousal and hormonal activity. Exercise can be stressful, especially if it is high intensity, for a long duration, or an important competitive event. As discussed in the following chapter, exercise also can serve as a stress reduction technique.

Selye (1975) characterized the state of physiological readiness to protect the body from environmental challenge as the general adaptation syndrome (GAS). The GAS is based on a three-part, sequential response to either psychological or physiological stressors: the alarm stage, the resistance stage, and the exhaustion stage. See Table 7.8 for a description of the characteristics of each stage.

According to the GAS, stress is a direct, nonspecific reaction of the body to any demanding environmental stimuli (Selye, 1975). Thus, the GAS is considered a *reactive model* of stress. This means that stress is a direct reaction to specific stimuli. Selye (1975)

Table 7.8
General Adaptation Syndrome (GAS); Selye, 1975

Stage	Name	Description
Stage 1	Alarm Reaction	Resistance is decreased
		Acute or immediate response to a stressor
		Death occurs if the stressor is sufficiently strong (e.g., severe burns and extreme temperatures)
Stage 2	Resistance stage	Intermediate stage
		Stress symptoms of Stage 1 nearly disappear
		If adaptation is compatible with the stress, resistance rises above normal
Stage 3	Exhaustion stage	Chronic, or accumulative effects of stress
		Ability to adapt to stressors is finite
		With continued exposure to the same stressor, the body eventually becomes exhausted.
		"The signs of the alarm reaction reappear, but now they are irreversible, and the individual dies" (Selye, 1975, p. 27)
		Emphasizes the seriousness of chronic stress

maintained that similar "undifferentiated" or "nonspecific" neuroendocrinological changes are associated with all stressors. In this model, stress results from increased cortical steroid output. Although Selye's (1975) claim of nonspecificity has been modified, his early research and writings spawned a huge, ongoing area of research (Lazarus, 1999).

The Fight-or-Flight Response

The great Harvard physiologist Walter B. Cannon noted in the late 1920s that stress greatly disrupts homeostasis in many systems of the body. Cannon investigated one particular aspect of the stress response, the neuroendocrine process, and coined the phrase "fight or flight" (Seaward, 1997b). The fight-or-flight response readies the body for muscular activity in response to a perceived threat. Modern threats include stimuli such as being in a car accident and facing a surprise quiz in class. In response to such threats, the pituitary gland at the base of the brain activates the adrenal glands to secrete adrenaline, cortisol, and other hormones. These hormones cause increased muscle tension, heart rate, and blood pressure and halt the digestive process.

Prolonged, or chronic, stress greatly detracts from our physical and psychological well-being. When stress is constant, or chronic, the body adapts to it and may channel the strain into one or more organ systems, and these bodily adaptations differ from one individual to another. As a result, each of us responds to stress in our own unique, intra-individual pattern. We may experience increased muscle tension and rapid heart rate. We also may have elevated blood pressure and an inability to concentrate. These individual patterns are identified as *stress profiles*.

Identity Disruption Model

The identity disruption model of stress explains why specific positive and negative events are not equally stressful to *all* individuals. According to this model, vulnerability to life stress is based on a variety of psychological characteristics, especially on dependency, achievement needs, and self-esteem (Wallis et al., 1983). The identity disruption model, as the name implies, suggests that events that are most stressful are those that are related to an individual's self-identity. Self-identity includes family, student/professional, sport, or personal aspects of ourselves.

The identity disruption model's two-step stress-illness process is "(a) life events create alterations in identity and (b) identity disruption has negative effects on health" (Brown & McGill, 1989, p. 1103). According to this model of stress, the more an event or stressor changes the way we think about ourselves, the more likely we will develop a stress-related illness (Brown & McGill, 1989).

A fascinating aspect of the model is that positive life events actually have detrimental effects on self-reports of physical health for individuals who have negative views of themselves (Brown & McGill, 1989). In other words, positive events such as scoring the winning shot in a basketball game can be very stressful to exercisers who see themselves as the least skilled members of a basketball team. Depending on whether the self-view is positive or negative, specific life events have differential stress-evoking effects, according to the identity disruption model. In a study of college students, Brown and McGill reported that the number of visits to a health center increased for students who had low self-esteem, and decreased for those with high self-esteem, as the number of positive life events increased. The identity disruption model supports the interactional view of stress. Hassles and life events are stressors only if an individual appraises them as such, and the appraisal depends on the person's feelings of dependency, self-esteem, and need for achievement.

Disparity or Relational Model

The disparity model of stress also emphasizes the role of *personal perception* in the stress process. However, this model includes many more components than personal perception (see Figures 7.3 and 7.4 for the many components). In the *disparity model*, a gap between the demands of a situation and the individual's personal capacities results in stress (Lazarus, 1999; Trumbull & Appley, 1986). The disparity model also is considered to be a *relational* model because it emphasizes the relationship between the stressor demands and the individual's resources for responding to the stressor. An imbalance between stressor and resources can result in either an *underload* or an *overload* of individual coping capabilities. Exercise can enhance coping capabilities by improving mood, self-concept, and physical and psychological energy levels.

Disparity and, ultimately, stress are caused by the commonly acknowledged *external* life events and demands and *internal* events. According to the disparity or relational model, stress results from a perceived disparity between a person's capabilities and the necessary response to a stressor rather than simply from the stressor itself. In conclusion, people are stressed when they must struggle with demands that do not match their resources and capabilities for responding. The situation of having *too many resources* and the opposite situation of having *too few resources* may both result in stress.

To further understand how exercise might influence the various stages of the stress process, it is necessary to examine the individual components. Refer to Figure 7.3 for the interacting factors in the disparity model.

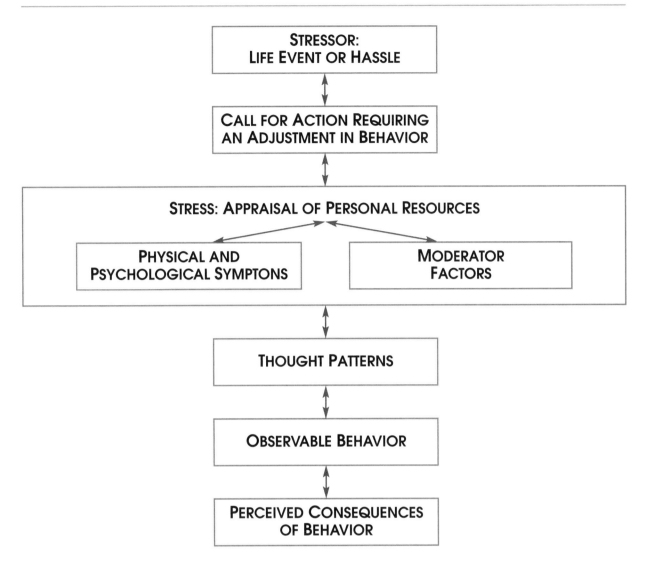

Figure 7.3. Disparity model of stress: Basic elements (Berger, 1983/1984; Sarason, 1980).

The eight basic components within the stress process include

- Occurrence of a stressor;
- Call for action and perception of the personal importance of the demand;
- Cognitive appraisal of ability and skills necessary for responding (these can be at conscious and/or unconscious levels);
- Physiological and psychological stress responses or symptoms;
- Personal or moderator characteristics;
- Thought patterns;
- Observable behavior; and
- Perceived consequences of the behavior.

The components within the stress process emphasize that stress occurs when a person's failure to meet the demand of the stressor is deemed important to the individual. Please refer to Figure 7.4 for additional details within the stress process.

The components in Figures 7.4 and 7.5 are not necessarily sequential and can interact repeatedly throughout the stress process as indicated by the bidirectionality of the arrows. The value of the disparity model is that it emphasizes multiple interactions between the *environment* or *stressors, the individual*, and a host of *moderating variables*. The disparity model highlights an interactional approach to stress, which is widely employed by many stress therapists, researchers, and exercise science specialists. Habitual participation in physical exercise influences a variety of psychological and social moderators that determine stress responses.

Exercisers, in comparison to sedentary individuals, seem to experience less stress as suggested in the next chapter on "Exercise as a Stress Management Technique." In reference to the stress process illustrated in Figure 7.3, exercisers tend to score lower on depression and anxiety, have a stronger commitment to a particular activity, and enjoy and even seek sensations and

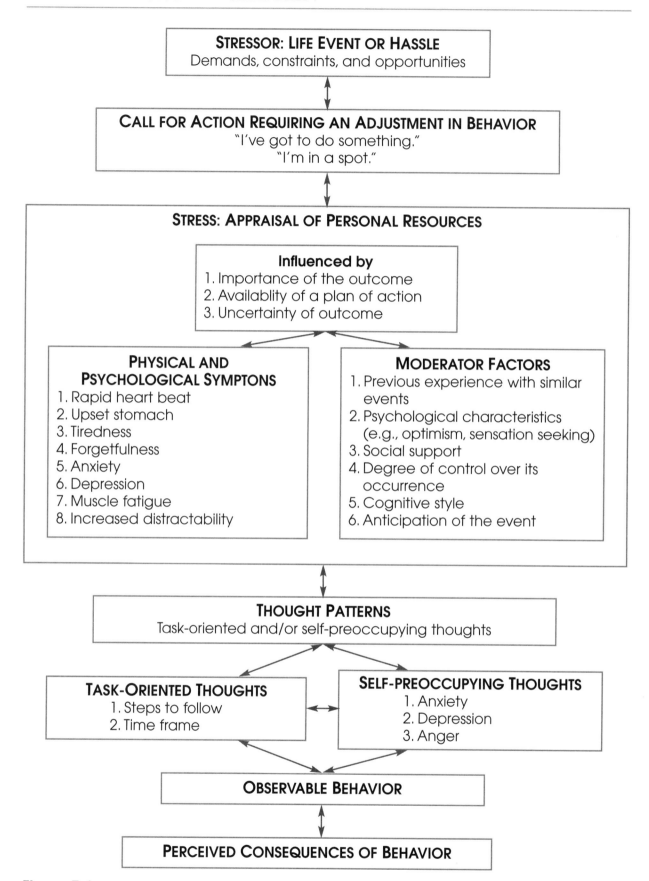

Figure 7.4. Disparity model of stress: Evaluation of capabilities in comparison to the demand of the stressor (Berger, 1983/1984; Sarason, 1980).

challenges. Exercisers also tend to have an internal locus of control and thus take control of hassles, uplifts, and life events. Many exercise participants can gain social support by participating in group activities. These characteristics of physically active people seem to carry over from exercise and sport environments to everyday life and have implications for stress management.

Conservation of Resources Model

The conservation of resources model bridges the gap between stressor-based models and cognitive models that emphasize personal interpretations of stressors. The conservation of resources model suggests that stress results from *a loss or a potential loss* of resources. S. E. Hobfoll has two useful resources on this subject: one book, *Stress, Culture, and Community: The Psychology and Philosophy of Stress,* and one article, "Conservation of Resources: A New Attempt at Conceptualizing Stress." Death and separation from a loved one, for example, are major losses and central elements in bereavement. Upon examination, many items in Tables 7.3 and 7.4 are loss events: death of a parent or spouse, divorce, trouble with in-laws, job loss, and minor law violation (loss of prestige, loss of friends). Resources include friends, family, and acquaintances as well as objects, personal characteristics, and physical and psychological energies (Hobfoll, 1998).

All types of personal resources counteract loss and form the conceptual base of the conservation of resources model. Resources include all items that are valued by the individual. Their loss is linked to stress; their gain is linked to enhanced well-being and even to eustress. According to Hobfoll (1998), we strive to obtain, retain, and protect our resources to sustain ourselves, our families, and our culture. Basic categories of resources include:

- *Objects* (money, jewelry, car, stereo, apartment, and house),
- *Conditions* (being physically fit, being an athlete, dating someone, being married, having a job, and enjoying seniority),
- *Personal characteristics* (physical appearance, mood, mastery, intelligence, grades, self-esteem, social support, and socioeconomic status), and
- *Energies* (time, effort, love, knowledge, and power). (Hobfoll, 1989, 1998)

According to this model, resources are objective items and do not rely on personal appraisals. Thus, stress is an objective event rather than a transactional or relational process.

Resources have *instrumental* (or inherent) *value* to us and *symbolic value* by defining to others who we are. You may consider your car and stereo equipment to be important resources. Having a well-defined physique is another resource that you may value. Instrumental values of these resources include a means of transportation, the opportunity to listen to preferred music, and physical strength. A car, stereo equipment, and a person's body would be worth a certain amount of money if they were marketed. These same resources also have symbolic values. For example, a car, stereo system, or attractive body may indicate that you are a worthwhile person. These items may indicate that you worked hard to purchase or develop these objects, or that your parents love you by giving these presents, or a host of other symbolic values.

The conservation of resources model suggests that when confronted with stressors, people strive to minimize their losses. Thus, as they age and become stressed about getting older and losing sex appeal, they might use exercise to offset the decline in appearance by having a firm, well-developed body or, alternatively, by purchasing a highly coveted sports car.

When not facing specific stressors, people strive to develop resource surpluses to offset future losses. Gathering surplus resources by improving one's appearance, increasing the number of friends, or earning more money—all result in enhanced well-being, or even eustress. According to the conservation of resources model, if people are poorly equipped to gain resources, they are particularly vulnerable to stress.

Physiological Toughness Model of Stress

This final model of stress is particularly relevant to exercise specialists because it includes the use of exercise as one way to increase physiological toughness. According to the physiological toughness model, there are two different types of physiological arousal: (a) arousal that arises from *challenges* and (b) arousal from *threats* of harm and loss. Dienstbier (1989) suggests that a pattern of intermittent arousal and recovery defines physiological toughness. *Tough* individuals respond to stressors effectively and view stressful situations as challenges. Those who are *less tough* view stressors as threats of harm and loss.

Challenges. If you are tough, challenges result in feelings of control and of "effort without distress." According to the physiological toughness model, challenges activate the "good" sympathetic nervous system (SNS)-adrenal-medullary arousal and result in increased adrenaline and noradrenaline. This SNS-adrenal-medullary arousal is associated with a host of desirable characteristics, many of which are the direct opposite of the stress response: emotional stability, improved performance in challenging or in stressful situations, enhanced immune function, retention of learning, lower initial catecholamine and cortisol base rates, and increased catecholamine availability (Dienst-bier, 1989).

Threats of harm. In contrast to challenges, threats of harm or loss activate the "bad" pituitary-adrenal-cortical responses and release adrenocorticotropin (ACTH) and ultimately cortisol. Elevated cortisol has been associated in numerous studies with negative situations and characteristics. Some of these include understimulation in activity-seeking Type A individuals, the mood disorders of anxiety and depression, anorexia, and poor ability to cope with illness (Dienstbier, 1989). Elevated cortisol levels also result in many undesirable consequences of stress such as coronary heart disease, poor immune function, ulcers, neuroticism, anxiety, depression, and other psychological problems.

Facilitating physiological toughness. Three types of events or activities are theorized to facilitate *toughness.* These events include (1) a person's early experience with stressors, (2) passive toughening (animal adaptation from exposure to shock and cold), and (3) active toughening, which consists of fitness training through regular aerobic exercise. With toughening experiences, threats are more likely to be viewed as challenges, and the negative effects of stress are avoided. An individual who has a "toughened" stress response has "sufficient energy to cope mentally and physically without great effort or exhaustion" (Dienstbier, 1989, p. 95).

Current Issues in Stress Theory: Prolonged Activation and Perseverative Cognition

In a theoretical article examining the stress-illness relationship, Brosschot, Pieper, and Thayer (2005) suggest that many stress theorists have failed to incorporate key elements within their theories. These needed elements in most theories include

- *Prolonged physiological activation* in response to stressors and
- *Perseverative cognition* that results in a person continuing to mentally focus on the stressors and entire stressful situation, and thus extend prolonged physiological activation.

The first element, *prolonged physiological activation,* results in the pathogenic state of stress that eventually may lead to organic disease (e.g., Seaward, 1997b; Ursin & Eriksen, 2004). Selye (1950) emphasized the prolonged activity or duration of the stress response. However, duration of the stress response has not been a prominent element in many stress theories or studies (Brosschot et al., 2005) until recently (e.g., McEwen, 1998; Linden et al., 1997; Brosschot & Thayer, 1998; Sluiter et al., 2000). Many stress theories and models such as *reactive models* emphasize that it is frequent

and strong responses to stressors, rather than duration of the stress response, that result in pathogenic wear and tear of organisms and in disease. The *duration of the stress response* includes a person's stress responses that may occur far in advance of the stressor and also continue long after it is over or concluded. Thus stress inventories that measure people's appraisal of past experiences with life events and hassles/uplifts focus on the past, but tend to ignore future stressors and the anticipation of them.

Perseverative cognition is the second often-neglected element of the stress process and has been defined as "the repeated or chronic activation of the cognitive representation of stress-related content" (Brosschot & Thayer, 2003, 2004). This cognitive process of perseveration, rather than the stressor itself, is a mediator of the stress-illness relationship. Perseverative cognition extends, or prolongs, activation of the stress response and ultimately results in illness (Brosschot et al., 2005). Stressors lead to prolonged activation when people cognitively perseverate about stressors for a period of time. This perseveration produces prolonged physiological activation of several bodily systems and increases the risk of disease. Common physiological responses and diseases associated with physiological activation include myocardial infarct, high heart rates, increased cortisol levels, slow blood pressure recovery, resting blood pressure levels, less Natural Killer cells, and higher cardiovascular activity.

Perseverative cognition includes (1) the personality trait of worry which leads to anticipatory worry, (2) rumination, the tendency to replay events, thoughts, and worries, and (3) anticipatory stress. Trait worry also can detract from sleep quality. This is a major health issue since sleep is an important and natural recovery period. Sleep provides opportunity for restoration to homeostasis, but it also is an opportunity for prolonged activation (Brosschot et al., 2005).

Stress Management

Due to the frequency of our stress responses, we need to know how to actively manage our stress levels to create and maintain our optimal levels (see Figure 7.2 for differences in optimal levels). The term *stress management* rather than *stress reduction* emphasizes the fact that **some stress is desirable**. "Management" indicates that stress may need to be increased or decreased. In reality, we wish to reduce stress only when it is so intense that it is unpleasant or produces undesirable stress symptoms. Optimal stress levels, as illustrated in Figures 7.1 and 7.2, provide us with energy and excitement. Stress management techniques enable each of us to live creatively with stress.

As an exercise science specialist, you probably will want to learn to monitor and regulate stress levels for your own optimal well-being and to be able to assist others in mastering some of the techniques. To become more knowledgeable with a variety of approaches, you will want to practice the various techniques until you feel comfortable with them. Practicing the techniques yourself provides invaluable insights into their effectiveness and the common procedures associated with their adoption.

As discussed in the next chapter, specific types of physical activity can either increase or decrease a participant's stress level. Thus, exercise is an ideal form of stress management. Swimming laps in a pool or going for a run, for example, can be stress reducing, especially if an individual enjoys the activity (Berger, Friedmann, & Eaton, 1988; Berger & Owen, 1983, 1988). These physical activities provide opportunities for peace and quiet and a time-out from a busy day. Participants can reflect on a variety of topics or can completely tune out the world while intermittently focusing on the movement sensations. A minimal level of enjoyment of an activity also may be a necessary requirement for stress reduction (Berger, 1994). An individual who participates in an activity that she or he greatly dislikes will reap fitness benefits, but is unlikely to find the activity stress reducing.

In contrast to noncompetitive exercise activities, a *competitive* game of basketball or a tennis match can provide thrilling competition and exciting challenges. In competitive activities, whether you have desirable or undesirable changes in stress when exercising may depend on factors such as your "need to win," whether you are ego involved or task involved, and the outcome of the game. In competitive types of exercise, you may experience eustress from winning or from responding to manageable challenges, or distress from losing and the subsequent questioning of your physical skills. As emphasized throughout this chapter, stress and challenges add excitement and, at times, eustress to our lives. Too much stress, however, is detrimental.

If you have too much stress, you need to do something about it before stress causes you to become ill or detracts from your full enjoyment of life. Distress is associated with minor health problems such as colds and the flu. Chronic distress is associated with more serious ailments and diseases such as anxiety, asthma attacks, depression, high blood pressure, heart disease, and even cancer.

The self-regulation of stress is based on accurate self-awareness of your stress level. Depending on your stress level, you may decide to adopt one or more of the coping and/or stress management techniques that are described briefly in the following sections. Coping techniques include changing your mental outlook on stress and on life in general. In contrast, stress management techniques involve actively practicing an established method on a regular basis.

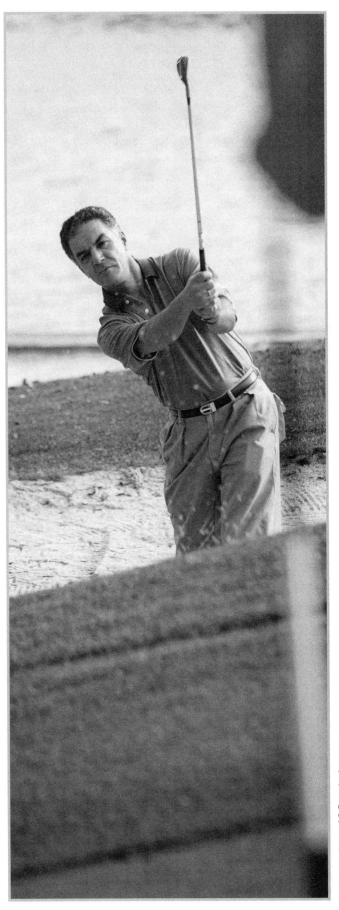

Coping Techniques

Coping is the everyday effort to manage stress; it includes a variety of approaches to change your thoughts about and interpretation of stressful situations. Coping can be defined as "the changing thoughts and acts the individual uses to manage the external and/or internal demands of a specific person-environment transaction that is appraised as stressful" (Folkman, 1991, p. 5).

Common coping approaches include:

- Acceptance of responsibility,
- Denial,
- Distancing,
- Escape-avoidance,
- Maintenance of a sense of humor,
- Optimism,
- Pharmacological treatment,
- Positive reappraisal of personal resources,
- Seeking of social support,
- Temporary escaping and taking time out,
- Thoughtful problem solving, and
- Use of religious faith.

Effectiveness of a particular coping strategy is dependent on the specific stress situation and its particular stage. A test or exam, for example, includes an announcement of its occurrence or a warning, the test-taking situation, a waiting period before grades are announced, and another time period in which you learn how you and your classmates did. Different coping techniques may be differentially helpful in these diverse stages of test taking (Lazarus, 1999).

A useful approach for coping with stress is to adopt the "Four Commandments of Contentment" (Hansel, 1979, pp. 80–89), which can be thought of as commandments for coping. The commandments illustrate a cognitive approach to coping with stress that can help you to change your stress-related thought patterns. The four commandments are as follows:

1. *Thou shalt live here and now.* This commandment helps you to decrease dwelling on the past and worrying about the future.
2. *Thou shalt not hurry.* This commandment provides time for the collection of thoughts and for living in the present.
3. *Thou shalt not take thyself so seriously.* This enables you to maintain your sense of balance and humor.
4. *Thou shalt be grateful.* This commandment encourages you to appreciate what you have, as well as what you do not have, which can contribute to a sense of peace.

Table 7.9
Specific-Effects Hypothesis for Relaxation Techniques

Technique Categories	Relaxation Techniques
Somatic approaches (body-mind)	• Biofeedback • Diaphragmatic breathing • Exercise • Massage • Progressive relaxation • Hatha yoga
Cognitive approaches (mind-body)	• Cognitive restructuring and reframing • Hypnosis • Meditation and the Relaxation Response • Psychotherapy and counseling • Stress inoculation • Thought-stopping
Behavioral approaches	• Assertiveness training • Changing Type A behavior patterns • Saying "No" to requests • Developing social support skills • Time management

Coping techniques interrupt the stress cycle in a variety of ways. They change habitual thought patterns, increase evaluation of personal resources, and change typical behavior patterns. Major functions of coping are (a) to manage a problem or stressor and (b) to regulate emotion (Lazarus, 1999). In conclusion, coping techniques enable stressed individuals to regulate their thought patterns and related emotions.

Stress Management Techniques

Regardless of our general level of stress or relaxation, it is important to be knowledgeable about and proficient in several different stress management techniques. As emphasized by Peper and Holt (1993) in *Creating Wholeness: A Self-Healing Workbook Using Dynamic Relaxation, Images, and Thoughts*, relaxation techniques "will help you to become an active participant in your growth/health process" (p. 4). Depending on your professional goals and whether you will be working with stressed individuals, you may need expertise in an even broader base of relaxation techniques. Relaxation training enables us to regulate the stress in our own lives and to provide training to others in exercise, sport, and rehabilitation settings.

You will need familiarity with a variety of stress reduction techniques to knowledgeably select, recommend, and teach them. Exercise specialists who use only one or two stress reduction techniques are limited in their effectiveness because they are unable to accommodate the specific needs of a client. Considerable information is needed to use the techniques appropriately for yourself or with your exercise clients or students. For in-depth descriptions of the techniques, you will need to locate several stress books and manuals that are available in your college or university library and preferably take a course in stress management. Common relaxation techniques identified in Table 7.9 include diaphragmatic breathing, meditation, hatha yoga, progressive relaxation, the relaxation response, and physical exercise (Seaward, 1997a).

A three-part specific-effects hypothesis approach outlined in Table 7.9 is an appealing guide for selecting a stress management technique (Davidson & Schwartz, 1976). According to the *specific-effects hypothesis*, a stress management technique from one of the following three categories has the greatest benefits for stress symptoms in that same category: somatic, cognitive, and behavioral.

Somatic techniques emphasize the body-mind relationship and focus on relaxing the body to relax the mind. These techniques are helpful in treating somatic symptoms of stress such as muscular tension, headaches, and digestive disturbances. *Cognitive techniques* focus on quieting the mind to relax the rest of

Table 7.10

Commonalties Within Meditation and Other Relaxation Techniques

Requirement	Purpose
A quiet place to practice	Provides freedom from distractions and interruptions
Sitting or lying in a comfortable position	Requires minimal muscular tonus Frees the mind to concentrate on the technique Facilitates a full 20 minutes of practice
A word, sound, or object to dwell upon	Encourages the "letting go" of thoughts by keeping the mind occupied
Passive attitude	Allows participants to disregard and dismiss distracting thoughts Facilitates a return to the initial focus on the technique
Regular practice	Maintains technique awareness and competency
Sessions of 20 minutes minimum	Permits uninterrupted practice Enables the technique to produce benefits

the body. These techniques are useful for reducing cognitive stress symptoms such as worry, anxiety, forgetfulness, and sleep disorders. *Behavioral techniques* assist you in changing your actions to modify your environment that might be stress producing. By changing your own behavior, you reduce your stress-producing activities. Saying "no" is a particularly effective behavior modification for reducing stress that results from overload.

Despite technique specificity, it is likely that the regular practice of stress management techniques affects a generalized relaxation response, which is opposite to the fight-or-flight response (Benson, 1984; Lehrer & Woolfolk, 1984). Relaxation results in the *trophotropic response*, which is characterized by decreased metabolic activity. The trophotropic response also is characterized by decreases in oxygen consumption, carbon dioxide production, heart rate, respiratory rate, and blood pressure. Relaxation also is accompanied by increases in skin resistance and electroencephalogram recordings of alpha wave activity (Benson, 1984). Most stress reduction techniques can be effective; however, they need to be practiced correctly and on a regular basis. See Table 7.10 for key elements that are common to many of the techniques, which differ widely in philosophical bases and methodologies. As noted in the table, most stress reduction techniques require a quiet place for practice; a comfortable body position in order to concentrate on the technique; repetitive focus on a word, sound, or muscular activity; adoption of a passive attitude toward intruding thoughts; and practice on a regular basis for a minimum of 20 minutes per session.

No single stress management technique is effective for all people. As an exercise specialist, you need to be acutely aware of an individual student's or client's responses to a stress management technique. You must be able to prescribe and teach a variety of approaches. For example, one person may hate the physical exertion in exercise, but thoroughly enjoy sitting quietly and meditating. In contrast, another individual may find sitting quietly for 20 minutes and practicing the relaxation response akin to "doing nothing," "wasting" time, and even producing stress. This person is an ideal candidate to use the active technique of exercise for stress reduction. Personal preference for a technique is an important consideration in selecting a stress management strategy.

Summary

There are numerous definitions of stress and distress. Many of the definitions employed in this chapter are highlighted in Table 7.1. Basically, stress is a dynamic interchange between the individual and her or his environment. Stress is a series of bidirectional interactions that occur within an individual in response to environmental events (stressors) that demand change and/or a response. A certain level of stress is desirable. Stress adds excitement and energy to our lives. In fact, regulating the amount of stress in our lives is an essential influence on our quality of life.

Stress has both psychological and physiological manifestations. Psychological and cognitive symptoms include anxiety, depression, muscular tension, forgetfulness, inability to concentrate, insomnia, and irritability or quickness to anger. Typical physiological responses include sweaty palms, rapid heart rate, change in breathing pattern, upset stomach, diarrhea, and physical exhaustion. Unrelenting stressors result in chronic stress and eventually overwhelm our adaptational reserves. Chronic stress results in a decreased quality of life and has potentially serious health consequences.

If you have the resources or abilities necessary to react to a situation in a satisfactory manner, an event is not stressful. When stressors exceed your resources, you experience distress. When you notice a disparity or an insufficiency of your personal resources for responding to a stressor, you tend to experience some of the psychological and physiological stress symptoms listed in Table 7.2. The stress process includes eight primary components in Figure 7.3:

- Occurrence of a stressor,
- Call for action and appraisal of the personal importance of the stressor,
- Appraisal of personal resources,
- Physical and psychological stress symptoms,
- Personal characteristics that moderate individual stress responses,
- Task-oriented and self-preoccupying thought patterns,
- Behavior, and
- Perceived consequences of behavior.

Theoretical models of stress capture various aspects of the process. These include Selye's (1975) general adaptation syndrome, the identity disruption model, the disparity or relational model, the conservation of resources model, and the physiological toughness model. These models emphasize complex interactions between the person and the environment or situation. Regardless of the model of stress employed, it is clear that stress is an ongoing, multifaceted process. Too often, we ignore stress until there is an obvious psychological or physical malfunction such as a panic attack, a severe headache, or a heart attack. Only after suffering considerable personal distress or physical breakdown do we seek assistance in dealing with stress. Ideally, use of a stress management activity such as exercise as described in the next chapter will prevent future stress episodes and enable us to use stress to enhance our quality of life. As noted by Dienstbier

(1989, 1991) in the physiological toughness model, habitual exercisers may experience less stress symptomatology and interpret fewer events as stressors.

The term *stress management* emphasizes that both too much and too little stress is unpleasant. Most of us use various coping processes that roughly can be described as problem and emotion oriented. Each of these approaches is effective in different stressful situations and in different stages of the stress process. Some specific coping factors include acceptance of responsibility, confrontational coping, distancing, escape-avoidance, positive reappraisal, and seeking of social support. If you are highly stressed, you might choose to employ a stress management technique in addition to coping behaviors. Stress management techniques are helpful in changing your stress responses and include techniques such as the relaxation response, progressive relaxation, positive self-talk, biofeedback, and physical exercise.

Can You Define These Terms?

conservation of resources model of stress

disparity or relational model of stress

distress and eustress

external and internal stressors

fight-or-flight response

general adaptation syndrome (GAS)

hassles and uplifts

identity disruption model of stress

intra-individual and inter-individual variation in stress

life events

physical toughness model of stress

specific effects hypothesis

stress

stressor

Can You Answer These Questions?

1. Why are there so many definitions of stress? Cite several of your favorite ones.
2. Have you or members of your family experienced any relationship between numerous life events and illness? Has exercise played any role in this relationship? Please elaborate.
3. What recent life events and hassles have added to your current stress levels?
4. What are the essential elements in your personal stress profile? Is there a particular sign that you note when you are highly stressed?
5. Compare a friend's intra-individual stress responses to your own. What are the major inter-individual stress differences between the two of you?
6. How are life events related to illness?

7. What role(s) might exercise play in the life event-illness relationship?

8. What are the differences and similarities between the reactionary and interactional models of stress?

9. Which model of stress do you find most appealing? Provide the rationale for your decision.

10. What are the major differences between coping responses and stress management techniques?

CHAPTER 8

Exercise as a Stress Management Technique: Psychological and Physiological Effects

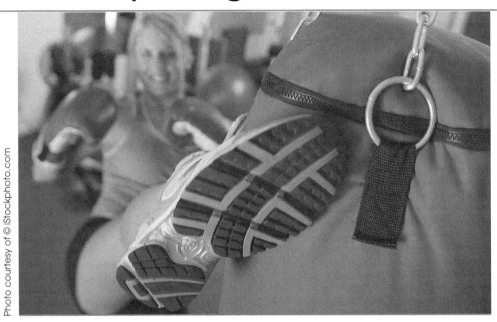

Photo courtesy of © iStockphoto.com

After reading this chapter, you should be able to

- Elaborate on the psychological and physiological benefits of exercise for stress management,

- Plan a study to examine the influences exercise might have on stress responses,

- Identify important factors influencing the relationship between exercise and stress reactivity,

- Explain the paradox that highly stressed individuals who could benefit from exercise as a stress management technique are less likely to exercise than their less-stressed peers,

- Elaborate on the role of hatha yoga in promoting stress reduction,

- Explore how exercise might moderate the life stress-illness relationship,

- Describe Dienstbier's (1991) toughness model of stress responsivity,

- Explain why the physiological and psychological responses to stressors often do not agree with one another, and

- Discuss exercise as a stress management technique for special populations including cardiac rehabilitation clients.

I am an old man who has known a great many problems, most of which never happened.

—Mark Twain

Life is either a daring adventure or nothing at all.

—Helen Keller

Introduction

Too much as well as too little stress contributes to distress and can have deleterious effects on our health and quality of life. As reviewed in the previous chapter, "distress" is shortened to the word "stress" in common usage and detracts from our mood states, daily performance, and health. Stress is associated with a high incidence of minor health problems and illnesses such as colds, flu, canker sores, cold sores, and chronic fatigue (Cohen & Williamson, 1991).

When stress continues for a prolonged period or occurs repeatedly, it can be associated with more serious health problems. Stress-related illnesses including asthma, high blood pressure, coronary heart disease, back pain, colitis, Epstein-Barr disease or chronic fatigue syndrome, and even cancer depend on an individual's genetic vulnerability as well as stress levels (Blascovich, & Katkin, 1993; Seaward, 1997a; Sternfeld, 1992). Psychological distress symptoms include anxiety, nervousness, depression, irritability, hostility, neuroticism, and personal unhappiness in general (Lovallo, 2005; Nelson & Burke, 2002). Pelletier (1977) estimated that between 50 and 70% of all disease and illness were stress related. Today, the estimates are an even higher—70 to 80% (Seaward, 1997a).

A variety of coping and stress management techniques are useful in reducing the deleterious effects of stress and may be differentially effective in reducing behavioral, cognitive, and somatic symptoms of stress. The techniques, however, do have broader, generalized relaxation effects. Exercise science specialists can help clients select a technique that is personally appealing and appropriate for specific stress symptoms. Choosing an effective method that is appealing and enjoyable has major implications for technique adoption and adherence.

Stress Management Approaches and Exercise

Somatic stress management techniques such as exercise are hypothesized to focus directly on alleviating physical stress symptoms such as muscle tension and increased heart rate (Davidson & Schwartz, 1976; Ghoncheh & Smith, 2004). Exercise psychologists and other movement specialists use a variety of stress management techniques to help people decrease their general stress levels and improve their exercise performance through the management of stress and anxiety. Stress management techniques, especially those with a somatic base, emphasize the dynamic relationship between body and mind. As emphasized in Chapter 7, exercise is an ideal stress management technique. It is one of the few stress management techniques that you can use to both raise *and* lower your ongoing stress level—depending on your needs. It also has desirable health-related side effects.

Using Exercise to Raise Stress Levels

Pursuing high-risk physical activities and competitive sport raises stress levels and decreases the boredom and apathy often associated with too little stress. Physical activities such as rock climbing, whitewater rafting, downhill skiing, and competitive exercise activities are exciting and can produce highly sought feelings of eustress, the thrilling form of stress.

Individuals with high needs for sensation and thrill seeking tend to gravitate toward high-risk and competitive activities. These activities provide desirable opportunities for stress production. In both high-risk and competitive physical activities, participants often practice and train at high intensity and for long periods of time to surpass their own previous performances and beat their opponents. Training and competing under the watchful eyes of coaches and fans are additional sources of stress. Individuals differ in their preferred level of stress and its myriad effects on their psychological and physical well-being. Thus, it is important that each person learn to self-regulate activities to maintain optimal levels of stress.

Using Exercise to Lower Stress Levels

In contrast to the stress-producing nature of some physical activities, other types, especially those that are noncompetitive, highly predictable, and performed at moderate intensity levels and for relatively short duration, tend to lower participants' stress levels (Berger, 1994). Exercise such as hatha yoga that require an inward focus, awareness of the present, and an emphasis on breathing would appear to be particularly related to stress reduction and relaxation. These types of exercise can be associated with psychological and physiological benefits that enable participants to cope with too much stress. As Berger has emphasized, however, the stress reduction benefits of exercise are not automatic. Thus, it is important to investigate and understand the multiple interactions between exercise and stress management.

Exercise and Stress: Complex Interactions

It is likely that the specific stress-related influences of exercise result from complex interactions among numerous factors. These factors include

- **The participants**, especially their gender, personality characteristics such as Type A behavior and hostility and trait anxiety, self-esteem, social interactions and support, and fitness levels (e.g., Johnson-Kozlow, Sallis, & Calfas, 2004; Lovallo, 2005; Nelson & Burke, 2005),
- **Type of exercise**: enjoyment, mode, intensity, frequency, and duration (e.g., Ghoncheh & Smith, 2004; Spalding, Lyon, Steel, & Hatfield, 2004),
- **The exercise environment** or setting, such as its evaluative aspects, competitiveness, social interaction, proximity to nature, etc. (e.g., Berger, 1994; Plante, Coscarelli, & Ford, 2001), and
- **The stressors themselves,** such as whether they are psychological or physical (e.g., Hong, Farag, Nelesen, Ziegler, & Mills, 2004; Lovallo, 2005).

The relationship between these factors and mood alteration is examined in Chapters 6 (Mood Alteration, Self-Awareness, and Exercise: Multiple Relationships), 20 (Exercise: What Type Is Best for Optimal Psychological Benefits?), and 21 (Exercise: Practice Guidelines for Optimal Psychological Benefits). It seems that exercise that is enjoyable, promotes abdominal breathing, and is relatively noncompetitive, predictable, and rhythmical is likely to promote feelings of stress reduction along with desirable mood changes that are conducive to altering an individual's perception of stress. The exercise probably should not be so intense or so long that it is physically depleting. However, the exercise does need to provide a training effect to facilitate ease of participation and enjoyment for the stress-reducing benefits.

Another way in which exercise may serve as a stress reduction technique is by enhancing self-concept and self-esteem (see Chapter 4, Exercise and Enhanced Self-Concept and Self-Esteem). Liking themselves and feeling good about themselves may change how exercisers perceive and react to stressors. People with positive self-concepts who experience stress would be less likely to appraise their capabilities and talents as insufficient to meet needed behavior. We are not aware of any studies that have investigated the relationship between exercise, self-concept, and stress directly. McInman and Berger (1993) did observe, though, that aerobic dance participants reported short-term changes in both their self-concept and mood states. These two benefits of aerobic dance appeared to be independent of one another, but both enhanced

mood and self-concept may be useful in responding appropriately to a variety of stressors.

Relative Effectiveness of Exercise

Exercise has been as effective as other, more traditional stress management techniques such as meditation, progressive relaxation, the relaxation response, and stress inoculation training (Bahrke & Morgan, 1978; Berger, Friedman, & Eaton, 1988; Long, 1993). In a recent comparison of yoga stretching and progressive muscle relaxation, each of the stress management techniques was differentially effective in reducing stress indices as measured by specific psychological measures (Ghoncheh & Smith, 2004). Accumulating evidence suggests that the benefits of exercise as a stress reduction technique are not greater than those of other techniques. The lack of superiority of exercise, however, does not decrease the value of its effectiveness as a stress management technique. Exercise does have several advantages over other stress reduction techniques. It can be stress- and eustress-producing and has numerous health benefits in addition to those of stress management.

Stress Management and the Physiological Benefits of Exercise

Among the various stress management techniques available, exercise is a personal favorite for many reasons. We seek a host of desirable benefits of exercising on a regular basis, one of which is stress management and the accompanying physiological benefits of decreased blood pressure, resting heart rate, and muscular tension that can be stress-related. We also desire the other physiological benefits of weight control; a decrease in body fat and incidence of osteoporosis; and increases in muscle definition, cardiorespiratory fitness, muscular strength, endurance, flexibility, and perhaps even in the length of life (e.g., American College of Sports Medicine, 2006).

To some individuals, the aging process can be stressful as they note changes in appearance, decreased physical capacities, and level of energy. As discussed in Chapter 19, exercise has desirable anti-aging benefits and can offset some of the stress associated with the aging process. Habitual exercise creates a more youthful appearance as evidenced by a relative lack of abdominal girth, well-defined muscles, and decreased body fat. Exercise also contributes to a youthful manner characterized by high energy and vigor. In addition, exercise influences many indices of physical decline that are associated with aging and that become obvious as we move through our 50s, 60s, and 70s. Habitual exercise increases maximum cardiac output, muscular endurance, strength, and flexibility and decreases osteoporosis (Spirduso, Francis, & MacRae, 2005). If you are in your early 20s, you probably are not worried about the physical decline associated with the aging process. Some of the exercise benefits that interest you probably include improved appearance, high energy, and stress management.

Stress Management and the Psychological Benefits of Exercise

As discussed throughout this text, many of the physical benefits of exercise are inseparable from the psychological benefits. Together, these benefits interact to give one the sensation of "feeling better." Exercisers can experience more positive mood states and thus fewer psychological stress indices as evidenced by lower levels of tension, tiredness, depression, and anger and higher levels of calmness and energy for several hours after exercising (e.g., Berger, 1994; Plante et al., 2001). They also feel more attractive and sure of themselves as a result of the physical changes of exercise to their bodies. In addition, exercisers tend to be more confident about their physical capabilities, and they have more positive self-concepts and more self-esteem than do non-exercisers.

Psychologically and physically, exercisers feel stronger and have more energy. Increased physical strength and endurance enable exercisers to participate in a wide variety of pleasant and enjoyable activities. Additional psychological benefits include such uplifts as experiencing peak moments and flow states, enjoyment of exercise sessions, increased awareness of personal meanings connected to exercise programs, increased self-awareness, and youthfulness, as well as stress management—the focus of this chapter.

Stress Indices Affected by Exercise

Habitual exercise, especially aerobic exercise, decreases a number of stress indices. For example, regular or chronic exercise usually results in decreases in tension, depression, anger and hostility, and fatigue as well as a lower resting heart rate, greater stroke volume, and lower systolic and diastolic blood pressure (American College of Sports Medicine, 2006). In addition, single exercise sessions have included increased brain wave activity, which may be related to feelings of enhanced psychological well-being (e.g., Crabbe & Dishman, 2004). A recent meta-analysis of 18 studies measuring brain electrocortical activity during and after exercise indicated that there is accumulating evidence for increased activity in the alpha frequency band of brain waves which often have been associated with reports of relaxation and enhanced mood states (Crabbe & Dishman, 2004). Results of the meta-analysis also indicated that there were exercise-related increases in beta, delta, and theta brain wave activity (see Table 8.1 for a listing of key stress indices that can be affected by habitual physical activity). As previously noted, the exact response to exercise is dependent on the participant's characteristics, exercise mode and training parameters, and the stressors themselves. Despite the complexity of the relationship between exercise and stress reactivity, it seems that exercise may result in a decreased response to a standard exercise workload and/or facilitate a fast return to resting baseline levels after exercising (e.g., Hong et al., 2004; Plante et al., 2001; Spalding et al., 2004).

Table 8.1
Common Stress Indices That May Be Modified by Exercise
(e.g., Crabbe & Dishman, 2004; Hong et al., 2004; Plante et al., 2001; Spalding et al., 2004)

- Aggression and hostility
- Anxiety and tension
- Atherosclerosis
- Brain waves or electrocortical activity
- Alpha frequency brain wave activiation
- Beta, delta, and theta wave activation
- Cardiovascular reactivity to psychological stress
- Catecholamine levels
- Plasma epinephrine
- Plasma norepinephrine
- Coronary heart disease
- Decreased calmness
- Depression
- Fatigue and tiredness
- Fear
- Natural killer (NK) cell numbers
- Plasma glucose and insulin levels
- Resting heart rate
- Systolic and diastolic blood pressure, a risk factor for cerebrovascular disease
- Target-organ damage

Current research concerning the influence of exercise on physiological stress responses has investigated two major aspects of the stress response. One is the absolute *extent* or *magnitude* of the stress response. Exercisers may not have the same elevations in blood pressure, heart rate, or circulating hormones as those of sedentary or less fit individuals. A second way that exercise might affect the stress response is to shorten the *duration* of the elevations and to facilitate a quicker return to baseline. Each of these possibilities has important implications for the relationship between stress and health by enabling the body to return to homeostatic functioning; thus, stress causes less wear and tear on the body. This chapter focuses on the current thinking and research related to exercise and stress management to provide a comprehensive picture of the role of exercise as a stress management technique.

Typical Studies of Exercise and Stress

To investigate the relationship between habitual exercise and the magnitude and/or duration of an individual's stress response, researchers generally conduct laboratory experiments. Basic steps in many of the studies are as follows:

- **Comparing two or more groups of participants.** Often these groups are habitual exercisers, those who are sedentary, and a control group.
- **Acclimation to the laboratory setting.** Participants become familiar with their surroundings and learn about the procedures that will be employed in the study. This acclimation opportunity enables participants to feel comfortable with the situation and to return to their normal baseline physiological levels if the experimental setting and/or procedures are potentially stress producing.
- **Completing a variety of demographic or personal background questionnaires.** The questionnaires reflect important characteristics of the participants such as age, marital status, prescription drug use, amount of exercise during a typical day or week, and other information related to the study.
- **Collecting baseline physiological and psychological responses.** These responses often include anxiety, anger, depression, fatigue, hostility, vigor, heart rate, blood pressure, muscle tension, and hormone levels that will be monitored throughout the study. The baseline data reflects the participants' scores in nonstressful situations.
- **Participating in one or more carefully planned stressful tasks.** An example of such tasks is counting backwards from 1,000 by 7s as rapidly as possible. To increase the amount of stress in the task, the researcher might indicate to the participants that

they are not doing as well as others in the study, ask the participants to speed up the counting, or provide a background metronome sound that is distracting.
- **Monitoring participants' stress indices during completion of the stressful task.** Typical measures include anxiety, aggression and hostility, depression, heart rate, blood pressure, catecholamines, and galvanic skin response.
- **Comparing the size and duration of the physiological stress responses of the exercisers to those of the sedentary participants.** This provides some idea whether exercisers have differing reactions to stress than do nonexercisers.

As indicated in the previous chapter on stress, it is difficult to measure stress responses. People have individualized response patterns across modalities, may respond differently to various types of stressors or laboratory stress tasks, and have stress reactions that vary in duration. After these precautionary remarks, let us examine the research that has been conducted in the area of exercise and stress responses. Individuals who exercise frequently and those who are physically fit either

- Have reduced or stronger psychophysical stress responses, or
- Recover more rapidly from various stressors (e.g., Crews & Landers, 1987; Dienstbier, 1989, 1991; Hong et al., 2004; Spalding et al., 2004).

Exercise and Magnitude of the Stress Response

Changes in Systolic and Diastolic Blood Pressure and Heart Rate

In a typical study examining the relationship between exercise and the magnitude of the stress response, mildly hypertensive men participated in a 10-week aerobic training program. They had *less systolic (SBP) and diastolic blood pressure (DBP) reactivity* to a challenging video game than did untrained men who also had mild levels of hypertension (Perkins, Dubbert, Martin, Faulstich, & Harris, 1986). Illustrating the complexity of the relationship between stressors and the stress response in this classic study, the same trained and untrained men also performed a mental arithmetic task that was stressful and did not differ in *heart rate responsivity* or in other stress reactions. These results highlight differences in the magnitude of physiological symptoms when performing different tasks that are stressful.

A recent, controlled study of exercise and cardiovascular reactivity to psychological stress focused on sedentary, but otherwise healthy, young women and men ($N = 45$), rather than on the typically investigated older adults with cardiovascular health concerns (Spalding et al., 2004). In support of a meta-analytic review of aerobic fitness and reactivity to psychosocial stressors (Crews & Landers, 1987), aerobic exercise had stress protective effects. Participants were between the ages of 19 and 22 years, were normotensive, and performed a stressful mental arithmetic task for approximately six minutes to provide a baseline set of measures indicating their reaction to psychological stress. Stress indices included the usual measures of systolic blood pressure (SBP), diastolic blood pressure (DBP), heart rate (HR), and rate-pressure product (RPP; a product of HR and SBP that indicates workload and myocardial oxygen consumption). After the initial baseline testing on the stress-producing task, the young women and men were randomly assigned to one of the three treatment conditions: Aerobic Exercise ($n = 15$), Weight Training ($n = 15$), or No-Treatment ($n = 15$). These initially inactive participants completed six weeks of supervised physical activity or no-treatment. Aerobic exercise sessions were at a fairly intense 70% to 85% of maximal heart rate, and participants completed three to five 20- to 30-minutes sessions a week for the six-week period. Strength training sessions were three to five times a week for six weeks in 40- to 45-minute sessions. The third group of participants had no-treatment. Participants then completed the stressful mental arithmetic task a second time. After the six-week period of exercise or no-treatment, results supported the stress-protective benefits of the aerobic exercise, but not of strength training as indicated by HR and RPP when performing the mental arithmetic task. Weight training had some influence on stress reactivity as indicated by the result that both aerobic training and weight training participants had lower SBP in response to the stressor than did the no-treatment participants. These impressive results suggest that aerobic exercise training in particular has a protective role in the age-related increases in hypertension and coronary heart disease by decreasing cardiovascular stress reactivity for people who participate in aerobic exercise early in life and continue aerobic exercise across their lifespan (Spalding et al., 2004).

Magnitude of the Stress Response: Increases in Mental Processing, but Few Changes in Emotional Reactivity

In a set of investigations examining the influence of an aerobic exercise session on both (1) emotional reactivity and (2) ability to perform a cognitive task utilizing working memory, there was little evidence that acute, aerobic exercise influenced emotional reactivity (Tomporowski et al., 2005). The exercise did facilitate mental processing. In the first investigation, nine men who were recreationally active performed a memory taxing task that required response-inhibition, the Paced Auditory Serial Additional Test (PASAT; Gronwall & Sampson, 1974). The men then rated the difficulty or workload of the task on the NASA-Task Load Index (TLX; Hart & Staveland, 1988) which is designed to measure changes in emotional states, or emotional reactivity. After completing the baseline PASAT and TLX and resting for 60 minutes, the men performed a 40-minute cycling session at 60% of VO_{2max}. Then, they once again completed the PASAT and TLX. Results indicated that the single, 40-minute bout of exercise improved the men's cognitive performance, but had little effect on their emotional reactivity as compared to baseline.

A second investigation employed a 120-minute cycling session at 60% to 75% VO_{2max} that was completed by ten highly trained women competitive cyclists who then performed a memory taxing, response-inhibition task, the PASAT (Tomporowski et al., 2005). After completing the task, the women rated the difficulty or workload of the task on the NASA-Task Load Index. Results indicated that the single, 120-minute bout of exercise improved the women's cognitive performance, and that ratings of Frustration decreased significantly. The exercise had little effect on their other ratings of emotional reactivity. In conclusion, these two investigations suggest that acute, aerobic exercise facilitates mental processing. The aerobic exercise, however, did not seem to blunt the negative psychological effects (i.e., the emotional reactivity to the taxing mental workload of the PASAT; Tomporowski et al., 2005). As with any non-significant findings, many factors, such as the specific exercise durations of 40 and 120 minutes and small number of participants, may explain the lack of change in emotional reactivity caused by the demanding mental task. The possibility of decreased emotional reactivity following an exercise session needs further investigation.

Magnitude of Differences: Intra-Individual Interactions Between Psychological and Physiological Responses to Stress

Within a particular individual, there often is a lack of correlation between physiological and psychological/behavioral changes in stressful situations. For example, Roskies and colleagues (1986) observed no changes in physiological reactivity to stressful laboratory tasks, even though there were psychological changes. In this study, men who were high in Type A characteristics or highly prone to stress participated in one of three stress management approaches for a 10-week period: cognitive-behavioral techniques, weight training, or aerobic exercise. Participants in the cognitive-behavioral stress management treatment group significantly reduced their Type A behavior as measured in a structured interview. Men who were in the weight-training program changed some of their Type A behavior, but participants in the aerobic exercise group showed no changes in their Type A behavior patterns.

This study emphasizes that there can be behavioral or psychological benefits even when there are no physiological changes as a result of exercise. Physiological and psychological responses to stress often appear to be independent. Sometimes there are psychological changes such as tension and depression in response to stressors, but no accompanying physiological changes. Other times, there are physiological signs of stress such as an increased heart rate, but no measurable psychological stress indices. There is considerable need for additional research in this fascinating area of exercise psychology in order to understand the apparent lack of a relationship between psychological and physiological stress indices.

Fitness Levels and the Magnitude of the Stress Response

An individual's physical fitness level may be related to his or her responsivity to psychosocial stressors. Studies in this area employ correlational designs in which the responses of people with high and low fitness scores are compared. As with all correlational research, the results should be interpreted with caution. People who differ in physical fitness also may vary on other influencing variables such as (1) personality (e.g., hardiness, Type A behavior, and self-efficacy) and (2) biological/genetic constitutional factors (e.g., low resting heart rate and low blood pressure). These variations could moderate their responses to stressors. In one study, both highly fit and sedentary men had similar cardiovascular and sympathetic nervous system responses to *novel* stressor tasks (Claytor, 1991). However, with repeated experience or overexposure to the tasks, fit individuals had an attenuated stress response as indicated by their arterial pressure and cardiac output.

There is further evidence that highly fit individuals in comparison to those who are sedentary have attenuated stress responses (Holmes & Roth, 1985; Hong et al., 2004; Keller & Seraganian, 1984; Sinyor, Golden, Steinert, & Seraganian, 1986). For example, when exposed to a stressful psychological test, highly fit women had comparatively lower elevations in heart rate than did women who were less fit (Holmes & Roth, 1985). Other studies also support an attenuated stress response in fit individuals. Highly fit women have reported lower diastolic blood pressure and psychological distress reactivity scores after performing a

mental arithmetic task than have women who are less fit (Long, 1991). In another study, physically fit men had higher levels of norepinephrine and prolactin, which could indicate a more efficient stress response during three stressful laboratory situations (Sinyor, Schwartz, Peronnet, Brisson, & Seraganian, 1983). The same physically fit men also had a more rapid return to baseline, thought to be indicative of psychological well-being, than did untrained men. Other investigators, however, have reported no differences in cardiovascular reactivity to stress for individuals differing in physical fitness (e.g., Roth, 1989).

Illustrating the complexity of the relationship between physical fitness and the magnitude of the stress response, there may be a difference between habitual exercisers (physically fit individuals) and less fit individuals as indicated by their responses to different types of stressors (Hong et al., 2004). Volunteers who were physically active according to their self-reports ($n = 24$) showed attenuated responses to a psychological stressor as evidenced by specific subsets of their lymphocyte levels including natural killer (NK) cells in comparison to their less fit counterparts ($n = 24$). The high- and low-fit participants performed two different stressful tasks: a 15-minute speech task (psychological stressor) and a 15- to 18-minute ramped bicycle ergometer exercise task performed at approximately 75% estimated maximal heart rate (physical stressor). Both tasks were stressful as evidenced by participants' increases in plasma epinephrine, norepinephrine, and numbers of lymphocyte subsets. The more physically fit participants had attenuated responses on selected lymphocyte subsets or indices in response to the speech stressor when compared with the less fit participants. Since there was little difference between the high- and low-fit groups in response to the exercise stressor, exercise seems to involve more complex mechanisms than psychological stressors. These cross-sectional results suggest that physical fitness levels may affect people's immune responses to a psychological stressor, but not to a physical stressor (Hong et al., 2004). Future studies are needed to assess fitness more objectively than the self-reports used in the study and to assess the intensity of the exercise in which participants habitually engage. Such studies will provide further insight into the effects of physical fitness on people's responses to a wide variety of stress indices including the immune regulation in response to various stressors.

Exercise and the Duration of the Stress Response

Prolonged activation of the autonomic nervous system puts wear and tear on the body and often has harmful long-term effects. If exercise-related cardiorespiratory efficiency promotes faster recovery from stress moreso for fit than nonfit individuals, then exercisers would have more time between stressors to maintain equilibrium. Abbreviated stress responses are highly desirable because there is less wear and tear on the body. However, relatively few investigators have examined this relationship.

Rapid Heart Rate Recovery

When comparing the stress responses of exercisers to those of sedentary individuals, exercisers have *higher* levels of norepinephrine and prolactin and more rapid heart rate recovery following the stressors than do untrained individuals (Sinyor et al., 1983). These differences indicate that exercisers have a shorter stress response or less physiological disruption than do nonexercisers. Other researchers have found no exercise-related benefits for responsivity to a laboratory stressor of mental arithmetic as measured by heart rate (Albright, King, Taylor, & Haskell, 1992; Roskies et al., 1986; Sinyor et al., 1986), cardiovascular reactivity as measured by EKG response, or blood pressure (Albright et al., 1992; Roskies et al.; Roth, 1989).

Aerobic Exercise Programs and the Duration of the Stress Response

Aerobic training may facilitate faster recovery from laboratory stressors. Testing this possibility, adult women and men were randomly assigned either to an exercise group, or to sedentary activities. The exercisers reported faster electrodermal recovery than did those in either music appreciation or yoga meditation (not exercise) groups (Keller & Seraganian, 1984). Yoga meditation was a control activity for expectancy effects because meditation often is employed as a stress reduction activity. Participants in each of the three activities met in 30-minute sessions and practiced 4 days a week for a period of 10 weeks to develop competency in each of the stress management techniques.

In addition, the participants performed two laboratory stress tasks during weeks 2, 6, and 10. In week 2, the three groups were nearly identical. In weeks 6 and 10, the exercisers had a quicker autonomic recovery from stress. Because the recovery time for participants in the other two groups remained unchanged, exercise was a superior technique for managing stress. Neither participants' expectancy of benefits nor the self-selection into an appealing group activity appeared to mediate the tendency for high levels of fitness to produce more rapid autonomic recovery from stressful laboratory tasks. A quicker autonomic recovery might allow people who are aerobically fit to cope with emotional stress more effectively than less fit individuals.

Fitness Levels and the Duration of the Stress Response

Levels of physical fitness may influence the duration of a variety of responses to stressful tasks, although the relationship is not always clear. Highly fit men between the ages of 20 and 30 years had different response profiles to three laboratory stressors than did those who were less fit (Sinyor et al., 1983). In addition to their higher levels of norepinephrine and prolactin early in the stress period, the highly fit men had more rapid heart rate recovery after the stressors and lower levels of state anxiety. This study by Sinyor et al. (1983) is one of the few in which physiological and psychological stress responses are similar.

Illustrating the complexity in this area of research, Long (1991) investigated the stress responses of heart rate, systolic and diastolic blood pressure (SBP & DBP), and blood levels of epinephrine, norepinephrine, and cortisol. Women between the ages of 18 and 48 years ($M = 30$) were separated into high and low fitness groups according to their scores on a submaximal bicycle ergometer test. After initial baseline testing, the women completed two stressful tasks, mental arithmetic and an "electrocardiogram quiz," for a total of 10 minutes. Their stress responses were measured after a 15-minute baseline period, the 10-minute stressor tasks, 5 minutes of recovery, and 30 minutes of recovery. Women who were more physically fit recovered faster on heart rate and norepinephrine measures than did those who were less fit. After adjusting for initial baseline differences between the two groups, however, there were no differences in recovery from the stressors. These results of Long (1991) differ from those other studies (Hollander & Seraganian, 1984; Sinyor et al., 1983) in which highly fit individuals have more rapid heart rate recovery to stress. Long (1991) completed additional statistical analyses to examine select subgroups of highly fit and poorly fit women. The highly fit women had an attenuated stress response in comparison to the less fit on diastolic blood pressure and on psychological distress. Again, there were no differences in duration of stress responses. These results suggest that the more efficient recovery to stress by highly fit individuals in other studies may be due, at least partially, to initial differences in fitness between the groups.

Acute Effects of Exercise on Stress Indices: Before and After an Exercise Session

Many researchers in the area of exercise and its influence on the magnitude and duration of the stress response have focused on the chronic exercise and stress indices that are measured at the beginning and end of an exercise program. Other researchers have examined the influence of differing aerobic fitness levels on stress responses. Still other researchers have investigated the influence of acute exercise, or single exercise sessions, on stress responses.

In a typical study of the acute effects of exercise, highly fit racing cyclists performed a stressful laboratory test (modified Stroop color task) 30 minutes after each of three laboratory conditions (Rejeski, Greg, Thompson, & Berry, 1991). The conditions included light exercise (50% of VO$_2$max for 30 minutes), heavy exercise (80% of VO$_2$max for 60 minutes), and a control activity. Testing was conducted once a week for three weeks. In these fit cyclists, a single exercise session influenced the magnitude, but not the duration, of their stress responses. After the 60 minutes of high-intensity exercise, the cyclists had significantly less change in mean arterial blood pressure and lower systolic and diastolic blood pressure after the Stroop task than they did after a control activity. After 30 minutes of light exercise, cyclists had significant benefits on two of the three blood pressure indices. They showed decreases in their mean arterial and diastolic blood pressure. There were no differences between the three activities in the magnitude of heart rate responsivity. There also were no differences between the exercise and control conditions on blood pressure and heart rate recovery when measured 5 minutes after the stressor.

Questioning whether exercising with another individual influenced the stress-reducing benefits of exercise, Thomas Plante and his colleagues (2001) examined the acute effects of a 30-minute exercise session on a stationary bicycle at a moderate intensity level of 60% to 70% of maximum heart rate. They randomly assigned participants ($N = 136$) to one of three exercise treatment groups: 1) exercising alone, 2) exercising in the presence of another person who also was riding a bicycle ergometer but not talking with that person, and 3) exercising with another person riding an ergometer and talking with that person. All three groups of exercisers reported decreased stress as indicated by significant increases in self-reported energy, and calmness and decreases in tiredness on the Activation-Deactivation Adjective Check List (Thayer, 1986) immediately after a single exercise session. Participants who exercised in the presence of another person—regardless of social interaction or talking—reported more calmness, but also more tiredness than participants who exercised alone. Plante and colleagues (2001) speculated that the increase in tiredness may be the result of increased competition and /or increased workload. The potential influence of exercising in the presence of another individual on the role of exercise in stress management, especially on calmness and tiredness, is an important topic worthy of further investigation.

Hatha Yoga and Stress Management

Hatha yoga is a specific type of exercise that focuses on psychological stress reduction. As illustrated on the April 23, 2001, cover of *Time* magazine, "Millions of

---

Table 8.2

Hatha Yoga Procedures for Relaxation and Body-Mind Integration
(Goyeche, 1979; Iyengar et al., 2005; Patel, 2003)

Procedure	Purpose
Maintenance of a variety of postures	Stretch major muscle groups and affect total bodily carriage
Practice of "head-low" postures	Increase blood flow to head
Ocular and vocal muscle stretching	Temporarily inhibit normal patterns of perceptual-cognitive functioning (this, in turn, is said to facilitate concentration)
Voluntary relaxation of breathing	Interrupt irregular breathing patterns and restore optimal diaphragmatic breathing
Practice of complete somatopsychic relaxation	An optimal period at the end of a yoga session

Americans are discovering this ancient exercise" ("Science of Yoga," 2001). In the feature article, Carliss (2001) explores the medical benefits of yoga and examines available scientific support for its effectiveness. Yoga is thousands of years old and thus is described as the oldest assemblage of exercises designed to enhance human health by integrating body, mind, and spirit (Patel, 2003).

Because of its holistic approach, yoga is of great value for stress management. The word *yoga* is derived from the Sanskrit root-verb *yuj,* which means, unite, control, or join together. Yoga literally means joining of body, emotions, and the mind (Hittleman, 1969; Patel, 2003; Vann, 1983). Most types of yoga systematically combine personal reflection, quiet observation, breathing exercises, and physical exercise in precise postures or *asanas*. Asanas promote steadiness, strength, suppleness, and spine flexibility (Patel, 2003, p. 12). Hatha yoga, the physical exercise form of yoga, incorporates the relaxation procedures highlighted in Table 8.2. These procedures include maintenance of asanas, inclusion of "head-low" postures, ocular and vocal stretching, relaxing one's breathing, and specific relaxation techniques employed at the end of a yoga session (Goyeche, 1979).

Components of Hatha Yoga

With its relative lack of mysticism and religious overtones, hatha yoga is the form of yoga most often practiced in the West. Hatha yoga aims at connecting the body to the mind and soul and at increasing communication among the body, mind, and soul (Iyengar, Evans, & Abrams, 2005). Hatha yoga is based on maintaining two major components: *asanas* or precise postures, and *pranayama* or the use of breath regulation to control vital energy. The asanas are specific body postures that are maintained for approximately eight to ten seconds. Pranayama, or breath/energy control, is designed to prepare the mind for meditation (Patel, 2003, pp. 12, 26). Hatha yoga is said to unlock participants' latent energies and to facilitate self-development (Patel, 2003, p. 12).

Asanas, or postures, within the practice of hatha yoga are thought to influence both cognitive and somatic functioning and thus are ideal for stress management. The asanas develop muscular flexibility, which seems to automatically decrease muscular tension. Tensing and relaxing specific muscles groups in each asana is somewhat analogous to the tensing and relaxing of specific muscle groups in Jacobson's (1976) stress management technique known as progressive relaxation.

Prana is the subtle universal energy or breath that "pervades all entities" (Patel, 2003, p. 26). *Pranayama* refers to energy/breath control, to the harmonization of

breath to movement, and the regulation of breath. Pranayama is another major component of hatha yoga. This component is most evident in such specific breathing exercises as alternate nostril breathing and the complete breath. In addition to the specific breathing exercises, however, there is a conscious awareness of breathing throughout the entire yoga session. Illustrating the importance of breathing, Finger and Guber (1984) suggest that "when doing postures let your breath be your guide. If it becomes harsh and jerky, you're overdoing it. Always keep your breath full and even . . . . Breathing is the key to understanding prana—our life force" (p. 20). Emphasizing the importance of pranayama and its benefits for stress management, Iyengar and colleagues (2005) suggest that

Breath is the vehicle of consciousness, and so, by its slow, measured observation and distribution, we learn to tug our attention away from external desires (vasana) toward a judicious, intelligent awareness (prajna) . . .

By drawing our senses of perception inward, we are able to experience the control, silence, and quietness of the mind. (p. 12)

Effectiveness of Hatha Yoga for Stress Reduction

Yoga, with its emphasis on body postures, breathing, and the mind-body-spirit connection, seems to be effective in reducing stress, enhancing mood, and treating a wide range of psychosomatic disorders (Carliss, 2001; Ghoncheh & Smith, 2004; Kabat-Zinn, 1982; Kabat-Zinn, Lipworth, & Burney, 1985). It also has been a successful approach to treating a variety of stress-related disorders such as asthma, migraines, chronic gastrointestinal disorders, and hypertension (Goyeche, 1979; Patel, 1973, 1975a, 1975b). Berger and Owen (1988, 1992a) found that participants in hatha yoga consistently reported acute benefits in mood. These benefits included decreases in state anxiety, tension, depression, anger, fatigue, and confusion.

Comparing the effectiveness of yoga stretching and progressive muscle relaxation for their differential positive psychological effects, rather than for the reduction of arousal or stress symptoms, Ghoncheh and Smith (2004) concluded that the two relaxation techniques were associated with differing psychological effects. Although the exact content of each relaxation technique as employed in the study is somewhat uncertain, it seems that yoga and progressive relaxation were differentially effective. Participants in five-week yoga stretching sessions reported significantly higher Physical Relaxation in the first week. As reported, participants in each of the two activities did not differ in their increases in the Energized or Aware categories at the beginning and end of the training sessions as measured on the Smith Relaxation States Inventory (Smith, 2001). Participants in the progressive muscle relaxation sessions reported higher scores on Disengagement and Physical Relaxation in week four, and higher scores on Joy and Mental Quiet in week five, than did the participants in yoga stretching (Ghoncheh & Smith, 2004).

Clearly there is a need to continue examining the differential effectiveness of yoga with its emphasis on yoga postures and breathing with other types of exercise for stress reduction and psychological well-being. Many yoga participants begin yoga practice for practical reasons such as coping with stress or a sports/exercise injury (Iyengar et al., 2005). However, as emphasized by B. K. S. Iyengar (Iyengar et al., 2005), one of the world's masters of yoga, in his recent book that is based on his 72 years of yoga practice, the yoga journey is to wholeness, inner peace, and ultimate freedom.

Yoga provides an opportunity for spiritual self-realization; for feelings of lightness, calmness, and joy; and an inward journey of self-discovery (Iyengar et al., 2005; p. xxi). These benefits of yoga are in direct opposition to the symptoms of stress. To explore your personal reactions to yoga, enroll in a hatha yoga class and complete the sequence of activities outlined in Case Study 8.1. It is important when exploring the benefits of yoga that you participate in more than one session, preferably five or six yoga sessions, in order to establish a beginning level of competence and to become comfortable with the activity. Completing the Case Study will provide you with some personal data for discussing the questions about the possible effectiveness in the use of hatha yoga as a relaxation form of exercise.

Potential Mechanisms Underlying the Yoga-Stress Relationship

Possible bases of hatha yoga's relaxation effectiveness include such underlying neurophysiological mechanisms as increased proprioceptive feedback, deconditioning of irrelevant muscular tension, greater oxygen consumption, and being with the moment. Yoga definitely encourages a high degree of somatic awareness, which is a first step in effective stress management. In conclusion, yoga is an effective, pleasant, simple, and inexpensive stress management technique that has many of the additional health benefits of exercise.

Exercise and Physical Fitness as Moderators of the Stress-Illness Relationship

Exercise may decrease the likelihood of illness associated with high levels of life stress (e.g., Brown, 1991; Brown & Siegal, 1988; Hong et al., 2004; Roth,

Wiebe, Fillingim, & Shay, 1989). In a well-designed, prospective correlational study of the relationship between exercise habits, stressful life events, and health, Brown and Siegel (1988) linked stressful life events to deteriorating health, but only for the adolescents who exercised infrequently. The undesirable impact of stressful life events on health decreased as the amount of exercise increased. This was true for both aerobic *and* anaerobic types of exercise.

Results of a subsequent prospective study support the possibility that physical fitness protects individuals from illness during periods of stress (Brown, 1991). This study used more objective measures of fitness and illness than did the self-reports employed by Brown and Siegel (1988). Fitness measures included performance on a submaximal bicycle ergometer test and a self-report. The two illness measures were the number of visits to a medical facility and a self-report inventory. A submaximal stress test is not a perfect measure of fitness, and visits to a medical facility may indicate a variety of things other than health, such as a low pain threshold. These measures, however, are less subject to a "response bias" and to forgetting than are the subjective measures used in many other studies.

Only the students who were low in physical fitness had increased illness associated with high life-stress scores. Further supporting the stress-buffering effects of exercise, highly fit students who had high stressful life-event scores did not have high illness rates. This study (Brown, 1991) is particularly sound because the relationship between fitness and illness was prospective. *Prospective* means that the life stress occurred during the fall semester in which the study began, and illnesses occurred in the subsequent spring semester. Of course, the results are not completely certain due to the impossibility of randomly assigning study participants to experimental conditions of high and low life stress.

Potential Causal Mechanisms

Both of the causal mechanisms for the fitness-illness relationship suggested by Brown (1991) and Brown and Siegel (1988) were psychologically based as reflected by

- Increased feelings of perceived control and mastery, and
- The restorative function of time-out from stressful circumstances.

Another study illustrates the complex relationship between fitness and illness (Roth et al., 1989). Perceived fitness (as measured by a paper-and-pencil inventory) and the psychological characteristic of hardiness were related to low illness rates in undergraduate students. Students who judged themselves to be fit, regardless of their actual fitness levels, had fewer ill-

CASE STUDY 8.1

Exploration of the Stress Management Effects of Hatha Yoga

Yoga is a gentle type of exercise based on asanas and pranayama and is conducive to relaxation. Because of its primary emphasis on stretching, flexibility, strength, and breathing, some participants in high intensity exercise find it difficult to participate in yoga. This case study encourages you to obtain personal experience with yoga to become more familiar with the activity.

Regardless of whether you have completed a yoga class or have knowledge of the activity, the case study is designed to assist you in exploring the value of yoga for your own use. By becoming familiar with this exercise mode, you will be able to form knowledgeable opinions, and possibly recommend yoga to your clients and students.

ENROLL IN A HATHA YOGA CLASS

A major requirement in this Case Study is that you enroll in a yoga class. You will need to attend and participate in *a minimum of three (and preferably five) hatha yoga sessions* to become familiar with the exercise format and also grow comfortable with the teacher and your own reactions. The need for sustained participation in yoga (even more than three to five sessions) reflects the view that the exercise portion of yoga (i.e., performance of the asanas and pranayama) is only the beginning to a *lifelong* turning of our awareness inward through the practice of yoga. As emphasized by Iyengar (2005), hatha yoga is much more than attending a few classes and mechanically performing a set of asanas. It is using the asanas to join or integrate the multiple components of our being. By participating in three to five yoga sessions, you will gain initial information about yoga and stress management that may be useful as you work with clients and students. As described by Iyengar (2005),

. . . we will discuss asana not in terms of the techniques of each position but in terms of the qualities and attributes that one must strive for in all asana and in life. As we perfect asana, we will come to understand the true nature of our embodiment, of our being, and of the divinity that animates us. And when we are free from physical disabilities, emotional disturbances, and mental distractions, we open the gates to our soul (atma). *To understand this, one must gain far more than technical proficiency, and*

one must do asana not merely as a physical exercise but as a means to understand and then integrate our body with our breath, with our mind, with our intelligence, with our consciousness, with our conscience, and with our core (italics added). In this way, one can experience true integration and reach the ultimate freedom. (pp. 22-23)

DATA GATHERING

Directions: Circle the number that indicates the level of the mood or feeling states you are experiencing.

Note: Make separate copies of this rating form for *each* of the days that you plan to attend and evaluate a yoga session.

Pre-Yoga Measures

Before going to the class and as close to the class session as possible, record how you feel by circling the appropriate number for each of the following feeling states:

Scale

1 = Low level
2 = Somewhat low level
3 = Moderate level
4 = High level
5 = Extremely high level

State	Level				
Anxiety or tension	1	2	3	4	5
Stress level	1	2	3	4	5
Depression	1	2	3	4	5
Anger	1	2	3	4	5
Fatigue	1	2	3	4	5

Total Negative Feeling States Score (sum of all numbers circled) _____

Enjoyment	1	2	3	4	5
Feelings of peace	1	2	3	4	5
Mental clarity	1	2	3	4	5
Vigor	1	2	3	4	5

Total Positive Feeling States Score (sum of all numbers circled) _____

CASE STUDY 8.1 (cont.)

Total Feeling State Score _____ (Positive Feeling States Score minus the Negative Feeling States Score)

Participate in the Yoga Class: Generally, a 60-minute session

Post-Yoga Measures

Within 30 minutes of the yoga session, preferably immediately before the world intrudes, record your post-exercise feeling states by circling the appropriate number.

Scale

1 = Low level
2 = Somewhat low level
3 = Moderate level
4 = High level
5 = Extremely high level

State	Level				
Anxiety or tension	1	2	3	4	5
Stress level	1	2	3	4	5
Depression	1	2	3	4	5
Anger	1	2	3	4	5
Fatigue	1	2	3	4	5

Total Negative Feeling States Score _____

Enjoyment	1	2	3	4	5
Feelings of peace	1	2	3	4	5
Mental clarity	1	2	3	4	5
Vigor	1	2	3	4	5

Total Positive Feeling States Score _____

Total Feeling State Score _____ (Positive Feeling States Score minus the Negative Feeling State Score)

CAPTURING YOUR YOGA EXPERIENCE:

(Additional Qualitative Data Collection)

To describe the essence of the yoga class completed, record the following after each session:

1. What did you enjoy about the class?
2. What aspects of the class presented a difficulty to you?

3. How able were you to perform the asanas?
4. Were you able to avoid competition with yourself? With others in the class?
5. What were your feelings of personal ease in the class?
6. What concerns did you have as you were in the class?
7. Do you have other pertinent observations about the yoga class?

DATA ANALYSIS

Analyze and discuss the following in regard to each of your yoga sessions. Provide as much information about each of your experiences.

1. Compute your **Total Negative Mood States Scores** for _each_ of the yoga sessions, and compare your post-yoga scores to the pre-yoga scores.
2. Compute your **Total Positive Mood States Scores** for _each_ of the yoga sessions, and compare your post-yoga scores to the pre-yoga scores.
3. Compute your **Total Mood States Score** for the _combined days_ by adding the Negative Mood States Scores and forming a Total Negative Mood States Score and subtracting from them your Total Positive Mood States Score.

DISCUSSION: Effectiveness of Hatha Yoga for Stress Management

1. Describe and elaborate on how the changes in mood states and your enjoyment of the activity changed (if at all) from the beginning to the end of a class session.
2. Discuss how your mood states and enjoyment might have changed from one session to the next as reflected by your post-yoga score, and then describe the factors that might have caused these changes.
3. Analyze and discuss whether you would consider practicing yoga on a more long-term basis and why.
4. Discuss whether you would recommend to your students or clients that they enroll in a yoga class. If so, to whom would you make this recommendation? Why?
5. Finally, discuss the key issues in your personal analysis of the stress management benefits of hatha yoga.

nesses. In contrast to the results of other studies (e.g., Brown, 1991; Brown & Siegel, 1988), self-reports of exercise participation were not related to illness. There also was no evidence that perceived fitness, current amount of exercise, or hardiness moderated the stress-illness relationship. Because studies focusing on fitness as a moderator of the stress-illness relationship contain a wide variety of variables and measurement approaches, it is not difficult to discern why the results of the studies disagree with one another.

Habitual exercise and fitness may decrease the likelihood of becoming ill during periods of prolonged stress by increasing the number of natural killer (NK) cells. NK cells provide a primary defense system against foreign materials in the body and can partially control foreign materials until the antigen-specific immune system begins to respond (Herberman & Ortaldo, 1981). Physical activity of varying duration and intensity is associated with increases in NK cells immediately after exercise (Brahmi, Thomas, Park, & Dowdeswell, 1985; Hong et al., 2004). In support of the protective role of exercise in the stress-illness relationship, people who have higher fitness levels have attenuated responses to a psychological stressor as indicated by their lymphocyte levels in comparison to those who have lower fitness levels (Hong et al., 2004). It is not clear, however, whether the attenuated lymphocyte responses to stress in regular exercisers has noticeable, real-life implications for the health-illness relationship (Hong et al., 2004).

A certain amount of exercise may have a positive influence on immunity. However, there can be "too much of a good thing." Exercise programs that exhaust the participant may compromise the participant's immune system by decreasing NK cells (Berk et al., 1990). For example, 10 experienced marathoners who exercised for three hours in the laboratory on a treadmill had decreased levels of NK cells (in comparison to their baseline levels; Berk et al., 1990). Their NK levels were significantly decreased 1.5 and 6 hours into the recovery period. Twenty-one hours after exercising, their NK-cell activity had returned to baseline levels. Thus, even highly trained individuals who run to exhaustion may show decreases in NK cells. Further research is needed to delineate the relationships between fitness level, exercise intensity, exercise duration, and increases and decreases in NK cells.

Conclusions: Exercise, Physical Fitness, and the Stress-Illness Relationship

Physical fitness and habitual exercise seem to moderate the relationship between life stress and illness. The illness-prevention benefits of exercise appear most helpful during times of high stress. Because exam periods are particularly stressful for college students, students should schedule exercise sessions during finals week and during other times of perceived stress. Moderate levels of exercise may attenuate the stress response to psychological stressors and also increase the level of NK cells and thus strengthen the immune system for most recreational participants.

In contrast to the stress-reduction benefits of moderate exercise, the exercise intensity and duration levels at which some highly motivated exercisers and competitive athletes exercise may compromise their immune levels. It is encouraging to note, however, that within 21 hours after highly trained marathon runners completed an exhausting 3-hour treadmill run (equivalent to a marathon), their natural killer cells returned to baseline levels (Berk et al., 1990). Marathoners and participants in other physical activities of long duration and high intensity would be well-advised to avoid people with colds and other contagious diseases the day following their exhaustive physical activity because of their lower defense abilities.

Exercise and the Toughness Model of Stress Responsivity

The toughness model of stress described in Chapter 7 separates stress into positive stress arising from *challenges* and negative stress as a result of *threats of harm and loss* (Dienstbier, 1989, 1991). Challenges may activate the sympathetic nervous system (SNS)-adrenal-medullary arousal system and increase circulating levels of adrenaline and noradrenaline. These psychophysiological responses result in a host of desirable exercise performance and psychological benefits. In contrast, threats of harm and loss activate the pituitary-adrenal-cortical arousal system, which releases cortisol and results in the unpleasant feelings of stress. The toughness model of stress proposes that stress management is synonymous with an increase in SNS-adrenal-medullary arousal rather than with arousal reduction.

According to the toughness model, habitual exercise is a major intermittent stressor that strengthens the individual and enables her or him to respond to all types of stressors with less psychological distress and with more highly skilled behavior. Exercise psychologists should be interested in the fact that Richard Dienstbier (1991), a psychologist at the University of Nebraska, recommends the use of exercise for stress management over and above the other stress management techniques such as the relaxation response, progressive relaxation, and cognitive restructuring. Parts of this appealing toughness model "are closely bound to replicable research, other aspects are somewhat speculative" (Dienstbier, 1991, p. 849).

Dienstbier (1991) theorizes that frequent exercise

serves as an *intermittent* stressor that over a period of time leads to the following increases in

- Availability of catacholamines for coping,
- Release of catecholamines in response to stressors, and
- Sensitivity of the physiological systems to catecholamines.

These neuroendocrine changes, associated with habitual exercise, result in improved coping, resistance to depression, emotional stability, and immune system enhancement.

Contrary to the common belief that attenuated catecholamine stress responses to laboratory stressors are desirable, Dienstbier (1991) suggests that individuals who have the larger rather than smaller increases in urinary catecholamines perform better on laboratory tasks. It is only when people either are severely taxed by exercise and overtraining or are stressed for *continuous periods of time* in their lives that they have continuously elevated base rates of catecholamine levels. These chronic elevations in catecholamines and increased pituitary-adrenal-cortical functioning (increased cortisol) are associated with psychological distress and low levels of performance. In contrast, rapid decreases (in addition to initial large increases) in urinary catecholamines after a stressor or challenge are associated with enhanced performance on laboratory tasks, emotional stability, and low levels of anxiety (Dienstbier, 1991).

Responding to the very important question "Why are catecholamine enhancement effects from exercise seldom found?" Dienstbier (1991) concluded that aerobically trained individuals do not show increased catecholamine capacity to *all* stressors. The specific laboratory procedures and methodology in studies of stress and exercise are crucial. Exercise-trained individuals do not demonstrate their increased catecholamine capacities when stressors are not taxing. This includes tasks of short duration, tasks that are familiar, and tasks that are unimportant to the participant. If the tasks are too taxing, both exercisers and nonexercisers respond with their full neuroendocrine capacities. The few studies that have shown increased catecholamine production from trained individuals to psychological stressors have employed stressor tasks that are 45 minutes in length or longer. Typically researchers use stressor tasks of 5 to 10 minutes. Dienstbier's (1989, 1991) toughness model is appealing and supports the effectiveness of exercise as a stress reduction technique.

Relationships Between Exercise and Stress Levels in Specific Populations

Participants in Cardiac Rehabilitation Programs

Traditionally, the focus of cardiac rehabilitation programs has been on employing exercise to improve multiple aspects of cardiac functioning to decrease the risk of disabling illness and death. These exercise programs have been successful in reducing the risk of mortality by as much as 20% to 25% for those who participate (Oldridge, Guyatt, Fischer, & Rimm, 1988). Health, however, includes considerably more than avoiding death and even returning to the level of physical functioning prior to a coronary event. Recognizing that health encompasses more than the absence of disease, directors of cardiac rehabilitation programs are initiating multifaceted aspects of health promotion in programs to improve both quantity and quality of life of patients.

In many cardiac rehabilitation programs, stress management classes are offered to assist participants in regulating their stress levels. These classes are important because stress and emotional distress are risk factors for ischemic heart disease and sudden cardiac death (Denollet, 1993a, 1993b). In addition, heart specialists are beginning to focus on the mood benefits of exercise in addition to its physical training effects

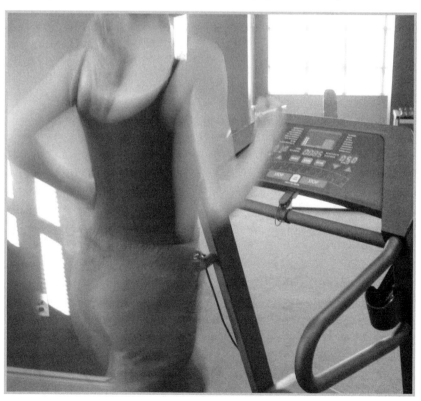

Photo courtesy © iStockphoto.com

for improving cardiac functioning. Stress emotions, especially negative mood states such as anxiety, depression, and anger, have been related to heart disease and coronary events (e.g., Kawachi, Sparrow, Vokonas, & Weiss, 1994; Ketterer, 1993). Thus, the exercise portions of cardiac rehabilitation programs provide dual benefits: the promotion of mood alteration as well as the cardiorespiratory conditioning to assist participants in reestablishing active, productive, and enjoyable lives.

Recognizing the need for cardiac rehabilitation programs to help participants improve their quality of life, researchers are investigating psychological benefits of cardiac rehabilitation programs. In a study of 60 cardiac patients, participants completed psychological and physical performance measures at the beginning and end of a 3-month rehabilitation program (Denollet, 1993b). Participants in the exercise program reported significant increases in positive affect, decreases in negative affect, and improvement in feelings of disability and well-being in comparison with cardiac patients who did not participate in the program. These psychological benefits are similar to those of a recent examination of the quality of life and mood states of participants in a phase II cardiac rehabilitation program (Engebretson et al., 1999).

The structured program included three physical conditioning sessions per week that initially were 10 to 15 minutes in duration and progressed to 30 to 45 minutes of continuous aerobic exercise. The 75-minute sessions included exercise as well as sessions on nutrition, medical education, and risk-factor reduction. When measured at the beginning and end of the 12-week, 36-session program, the men and women reported less distress as indicated by decreases in Tension, Depression, and Total Mood Disturbance and increases in Vigor on the POMS. Participants also reported enhanced quality of life as evidenced by improvements in physical functioning, energy, and health perceptions. Exercisers who were high in trait anxiety were especially responsive to the structured rehabilitation program. Thus, participants in cardiac rehabilitation programs who are high in trait anxiety should be targeted in the future with treatment packages that include mood and stress management skills and more frequent medical monitoring.

Patients with Chronic Obstructive Pulmonary Disease

The stress management benefits of exercise are of value to individuals with chronic health problems. Men and women with chronic obstructive pulmonary disease often have emotional distress—especially anxiety and depression—that is associated with limita-

tions in activities of daily living (Emery, Schein, Hauck, & MacIntyre, 1998). Participants who were randomly assigned to one of three separate treatment groups met daily for a five-week period. The treatment groups included a variety of components including exercise and stress management:

- **Group 1.** *Exercise sessions* of 45 minutes each, and weekly one-hour *stress management sessions* on progressive muscle relaxation and strategies to reduce negative emotional consequences of cognitive distortions, and one-hour *education sessions* focusing on medications and other topics related to the disease;
- **Group 2.** *Stress management* and education sessions but no exercise; or
- **Group 3.** *Wait-list controls.*

The exercisers reported reductions in anxiety and depression, demonstrated improved cognitive performance, and increased their cardiopulmonary endurance. These changes were not observed in the other two groups. These mood, cognitive, and physiological benefits for the combined treatment group in patients with chronic obstructive pulmonary disease were impressive. Exercise and stress management techniques together may provide important contributions to the quality of life of individuals with chronic health problems with which they will be living for a considerable number of years.

Paradoxical Relationship Between Stress and Exercise Participation

Highly stressed individuals need to practice stress management and coping techniques to lower their stress levels and perhaps experience fewer illnesses and a higher quality of life. Although exercise is an ideal stress management technique, individuals who are experiencing high levels of stress in their lives may be less inclined than others to exercise on a regular basis (e.g., Johnson-Kozlow et al., 2004; Kouvonen et al., 2005; Oman & King, 2000). This paradoxical relationship—the greater the need to exercise to reduce stress, the less likely individuals exercise—may reflect a variety of factors that need investigation. One factor may be a lack of awareness or understanding of the stress-reducing benefits of exercise. Other factors may include the conflicting time demands often associated with resolving life stressors and daily hassles, or the low energy levels and fatigue that is experienced when stressed. As reflected by the following studies, the dynamics underlying the relationship between experiencing high levels of stress and subsequent physical activity is an area in need of continued investigation.

Work-Related Stress and Decreased Physical Activity

In a large cross-sectional study of 46,573 Finnish workers (37,530 women and 9,043 men) between the ages of 17 and 64 years, higher work stress was associated with lower levels of leisure time physical activity (Kouvonen et al., 2005). Participants were classified into the following work-stress categories to investigate the relationship of job-related stress, as indicated by job control and work demands, to exercise participation. The resulting categories were as follows:

- **High strain** as evidenced by low job control, and high job demands,
- **Low strain** as evidenced by high job control, and low job demands,
- **Active jobs** as reflected by high job control, and high job demands, and
- **Passive jobs** reflected by low job control, and low job demands.

Participants completed inventories to indicate the average amount of time spent each week in leisure time activity and in journeying to and from work during which the exercise intensity as at least the intensity of vigorous walking, jogging, and running. Their time spent in equivalent leisure time exercise activities each week was multiplied by the activity's typical energy expenditure as expressed in metabolic equivalent tasks (METs) to form a MET index, the sum of leisure MET hours/week. Separate analyses were conducted for men and women, for three socioeconomic groups, and for three age groups: ages 17 to 34, 35 to 50, and 50 to 64 years.

Results indicated that leisure time exercise was higher for men than for women, decreased with age, and was lowest for manual workers and highest for lower socioeconomic non-manual employees (Kouvonen et al., 2005). Although the findings were complex, leisure time exercise decreased primarily for individuals who had low job control (i.e., those categorized as high job strain or as passive). This relationship between low job control and low levels of leisure exercise was evident regardless of whether their jobs had high or low task demands. In addition, males and older workers who had active jobs (high in control and high in demands) reported lower leisure time exercise (Kouvonen et al., 2005). As the authors concluded, the associations were not explained by other correlates of physical activity such as socioeconomic status, marital status, or trait anxiety.

This study on work-related stress suggests that people who are most stressed and need to exercise are less likely to exercise than their less-stressed counterparts (Kouvonen et al., 2005). Facilitating their participation in exercise activities in worksite health promotion programs and in leisure time may help interrupt the decline in exercise activities in response to high stress and to lower job strain and stress from low job control. Such worksite health promotion programs are needed to address the paradox that individuals who need to exercise the most tend to be the least likely to exercise in their leisure time.

Intervention Designed to Interrupt the Relationship Between Life Stress and Decreased Physical Activity

Based on the undesirable link between high stress and decreased exercise, Johnson-Kozlow and her colleagues (Johnson-Kozlow et al., 2004) designed an exercise intervention course for university seniors about to graduate to facilitate their participation in physical activity, especially when feeling stressed. The course included specific instruction in the use of physical activity as a method of stress management, emphasized the scientific data suggesting that exercise can reduce the physiological and psychological symptoms of life stress, and was based on the transtheoretical model of exercise adoption and adherence. Course content also was designed to emphasize the multiple benefits of exercise, enjoyment of physical activity, goal setting, and relapse prevention. Johnson-Kozlow and her colleagues randomly assigned students to one of the two three-month courses and compared the effectiveness of the exercise intervention course to a comparable control course that focused on general health topics.

Results indicated that male students in the exercise intervention course who had high levels of negative life stress on the Life Experiences Survey (Sarason, Johnson, & Siegel, 1978) during the past year were more active than men in the same intervention class who had lower levels of negative life stress when measured nine months after the conclusion of the three-month course (Johnson-Kozlow et al., 2004). Since highly stressed individuals generally exercise less than those who are less stressed, these results suggested that the intervention class designed to help students use exercise as a stress management technique was successful—at least for men who subsequently experienced high levels of life stress. Clearly the relationship between ongoing stress levels as indicated by negative life events and hassles, and the use of exercise as a stress management technique, is complex. Additional research is needed to determine how to assist women as well as men and other subsets of the population who have high levels of stress in employing exercise as a stress management technique.

A Novel View of Stress: Imbalance Among Physical, Mental, Emotional, and Spiritual Components of Health

Stress may be more than a reflection that our personal resources are inadequate to address our many needs and life tasks. Stress may be a reflection that we "believe in one way and live in quite another. Our stress may be an issue of personal integrity rather than time pressure: A function of the distance between our authentic values and how we live our lives" (Seaward, 1997b, p. ix).

Brian Seaward, a faculty member at the University of Colorado and a noted stress researcher and stress therapist, suggests that the view of stress as a response that produces wear and tear on the body is mechanistic. Human beings certainly are more than machines. Although stress does include wear and tear on the body and reflects an inability to cope with demands, it may be something more. Stress may result from "a feeling of separateness from God, a feeling of being disconnected from our divine source" (Seaward, 1997b, p. 11). Seaward conceptualizes stress with the following statements:

- Stress is tension between divine will and free will.
- Stress is tension between ego and soul.
- Stress is coming to terms with the responsibility to venture in uncharted territories.
- Stress is resistance to living the present moment.
- Stress is learning to employ the power of spirit through love at times when it seems there is none left to give.
- Stress provides the greatest opportunity for the growth of the soul (p. 55).

Stress may reflect an imbalance of mind, body, and spirit as suggested by Seaward (1997b) in his thought-provoking book *Stand Like Mountain, Flow Like Water*. The book title reflects the message that standing like a mountain imparts a feeling of stability. Moving like water indicates the need to go with the flow, rather than resisting and trying to change things over which we have no control. To flow like water implies the ability to persevere, yield where necessary to gain strength, and move on once again. What this ageless wisdom advises is to have strength and security in your own being, like a mountain, yet at the same time hold the fluidity of moving water (Seaward, 1997b, p. 8).

An underlying theme in Seaward's (1997b) book is that a cause of stress is losing a sense of our soul. Activities such as exercise—when practiced with a sense of awareness (especially hatha yoga)—meditation, and prayer can help to reduce feelings of stress. Stress is exacerbated by an imbalance. Seaward (1997b) suggests that balance is the ability to achieve a sense of symmetry in our life. Balance is a learned skill that must be practiced regularly with the constant recognition of our spiritual essence (Seaward, 1997b). This view of the spiritual elements within stress emphasizes the need for a broad psycho-spiritual-physiological approach to stress management.

Relative Effectiveness of Exercise in Comparison to Other Stress Management Techniques

Investigators have compared the chronic effects and relative effectiveness of aerobic exercise with a variety of other stress management techniques. In comparisons of stress management techniques such as exercise, the relaxation response, progressive relaxation, and cognitive appraisal, participants usually are monitored on a variety of measures. These measures often include tension, depression, aggression, heart rate, systolic and diastolic blood pressure, and galvanic skin response at the beginning and end of the studies. Most techniques tend to be associated with changes on one or more of the parameters (e.g., Berger et al., 1988; Ghoncheh & Smith, 2004).

One problem with studies comparing only the physiological changes is that it is difficult to conclude that the results, although significant, reflect changes in ongoing levels of stress. Exercisers usually have lower heart rates and systolic blood pressure and stronger cardiorespiratory system pressure after three to six months of training programs as a result of habitual training. However, it is not clear that these changes reflect a greater ability to respond to psychological stressors in a more efficient manner. If so, the studies reviewed earlier concerning magnitude and duration of physiological stress responses for exercisers and sedentary individuals should report significant differences between groups more often. The improved physiological indices associated with habitual exercise are not synonymous with the cognitive experience of less stress.

Studies that include measures of both the physiological and psychological stress indices associated with exercise often have conflicting results. In some studies, there are many psychological changes, but few physiological changes associated with exercise (e.g., Blumenthal et al., 1989; Roth, 1989). In other studies, there are more physiological than psychological effects associated with exercise (e.g., Boutcher & Landers, 1988). It seems that each of us has diverse stress profiles and that our physiological responses often are independent of our psychological responses. Intuitively, our physiological and psychological responses to exercise and to stress should agree with one another; they often do not. Including both physiological and psychological parameters in a single study of exercise and stress seems to muddle rather than enhance our knowledge about exercise and stress management. Additional studies are needed to shed light on these apparently disparate responses.

A study of habitual exercisers and sedentary individuals illustrates the complexity of a dual approach to investigating exercise and stress indices (Boucher & Landers, 1988). Exercisers were highly trained adult males who habitually ran 30 or more miles per week for the two years prior to the study. They also had completed a 10-km race in under 36 minutes within the last year. In this study, the 15 runners and 15 sedentary men performed two tasks: running on a treadmill for 20 minutes at high exercise intensity (80 to 85% of their maximal age-adjusted heart rate) and the control activity of reading the *Readers' Digest* for 20 minutes while resting in a chair. Physiological measures (heart rate, electroencephalography [EEG], and systolic and diastolic blood pressure) and psychological measures (state anxiety and mood) were recorded during the 21 minutes before and after each of the two tasks. Runners and the sedentary men differed on heart rate, but not on systolic or diastolic blood pressure or on state of alertness as indicated by alpha brain-wave activity. Only the habitual exercisers reported decreases in state anxiety after the high-intensity jogging. Surprisingly, there were no changes for either runners or sedentary individuals on mood scores after the exercise. Because other studies have found acute changes in state anxiety and mood after less-intense exercise for all levels of participants, these results seem to indicate that high-intensity exercise can inhibit the benefits. The sedentary men who exercised reported no psychological benefits; the serious runners reported reduced state anxiety, but no other mood effects.

Summary

The results of studies examining the influence of acute and chronic exercise on a variety of psychological and physiological stress indices emphasize the difficulties in coming to solid conclusions in this area of investigation. The discrepancies in the results are difficult to interpret, because of interstudy differences in the exercise stimulus (acute and chronic programs; frequency, duration, and intensity of the exercise), participants' fitness characteristics, the dependent variables measured, and the timing of the measures (magnitude and duration of the responses). The nature of the stress tasks and the timing of a stressor in relation to the exercise also make it difficult to compare the results of one study to another. Emphasizing the complexity of the exercise-stress relationship, subjective levels of psychological stress may be independent of the psychological indices.

Despite the complexities in the area of stress, it seems that individuals who exercise frequently or those who are physically fit, or both, may have reduced stress symptoms. Aerobic exercise in particular seems to have numerous benefits that can affect cardiovascular reactivity to psychological stress (Spalding et al., 2004). More specifically, exercisers seem to

- Have attenuated (or more pronounced) psychophysical stress responses (Dienstbier, 1989; Holmes & Roth, 1985; Hong et al., 2004; Rejeski et al., 1991; Rejeski, Thompson, Brubaker, & Miller, 1992; Spalding et al., 2004),
- Recover from stress more rapidly (Crews & Landers, 1987; Keller & Seraganian, 1984; Spalding et al., 2004),
- Have less illness when experiencing many negative life events (Brown, 1991; Brown & Siegel, 1988), and
- Occasionally increase their stress levels by overexercising and triggering an immunosuppressive response (Mackinnon, 1992).

Despite these stress-reducing benefits of exercise, individuals who are highly stressed tend to participate in less leisure-time exercise than their less-stressed peers (Johnson-Kozlow et al., 2004; Kouvonen et al., 2005; Oman & King, 2000). Thus exercise programs are needed that are designed to address this paradox: the greater the need for exercise for stress reduction, the less likely the individual is to participate.

Can You Define These Terms?

acute exercise

asana

chronic exercise

duration of the stress response

hatha yoga

magnitude of the stress response

paradoxical relationship between stress and
leisure-time exercise

physiological stress indices

prana

pranayama

psychological stress indices

psychophysiological responses

quality of life

spiritual components of stress

stress responsivity

toughness model of stress responsivity

Can You Answer These Questions?

1. What are some of the psychological and physiological benefits of habitual exercise?

2. Why might habitual exercise affect an individual's ongoing levels of stress?

3. What type of study do you think is needed to further our understanding of the exercise-stress relationship? Explain whom you would select as subjects, the procedures followed in the study, types of measures that you would use, and the results you would expect.

4. Why does hatha yoga seem to be a particularly effective exercise mode for stress reduction?

5. Why might exercisers differ from nonexercisers in either the magnitude or duration of physiological stress indices?

6. How does the toughness model of stress responsivity predict that exercisers will respond to stressors?

7. Do exercisers have as much illness as sedentary individuals? Please explain your answer.

8. What factors contribute to the contradictory results concerning the possible influences of exercise on stress responsivity?

9. How might a primary cause of stress be loss of a sense of our soul?

10. Why might exercise serve as a particularly useful stress-management technique for people with health problems such as those with coronary artery disease?

11. Can you explain the paradox that highly stressed individuals (who can benefit the most from the stress-reducing effects of exercise) tend to exercise less than their less-stressed counterparts?

12. How would you design, promote, and supervise an exercise program to encourage highly stressed individuals to participate in leisure-time exercise?

text. We can learn not to aggress in certain environments, although this does not mean that the trait or tendency is not present.

Some theorists use the word *type* to refer to a collection of traits. Within the type, traits are activated to varying degrees in response to different environmental stimuli.

Origins of Personality

- What are the origins of personality?
- Do we inherit traits, or are they acquired during our lifetime?

Recently, geneticists have been attempting to show that coded information in our genes substantially influences the strength of personality traits. Some individuals, therefore, may be "programmed" with behavioral inclinations. Evidence in support of genetic/behavioral links continues to be found, particularly in animal studies (Bouchard & Lochlin, 2001; Johnson, McGue, & Kreuger, 2005).

Two appropriate issues require attention:

- Do traits make their existence known throughout all situations?
- Are they enduring?

These questions continue to generate much discussion and disagreement among psychologists and a number of theories (none of which is definitive, however) offer possible clarifications. Table 9.1 provides a sample scenario that differentiates among four such theoretical approaches.

Trait theory. In spite of the aforementioned caveat about the predictability of behavior through the exclusive use of personality trait scores, some authorities believe that behavior is indeed fundamentally a function of traits that are stable and endure throughout all or most situations. *Trait theorists* (see the studies and writing by such investigators and theorists as Cattell, Eysenck, and Guilford for examples of work based in trait theory) maintain that traits appear very early in life and are not easily manipulated. A considerable body of evidence strongly suggests that some personality traits continue to develop after childhood, with a considerable amount occurring in young adulthood (Helson, Kwan, John, & Jones, 2002; Roberts, Robbins, Caspi, & Frzesniewski, 2003). However, traits vary in both the extent and complexity of change. What accounts for this change? Some personalogists take the position that we (humans) harbor genetic *predispositions to change* in particular ways. Supposedly, as we age our dispositions to undergo trait alterations express themselves. The Five Factor Theory (McCrae & Costa, 1994) proposes that personality trait development is largely a genetic phenomenon. A contrary view is offered by other scientists who argue that experiential forces (cultural) account for the changes (Roberts, 1997). It is this latter perspective that appears to receive considerable research support (Roberts, Wood, & Smith, 2005). Perhaps the most acceptable resolution to this debate is to conclude that environmental variables influence the genetic tendencies.

Some theorists allege that traits are transmitted genetically or at least have a hereditary connection. They have devised trait personality tests that yield profiles of an individual's behavioral dispositions, although, as the renowned psychologist Cattell (1973) observed some time ago, traits need not be assessed exclusively by verbal reports or pencil-and-paper instruments. Observations conducted in the real world or laboratory settings may also be helpful. If such approaches are properly constructed and applied, they should contribute to an understanding and prediction of all kinds of behavior, including exercise.

Whereas traits are supposedly stable (enduring), the word *state*, on the other hand, refers to temporary feelings of a brief and changeable nature. For example, a person may briefly feel anxious in a particular circumstance, and thus experiences a *state* of anxiety. However, one who is often anxious and who scores high on a test of anxiety may be said to have high *trait anxiety*. This would be in contrast to someone who briefly feels anxious and has low trait anxiety. *Traits* are stable over long periods whereas *states* are not. Another way of characterizing this comparison is to say that trait anxiety is a general predisposition to experience fluctuating states of anxiety. For a thorough analysis of traits and states, consult Spielberger's book, *Anxiety: Current Trends in Theory and Research* (1972).

Until recently, agreement was lacking among personality scientists as to what constitutes basic personality structure and there are varying opinions about how many factors exist within an individual's personality. Some psychologists, such as S. B. G. Eysenck (1983), argue that there are but three components. In contrast, Cattell, Eber, and Tatsuoka (1980) believe the number of personality factors to be 16. Currently, many experts consider a five-factor model to be the best representation of personality.

For examples of this position, see Digman's "Personality Structure: Emergence of the Five-Factor Model," McCrae and Costa's "Personality Trait Structure as a Human Universal," and Smith and Williams's "Personality and Health: Advantages and Limitations of the Five-Factor Model."

In this model, the following dimensions (traits) are included:

a. neuroticism or emotional stability,
b. extraversion,

c. openness to experience,

d. agreeableness, and

e. conscientiousness.

Despite its current popularity, the Five-Factor Theory (FFT) is not without its ardent detractors (Mayer, 2005). For instance, in a recent critique and evaluation of the model, Roberts, Wood, and Smith (2005) suggest that little support exists for the FFT. Nonetheless, the FFT has garnered enough recognition among personologists to merit inclusion and consideration here.

Other personality traits such as hardiness (strong sense of commitment, control, and challenge), dispositional optimism (generalized expectation that good things will happen), and health locus of control (belief that one's health is under personal control) have been related to health and fitness. These traits have been hypothesized to account for strong or weak responses to painful (discomforting) stimuli during exercise, willingness to enter an exercise program for the first time, ability to get along with other participants, and possession of adequate self-discipline to remain in the exercise program.

Situational approach. In contrast, other theorists place greater emphasis on *situational influences*, such as the particular role a person believes he or she is fulfilling at a particular time. For instance, when participating in a group discussion of politics, a reticent person may try to influence the group's level of cohesion or bestow order in a setting that is becoming increasingly heated. Although not inclined to do so in other situations, she may become more assertive in an attempt to exercise leadership. In other words, those who believe in the predominant influence of the *situation* feel that behavior changes in accordance with what is happening in the environment (Mischel & Shoda, 1995). According to this approach, personality traits alone account for only modest amounts of behavioral variation.

Interactionist approach. Interactionists believe that a combination of personality traits and situational factors accounts for behavior. They believe that traits, as they exist in an individual's psychology, countermand one another, modify each other, and interact with various aspects of the environment and one's perception of the reason for being in it (Endler & Magnusson, 1976). The interactionist explanation currently enjoys considerable favor among psychologists working in the area of personality; however, it too is not immune to criticism.

Fischer and Zwart look closely at the interactionist approach in "Psychological Analysis of Athletes' Anxiety Responses," as do Vanden Auweele, De Cuyper, Van Mele, and Rzewnicki in "Elite Performance and Personality: From Description and Prediction to Diagnosis and Intervention."

Very few psychologists deny the existence of traits. Similarly, few believe traits to be the exclusive determinants of behavior. Thus, because the interactionist approach allows for both views, it is considered to be most helpful and sound.

Psychodynamic approach. In attempting to clarify the bases of personality, some authorities emphasize subconscious forces that act upon behavior. The *psychodynamic theory* of personality, perhaps the oldest, maintains that unresolved unconscious problems—notably, psychosexual problems—contribute to an individual's personality. Some of these may relate to incidents that occurred many years in the past and may have been repressed or buried in low levels of awareness. Other incidents may be recognized but not fully understood. Thus, personality may be clarified in terms of a person's individual struggle to resolve his or her drives or conflicts. Certain behaviors contribute to this resolution and eventually become preferred or frequently exhibited. In this way, the renowned patriarch of psychoanalysis, Sigmund Freud, accounted for behavioral tendencies. Extended one-on-one discussions between professional consultants and their clients would be necessary to encounter unconscious or inaccessible motives and inhibitions for behavior.

According to Freud, whose ideas represent the basis of the psychodynamic approach, personality comprises three major components: id, ego, and superego. Freud viewed the *id* as the personality's biological entity, containing its sexual and primitive urges. It moved the individual towards pleasure and away from pain. The *ego* was considered by Freud to contain

Table 9.1
Characteristics of High and Low Sensation-Seekers

1. High sensation-seekers appraise many situations as less risky than do low sensation-seekers.

2. When risk appraisal of high and low sensation-seekers is equivalent, high sensation-seekers report a reaction of less anxiety and more positive affect or sensation-seeking state arousal.

3. The difference between high and low sensation-seekers on anxiety and sensation-seeking states i less in low-risk than in high-risk situations.

4. For high sensation-seekers, particularly males, there is little increase in anxiety and little drop in sensation seeking in response to high-risk situations in terms of the model proposed.

CASE STUDY 9.1
Mary's Locker-Room Behavior

Different Theoretical Approaches: Different Explanations

Mary is dressing in her exercise club's locker room. Another woman whom she has never before seen has just showered and towel dried herself. She now proceeds to splash talcum powder on herself, much to Mary's annoyance, because Mary's jeans and recently cleaned sweater that she has just removed and was in the midst of hanging up in her locker are also being powdered, although apparently unintentionally. Mary is bothered by this and remarks to her neighbor, "Please watch what you are doing. You are getting that stuff all over my clothes." Mary's neighbor tells her to stop whining—that these things are expected in locker rooms. Words are exchanged, followed by shouting and shoving. Mary grabs the canister of powder and dowses the other woman, who, in turn, throws Mary's sweater on the damp locker room floor. Other women intervene and restore order.

Trait Theory Approach

Mary's tendency to aggress is strong. She is also high in the trait "assertiveness." She always behaves in similar fashion. She often argues and frequently engages in shoving bouts with others. This is the way she is. She is, by nature, very assertive and tends to lose her temper.

Situational Approach

Mary would not behave in this fashion in other locales. She perceives the locker-room environment as an acceptable place for altercation. The constraints she would abide by in other environments do not temper her actions in this setting. She believes that it's OK to fight in the locker room. She would never exhibit such behavior elsewhere.

Interactionist Approach

Mary came to the exercise club in a state of heightened anxiety and frustration. She received a very poor grade on an important exam and felt that her teacher's comments on the paper were uncalled for and wrong. The other woman's inconsiderate behavior was the last straw. Mary "lost it."

Psychodynamic Approach

Mary's readiness to argue and willingness to engage the other woman in altercation is related to forces operating at lower levels of her awareness. Perhaps the sweater sprinkled with powder has special meaning to her—meaning that she is not presently in touch with. Perhaps it is reminiscent of a gift that she received as a child from a beloved relative. Perhaps the powder itself triggers memories of infancy that have been buried in Mary's storage depot of unpleasant experiences.

---

unconscious and conscious elements that fought to maintain civility in the individual, to engage in logical thinking, and to keep the id under control. Lastly, Freud saw the *superego* as the force in his personal model that enables a person's behavior to be compatible with society's moral values; in other words, the superego serves as the person's conscience. It enables the individual to understand and interpret societal rewards for appropriate behavior.

Although many of the original Freudian concepts are no longer in vogue, contemporary psychiatrists and psychologists still find some of them to be useful. The importance of Freud's emphasis upon sexuality, for example, is greatly diminished today; however, his belief in the criticality of early childhood experiences largely remains acceptable.

The Relationship Between Exercise and Personality

Having completed a brief discussion of what the term personality means and what issues and conflicts it engenders among experts, we may now turn to the essential concern of this chapter: namely, the relationship between exercise behavior and personality. Conventional wisdom suggests that a combination of heredity and very long-term learning resulting from the interaction of people and their environments accounts for most of human behavior. Although we do not possess an "exercise-tendency" trait, can exercise induce changes in personality? One researcher in the field, Dienstbier (1997), responds to this question with a resounding "yes." He posits that exercise may very well influence personality through four *mediators*: physiological changes, perception of physical change, changes in patterns of socialization and living, and changes in expectations. Although Dienstbier acknowledges that it is difficult to examine these mediators in sound research frameworks, he concludes that they account for allegations that exercise does exert an influence on personality. In particular, he focuses upon running as the exercise of choice. A brief discussion of these four mediators follows.

Physiological Changes

It is well established that physiological changes accompany short- and long-term involvement in exercise. Dramatic alterations in cardiovascular function, cellular biochemistry, respiration, and hormonal and enzymatic production usually accompany exercise. These changes may be associated with alterations in mood and temperament shifts.

> Yeung (1996) looks closely at the interaction between physiological change and state change in the article "The Acute Effects of Exercise on Mood State."

Although some changes may be of short duration, others may endure. Some authorities view these effects upon psychology as personality changes. Among the first to discuss these alleged effects was Cureton (1963). Although an exercise physiologist, Cureton was interested in the effects of exercise upon psychological states. After observing that scores on eight factors of Cattell's Sixteen Personality Factor Questionnaire (Cattell & Eber, 1961) correlated positively and significantly with an intense treadmill run, he concluded that personality is responsive to physical training due to changes that can be made in the autonomic nervous system and in cardiovascular condition. It is, however, questionable if the more deeply embedded, or core, personality traits would be modified during or as a result of a brief, although intrinsic, episode of exercise, as Cureton's findings imply.

Perception of Physical Change

Overt physical changes involving redistribution of body weight, reduction of stored body fat, and increased energy levels associated with regular participation in exercise regimens are likely to result in improved body image. When you believe that your appearance has improved and feel that your functioning has changed for the better, your self-concept may very well improve—it becomes more positive, and positive self-concept has been shown to be linked with general psychological health (Sonstroem, Harlow, & Josephs, 1994). These causal relationships enable

Dienstbier (1997) to reach the conclusion that exercise (running) indeed has an impact on personality.

Changes in Patterns of Socialization and Living

This mediator refers to new relationships fostered by exercise and the lifestyle changes it initiates. New social relationships may be forged as a result of being part of new environments (e.g., health clubs, jogging groups, new contacts while skiing). When you become committed to a regular exercise program, your schedule for the day may undergo revision. You, therefore, meet different people and move in different circles, perhaps all in new places. The positive effects of long-term participation in exercise programs are also likely to result in enhanced ability to carry out normal daily tasks and roles. Physical activity is associated with improved function among relatively healthy persons as well as among those with chronic illness. Those who exercise regularly achieve improved levels of physical fitness (readiness to meet specific sets of physical tasks). Physically fit individuals are capable of expanding their range of activities and, consequently, the number of persons with whom they interact. Because exercise has opened new doors for them, participants interact with their social environment differently; that is, their behavior has changed.

Changes in Expectations

Exercise is often portrayed in such a positive light (for example, "Running is good for you") that participants actually anticipate desirable structural and behavioral change. The exerciser believes this and integrates the notion into his or her system of beliefs to the extent that a placebo effect operates.

It is worth repeating at this point that first-order, or core, personality traits are not likely to change due to exercise participation; however, behavioral tendencies (those that are role related or learned) may indeed be altered according to the dynamics identified by Dienstbier (1997). In other words, an interactional approach is understandably useful in clarifying variations in some behavioral tendencies.

Personality and Level of Fitness

Very little evidence is available that scores on personality tests predict physical fitness. However, results from some older studies conducted in the 1960s and '70s have suggested that certain traits are associated with membership in groups designated as high fitness. Each of these studies used Cattell's Sixteen Personality Factor Questionnaire (Cattell & Eber, 1961), a time-honored personality inventory that has been incorporated in a large number of sport and exercise psychology studies. It must be noted, though, that these studies are old and characterized by methodological weaknesses that minimize the value of their results. For instance, the length, type, and intensity of the fitness training programs varied, as did the definitional approach to levels of fitness. Nonetheless, McClenney (1969) reported that college-aged men, identified as "high fit," scored higher on group dependence and desire for social approval than did subjects designated as "low fit." Also, the low-fit subjects scored higher on self-sufficiency and independence with a desire to make decisions and take action of their own.

In another study, Tillman (1965) found that high-fitness groups tended to be more extroverted, more dominant, and more socially oriented than did members of low-fitness groups. Ismail and Trachtman (1973) observed high-fitness group members to be higher than low-fitness group members in emotional stability, imaginativeness, guilt proneness, and self-sufficiency. What remains unresolved, to date, is this question: Is the personality of the highly fit exerciser a consequence of his or her physical fitness, or are individuals high in certain traits to be found in greater numbers in groups identified as highly fit?

Personality and Exercise Adherence

A paramount problem for exercise leaders and those who organize and administer exercise programs is participant *adherence*—meaning the longevity of exercise involvement. Sizable numbers of those who enter exercise programs disengage shortly thereafter (Dishman, 1993; U.S. Department of Health and Human Services [DHHS], 1996). This is also true with regard to children (Douthitt, 1994). In Chapter 12, the extent of the dropout problem and suspected reasons for its high incidence are discussed.

A number of social influences have been associated with exercise adherence, such as family support and task cohesion.

To read more about this topic, see "Social Influence and Exercise: A Meta-Analysis" by Carron, Hausenblas, and Mack (1996).

The term *cohesion* refers to the "sticking together" of group members. In the sense in which we use it here, reference is made to the inclination of some exercisers to drop out of their program when social support derived from group membership wanes because the group loses its cohesive potency. Therefore, in order to adhere, some exercisers need interaction with others (Crone-Grant & Smith, 1999). Perhaps their personalities require positive evaluations of the exercise environment and its social characteristics before a comfort level (low amounts of nervousness and anxiety) adequate for adherence is secured.

For more on this, see Terry, Lane, Lane, and Kehohane's "Development and Validation of a Mood Measure for Adolescents: POMS-A" (1999).

Attitude has also been suggested as a correlate of adherence (Dzewaltowski, Noble, & Shaw, 1990; Kimiecek, 1993) and attitude, or the perspective we hold about situations, is likely to be a function of personal values as well as personality. Here, our primary focus is on personality traits that may interfere with or promote exercise adherence.

Locus of Control and Adherence

When behavioral outcomes are typically attributed by a person to external (outside the self) forces such as luck, other individuals, or simplicity/complexity of a task, an *external* attributional style is said to prevail. When event outcomes are usually viewed as being a result of personal effort or ability, the attributional style is said to emphasize *internal* control. The tendencies to ascribe behavioral outcomes to internal or external controlling factors reflect one's *attributional style*, which may also be considered a personality factor. Results of some studies indicate that attributional style may be linked with exercise adherence. For instance, individuals with internal styles tend to adhere to physical activity of the "free-living" kind more than do those with an external locus of control (Dishman & Steinhardt, 1990). A *free-living* exercise program is exemplified by unobserved behavior of an aerobic nature that is characterized by rigor and regularity. Examples include climbing stairs rather than using an elevator and walking rather than riding a bus. In other words, a person who is exercising in a free-life manner is not responding to group or leader motivational attempts in a formally organized setting. Rather, that individual incorporates appropriate principles of exercise into everyday activities.

Neuroticism and Adherence

Neuroticism is a trait included in many personality inventories. Persons scoring high on the neuroticism scale frequently complain of vague somatic problems and tend to worry excessively.

Potgieter and Venter (1995) classified 116 subjects as either adherers or dropouts on the basis of their exercising at a facility for a period of more than one year. Dropouts were observed to have significantly higher neuroticism scores on the Eysenck Personality Inventory than those of adherers. This may explain their dropping out of an exercise program. Neuroticism has been fairly well demonstrated to be negatively related to exercise participation and adherence.

Yeung and Hemsley (1997) discuss this in "Personality, Exercise and Psychological Well-Being: Static Relationships in the Community."

High levels of neuroticism may also be linked to reliance on inappropriate coping strategies during rehabilitation from injury. According to some research findings, neuroticism is positively related to rehabilitation strategies considered to be emotion-focused rather than problem-focused strategies.

See the investigation by Grove, Bahnsen, and Eklund, written up as "Neuroticism, Injury Severity, and Coping With Rehabilitation."

Among such emotional coping strategies are denial, mental disengagement, and emotional venting whereby the neurotic and injured individual deals with the injury by resorting to elevated levels of feelings. Overreliance upon such coping approaches may cause denial, mental disengagement, etc., to become dysfunctional strategies, particularly when used over extended periods of time.

Zeidner and Saklofske's (1996) "Adaptive and Maladaptive Coping" looks at just such issues.

This suggests that personality, especially the trait neuroticism, may influence rehabilitation from exercise-related injury.

Another aspect of neuroticism's relationship to exercise is its link with trait anxiety—a personality trait that refers to tendencies to respond stressfully or anxiously to many environmental stimuli. In turn, trait anxiety has been shown to be positively related to scores on neuroticism.

A. F. Jorm (1989) does this in "Modifiability of Trait Anxiety and Neuroticism: A Meta-Analysis of the Literature."

In addition, trait anxiety may also be related to injury.

As C. H. Kelly (1971) investigates in "Stress, Trait-Anxiety, and Type of Coping Process."

Also, high neuroticism scores (Eysenck Personality Questionnaire) have been shown to correlate with compulsive or excessive exercise, referred to as "exercise dependence" (Thompson & Blanton, 1987).

Additional support for considering personality in exercise contexts is provided by Courneya and Hellsten (1998). They used the five-factor model (discussed pre-viously) to examine neuroticism, openness, extraversion, agreeableness, and conscientiousness in relation not only to exercise behavior, but also to motives, perceived barriers (psychological inhibitors to exercise participation), and preferences for exercise context and structure in undergraduate college students. Extraversion and conscientiousness correlated positively, whereas neuroticism (a barrier) was negatively related.

It appears that personality information, when used wisely and judiciously, may be useful in understanding the exercise motives and barriers. Such understanding might enable professionals to match exercise programs with participants' needs and thereby maximize adherence.

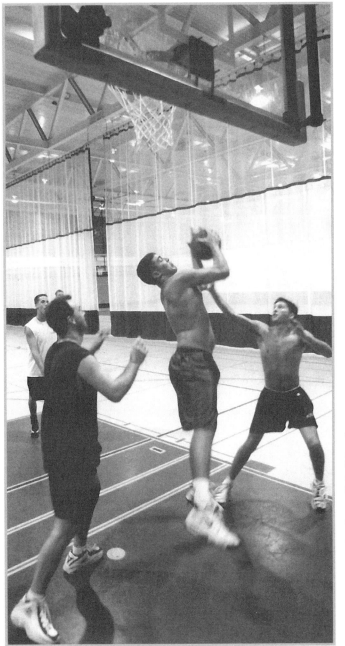

Self-Competency and Adherence

A relationship may exist between the way in which individuals continue to participate in an exercise program and the view they hold of themselves as competent people. A study conducted by Douthitt (1994) produced interesting findings pertinent to adolescent subjects. She observed a meaningful link between aspects of *self-competency* (i.e., perceived physical appearance; Harter, 1990b) and adherence. That is, those adolescents with low perceived competence scores tended to adhere better to exercise programs, suggesting the motive to improve appearance. Douthitt also examined the value of personality/sport congruence in predicting adherence. *Personality/sport congruence* refers to the hypothesized match between an individual's personality and the particular kind of exercise in which he or she is involved. Douthitt tested 132 male and female physical education high school students on an instrument that measures the congruence of personality to exercise adherence—The Psychosocial Activity Dimensions Profile (Gavin, 1987). Results indicated that the more a particular form of exercise matched a subject's personality, the more likely he or she would adhere to an exercise regimen. These interesting findings may encourage those planning an exercise program to consider their personality characteristics (weak as well as strong) before deciding upon the nature of their regimen.

A line of research pursued by Eklund and colleagues (Eklund, Mack, & Hart, 1996) has emphasized the perceptions held by exercisers about their bodies in relation to their involvement in exercise. *Social physique anxiety* is the term Eklund applies to concern about physical appearance. Individuals high in social physique anxiety are inclined to conceal their body from other exercisers or engage in exercise in order to improve their physical appearance (Crawford & Eklund, 1994; Eklund & Crawford, 1994).

Self-Motivation and Adherence

Dishman (1982) has constructed a test that he believes reveals a person's inclination to adhere to an exercise regimen. In effect, this instrument (Self-Motivation Inventory; SMI) assumes the existence of the personality trait *self-motivation*, which, when embedded in the psychology with considerable strength, enables high levels of adherence. Dishman (1993) believes that adherence to exercise is a function of one's trait measure of self-motivation that interfaces with other personal abilities and skills, but is independent of situational reinforcements. This trait, therefore, suggests that exercisers may reinforce themselves or put gratification on hold (for some future time). Dropout from exercise programs is a formidable problem for those attempting to encourage exercisers to enter and sustain adequate motivation for adherence. According to Dishman (1982), self-motivation includes self-regulatory skills such as goal setting, self-monitoring of progress, and self-reinforcement. Self-motivation also interacts with characteristics of the exercise program (high or low intensity) and the social environment in which the program takes place. Those exercisers with relatively higher levels of self-motivation who are able to self-regulate well, set personal goals effectively, and provide their own reinforcement for adhering are likely to remain in their exercise programs. In addition, Dishman and Steinhardt (1988) suggest that persons high in self-motivation may leave a supervised program in order to enter and maintain a personal program. That is, they feel they can "do it themselves."

> Of the many examples, see Knapp, Gutmann, Squires, and Pollack's "Exercise Adherence Among Coronary Artery Bypass Surgery (CABS) Patients" or Olson and Zanna's Report to the Government of Ontario, Canada, Ontario Ministry of Tourism and Recreation, entitled "*Predicting Adherence to a Program of Physical Exercise: An Empirical Study,*" or Snyder, Franklyn, Foss, and Rubenfire's "Characteristics of Compliers and Non-Compliers to Cardiac Exercise Therapy Programs."

Although the SMI has been validated through a number of studies, Knapp (1988) has raised some concerns about it.

According to Knapp, the SMI may actually assess skills acquired by individuals that permit them to continue with their exercise program despite absence of reinforcing cues. They adhere because of their conviction that exercise is the right thing for them to do. With this observation, Knapp argues that scores on the SMI may indeed be predictive of exercise adherence by assessing specific skills rather than a personality trait. Also, self-motivation, as defined by Dishman (1982), was not found to be a predictor of adherence in adolescents (Douthitt, 1994). This may suggest that self-motivation is not a core trait and is more heavily influenced by learning and experience than are first-order traits. Perhaps self-motivation is still undergoing development in adolescents.

Type A Behavior

A person who has tendencies to be competitive and hostile and who typically operates under a substantially high sense of urgency is said to demonstrate *Type A* behavior. The pattern indicates strength in certain personality traits but is also believed to be a function of learned behaviors. Those with contradictory or opposite behavioral inclinations (e.g., low competitive drive) are considered to be of the *Type B* pattern. Blumenthal et al. (1988) were able to demonstrate that participation in a program of regular exercise helped Type A individuals significantly reduce cardiovascular reactions to mental stress. Such persons may ultimately benefit from better health because their tendencies towards competitiveness, hostility, and urgency are frequently accompanied by cardiovascular turmoil that may be somewhat countermanded by exercise. According to Blumenthal et al., it is the elevated and internally directed anger-hostility, in particular, that is the primary component of the Type A behavioral profile and that contributes to cardiovascular disease. Exercise, then, may not only potentially alter mood in positive ways (see Chapter 6), but may also curtail harmful reactions to stress that influence cardiovascular health.

Personality and Risk-Taking Behavior

In 1964, psychologist Marvin Zuckerman (1979a, 1979b, 1983a, 1983b, 1994) formulated the notion of *sensation seeking* as a personality trait and believed that humans seek to find a state or level of stimulation in their immediate environment that satisfies their particular need. After observing individuals who could not be content for a few hours or days lying in a comfortable, dark, soundproof room, Zuckerman (1979a) concluded that some people are driven to seek novel experiences. He studied reasons for this and, ultimately, produced his well-known sensation-seeking hypothesis, which proposes that some individuals possess stronger inclinations than others to become involved in risk-taking behaviors. Stimulus seeking, therefore, is a personality trait and, like all others, is normally distributed within all of us. It may very well account for a share of the motivation to enter and sustain participation in an exercise program. More recently, Zuckerman (1994) revised his definition of sensation seeking to read as follows: "the seeking of varied novel, complex and intense sensations and experiences and the willingness to take physical, social, legal and financial risks for the sake of such experiences" (p. 3). These characteristics are believed to have a biological basis, and Zuckerman argues that biological disposition, reactivity, and the presence of biological correlates of sensation seeking are, in fact, genetically determined.

Evidently, some persons have stronger needs for stimulation than do others. Some of us tend to become overloaded with very few stimuli, whereas others have nervous systems that actually thrive on very substantial quantities. After becoming familiar with our personal stimulus-seeking needs, we pursue an "optimal" level; this self-perceived zone of stimulus comfort determines the intensity and direction of our volitional

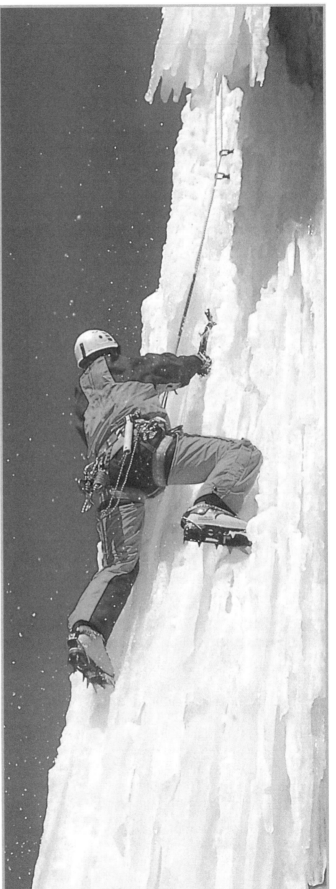

behavior. Thus, the choice to participate in exercise represents a conscious and strategic determination to satisfy personal stimulus needs. One specific dimension of Zuckerman's stimulus-seeking construct, *risk-taking behavior*, may be particularly applicable to adherence in programs of physical activity.

The term *risk* refers to the perceived uncertainty of a behavior's outcome. When a situation provides black or white, dichotomous and antithetical probabilities, including success-failure, winning-losing, injury-safety, or acceptance-rejection, then the condition of risk prevails. Risk, therefore, has a "probabilistic" nature.

See the book *Risk and Gambling* by J. Cohen and M. Hansel (1956).

Individuals who are high in sensation seeking are high risk-takers who are willing to take physical and social gambles for the sake of experience (Zuckerman, 1979b). In sum, risk-takers accept and are even attracted to the conditions implied by uncertain outcomes of a given situation (Niemand, 1978). However, the perception of risk is subjective and, therefore, varies considerably among individuals. Young automobile drivers between the ages of 16 and 24 are more likely to engage in high-risk driving behaviors and are, consequently, involved in more traffic accidents than are their older counterparts. Differences in perceptions about what constitutes a risk to physical safety thus separate the two groups.

As shown by Jonah and Dawson (1987) in "Youth and Risk: Age Differences in Risky Driving, Risk Perception, and Risk Utility."

It is precisely such variability in the perception of "risky situations," as well as inconsistencies in the definition of the term "risk," that may account for discrepancies in the risk-taking literature.

According to Zuckerman (1983a), high sensation-seekers tend to view many life activities as play. Such individuals cognitively restructure available stimuli in order to satisfy sensation-seeking needs. For instance, crossing a crowded inner-city street in defiance of the traffic signal's message, "Do not cross," may be interpreted by a high sensation-seeker as challenging or fun. Zuckerman (1983a) suggests that rough play among children is the first expression of sensation-seeking behavior, and as they grow older, formalized play (sport) becomes a natural outlet for their sensation-seeking needs. In this manner, strong sensation-seeking needs may be satisfied by individuals (adults as well as children) when they reframe ordinary situations or attach personal value of a risk-taking nature to stimuli that originally did not offer such potential. See Table 9.2 for typical characteristics of high and low sensation-seekers.

In sum, it may be concluded that individuals high in sensation seeking tend to pursue the most novel, complex, exciting, and risky experiences. In contrast, those who are low in sensation seeking require little stimulation of this kind, and individuals who are in the middle of the above extremes, seem to require some of both kind of experiences. Furthermore, midrange individuals would seek participation in medium-risk situations but would score higher on a measure of sensation seeking than would those who choose very low risk, or safe sports. Admittedly, very few studies have compared medium and low risk-taking subjects. Those studies that have been conducted exclusively use male subjects, probably because there has been little opportunity for females to participate in contact sports such as rugby, wrestling, lacrosse, boxing, and football (Durden, 1994).

Avoiding the Negative Effects of Risk-Taking Behavior

Exercisers who are inclined to enter high-risk situations should take precautions in order to avoid injury (Table 9.3 presents a questionnaire to aid in understanding your personal readiness for participation in physical activity from the standpoint of risk management). Following are guidelines intended to assist persons who advise, coach, counsel, or teach exercisers, or exercisers themselves with notable risk-taking inclinations.

Basic guidelines. Having determined that you, or someone with whom you are professionally involved, is high in risk taking or sensation seeking, there are precautions to exercise that are likely to reduce the frequency and intensity of injury. Although you may already be familiar with these guidelines, they deserve mention here so that readers may affirm the wisdom of considering and incorporating them into their preparation for exercise:

- Include a warm-up and cool-down in the program.
- Progress slowly and steadily (include at least one day a week of rest).
- Alternate heavy and light days of exercise.
- Pay attention to body signals.
- Be active all week (avoid being only a weekend exerciser).
- Use proper equipment and attire.
- Perform approved exercises and use proper form.

Extraversion and Exercise Participation

H. J. Eysenck's (Eysenck & Eysenck, 1991) personality theory complements the sensation-seeking ideas of Zuckerman. Eysenck, an internationally renowned psychologist, has long argued that we seek situations that are congruent with our personalities. Therefore,

Table 9.2
Self-Test: How Safety Conscious Are You?

Answer these questions to find out whether you are now doing everything reasonable to prevent exercise-related injury.

A. General Guidelines for Preventing Exercise Injuries

   1. I warm up before every workout and cool down at the end of each workout.

      Yes   No

   2. I increase my workload gradually.

      Yes   No

   3. I exercise consistently throughout the week, not only on weekends.

      Yes   No

   4. I wear appropriate clothing and use proper equipment for the activity in which I participate.

      Yes   No

   5. I use proper form when performing my activities.

      Yes   No

   6. I am knowledgeable about activities that have a high potential for injury and attempt to avoid unnecessary risk.

      Yes   No

   7. I pay attention to the signals (pain) that my body provides and act accordingly.

      Yes   No

B. Preventing Environmental Injuries and Accidents

   8. I take precautions related to the physical environment before engaging in outdoor activity.

      Yes   No

   9. I never swim alone.

      Yes   No

   10. I always wear a helmet when I cycle.

      Yes   No

C. Treating Sport and Exercise Injury

   11. When I suffer a minor injury, I discontinue the activity so that I can heal.

      Yes   No

   12. When I suffer a sport- or exercise-related injury I consult a health care professional to obtain diagnosis and treatment.

      Yes   No

Scoring

Give yourself 1 point for each "Yes" answer.

If you have accumulated 12 to 13 points, you are managing your activity risk adequately.

If you have accumulated 10 to 11 points, it is necessary for you to fine-tune your activity risk management.

If you have accumulated 8 to 9 points, it is necessary for you to restrategize your approach to activity risk management.

If you have accumulated 7 points or fewer, you may be at high risk for activity-related injury.

those who are high in extraversion—a trait included in Eysenck's Personality Inventory (H. J. Eysenck & Eysenck, 1964)—are inclined to gravitate to activities such as sport and exercise because it is there that they find the excitement and sensory stimulation that they require. Extraverted individuals are inclined toward outwardly directed behaviors. They pursue environments that contain other persons with whom they may interact, they enjoy being stimulated, and they desire excitement. Two Japanese researchers, Arai and Hisamichi (1998), have also reported higher scores on extraversion in a sample of 22,448 exercisers (ages

40–64 years) in contrast to nonexercisers. It may be that personality traits and not cultural factors are better predictors of exercise behavior.

Summary

All too many studies that focus on personality and sport behavior have been published. This is not the case with exercise, however. The literature dealing exclusively with exercise requires considerably more development. Consequently, there is much that is unclear about personality determinants of exercise behavior.

The term *personality* refers to behavioral tendencies. Some theorists are steadfast in their belief that these tendencies are good predictors of behavior and that adherence to exercise regimens or failure to adhere to exercise programs is a function of trait strengths or weaknesses. This approach is in contrast to other ways of understanding personality. For instance, some theorists believe that situational influences are predominant in determining behavior. In their view, traits are subservient to situational demands. Thus, exercise behaviors are a function of the role the exerciser believes she is fulfilling or the goals she is pursuing. Those forming an interactionist position believe that traits play off one another and also interact with specific aspects of the physical and social environment. An alternative way of explaining personality places an emphasis on unresolved conflicts and experiences from the past that have been repressed or buried in lower levels of consciousness.

Exercise may influence second-order personality traits by inducing the following four changes: physiological changes, perception of physical change, changes in patterns of socialization and living, and changes in expectations. It remains unlikely that first-order personality traits are affected by exercise; they are rather resistant to change in all areas of behavior.

A number of personality traits have been related to exercise adherence, including locus of control, self-competency, self-motivation, personality/sport congruence, and neuroticism. One's tendency to adhere to an exercise program may depend upon the strength of these personality traits as they exist in each individual.

The personality trait *sensation seeking* is inherent in much of exercise behavior. The term *exercise*, as used in this chapter, refers to movement involving large muscles of the body engaged in vigorous activity. Sport is a form of exercise that incorporates competition that, in turn, emphasizes success, victory, and excellence over others. We withdraw from exercise for many reasons, among them being concerned about injury. Despite careful preparatory measures, exercisers and sport participants do incur injury.

Risk suggests uncertainty in outcome. In the context of exercise or sport, this implies probability; that is, participants are unsure about what will occur. One is thus unsure of who will succeed, win, or excel.

Individuals who score high on a personality trait conceptualized by Marvin Zuckerman, known as sensation seeking, are high risk-takers and tend to pursue novel, complex, and exciting experiences. Such persons are comfortable with conditions of uncertain outcome or, indeed, even seek them.

Irrespective of the degree to which you are high or low in sensation seeking or the degree to which you are inclined to choose risky sport and exercise options, precautions should be taken prior to participation. General guidelines are thus provided in order to reduce the likelihood of incurring sport- and exercise-related injury.

Can You Define These Terms?

cohesion

core trait

ego

exercise adherence

first-order trait

id

interactionist approach

locus of control

neuroticism

personality

personality/sport congruence

personality core

personality traits

personality type

psychodynamic approach

risk

risk-taking behavior

sensation seeking

situational approach

stable trait

superego

trait theory

Type A behavior

Type B behavior

unstable trait

Can You Answer These Questions?

1. Identify and briefly discuss four theoretical approaches to understanding personality.
2. Are personality traits exclusive determinants of exercise behavior? Explain.
3. Is long-term participation in an exercise program likely to change one's personality? Explain.
4. What personality factors may influence exercise adherence?
5. Distinguish between Type A and Type B behavior. How might exercise affect an individual described as Type A?
6. How does extraversion relate to exercise participation?
7. Are high sensation-seekers likely to appraise many exercise situations as less risky than low sensation-seekers are? Explain.

CHAPTER 10

Exercise-Related Injury: Understanding and Coping

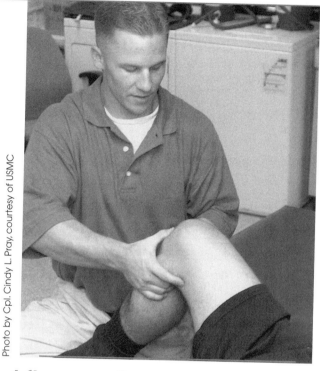

Photo by Cpl. Cindy L. Pray, courtesy of USMC

After reading this chapter, you should be able to

- Define injury,

- List and elaborate upon reasons for exercise injury,

- Discuss the computer information-processing model and its relationship to cognitive processes involved in exercise,

- Define malingering,

- Discuss why malingering is difficult to identify,

- Identify ways in which to help malingerers and injured exercisers, and

- Expand upon various aspects of pain and pain management associated with exercise injury.

Introduction

As we have so far argued or suggested in previous chapters, exercise is a popular, valuable, and necessary experience for all of us—young, middle-aged, or elderly. Although authorities bemoan the fact that too many of us do not exercise enough, millions of Americans participate and do so regularly and enthusiastically. Exercise is a popular form of leisure activity engaged in by many individuals for weight regulation and various long- and short-term health benefits. Its positive social, mental, and physical consequences are well established throughout this book and elsewhere. Because exercise may involve rigorous, strenuous, and often explosive activity done repeatedly for extended periods of time, physical injury is one of its frequent consequences. In people who are inadequately prepared for vigorous, sustained physical activity, or in whom skill levels are insufficient, the potential for injury is high. If all forms of physical exercise, including sport activities, are considered, as many as 15 million injuries occur per year in the United States (Heil, 1993).

Injury is an impediment to the accomplishment of long- and short-term exercise goals. It also may require that the exerciser establish new and different goals that place a premium on rehabilitation. Rather than attending to gains in strength, endurance, or flexibility, the injured exerciser's primary focus becomes redirected toward repair of damaged tissue. Rehabilitation regimes (which often involve exercise, but of a different kind) become paramount and displace prior exercise goals.

Positive outcome may conceivably result from exercise injury. For instance, one may meet new and empathetic friends in the physical therapist's or physician's waiting room. Exercise injury and resultant absence from work, school, or other regular activity may underscore the appropriateness of changing one's prior type of physical activity. The middle-aged runner may switch to cycling or swimming upon reinjuring her knee for the fourth time. Nonetheless, the negative consequences of injury far outweigh the possible desirable results. Although not by any means a certainty, injury assuredly looms as a likely outcome of regular and rigorous physical exercise.

What Is Injury?

For our purposes, *injury* means trauma to the body or its parts that results in at least temporary, but sometimes permanent, physical disability and inhibition of motor function. A fine line separates injury and discomfort (a feeling associated with injury), but the latter alone need not result in impaired movement. Acute discomfort or pain is typically—though not always—indicative of injury. Also, it is not necessarily true that immediate pain or discomfort accompanies injury.

Stiffness and soreness may result from a fall or excessive exercise without injury being present or without necessitating withdrawal from activity. Professional analysis from medical personnel is often required in order to establish the presence of injury. Among the diagnostic procedures used by physicians and athletic trainers are X-rays and imaging information (e.g., magnetic resonance imaging or MRI) as well as a multitude of other assessment procedures involving reporting pain upon use of a body part, observing swelling, and noting discoloration.

From a definitional perspective, *exercise injury* frequently incorporates the element of length of time of inability to participate in physical activity. Some authorities may designate a period of one, two, or three days of incapacitation as a criterion. Since researchers use different durations in their operational definitions, many reported research findings are not easily generalized from one study and sample to another. For our purposes, I offer the following definition of exercise injury: *Debilitation resulting in the inability to function as competently as before the occurrence of physical trauma during exercise participation.*

Reasons for Exercise Injury

Almost any cause of exercise injury may be located in one of the following categories:

1. Inappropriate exercise prescription,
2. Faulty execution of movement,
3. Personal psychological attributes or states (body image; perception about self),
4. Subconscious factors (psychodynamic), and
5. Environmental factors.

Recognizing and managing these five factors will help us avoid or mitigate injury.

Inappropriate Exercise Prescription

The *number of exercise sessions* per week (or per day in the case of highly trained exercisers with competitive goals or interests in more than one exercise modality) must be carefully strategized. In turn, a number of factors should determine the frequency of participation. Exercise done too frequently is likely to increase the probability of injury, especially during early stages of physical growth (i.e., young children) or for elderly exercisers, who tend to require longer intervals of rest between bouts of exercise. However, exercise that is not frequent enough may not have the desired training effects, as for instance might be the case with a program that only requires participation once a week or once every 10 days. Apparently, the physiological systems (respiratory, cardiovascular, excretory, etc.) and tissues (muscle, connective, etc.) involved in training are not likely to be altered by exercise that is that infrequent. Therefore, for optimal results, the American College of Sports Medicine (Pate et al., 1995; Schnirring, 1998) recommends that moderate-intensity exercise be performed 30 minutes every day, even if that 30 minutes is an accumulation of multiple short bouts of moderate-intensity exercise.

> Moderate-intensity exercise, for example, is the equivalent of a brisk 2-mile walk.

The *intensity* or *rigor* with which the exercise is performed must also be thoughtfully determined in order to avoid injury. Once again, maturational considerations deserve attention (maturation refers to advancement towards ultimate growth for a particular person) Individual exercise goals also merit attention here. Questions such as "What do I wish to accomplish?" and "How much resistance [e.g., weight on the barbell] is appropriate, realistic, and safe for me to handle?" deserve honest answers. All too often, failure to raise such questions or responding to them incorrectly due to naiveté or a poor understanding of personal capacities and limitations increases the likelihood of injury. An appropriate way to determine intensity of exercise is to incorporate the concept of Target Heart Rate (THR = 220—age (0.7) and THR = 220—age (0.85); American College of Sports Medicine, 1991).

Duration of the exercise bout is yet another issue to be insightfully resolved in order to assure safe and injury-free exercise. "Shall I exercise for a half hour, an hour, or an hour and a half?" Overextending the length of the exercise session may severely stress those body parts (limbs) or systems that are key participants in the activity. Tissue damage, inability of waste products to be dissipated, and undue fatigue may result. Muscular fatigue and depletion of energy sources are precursors to exercise injury.

Rest. Rest means desisting from an activity for a period of time sufficient to replenish fuel supplies necessary for specific muscular function and dissipating waste products that have accumulated as a result of exercise. Resting does not necessarily require lying in bed or even being seated. Switching from one physical activity to another and thus alternating different kinds of exercise can be restful. A schedule that includes jogging on one day, swimming the next, and cycling or walking on the third day is an example of *cross-training* and may satisfy the need for rest. The antithesis of rest is *overtraining*, which may facilitate injury.

A convenient way to recall and attend to these important considerations is with the acronym FIT: **F** for frequency, **I** for intensity, and **T** for time (duration). By considering the issues represented by each of the three letters in the FIT acronym, appropriate decisions may be made about exercise prescription.

Faulty Execution of Movement

Exercisers may also injure themselves by moving improperly. When the body moves inefficiently or incorrectly, it becomes more susceptible to injury. Erroneous movement—movement defying proper biomechanical procedure—may result in inappropriate torque (rotational force), strain on connective tissue (tendons and ligaments), and stress on parts of the skeletal framework. In other words, improper exercise movements may lead to injury.

Personal Psychological Attributes or States

The psychology of the exerciser may be another factor that contributes to injury. For instance, heightened physiological activation associated with emotions may make it difficult for the exerciser to focus attention, which, in turn, may cause poor reactions to things that are happening in the immediate area. Thus, the angry exerciser may be oblivious to internal or external cues that it is "time to stop" or "slow down." Anxiety or worry may tap into limited cognitive resources and result in reduced attention to specific exercise tasks and demands. Our capacity to interpret environmental stimuli, attach meaning to them, render judgments, and make decisions (all cognitive functions) is not infinite. Although models for multichannel information processing have been proposed and some support has been established for them, a limit undoubtedly exists as to how many stimuli may be efficiently processed at any one time (although this limit is difficult to identify).

Efficacy predictions may also bear upon one's readiness to perform exercise. *Efficacy* refers to the degree to which we believe we are prepared to satisfy tasks that confront us. Low confidence levels or hesitancy in predicting successful movement outcome may interfere with making correct judgments about how and when to use the body in a safe and proper fashion.

Researchers who use psychology to study exercise injury tend to pursue one of two pathways, focusing on either injury causation or injury recovery. Much early work was on the causes of injury, and studies were designed with an eye toward predicting exercise-related (predominantly sport) injury (Pargman, 1999). However, more effort recently has been devoted to describing and developing methods for improving injury recovery, and this line of research has yielded useful and reliable findings. One profitable area has been *compliance,* wherein attempts have been made to identify psychological factors that account (at least in part) for adherence to rehabilitation programs. Most of what has been reported along these lines, however, is anecdotal.

For a good example of this, see "Psychological Rehabilitation and Physical Injury: Implications for the Sports Medicine Team," by D. M. Wiese and M. R. Weiss.

A few older studies have looked at exercise adherence in terms of locus of control (discussed in Chapter 12). *Locus of control* is a stylistic orientation involving a tendency to attribute behavioral outcomes to personal causes such as ability or effort. This represents an internal locus. Out-of-person attributions such as luck or weather are typically made by those with external orientations. These studies concluded that when exercisers were informed of healthful benefits of participation, investigators observed a significant positive relationship between internal locus of control and exercise. As Pargman tells us, "Because injury rehabilitation involves a high level of adherence (to exercise and physical activity) locus of control may be linked with injury recovery success" (p. 7). Duda, Smart, and Tappe (1989) and Fisher, Domm, and Wuest (1988) reported that self-motivation was an important factor in adherence to programs of rehabilitation.

Despite the above comments that imply doubt about using psychological variables to predict exercise injury, Williams and Andersen (1998) have proposed an attractive model that incorporates psychosocial factors that bear upon sport injury.

The model integrates cognitive, psychological, attentional, behavioral, intrapersonal, social, and stress history variables in an attempt to predict injury. To date, it has been applied almost exclusively to sport, but it also deserves consideration in the area of exercise. Of paramount importance in the Williams and Andersen (1998) perspective are the participants' history of total life stress, stress-coping resources, and stress responses. Essentially, the model implies that individuals who are able to manage stressful situations or interpret certain environmental stimuli as being nonstressful may avoid exercise-related injury. For this reason, the Williams and Andersen model is considered a *cognitive appraisal model of injury prediction*. We therefore propose that if the word "exercise" is substituted for "athletic" in the model (see the box on the extreme left side of Figure 10.1), then those dealing with or worrying about exercise-related (anxiety) would be relatively more vulnerable to injury. Persons with personality components that tend to make them anxious (e.g., trait anxiety—see Chapter 5) would be inclined to appraise environmental and exercise-related stimuli as being stressful. Axiomatically, injury itself is a source of stress, and resulting anxiety may, in turn, fuel additional injury or interfere with rehabilitation. As injured athletes have been shown to experience heightened levels of tension, anger, depression, confusion, and fatigue and

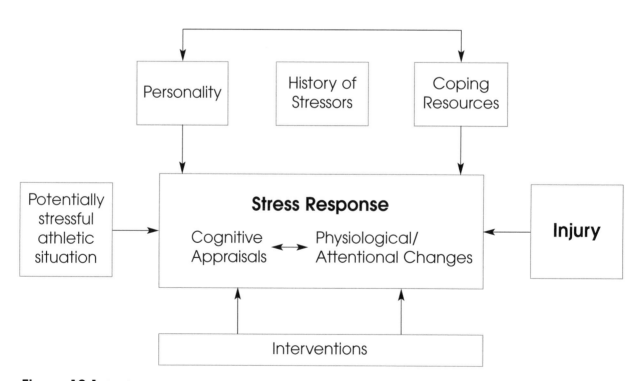

Figure 10.1. Revised version of the stress and injury model.
Note: The original model did not have the bidirectional arrows between personality, history of stressors, and coping resources.

decreased levels of vigor and self-esteem, so may be the case with injured exercisers.

For a closer examination of this topic, see "Sport Injury and Grief Responses: A Review" by Evans and Hardy.

Additional psychological factors that may be associated with injury incidence are self-perceptions, including self-concept and body image. Self-views fluctuate, and if they involve inaccurate perceptions and judgments about the ability to satisfy certain task requirements, they may cause doubt. In contrast, they may also result in overconfidence. Either outcome may set the stage for injury. Misplaced confidence in a whitewater rafter's readiness to tackle a particular course or an incorrect assumption that one can indeed bench press a large amount of weight may predispose to injury. Self-perceptions undoubtedly play an important role in injury rehabilitation as well. Later in this chapter we will discuss cognitive appraisal, or how an injured exerciser understands the severity, nature, and consequences of an injury. Incorrect judgments about readiness to return to exercise after injury, based on inflated self-confidence, may lead to unfortunate reinjury.

Whenever feasible, exercise leaders should examine the confidence and self-perceptions of participants in their programs with an eye towards realism. Some exercisers may not hold accurate views of their preparedness to satisfy certain exercise demands. Their assertion that "I can do it" may not always be correct.

Some twenty-five years ago, Yaffee (1978) suggested that injury (not necessarily exercise or sport injury) could be understood by considering the injured individual's self-concept. And indeed, Lamb (1986) was able to report a significant inverse relationship between self-concept and injury frequency in sport. Pargman and Lunt (1986) also reported a negative correlation between self-concept and injury severity in freshman collegiate football athletes. This suggests that athletes or exercisers with weak self-views and doubt about their personal resources (in physical, social, and intellectual matters) but who nonetheless persist in executing the exercise tasks confronting them despite the formidable challenges they present may be vulnerable to injury. However, despite such reported linkages between injury and psychological variables, it is appropriate to conclude that psychological factors alone are not likely to be the most influential cause of exercise injury. Other factors that may have tangential psychological implications may contribute to a far greater extent. An example of such a factor would be overuse, which may indeed have a psychological foundation. Why is the exerciser participating to an abusive extent? Or why is the individual responsible for the activity prescription assigning improper frequencies and intensities? Such factors that may be responsible for injury and have psychological overtones are not endogenous to the exerciser.

Anderson and Williams' Stress/Injury Model. A model that clarifies injury in sport may also have value in explaining psychosocial factors underlying exercise injury.

This model emphasizes what participants are thinking during physical activity. Those who are cognitively focused upon stress-related issues may be vulnerable to injury since stress buildup compromises coping ability. Thus the result may be fatigue or injury. The flipside of this speculation is that exercisers who manage stressful situations well or who tend to interpret environmental exercise stimuli as non-stressful would succumb to injury with lower frequencies. Again, the Anderson/Williams' Model is designed to explain a possible connection between stress-coping resources and stress responses and sport injury. It is, however, speculatively applied here to exercise in that the two physical experiences overlap in many of their basic elements.

Risk-taking/stimulus-seeking behavior. Mastery of risk is a thrill that makes many forms of physical activity very exciting.

See Tricker and Cook's *Athletes at Risk: Drugs and Sport* for several discussions of the thrill of risks on the part of athletes.

Through years of study, Zuckerman (1979a, 1979b, 1983a, 1983b, 1994) has concluded that all of us have individual risk-taking needs and interests. Some individuals prefer to deal with their private worlds with low levels of risk; others prefer, seek out, and gravitate to high-risk situations. Environmental demands involving issues of physical safety are physiologically, cognitively, and emotionally arousing. That is, we respond with different levels of arousal and with varying degrees of intellectual depth to various kinds of situations and challenges. According to Zuckerman (1979a, 1979b, 1983a, 1983b, 1994), some of us thrive on heightened arousal and seek it; others do not—their preference is for situations characterized by low degrees of stimulation, including risk. We may speculate here that exercisers with very high arousal requirements (where they feel comfortable) may be willing to risk safety in deference to this need. Thus, they may frequently put themselves in harm's way and be more vulnerable to exercise-induced injury than would those with lower arousal requirements. This may be viewed as a form of self-abuse through exercise or an attempt to exercise in ways that are otherwise unsafe.

Subconscious Factors

Another category of causal influence upon exercise injury may be of the subconscious variety. The speculation is that the bases for injury are psychiatric in nature. Thus, certain stimuli operating at low levels of consciousness might provoke behavior or thought that precipitates injury. However, the participant remains unaware of the underlying motives. Repressed or deeply submerged undesirable experiences, emotions such as guilt, or shameful and unacceptable thoughts may become activated, roil, and bubble. In their activation, they bear upon behavior, including exercise. They may accordingly interfere with the correct execution of motor response or influence sensory function. A consequence may be injury. An extension of this reasoning leads to the conclusion that some exercisers may actually seek injury as a form of penance or retribution for their repressed, regrettable thoughts or past experiences. In other words, undue risk-taking or

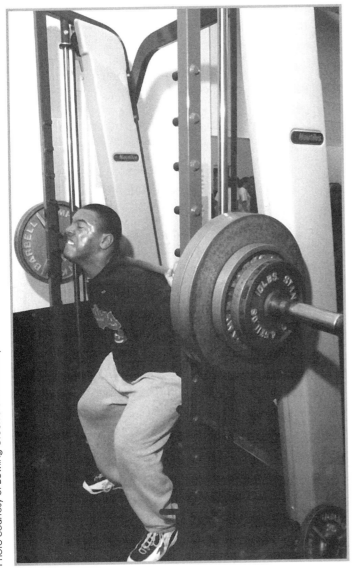

overtraining may be a result of unresolved unconscious turmoil. There have been published papers in which such dynamics are discussed.

See Nagel's article, "Injury and Pain in Performing Musicians: A Psychodynamic Diagnosis," for one example.

They are, however, few in number and presently provide fascinating reading and interesting speculation.

Environmental Factors

Injury may be caused by unwise decisions about where and when to exercise. Air temperature, humidity, and inclement weather conditions associated with heavy rain, snow, wind, and ocean water turbulence are in Mother Nature's hands. We, however, are responsible for decisions about the clothing (e.g., footwear) and equipment we wear and use while exercising under such conditions. Moreover, the decision to exercise at all in such environments is something that is under our control. Certainly, skiers, rock climbers, scuba divers, and skydivers must evaluate environmental situations and make prudent decisions about participation. If not, injury looms as an authentic consequence.

Often, the term *accident* is applied to trauma resulting from unforeseen causes. This might be exemplified by the unfortunate dropping of a barbell upon an adjacent trainee's foot or twisting and severely spraining an ankle when tripping on a tree root while jogging on a forest path. These unfortunate outcomes are due to happenstance, but banging one's head on a submerged boulder and incurring a concussion while diving into a lake where "No Swimming or Diving Permitted" or "No Lifeguard on Duty" signs are amply posted is avoidable. Such trauma as we discuss it here is not a function of accident but rather of poor decision making. Tragedies of this sort may indeed be anticipated. We make a case here for thoughtful, responsible, and prudent decision making accompanied by self-regulation—that is, the will and ability to resist entering into improper experiences. Proper choices associated with exercise location and environmental conditions decrease the probability of injury (see Figure 10.2).

Cognitive Considerations

Choice is a product of thinking, solving problems, and making judgments. We do these things in accordance with knowledge we acquire as a result of experiences. Developmental psychologists such as Piaget (1932/1965) have concluded through their research that the ability to reason and solve problems has a developmental basis. That is, children pass through stages en route to adulthood, and in doing so, their cognitive functions are expected to change and improve. Very young children, for example, have great difficulty

INJURY

◄------ No Control --- Much Control -----►

| Happenstance (Involves accidents) | Poor Decisions (Involves choices) |

♦ Cable snapping while water skiing

EXAMPLES

♦ Decision to water ski at night without lights and getting struck by the boat's propeller

♦ Being stung by a ray while swimming in the ocean

♦ Swimming despite life-guard's warning about stingrays

MEDIATORS
♦ Risk-Taking Level
♦ Cognitive Development

Accidents dependent upon:
♦ Laws of Probability
♦ Mechanical Errors (equipment failure)
♦ External Causes—Other

Choices dependent upon:
♦ Cognitive Factors (judgments, decisions, thought processes)

Figure 10.2. Decision making and exercise injury.

dealing with abstract ideas and hypothetical circumstances. They are usually unable to think reversibly or futuristically. Therefore, it may be difficult for them to associate causes of past injuries (a fall or improper use of equipment) with currently prevailing high probability of injury. Even adults may be located in different stages of cognitive abilities, making it difficult for them to anticipate imminent danger. Piaget has described the highest stage of cognitive development (Stage of Formal Operations) as being a stage in which individuals understand, for example, how billiard balls rebound off the side of the table or how a basketball may rebound off the backboard in accordance with the angle of incidence (the exact same angle at which the ball struck the table or backboard), but not all adults enter this stage and thus have difficulty resolving cognitive challenges that involve such reasoning.

If, therefore, we expect exercisers to make safe choices and proper decisions about when, where, and how to exercise, their activities should be selected (particularly in the case of children) in recognition of cognitive as well as physical developmental characteristics. A child may appear to be physically suited for an activity because of growth and level of maturation. However, sophisticated decision making may be innate to the activity. Whitewater rafting or kayaking requires quick decision making for which most young children are not yet developmentally prepared. Adult

skiers and judo participants may also commit tactical errors due to poor judgments about when to move or turn that may result in injury. Achievement of adulthood does not, by any means, confer attainment of the highest stage of cognitive development. Selection of safe and appropriate exercise forms should take into consideration reasoning, problem-solving, and decision-making capabilities of the participant.

The Computer Information-Processing Model

Some psychologists who study learning have produced a model that attempts to clarify how knowledge is acquired. Because we argue that injury avoidance involves making appropriate decisions, let us see how this computer information-processing model (CIP) works. It should explain how exercisers become knowledgeable so that they are able to make safe choices.

Again, when the model's various elements are unsatisfied (see Figure 10.3), incorrect or inadequate knowledge acquisition may occur. Correct or safe exercise decisions become less likely, with injury being an unfortunate consequence.

The dots on the extreme left side of the model represent environmental stimuli that may be understood as changes in the physical environment. A hand clap changes the sound wave structure of the environment

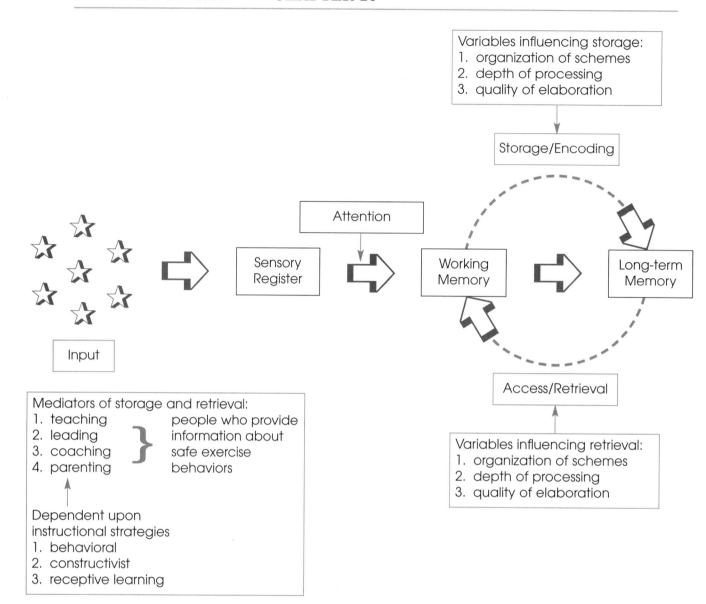

Figure 10.3. Computer information-processing model.

and is, therefore, a stimulus. The image of a bird flying overhead creates a visual environmental change and is, thus, another example of a stimulus. Ears, eyes, nose, and other specialized organs of sensation are designed to funnel stimuli into the central nervous system. Hence, reference is made to our various senses such as smell, vision, hearing, taste, touch, and kinesthesis. During exercise, some organs of sensation tend to be more critical than others. For instance, in a gross motor activity such as exercise, vision and *kinesthesis* (knowing where the body and its parts are in space) are likely to be all-important, whereas smell or taste is usually not.

The model proposes that environmental stimuli arrive at a hypothesized brain center for initial pro-

cessing—the sensory register. In a very short time, perhaps no more than 2 or 3 seconds, the incoming stimuli are sorted and roughly interpreted. Then they are shunted to the working memory part of the brain for higher-level treatment, where more fully developed meaningfulness is attached to the stimuli. Past experience is applied in this effort. Incoming material is categorized, sorted, and some of it culled or discarded. Only a small amount of information can be actively dealt with in this fashion, however, repetition (practice) can extend the amount of time the information remains active in the short-term or working memory. From the short-term or working memory, information travels to the long-term memory. Here, according to some experts, this information is stored

See the article "On the Permanence of Stored Information in the Human Brain," by Loftus and Loftus, and the book, *Educational Psychology: A Practitioner-Researcher Model of Teaching,"* by Parsons, Hinson, and Sardo-Brown, for some of the work of the experts.

permanently. Thus, everything that reaches long-term memory is filed away; the more information an exerciser has in her long-term memory repository, the more she knows about how, when, and where to exercise. She has learned about exercising safely. Information-processing efficiency is undoubtedly influenced by neuroanatomical factors that vary from person to person. The manner in which individuals attend to environmental stimuli is also variable. This means that we differ in how we process information.

There are additional components of the model. For example, how do instruction and guidance enter the model? Are there factors that may inhibit smooth processing?

Encoding. An exerciser moves volitionally or when inspired to do so by circumstances, suggestion, or command from others. He may do so ballistically, explosively, artfully, gracefully, skillfully, and accurately. Of course, his movements may also be clumsy, inaccurate, unsafe, ill conceived, or too slow/too rapid. Feedback from someone or some source in the environment interacts with the stored knowledge that has made its way from long-term memory back into the working memory. Environmental impact thus modifies the knowledge. When information about the quality of the recently executed behaviors is returned to long-term storage, it has been changed—hopefully improved and enriched. This ongoing process is known as *encoding*. Its implications for teaching and coaching are important in that leadership provides input into the encoding process. Corrections and reinforcement of correct movements provide structure to the information going from working memory into long-term storage. On subsequent occasions when knowledge about how and under what circumstances movement is to occur becomes necessary, the exercisers possessing fully elaborated bundles of information about the activity (schemes) are well prepared to act. Those with neatly organized, logically encoded schemes enjoy facility in retrieval. They can pull up the stored material more easily and quickly. Such people benefit from tricks and devices that enable logical storage and speedy accessing.

Acronyms and other mnemonic devices help facilitate logical storage and speedy accessing.

Exercise leaders should encourage use of these memory-recall techniques when teaching safe and cor-

rect procedures for exercisers. For instance, boat safety rules and procedures can be stored and recalled by use of an acronym wherein each letter of the acronym is the first letter for a word or phrase. Then, the boater need only retrieve one word or phrase (the acronym) that contains clues (first letter of each item) to all parts of the checklist (see Figure 10.4).

Inhibition. Sometimes new information making its way from the working memory to long-term memory

When going **OFFSHORE**, be sure to remember some important boating equipment.

O il

F uel

F irst aid Kit

S unscreen

H at

O ars

R adio Communication

E mergency Flares

Figure 10.4. Use of acronym for recall of safety issues in boating.

is blocked or interfered with due to attempts to activate and bring forth old information from storage. According to the CIP model, this interference is known as *retroactive inhibition* (when old material interferes with the acquisition of new material). Conversely, incoming information making its way through the processing channels may inhibit the retrieval of old knowledge. This is referred to as *reactive inhibition*.

So, injury avoidance during exercise entails sound decision making and proper judgment. Good choices are predicated upon knowledge gained through prior experience that is stored and available through information processing. Poor decisions about various aspects of exercise participation increase the exerciser's vulnerability to injury. Those who guide exercise behavior should, therefore, understand and monitor this processing. Good teaching and appropriate intervention may influence the storage and access of pertinent exercise-related knowledge. To be safe

CASE STUDY 10.1

Safety Concerns: Making Correct Decisions to Avoid Injuries and Fatalities

Consider the following tragic scenario described in a letter to the "Dear Abby" column of a local newspaper (Saturday, June 24, 2000, *The Atlanta Journal—Constitution*):

> On a lovely day in June 1986, my husband who couldn't swim but refused to wear a life-jacket, took our 3-year-old son, "Ronnie," fishing in the new "unsinkable" boat I had bought to protect them. My rule from day one for Ronnie was "no lifejacket, no water."
>
> While they were fishing, my husband somehow fell out of the boat. Ronnie went into the water to look for his father. He couldn't find him. Ronnie floated aimlessly for an hour before a wonderful teenage boy spotted him and rowed to his rescue.

> Had I not insisted that my son wear a life-jacket, I would have tragically lost both my husband and Ronnie.
>
> My husband was an adult who had a right to make his own choices in life. However, those choices ended his life far too soon.
>
> Our son could not make his own choices. As a parent, I made them for him. Fortunately, I made the right ones to protect him.

From "Mom's Rule on Life Jackets Saves Her Young Son's Life," by "Another Careful Mother in Washington," *The Atlanta Journal—Constitution,* June 24, 2000, p. C7. Copyright 2000 by *The Atlanta Journal-Constitution.* Reprinted with permission.

and injury free, exercisers should be made aware of proper training and participatory procedures. Case Study 10.1 presents the tragic tale of a man who chose to ignore safety standards.

Malingering

Malingerers are those who claim injury and incapacitation when, in reality, none has occurred. For any number of reasons, despite having made a commitment to exercise, an individual seeks to desist. She no longer derives satisfaction from attending aerobic dance or tae bo classes, or he finds his daily jog boring, too time-consuming, or stressful. He wants out, but finds no face-saving way of breaking his well-advertised (in his community of friends and associates) commitment to exercise. There is anxiety that fellow exercisers will view him as undisciplined and weak, or as a "wimp" or "wuss." If participation was motivated originally by an interest in losing or gaining weight or recovering from illness (e.g., bypass surgery), then disengagement may be met with disappointment or perhaps disdain from relatives, good friends, and loved ones who wish only the best for the participant. A claim of injury and, therefore, the inability to continue exercising provides a convenient pathway to cessation of exercise, for injury is universally respected, feared, and accepted as a legitimate reason to stop.

Because it is extremely difficult to be assured that a person is malingering, this condition is hard to study and, consequently, poorly understood.

See Rogers's article "Development of a New Classification Model of Malingering."

Athletic trainers, physicians, physical educators, and exercise leaders who work with clients claiming injury must speculate with caution about malingering. It is probably best to give benefit of doubt to claims of incapacitation rather than risk legal suit, further damage (if, indeed, injury prevails), or loss of reputation and confidence in the caregiver's skill and professionalism. Malingering and the confusion surrounding it are not restricted to exercise. The workplace, in general, and the domain of sport, in particular, are common areas for its occurrence. In both domains, malingering is problematic and costly.

See the work done by Lees-Haley ("Psychological Malingerers") and Rotella, Ogilvie, and Perrin ("The Malingering Athlete: Psychological Considerations").

Sometimes malingerers use short-term strategies that temporarily help them resolve problems on a one-shot basis, but often, malingering becomes a pattern, repeatedly invoked if competent professional intervention is not forthcoming. The malingerer is aware that others have difficulty in addressing the issue of his questionable injury claim. He understands that faking symptoms of pain and inability to exercise properly or adequately is extremely challenging for medical authorities and others to deal with, even in the absence of hard, cold evidence to the contrary (results of X-ray, MRI, physiological tests, etc.).

Malingering poses so many challenges to trainers, teachers, coaches, and exercise leaders that its diagnosis is a substantial challenge. Because confirmation of faking, discomfort, and functional incapability is so difficult to establish, arriving at an approximation of

the number of individuals who resort to this kind of behavior is practically futile. Nonetheless, it appears to be widespread.

For studies of malingering, see Brink (1989), Labbate and Miller (1990), Rotella et al. (1999).

CASE STUDY 10.2 — *Alan: An Exercise Malingerer*

Alan, a 20-year-old college senior registered for a fitness class offered by his university's physical education department. Because he tended to be physically inactive and was 40 pounds overweight, Alan's physician strongly encouraged him to pursue regular exercise along with a dietary program of restricted daily calories. Alan's parents urged him to follow the doctor's prescription to lose weight and "become fit." Alan, with some reluctance, signed up for the physical education class because he believed it would appease his parents and relieve the concerns about his health, while providing evidence that he was compliant with his physician's recommendation. Alan had, however, never enjoyed exercise and, as a young child, resisted all efforts encouraging him to play sports.

At first, the demands required of class participants were not very challenging, and Alan was able to satisfy them with modest effort. Each session began with brisk walking for about 15 minutes followed by a prescribed routine of stretching exercises and calisthenics (push-ups, sit-ups, etc.). At the sixth class meeting, a particularly demanding program known as circuit training was introduced to the class. This program required that participants execute three rounds of less than their maximum number of repetitions of each exercise, but as rapidly as possible while maintaining correct form. When participants completed the third round, the instructor provided the number of minutes that had expired since they began. The strategy required that participants strive to complete their three rounds of exercises in a shorter time each time the class met. For example, if Alan finished his three rounds of chin-ups, push-ups, sit-ups, bench presses (at submaximal numbers of repetitions) on one day in 32 minutes, his goal was to improve (decrease) his time on subsequent days. This striving to reduce the time required for completion was taxing to the cardiorespiratory system and would,

therefore, account for positive changes in aerobic fitness. Muscular endurance and strength would also improve because participants were executing exercise or movements designed to accomplish this.

As the weeks went by, Alan found the class meetings to be difficult, embarrassing, and aversive. He began to dread each session and felt demeaned by the instructor's unrelenting cajoling to "pick it up," "move it," and "faster, Alan, faster." Alan was convinced that the instructor was unfairly picking on him. He wanted out and decided to drop the class. He knew that his parents would view this disapprovingly and that his physician, who had attended to Alan and his entire family for many years, would be disappointed in his patient's apparent inability to carry out a prescribed course of action.

Over the years, Alan had resorted to feigned illness as a reason to be excused from school exams, music lessons, and accompanying his family to social functions that he wished to avoid. So Alan claimed that a painful shoulder would prevent him from further involvement in exercise. He petitioned the instructor to excuse him from physical activity, but yet maintain enrollment in the class. The instructor grimaced, insisting that the class's essence was regular physical activity. Alan dropped the course and identified his "injury" as the reason. He had learned from past experiences that a claim of injury would get him off the hook. Upon his parents' insistence, Alan was examined by his physician, who, after finding no shoulder problem, sent him to an orthopedic specialist. X-ray and other tests revealed no structural, neural, or muscular deficit. Alan's strategy, consciously falsifying injury in order to address a situational problem, once again paid off. He was very content to be referred to by former classmates on campus as the guy who hurt his shoulder in PE and had to withdraw. Alan is a malingerer.

Although many of its underlying motives remain elusive, one salient characteristic of malingering distinguishes it from other forms of feigned illness. It typically has a clearly defined goal. Malingerers are responding to specific, undesirable or unpleasant circumstances from which they seek disengagement and relief. Exercise, perhaps because of its demands of regularity and rigor, may be stressful to the point that it becomes unpleasant and aversive—something that the erstwhile participant may seek to avoid. Claiming injury when indeed it does not exist is the consciously chosen strategy.

Malingerers then establish a set of symptoms that they publicize to others (i.e., to exercise leaders and peers). Despite the unavailability of medical support, they steadfastly adhere to their claim of disability. No physiological system remains immune from mimicked dysfunction.

Many years ago, Ogilvie and Tutko (1966) discussed *need for attention* as a prominent cause for malingering. They were among the first to address this behavior in the context of physical activity. Although their analyses focused upon athletes, exercise malingerers may be motivated similarly. Deception, as abrasive as the term may be, with various creative twists, is part of malingering syndrome. As Ogilvie and Tutko claim, the need for attention overshadows the need to perform (in this case, exercise). Because the malingerer is very much aware of her deception, she labors under the fear of being exposed. Therefore, she remains alert to challenges and expressions of doubt about her alleged injury or illness and is always prepared to mount a sturdy defense of her claims. She steadfastly sticks to her guns and wards off and denies advice that she is really okay in view of the absence of legitimately medically supportable causes.

Malingering may be viewed as a learned behavior; that is, individuals acquire malingering skills. Whether or not learning is explained or understood from behavioral perspectives (reinforcement, punishment, etc.) or from cognitive perspectives (higher-order thinking and problem solving), somehow, somewhere, the malingerer has learned to use deceptive strategies that she now applies to exercise-related injury and disability. She has learned to fool others, including trainers, therapists of various persuasions, and physicians. Modeled behavior and previously utilized malingering that has in some way been rewarded may underlie the acquired attitude that lying is an acceptable strategy. Again, we emphasize the complexity of malingering. Undoubtedly, a multitude of environmental factors contribute to the development of malingering behavior. A need for attention, interacting with a wish to disengage from physically demanding activity, is a likely antecedent to acquiring the habits of deception and cheating. Those who apply these skills to exercise and other forms of physical activity undoubtedly have succeeded in using similar strategies in other areas of life (e.g., school and vocational environments). Case Study 10.2 presents the story of Alan, a young man exhibiting malingering from exercise.

Help for Malingerers

Leading malingerers to behavioral change is a substantial challenge for the teacher, trainer, coach, or psychologist. Malingerers employ dishonesty in their misrepresentation of illness or injury and do so convincingly and steadfastly. In some fashion, the malingerer believes that the deception will result in positive outcomes and that such gain would outweigh the costs of lying and faking. Helpers should, therefore, try to identify and understand the pressures, anxieties, or fears that are behind the motive to malinger. Another important aspect of helping is to get the malingerer to agree to a program of rehabilitation that has well-defined goals. Helpers should insist upon establishment of the program's length and specific requirements necessary for rehabilitation from the alleged injury. Reinforcement should be provided for compliance with these steps. In addition, use of the term *malingerer* should be carefully avoided because it may inspire denial reaction and stronger and more dramatic claims of nonexistent illness or injury.

Help for the Injured Exerciser

Earlier in this chapter, two potential applications of psychological theory were identified for use in exercise injury. The first focused upon predicting and thereby preventing injury. We now turn our attention to the second application, that is, recovery from exercise-related injury. It is this application of psychology that currently receives most of the attention from researchers and thus continues to generate a substantial amount of helpful findings. The subsequent sections present five rehabilitative approaches or emphases—namely, social support, team approach, imagery, modeling, and cognitive appraisal.

Social Support

The word "social" implies involvement with others. *Social support*, in the context in which we use it here, suggests that other persons, namely, friends, peers, relatives, etc., play a vital role in the debilitated individual's confrontation with and management of injury. Those who are close to injured persons and concerned about their predicament are in a position to offer assistance and support. Their service includes providing advice, resources, assistance in completing tasks, and assurance that injury has not caused deprivation of self-worth. As Richman, Rosenfeld, and Hardy (1993) conclude, social supporters provide emotional, informational, and material assistance.

Exercise injury, in one way or another, does involve some form of deprivation, and deprivation, in turn, may precipitate at least two undesirable outcomes: (a) loss of fine or gross motor function and (b) stress and anxiety (i.e., the perception of temporary or long-term reduction in personal resources and the worry that it causes). In view of these outcomes, injured individuals may seek help from caring others who can be of assistance by providing words of comfort, encouragement to accept and follow medically prescribed rehabilitative advice or treatment, and making available the well-known "shoulder to cry on."

Exercisers often pursue fitness or performance goals with well-defined endpoints that they are eager to attain within a predetermined timeframe. Injury upsets such plans, causing inhibition of goal attainment with frustration as a consequence (see Figure 10.5). Support from others may, therefore, take the form of goal evaluation and goal reestablishment. Peers in whom the injured party has confided may be

helpful in encouraging and persuading him or her to reconstruct the chronological framework for the training goal and putting long-term consequences of the injury into a realistic perspective.

For examples of this, see Hardy, Burke, and Crace's chapter, "Social Support and Injury: A Framework for Social Support-Based Interventions With Injured Athletes" and Richman, Rosenfeld, and Hardy's "The Social Support Survey: An Initial Evaluation of a Clinical Measure and Practice Model of the Social Support Process."

However, as Sarason, Sarason, and Pierce (1990) indicate, if the help is to be authentic, the injured individual must view the proffered assistance as beneficial. Only then can the result be physically and psychologically advantageous.

Hardy and Crace (1991) have proposed eight distinguishable dimensions of social support.

A balance is necessary between the recipient's need or requirement for support and the amount and nature of the support provided.

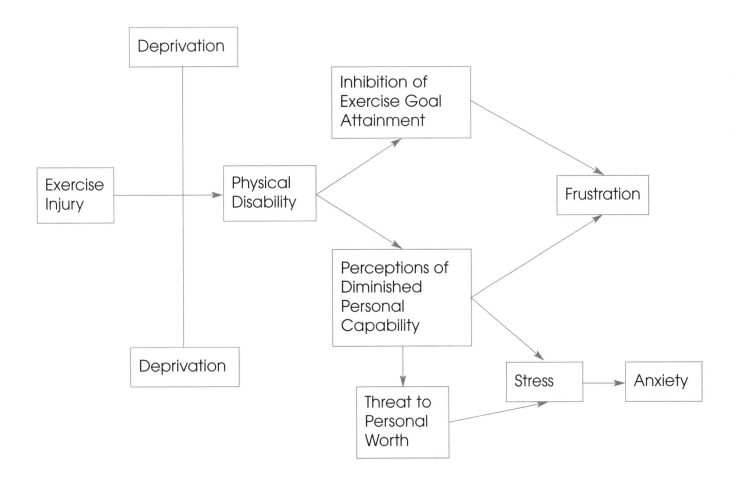

Figure 10.5. Physical and psychological change due to exercise-related injury.

Table 10.1
Eight Dimensions of Social Support

Dimension	Definition
1. Listening Support	Behaviors that indicate people listen to you without giving advice or being judgmental
2. Emotional Support	Behaviors that comfort you and indicate that people are on your side and care for you
3. Emotional Challenge	Behaviors that challenge you to evaluate your attitudes, values, and feelings
4. Task Appreciation	Behaviors that acknowledge your efforts and express appreciation for the work you do
5. Task Challenge	Behaviors that challenge your way of thinking about your work in order to stretch you, motivate you, and lead you to greater creativity, excitement, and involvement in your work
6. Reality Confirmation	Behaviors that indicate that people are similar to you—see things the way you do; helps you confirm your perceptions and perspectives of the world and helps you keep things in focus
7. Material Assistance	Behaviors that provide you with financial assistance, products, or gifts
8. Personal Assistance	Behaviors that indicate a giving of time, skills, knowledge, and/or expertise to help you accomplish your tasks

For more information, see Rook's "Detrimental Aspects of Social Relationships: Taking Stock of an Emerging Literature."

The recipient may feel pressure to abide by recommendations felt to be inappropriate or feel that he is being controlled by the social support (Goldsmith, 1994). Hobfoll and Stephens (1990) suggest that the longer the injury effects last, the more emotional support is appropriate. Sarason et al. (1990) believe that the rigor or intensity of the support should be a function of the supporter's closeness to the injured—the closer the relationships, the greater the intensity. Negative outcomes may be a consequence to recipient and provider, as well as to their relationship, when inappropriate support is rendered.

Suggestions for providing support. When one is providing social support to an injured exerciser, the following recommendations should be followed. First, the social supporter should have a clear and accurate understanding of the injury. Without such insight, it is difficult to establish credibility as a supporter. It is also important that the injured person perceive the helper's understanding and empathy. The supporter must make an effort to project those qualities.

Those who step forward as agents of support must also reflect upon their own motives and strengths. As Gottlieb (1988) implies in his analysis of what he refers to as support interventions, it is necessary for helpers to appreciate their own needs and reactions to distressed (i.e., injured) individuals. Hardy et al. (1999), therefore, caution the support provider to "know thyself" (p. 186).

Feedback offered by the helper should be authentic and emphasize daily or short-term rehabilitative goals rather than final rehabilitative programmatic outcomes. Social support should also acknowledge the injured person's need for emotional uplifting. Support devoid of this critical component is likely to be ineffective.

Injured exercisers should be encouraged to make self-assessments whereby they objectively and honestly examine their own rehabilitative progress. A considerable effort on behalf of the social supporter may be necessary for this to occur because injured individuals may not be inclined to do this.

Another point worthy of consideration when attempting to support injured exercisers has been elaborated upon by Weiss and Troxell (1986) and Wiese and Weiss (1987). They remind us that the injured exercisers can benefit from interacting with other injured persons who are able to empathize and understand the experiences of injury and the accompanying sense of deprivation. Small group sessions presided over by the main agent of social support can be arranged where ideas and feelings about injury are discussed and shared.

Social support provided by caring physicians, physical therapists, relatives, friends, and others who have sustained a similar injury can go a long way in alleviating stress associated with rehabilitation. However, total reliance upon others is to be avoided. A good measure of rehabilitative success must remain the responsibility of the injured person herself. To relieve her entirely from this obligation is incorrect. Social support is not a cure-all for injury rehabilitation, although it is certainly an essential element.

The Team Approach to Helping the Injured Exerciser

In the previous section, the value of social support in assisting the injured exerciser's rehabilitation was considered. The purpose of this section is to elaborate upon the ways in which individual supporters may integrate their efforts to form a team approach. In particular, we focus upon these so-called team members (i.e., physicians, physical therapists, psychologists), describe the professional attributes that enable their contribution to the team effort, and then overview specific ways in which their contributions may be rendered and integrated.

The physician. Primarily trained to analyze symptoms, diagnose their nature (including physical injury), prescribe appropriate remedial strategies, and monitor recovery progress, physicians play a primary role in injury rehabilitation. A visit to the physician is frequently made when injury impedes function, does not subside for a few days, or is associated with serious pain.

Physicians with training and experience in sport and exercise issues are said to specialize in sports medicine. Their interests also center on injury avoidance and preparation of participants for safe and optimal exercise behavior (conditioning). Many sports medicine physicians receive professional training in orthopedic, rehabilitative, or physical medicine. At the elite sport levels, team physicians are common and are typically available on the field of play (the so-called "team doctor"). Often, this physician's intervention is immediate or on the spot. This ready availability of the physician is not typical of most exercise environments.

Leisure-time exercise activities are also often executed in solitary areas where medical facilities and personnel are conspicuously absent. Examples would be kayaking, canoeing, rock climbing, snorkeling, skiing, lake or ocean swimming, in-line skating, ice skating, and wilderness backpacking. Sometimes, these activities take place in the company of others; often, they do not. At any rate, when exercise-related injury occurs, particularly when it involves pain or some form of incapacitation, the physician's services are sought. In the team concept, the physician's role is prominent. It is he or she who, after rendering a diagnosis, prescribes medication and further diagnostic tests, or, when indicated, recommends service from a sport/exercise psychologist or physical therapist.

The physical therapist. After consulting with a physician, the injured exercisers may be referred to a licensed physical therapist who initiates an organized regimen of treatment. This may take the form of carefully defined movements against progressively increasing resistance or stretching routines implemented with the aid of specially designed equipment. Sometimes exaggerated applications of heat or cold (ice, whirlpool bath, etc.) are incorporated on the treatment plan. On occasion, the physical therapist may also provide instruction about protective ways of moving. This may be necessary due to limitations related to reduced range of motion or inflamed or damaged connective and muscle tissue. The educational approach may also be valuable in that it clarifies the role of anatomical body parts that have been compromised. Models, illustrations, diagrams, and videotapes are frequently incorporated as instructional tools. With an understanding of "what's going on with my shoulder," the injured exerciser's readiness and motivation for understanding the prescribed therapy may be enhanced. The therapy administered by the physical therapist should also establish, with the client's participation, goals for recovery that are sensible and safe.

When and if compliance with the strategized rehabilitation program is a problem for the patient, possibly due to motivational, mood, or other psychological issues, the physical therapist may recommend involvement of yet another member of the rehabilitation team—the sport or exercise psychologist or counselor. The services of this team member may also be indicated if the injured exerciser has difficulty in accepting the severity or significance of the injury.

The sport or exercise counselor. The counselor or psychologist (legally protected terms; see Chapter 2) directs efforts towards alleviating despair, depression, anger, anxiety, and other moods that negatively influence adherence to or progress in rehabilitation regimens. Other objectives of psychological interventions include helping the injured prepare for various challenges associated with surgery or coping with the reality of long-term or permanent disability. Part of the counselor's effort is directed toward understanding the importance of exercise and the significance of its exclusion (short- or long-term) from the client's life. Counselors and psychologists may, in addition, teach injured exercisers various relaxation stress-management techniques. It may be necessary to refer injured exercisers for psychiatric help if the disability is causally related to severe depression, exercise addiction, personality, or eating disorders.

> D. M. Wiese-Bjornstal and A. M. Smith discuss techniques and approach in "Counseling Strategies for Enhanced Recovery of Injured Athletes Within a Team Approach."

If slightly modified, an instrument developed by Smith (1996) for use with athletes may serve nicely with exercisers. The instrument, the Emotional Response of Athletes to Injury Questionnaire (ERAIQ), has been shown to correspond with the depression, tension, and anger scales of the Profile of Mood States (POMS; McNair, Lorr, & Droppleman, 1971; see Chapter 5). It is also useful in providing information about the injured person's support system and personal projections about return to exercise activity.

A coordinated attempt among various health professionals strengthens the therapeutic effort to assist injured exercisers. Such unity need not, of course, be restricted to physicians, physical therapists, and counseling psychologists. Nurses, chiropractors, and nutritionists also may make valuable contributions. Some injuries in certain exercisers would benefit from rehabilitation teams of various sizes and constituencies. Too many cooks may indeed spoil the proverbial broth, but on the other hand, a well-composed team with competent, experienced, and caring members is in excellent position to provide optimal assistance to injured exercisers.

Imagery

During the past two decades, mental imagery has received a considerable amount of attention from health professionals working with ill and injured clients.

> For examples of this, see Achterberg, Kenner, and Lawlis (1988), Evans, Hardy, and Fleming (2000), Nicol (1993), and Varni, Jay, Masek, and Thompson (1986).

To understand its applications and potential contribution to rehabilitation, it is helpful to appreciate two things: (a) the limitations of imagery and (b) the efficacy of mind-body integration.

Imagery is a covert activity. Instead of experiencing an event overtly—that is, in the real or material world—the so-called "mind's eye" or "mind's ear" is where the event takes place. Thus, we image the happening by activating mental processes associated with our organs of sensation (vision, smell, taste, hearing, etc.). Individuals who have acquired imagery skills are able to invoke sensations that are felt, heard, and seen in the mind rather than in a truly physical fashion. It may be said that whatever we can experience overtly, we can also experience covertly.

Mental imagery has been used successfully by athletes as a means of relaxing prior to, during, or after competition.

> For examples, see Barr and Hall (1992), Ryska (1998), and Wrisberg and Anshel (1989).

When trial-by-trial repetition of a skilled act is imaged, the term *mental practice* or *rehearsal* is applied. Mental practice, although not effective enough to displace physical practice, has more or less been shown to play an adjunctive role in skill acquisition and refinement. In combination with physical practice, it results in augmented performance (Feltz & Landers, 1983). Imagery and mental practice techniques must be learned, and not everyone develops competency in their use. Some individuals have great difficulty in imaging and simply cannot do it. A number of tests are available that assess one's imaging capabilities. One such instrument, the Movement Imagery Questionnaire (MIQ) by Hall and Pongrac (Hall, Pongrac, & Buckholz, 1985), is particularly appropriate for use with athletes and exercisers because it requires the subject to image body positions and movements. One of the authors of this text used the MIQ to determine the number of female athletes at his university who could achieve a passing score (according to Hall) on the test. Of approximately 100 athletes, only 22 achieved the score indicative of marginal ability to image.

Our purpose in discussing imagery here is to propose its applicability to injury rehabilitation, particularly the rehabilitation of injured exercisers.

Guided imagery. Guided imagery involves leadership that directs the visual, auditory, and kinesthetic mental construction of the sensory experience. After guiding the injured party to a state of muscular relaxation, the leader offers suggestions and encouragement to the injured party to imagine that she is in various phases of leading. The client is asked to imagine disengagement from negative thought, that is, fear of not recovering and returning to action, the fear of reinjury, and the fear of pain.

Mind-body integration. Use of the term *mind-body* suggests an interface between the brain and the body's organs and systems. In the organism's quest for biochemical, structural, and functional integrity and balance, mental and physical operations occur interde-

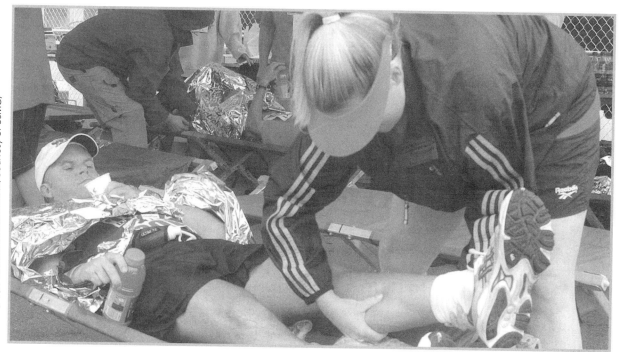

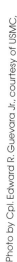

pendently. Thinking and associated feelings are, if not entirely determined, then certainly influenced by sensations emanating from various body parts. With the exception of reflexive movement and highly automated actions entrenched in neuromuscular patterns, meaningful motor function is very much dependent upon cognitive activity. The brain and body are locked in immutable partnership. Thinking precedes, accompanies, and follows movement. We move and think, think and move.

Can this relationship augment injury rehabilitation? As we reach for an answer to this question, let us consider results reported from the research literature. Some available findings provide evidence that imagery inspires positive immune system responses. The immune system is in the vanguard of our defense against invading pathogens. Immunological forces quell effects of harmful infections, some of which are debilitating. Sprained ankles, stretched ligaments, and pulled muscles are not exclusive disabling conditions that account for withdrawal from exercise programs. To this list, infections and tumors must be added.

Such results can be found in papers by Achterberg ("Enhancing the Immune Function Through Imagery") and AuBuchon ("The Effects of Positive Mental Imagery on Hope, Coping, Anxiety, Dypsnea, and Pulmonary Function in Persons With Chronic Obstructive Pulmonary Disease") and Post-White ("The Effects of Mental Imagery on Emotions, Immune Function and Cancer Outcome").

Many researchers have observed the beneficial effects of imagery use during rehabilitation from various illnesses as well as injury (Gaston, Crombez, & Dupuis, 1989; Hanley & Chinn, 1989; Korn, 1983). Older studies have shown that various physiological responses, such as salivation (Barber, Chauncey, & Winer, 1964), pupil size (Simpson & Pavio, 1966), increased heart rate (May & Johnson, 1973), gastrointestinal activity, and skin temperature (Barber, 1978) are amenable to the influence of imagery. When we consider these reported observations, we may comfortably conclude that injury rehabilitation, which is dependent upon such similar physiological responses, is conceivably facilitated by guided imagery that is strategically applied.

Modeling

The use of *modeling* (observational learning) is not new in sport and exercise (McCullagh, Weiss, & Ross, 1989). Effective coaches and instructors have used this strategic approach to teaching motor behavior since time immemorial. As Flint (1991) has suggested in her innovative doctoral dissertation, for those who have not experienced a debilitating, physical activity-related injury, an essential part of recovery encompasses coping with the requirements of the rehabilitation regimen. Recovered exercisers are excellent models to observe and emulate. In other words, the injured party can see the outcome of rehabilitative effort: "Someone else has been there, done it, and recuperated. It can be done . . . I can do it!"

Bandura (1986) is well-known for his efforts in describing and clarifying the theoretical bases of the modeling-behavior relationship. Not only behaviors, but also attitudes, may be acquired or modified by this instructional tool. When the injured exerciser is able to identify with the model, the motivation to attend to his or her behavior or projected attitudes is strengthened. Thus, careful selection of the model is essential to the effectiveness of this approach. Models should, therefore, be as similar as possible to the rehabilitating exercisers. Models may demonstrate the use of coping skills, high self-efficacy, and positive thoughts. They may also show the correct manner in which special therapeutic exercises are to be performed.

Cognitive Appraisal

With determination and effort, injured individuals may be able to reappraise and restructure the unfortunate consequences of their trauma. Competent counselors may assist the exercisers in this regard by encouraging a search for positive outcomes and ways in which personal growth has been a consequence of the injury. Such reframing is not likely to occur easily or quickly, but after the injured exercisers are helped to disengage from negative thoughts, they are taught to focus instead upon positive, supportive events and circumstances, such as the exceptionally high quality of medical care they are receiving or the new acquaintances and friends made in the physical therapy clinic. The recuperating exerciser may develop a new and strong affinity for someone who previously was only a jogging partner or fellow member of her aerobic dance class. Now, because of her empathetic overtures, frequent visits and telephone calls, and clear indicators of concern about the injury, she has become a valuable friend.

The chapter, "The Paradox of Injuries: Unexpected Positive Consequences," by E. Udry looks at some of the unexpected benefits of sports injuries.

It may be difficult to identify positive consequences of injury, and the reframing referred to above may also prove to be a challenge, but psychological development may be enhanced by concerted efforts at cognitive appraisal. Counselors who employ this approach must take care not to patronize the injured exerciser by artificially emphasizing the "great things that can result from your injury." Insincerity of this kind may reduce credibility of the well-intentioned counselor (or, for that matter, friend or fellow exerciser) and be counterproductive.

Pain

Engagement in rigorous, regularly done physical activity increases the probability of damage to body parts. Injury is not a necessary consequence of exercise—it may certainly be avoided—but it is a common result. Among the typical concomitants of exercise-related injury are swelling, skin discoloration, and decreased mobility and range of motion where bones meet bones (joints). These telltale signs are usually hurtful and often necessitate consultation with medical authorities. This hurt is referred to with the term *pain*, which, although largely physical in essence, also has an established psychological basis. Because our primary concerns in this book are focused upon exercise psychology, we now direct our attention to pain associated with exercise-related injury with a view toward cognitive and affective factors.

Throughout the body, in various locations such as in the skin, intertwined with muscle fibers and adjacent to bone and other tissues and organs, are to be found highly specialized aspects of the nervous system that serve as pain receptors. When activated through pressure exerted by collected body fluids in the area (e.g., blood, lymphatic fluid) or as a result of physical trauma, these receptors automatically send electrochemical messages via the peripheral nervous system and spinal cord to specialized brain centers. The speed with which the messages flow varies with the location of the receptors and their anatomical characteristics. Once the messages reach specialized brain centers, they are quickly processed, interpreted and assessed. In effect, attempts are made to attach meaning to sensations. This processing function is under the auspices of a part of the nervous system known as the *nociceptive system*. Loeser (1982) has provided a conceptual model of pain that graphically portrays the steps or phases through which pain is experienced (see Figure 10.6).

First comes the electrochemical (physiological) process referred to above wherein environmental stimuli are sensed by pain sensors (*nociception*). Next comes the attempt to interpret the sensation—to understand the importance of the pain in terms of its specific context (*perception*). Then, a higher degree of objectivity is reached as the injured person achieves an understanding of the pain's significance (*meaning*). Finally, *action* is taken. The injured exerciser chooses behaviors or attitudes that are consistent with her interpretation of pain.

Prior Experience and Pain Processing

One's experiential background is the basis for the processing and interpretation of pain. Different exercisers may interpret the same or similar pain stimuli in different fashion due to dissimilar histories of injury. As Heil and Fine (1999) write, "Pain is essentially a private intrapsychic experience" (p. 17). In one case, the pain may be associated with stubbing a toe on a submerged rock while launching a canoe. The canoeist may have banged his toe on numerous prior occasions in similar situations. He understands the cause of his pain and is able to tolerate it at a high level. His interpretation of the pain stimulus is reduced to "It's OK; it's nothing." His counterpart, however, having never canoed or even banged his toe before, experiences this for the first time, and reacts anxiously. He does so at a comparatively low tolerance level, and anxiety often mediates a worsening or amplification of the pain sensation. This point may be further exemplified by the case of veteran runners who, because of their years of participation, have incurred a variety of aches and pains. They have come to understand what particular agonies mean and are, therefore, able to identify certain of them as serious or inconsequential. Their prior experiences influence the manner in which they proceed to attach meaning to the pain stimulus (perception). Perception is a psychological process that represents the deciphering or clarification of incoming environmental stimuli.

Melzack and Wall (1965) have developed a theoretical depiction of pain stimulus processing that they named the "gate control theory of pain." These researchers hypothesize that along the spinal column are located checkpoints or gates through which pain stimuli must travel en route to the brain for processing. At times, these gates are open or closed, depending upon a number of physiological influences (e.g., hormonal, such as the body's opiates and neurotransmitters like endorphins and serotonins) as well as psychological influences. Consequently, the message flow is either blocked or permitted to proceed. Those stimuli that do not pass through the tollbooths dissipate or fade until they become ineffective. They never enter the brain's processing factory and, therefore, never "cause pain." In addition, some processing or interpretation of stimuli may occur at the gates themselves, interpretation that is believed to be influenced by psychological variables. Prior experience and memory alone are not exclusively involved in opening or shutting the gates or in the information-processing events.

Emotions, or present state of mind, also serve as mediators in spinal gating. An enraged person or an individual in the throes of guilt or high levels of frustration may be susceptible to the opening of relatively more numerous gates and, therefore, feel a heightened sense of acute (short-term) pain. As we noted previously, anxiety also tends to magnify pain because, among other things, it tends to elevate muscular tension that, in turn, may further aggravate pain receptors in the muscle tissue. Chronic pain is a long-lasting experience likely to involve sustained bombardment of pain stimuli that continue to be perceived in unaltered fashion—that is, as harmful, dangerous, and negative. Chronic pain does not go away. So then, pain stimuli are interpreted in keeping with physiological, emo-

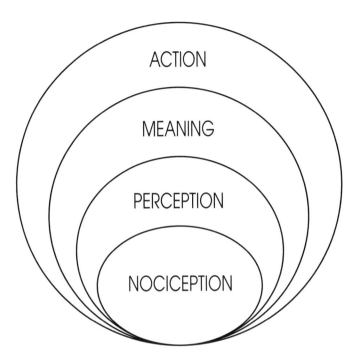

Figure 10.6. A conceptual model of pain. From "A Multifaceted Model of the Components of Pain," by J. Loeser, 1982, found in *Chronic Low Back Pain* (p. 146), by M. Stanton-Hicks and R.A. Boas, New York: Raven Press. Reprinted with permission.

tional, and an array of other cognitive inputs that reach the brain's perceptual centers at the same time. It is a malady that starkly integrates mind and body.

Pain Management

Because pain can be such a powerful, stressful, and disruptive experience, it often accounts for withdrawal from many daily activities, including exercise. It is important for exercisers to be aware of techniques and strategies designed to manage pain so that they may make good choices and react insightfully to treatments prescribed by knowledgeable, well-trained professionals. We do not suggest here that this brief section prepares you to implement the pain management methods we will identify. However, most of you are, or will eventually be, exercise leaders or exercise participants. You would, therefore, do well to be aware of and understand the value of some of many pain management treatments advocated by trainers, therapists, and physicians. The strategies selected for discussion here are in keeping with this book's focus, namely exercise psychology and, thus, we emphasize psychological applications.

To begin, let us acknowledge that there does not seem to be a significant relationship between pain intensity and the seriousness of the injury; it is the personal meaning of pain as interpreted by the injured person that appears to dictate the degree of suffering. For instance, Heil and Fine (1999) provide a list of pain elements that account for high degrees of tolerance (the higher the tolerance, the better an individual is able to cope with pain). Slightly modified, these elements may be applied to exercise. When necessary, the item is followed by a brief extension for clarification:

1. The expectation that pain can and will be tolerated.

    Most participants generally understand that discomfort and pain are part of vigorous physical activity, although the cliché "no pain, no gain" is nonsensical. If some form of pain is anticipated, then its perceived intensity is likely to be reduced.

2. A strong goal orientation.

    Exercisers who are involved in regular, rigorous physical activity are likely to be abiding by well-defined goals that serve to inspire their participation as well as favorably influence pain perception. Goals are powerful motivators and are discussed in considerable detail in Chapter 13.

3. Absorption in the "work in progress," that is, a focus on exercise more so than pain.

    Serious-minded exercisers tend to become so involved in their activities that their attentional focus narrows. Their concentration is centered on physical activity so they may therefore entirely exclude pain sensations or relegate them to a subordinate level. In this way, the stimuli associated with exercise become prominent or more important and override pain.

4. The assumption of limited pain duration.

    According to Heil and Fine's (1999) analysis, pain associated with exercise is likely to be of relatively short duration—or, as they put it, "pain control is more easily attained when there is an end in sight" (p. 17). By this Heil and Fine suggest that if the exercisers can see light at the end of the tunnel, they can more easily sustain pain control. If they understand, for example, that after a long hard workout or after a week of rest, discomfort will subside, their tolerance level can be maintained at a reasonably high level.

Let us now consider some specific pain-management approaches that relate to the above-mentioned elements that account for high levels of tolerance. Again, our interests here are with psychological strategies, although other kinds (chemical, electrical stimulation, acupuncture, massage, heat, cold, interventions, etc.) have been shown to be effective as well.

Psychological considerations. Injured exercisers may experience mood change during their incapacitation. This may occur for various reasons: the need to desist from enjoyable activity; deprivation of social interactions associated with their exercise participation; anxiety about diminishing skill/fitness levels or weight gain during abstinence from exercise; or distressing pain associated with the injury. Among these mood changes are increased anger, frustration, anxiety, depression, and tension. The severity of such disturbance is likely to relate to the degree of personal investment in exercise. Those who exercise more are relatively more dependent upon physical activity. Their identity may become tightly entwined with exercise that takes increasing priority over other activities. They may be more vulnerable to these negative shifts in mood.

One way of addressing undesirable mood alterations associated with pain is counseling. Before explaining how counseling accomplishes this, let us briefly discuss the meaning of the term *coping*, for it is this kind of behavior that effective counseling essentially addresses. Coping is learned behavior designed to alter specific demands coming from both internal and external environments. The perceptual phenomenon we have been discussing (pain) is precisely this— an internal demand that is interpreted as challenging, taxing, and something that exceeds the individual's personal resources. When such demands are converted into opportunities for growth or something positive rather than adversarial, debilitating, or negative, we say that the person is *coping* with his or her pain.

For more on this, see Tunks and Bellissimo's article "Coping With the Coping Concept: A Brief Comment."

We learn to do this. Coping is skillful, and counseling strategies are typically designed to teach such skills. Coping may be considered as occurring in three progressive stages:

1. Appraisal stage, wherein the client is helped to understand the demand's meaning and identify available ways of changing or meeting them;
2. Problem-focused stage, wherein the real challenges or particular aspects of the demands and their consequences are confronted and solutions and resources identified; and
3. Emotion-focused stage, wherein feelings stimulated by the demands are managed.

The competent counselor might introduce a goal-setting program to the injured exercisers and construct a system whereby accurate feedback about rehabilitation progress would be forthcoming. Exercisers are likely to respond positively to this approach because they probably are already employing some form of goal setting in their training (Wiese-Bjornstal & Smith, 1999).

Relaxation and training in guided imagery are additional counseling interventions used to lower anxiety levels and modify the intensity of pain stimuli. The term *guided imagery* refers to the counselor's constructing and shaping the images employed by the injured person. This may entail any of a number of relevant pictures formulated in the mind's eye of the exerciser. The counselor thus helps the exerciser envision himself proceeding through a rehabilitative series of difficult stretching movements or mastering certain skills necessary for using crutches or a wheelchair.

Cognitive restructuring, or changing negative thoughts to positive ones, and modeling, or using videotapes of other previously injured and rehabilitated exercisers, are examples of other strategies employed by counselors.

Adherence to Rehabilitation Programs. Injury is common among inveterate exercisers. Although medical science offers effective regimens designed to rehabilitate stricken aspects of the neuromusculo-skeletal systems, adherence to such programs is problematic for some individuals. A number of psychological variables have been examined as possible correlates of adherence. Among these are personality (Grove & Bianco, 1999); self-motivation and social support (Duda, Smart, & Tappe, 1989); and type of coping strategy (Brewer, 1994). Dispositional optimism in relation to coping style may also be linked to adherence and rehabilitation (Scheier & Chover, 1992). Optimists attempt to make the best out of difficult situations and therefore may adhere well. Optimists tend to deal well with adversity and view their situations in a positive way.

Summary

Injury is a common consequence of rigorous physical activity, and although its physical aspects are often addressed, its psychological dimensions receive much less attention. This chapter examines psychological correlates of exercise injury relative to prediction/avoidance as well as recovery/rehabilitation.

Injury among exercisers is often due to poor decision making and incorrect interpretation of relevant environmental stimuli. Stressors associated with rigorous physical activity and the emotional responses they generate may interfere with perceptual processes. Other psychological factors that may influence decision making relative to frequency, intensity, mechanical performance, location, and type of exercise are self-concept, body image, and risk-taking tendencies.

The way in which these psychological factors may interfere with injury is suggested by the computer information-processing model, which describes the treatment and storage of incoming environmental stimuli. Stored memories are accessed efficiently from long-term memory storage when they are encoded with strategies known as mnemonic devices.

Exercisers who claim injury when none exists are known as malingerers. It is difficult to know when an exerciser is malingering, and instructors should exercise caution before making such a diagnosis. Malingerers are typically motivated to withdraw from regimens of physical activity and use claims of injury as an escape mechanism. They usually learn to use their deceptive strategies and are likely to have succeeded in employing similar techniques in other areas of life.

Among the established ways of helping injured exercisers is social support or support from others such as family members, peers, teachers, trainers, and coaches. Those who provide social support should have a clear understanding of the injury and also reflect upon their own capabilities and motives. Social support should also acknowledge the injured person's emotional needs and focus upon short-term rehabilitative needs.

Physicians, trainers, physical therapists, as well as sport and exercise counselors compose a team that develops integrated strategies for the rehabilitation program. Such coordination strengthens the effort and provides optimal assistance.

Specific techniques designed to help injured exercisers that have been discussed in this chapter include imagery, cognitive appraisal, and modeling. Imagery involves use of the so-called mind's eye (and other senses) to create a covert experience—that is, not real but virtual in nature. Thus, for example, the injured exerciser imagines his or her participation in rehabilitative procedures. Cognitive appraisal techniques involve restructuring thoughts about negative aspects and consequences of the injury. In other words, the exerciser reinterprets the injury experience in a positive light. She emphasizes helpful aspects of the injury. Finally, modeling uses recovered exercisers as persons with whom the injured individual can identify. It is important to carefully select models who are as similar or whose injury is as similar as possible to that of the rehabilitating individual. Attitude as well as participation in the procedures of rehabilitation may be modeled.

Can You Define These Terms?

compliance

computer information-processing model

coping

cross-training

efficacy

encoding

FIT

imagery

injury

kinesthesis

locus of control

malingering

meaning

modeling

nociception

perception

reactive inhibition

retroactive inhibition

risk taking

social support

Can You Answer These Questions?

1. How does the NCAA prefer to define injury?
2. How might an inappropriate exercise prescription lead to exercise injury?
3. What is an alternative view of rest that is not necessarily consistent with the traditional definition of rest?
4. How do personality variables (e.g., as included in the Williams and Andersen (1998) model) interact with exercise injury?
5. What is meant by environmental factors, and how might this area moderate exercise injury?
6. Briefly elaborate upon the components of the computer information-processing model.
7. Why must one be cautious in attempting to identify malingering?
8. What are five rehabilitative approaches to consider when helping an injured exerciser?
9. What professionals make up the team approach to helping injured exercisers?
10. Describe mental imagery and its use for injured exercisers.
11. Does perception of pain differ across individuals? Explain.
12. What pain elements may account for a higher level of tolerance among individuals?

CHAPTER 11

Models of Exercise Behavior

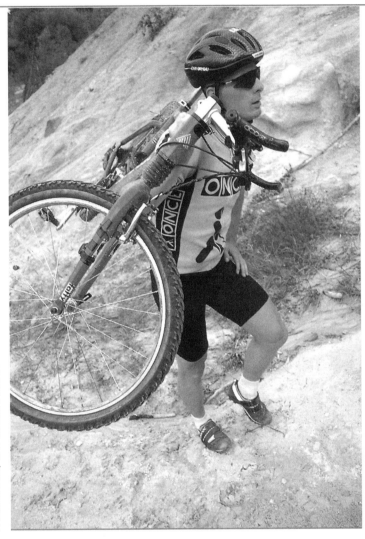

Photo courtesy of © Media Focus LLC

After reading this chapter, you should be able to

- Discuss the reasons for physical inactivity and

- Discuss models of exercise behavior including
  —health belief model,
  —theory of reasoned action,
  —theory of planned behavior,
  —self-efficacy theory, and
  —transtheoretical model.

Introduction

We know from looking around us that all sorts of people seem to be exercising in an attempt to look and stay young and to feel better. In most department stores, you can find athletic sportswear in vogue, not only for sport and physical activity but also for leisure and even work apparel. In addition, there seem to be more and more fitness clubs opening up where you can work out on your own or in a class to become fitter and leaner, but the fact is that most Americans do not regularly participate in physical activity. In fact, there is widespread consensus that physical inactivity during leisure time is a burden on public health in the United States and many other countries (NIH Consensus Conference, 1996). It should also be noted that in recent years, guidelines for physical activity have, in a sense, become more stringent—specifically, past guidelines emanating from the American College of Sports Medicine suggested 3–5 times a week of vigorous activity (vigorous activity being 60%–70% of maximum VO^2) for at least 20 minutes that was aerobic in nature. The most current guidelines suggest 4–7 days a week of moderate physical activity (although most preferably all days) of 30 minutes or more in bouts of at least 10 minutes in duration at an intensity similar to that of brisk walking. So staying physically active for health benefits is becoming even more difficult.

This increase in physical inactivity over the past two decades has been noted by the United States Department of Health and Human Services (USDHHS; 1996, 2000). Along these lines, the USDHHS has developed a preventive orientation in public health policies, promoting regular participation by children and adults in exercise and physical fitness as a major health objective for the nation. However, it should be noted that physical activity levels differ significantly across countries ranging, for example, from 16% of people being sedentary in Finland to 43% in Canada. In addition, such participation has been identified as a behavioral orientation, and literature exists to suggest that habitual physical activity can positively influence a broad range of health conditions, both physiological and psychological (Carron, Hausenblas, & Estabrooks, 2003; Dishman, 1994). Specifically, physical activity affects many aspects of health, including protection against early death, coronary heart disease, hypertension, diabetes mellitus Type 2, osteoporosis, colon cancer, depression, and anxiety (USDHHS, 1996). As previously noted, despite these benefits, much of the population is sedentary and underactive. For example, Caspersen and Merritt (1995), in investigating physical activity trends in 26 states, found a significant increase in physical inactivity, and they concluded that most people did little or no regular physical activity intense enough and long enough to receive health benefits. In addition, more recently, King et al. (1999) surveyed over 2,000 women over the age of 40 and found that slightly fewer than 60% of those surveyed rated themselves as inactive. Some of the specific data from the USDHHS (1996) and King et al. that underscore this lack of physical activity is provided below:

- Physical activity levels begin to decline at about 6 years of age and continue to decline throughout the life cycle.
- Fifty percent of youths 12–21 years of age do not participate regularly in physical activity.
- Twenty-five percent of children and adults report no vigorous physical activity, and another 35% do not exercise enough to meet the levels of participation recommended for health and fitness.
- Fifteen percent of adults participate in vigorous exercise regularly (three times a week for at least 20 minutes).
- Ten percent of sedentary adults are likely to begin a program of regular exercise within a year.
- Physical activity for both boys and girls declines steadily throughout adolescence from about 70% at age 12 to 30–40% by age 21.
- Physical inactivity is more prevalent among girls than boys (13.8% vs. 7.3%), among African American youth than white youth (15.3% vs. 9.3%), and among African American girls than white girls (21.4% vs. 11.6%).
- Among Americans, 64% were seen as overweight or obese in 2004.
- Sedentary behavior is more prevalent for women than for men (30.7% vs. 26.5%) and for less affluent than for more affluent individuals (41.5% vs. 17.8%).

Therefore, despite the overwhelming evidence of the positive effects of regular physical activity both physiologically and psychologically, most people still do not exercise on a regular basis, and those who try tend to drop out of exercise programs within 6 months. Maintenance is a particularly noteworthy endeavor given that individuals must continue to be physically active to sustain full health benefits. In the respect that there is a high relapse rate in exercise programs, exercise is like dieting, quitting smoking, or cutting down on drinking alcohol. That is, people intend to change a habit that affects their health and well-being negatively. In fact, fitness clubs traditionally have their highest new enrollments in January and February after sedentary individuals feel charged by New Year's resolutions to turn over a new leaf and get in shape (Dishman, 1994). Along these lines, the marketing of exercise has accelerated in North America in a mass persuasion campaign, with heavy media advertising from sportswear companies. Despite these efforts, people will drop out. So, why do people start an exercise program in the first place, and why don't they stick with it once they start?

Theoretical Models of Exercise Participation

One way in which we can better understand the reasons for adopting and eventually maintaining an exercise program is through theoretical models of exercise participation. Although identification of specific factors related to exercise participation and adherence is useful from an epidemiological point of view, theoretical models can underscore and identify the reasons why people participate in the first place and how they might continue participation (Culos-Reed, Gyurcsik, & Brawley, 2001). These models can also specify the workings of specific variables and factors related to exercise initiation and adherence and provide a rationale as to how the exercise process actually works. Consequently, understanding these models should help us understand how to intervene to get more people to start and continue exercising. Although many models have been put forth, we have chosen the ones that have generated the most research or support with regard to predicting exercise behavior.

Health Belief Model

The health belief model (HBM; Becker & Maiman, 1975) has been one of the most widely recognized and enduring theoretical models associated with preventive health behaviors (e.g., Bond, Aiken, & Somerville, 1992; Hayslip, Weigand, Weinberg, Richardson, & Jackson, 1996; Knapp, 1988; Rosenstock, 1974). The model is usually considered psychosocial in nature and was developed to help predict compliance and preventive health recommendations. This model assumes that people anticipate negative health outcomes and have the desire to avoid these outcomes or reduce their impact.

The basic components of the Health Belief Model are derived from a well-established body of psychological and behavioral theory whose various models hypothesize that behavior depends mainly upon two variables: (a) the value placed by an individual on a particular goal, and (b) the individual's estimate of the likelihood that a given action will achieve that goal (Janz & Becker, 1984). More specifically, this model proposes that the likelihood of adopting a behavior appropriate to the prevention or control of some disease depends on the individual's perception of a threat to personal health. In addition, the individual has a conviction that the recommended action will reduce this threat along with proper cues that might trigger appropriate reactions (see Figure 11.1). In essence,

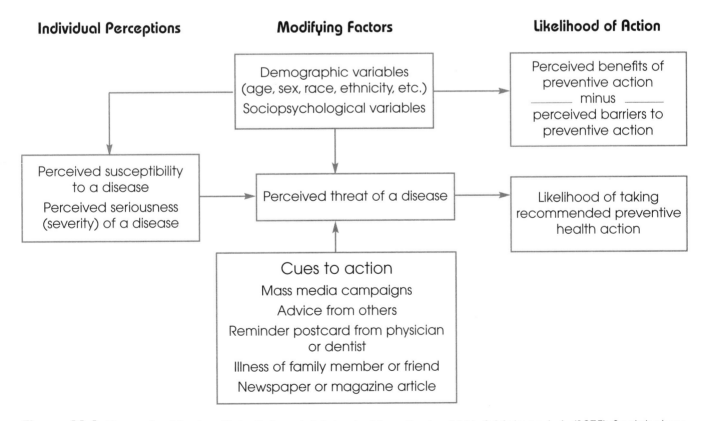

Figure 11.1. Elements of the health belief model. Adapted from Becker, M. H., & Maiman, L. A. (1975). Sociobehavioral determinants of compliance with health care and medical case recommendations. *Medical Care, 13,* 10–24.

readiness to undertake a health regimen such as exercise depends upon the following:

1. At least moderate motivation to make health issues salient (e.g., concern about health or illness, willingness to accept direction).
2. Evaluation of the illness threat (e.g., perceived susceptibility or vulnerability to serious health problems, or existence of current serious health problems).
3. Belief that the potential or existing problem is preventable or controllable (i.e., that exercise might yield physical and psychological remedial or preventative benefits).
4. Belief that participation in an exercise program will reduce the threat of illness.
5. Presence of cues that trigger or elicit action, making the individual aware of feelings about the need to improve health (e.g., demographic factors like age, ethnicity, and gender; structural factors such as cost and complexity; attitude about the exercise regimen; mass media campaigns; illness of a family member or friend; newspaper articles; reminder postcard from physician; or advice from others).

Relationship to exercise. One question that should be asked about any theory of behavior change is how well it has helped predict this change in behavior. A great deal of research has accumulated concerning the utility of the HBM constructs (e.g., perceptions of vulnerability to disease, cues to action, perceived barriers to exercise, and perceived benefits of exercise) as they relate to compliance with medical regimens and exercise adherence (e.g., Becker, Nathanson, Drachman, & Kirscht, 1977; Hayslip et al., 1996; Oldridge & Streiner, 1990). A comprehensive review of 46 studies by Janz and Becker (1984) found that the concepts of perceived barriers, perceived benefits, and perceived susceptibility were most useful in predicting health-related behaviors across the studies. However, it should be noted that most of these studies focused on younger populations and more research is needed with middle-aged or elderly persons whose ability to engage in vigorous physical activity may be limited.

Interestingly, several cross sectional studies (e.g., Slenker, Price, Roberts, & Jurs, 1984; Sommers, Anders, & Price, 1995; Taggert & Connor, 1995) found that perceived barriers were especially strong determinants of physical activity behavior. For example, perceived barriers were the most important factor discriminating joggers from non-exercisers. Some common barriers to undertaking physical activity includes inconvenience of facilities, perceived lack of time, low motivation, expense, injury, and discomfort (e.g., muscle soreness). These barriers may cause people not to engage in physical activity (or other healthy behaviors) even if they acknowledge the severity of their condition (e.g., obesity) and believe they are at risk for developing this condition.

Although some success has been found in using the HBM to predict exercise behavior, to date, the results would have to be considered inconsistent (Godin, 1994). This is the case whether one is studying people with or without a diagnosis of a disease. However, it should be noted that the HBM is concerned primarily with perceptions of disease; thus, it was not originally developed to study exercise behavior. Because the model focuses on health behaviors, and we know that health is only one of the reasons that people exercise, it is likely that results would be inconsistent regarding the prediction of exercise behaviors. Nevertheless, the HBM has provided the field with some important variables (variables used in other models), and by testing this theory, we have learned a great deal about exercise behavior.

Theory of Reasoned Action

The primary goals of the theory of reasoned action (TRA; Ajzen, 1985; Fishbein & Ajzen, 1975) are to understand and predict social behaviors at the level of individual decision making. The theory maintains that people are usually rational and that they consider the implications of their behaviors before deciding to engage in them—thus, the title "Theory of Reasoned Action." In this model, the basic assumption is that most social behaviors are voluntarily controlled and that *intentions* are considered to be the best predictors of actual behavior. In essence, barring unforeseen events, people are expected to behave in accordance with their intentions. Thus, if you have a strong intent to go for a run later today, you are likely to go for that run. In the TRA, intentions are the product of two basic determinants: (a) an individual's *attitude* toward a particular behavior and (b) what is normative regarding the behaviors (*subjective norm*). For some behaviors, the attitude is the major determinant of intentions, whereas for other behaviors the normative component is dominant (see Figure 11.2).

An individual's attitude toward the behavior is usually based on that person's positive or negative evaluation of performing the behavior. Generally speaking, people have between 5 and 10 readily identified beliefs with respect to a given action. So, for instance, an individual may believe that regular physical exercise will reduce weight, improve physical fitness, lower the risk of a heart attack, improve mood, and take time away from the family. As individuals shape their behavior, they evaluate the consequences attached to these beliefs in making a final decision on whether to exercise or not.

The second determinant of intention is called the subjective norm and is the product of beliefs about others' opinions and the individual's motivation to comply with others' opinions. In essence, it is how a

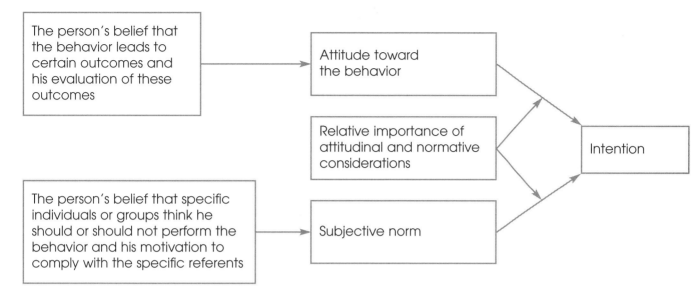

Figure 11.2. Theory of reasoned action. Adapted from Ajzen, I., & Fishbein, M. (1980). *Understanding attitudes and predicting social behavior.* Upper Saddle River, NJ: Prentice Hall, p.100.

person perceives social pressures to perform or not perform a specific behavior. Similarly, subjective norms may exert pressure to behave in a certain way despite the individual's attitude toward a particular behavior. If, however, an individual evaluates a behavior positively and believes that others think he or she should perform it, then typically the individual will engage in the behavior. For example, if you were a nonexerciser and believed that other significant people in your life (e.g., spouse, children, friends) thought you should exercise, then you might wish to do what others wanted you to do. This results in a positive subjective norm for exercising, an intention to exercise,

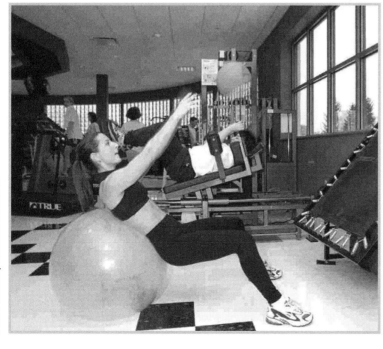

followed by actual exercise behavior. It is interesting to note that unlike many behavioral theories, TRA does not directly incorporate demographic elements, personality characteristics, social roles, and other external variables. These are seen as potentially important, but only to the extent that they influence a person's attitudes or perceptions of norms (Ajzen & Fishbein, 1980).

The basic assumptions underlying the TRA have been verified frequently. For example, Cooper and Croyle (1984) in their review of attitude change conclude that the TRA has been the basis for much of the progress in the field of social psychology. Similarly, in a meta-analysis of 87 studies (Sheppard, Harwick, & Warshaw, 1988), results indicated that behavioral intentions were a critical variable in the prediction of actual behavior. A number of studies have applied TRA to the study of exercise behavior (for reviews, see Godin, 1994; Godin & Sheppard, 1990). Results from these studies reveal that, although TRA has been very helpful in clarifying the decision-making process that underlies exercise behavior, it has only been of modest value in predicting exercise behavior. Moreover, the assumed determinants of intention, attitude toward behavior, and social norms have not predicted behavioral intention with any consistency. In part, this is due to the influence of some external variables (e.g., past behavior, exercise habit) on intention. This lack of behavioral prediction led the authors to develop a newer theory building upon the TRA.

Photo courtesy of Healthworks, Inc.

Theory of Planned Behavior

This theory (Ajzen & Madden, 1986) is an extension of the theory of reasoned action (Ajzen & Fishbein, 1975). Specifically, the theory of planned behavior extends the TRA by arguing that intention could not be the sole predictor of behavior. For example, it has been suggested that the longer the time interval between intention and behavior, the more likely intention will change as new information is received. This would result in a weaker relationship between intention and action. For example, Courneya and McAuley (1993) measured the behavioral intention to exercise in the short-term (two days) and in the long-term (four weeks). Results revealed that short-term intention was a better predictor of exercise behavior than long-term intention.

In addition, a second way the intention-behavior relationship is diminished is in situations in which people's control over the behavior might be incomplete. In essence, one of the authors of TRA (Ajzen, 1985) observed that the TRA was particularly valuable when describing behaviors that were totally under volitional control. Control is concerned with the extent to which nonvolitional internal and external factors interfere with an individual's attempt to perform a behavior. Most behaviors, however, fall somewhere along a continuum that extends from total control (e.g., making the decision on whether to jog or not) to complete lack of control (e.g., the weather). To take into account such barriers, real or perceived, the concept of perceived behavioral control was added to the original model.

Thus, in addition to the notions of subjective norms and attitudes, the theory of planned behavior states that *perceived behavioral control*—that is, people's perception of their ability to perform the behavior—will also affect behavioral outcomes. For example, even if a person has a positive attitude and subjective norm regarding exercise, if the person believes that she does not have the ability or opportunities to exercise, then her intention to exercise will likely be weak. In essence, to accurately predict behavior over which people have limited control, we must not only assess behavioral intention but also estimate perceived behavioral control. In addition, perceived behavioral control can affect behavior directly instead of simply affecting behavior through intentions as do the other variables from the TRA. A schematic diagram of the theory of planned behavior is presented in Figure 11.3.

As seen in this diagram, the three conceptually independent variables of attitude, subjective norm, and perceived behavioral control interact simultaneously to determine behavioral intention. In essence, the theory of planned behavior predicts that the more resources and opportunities individuals believe they

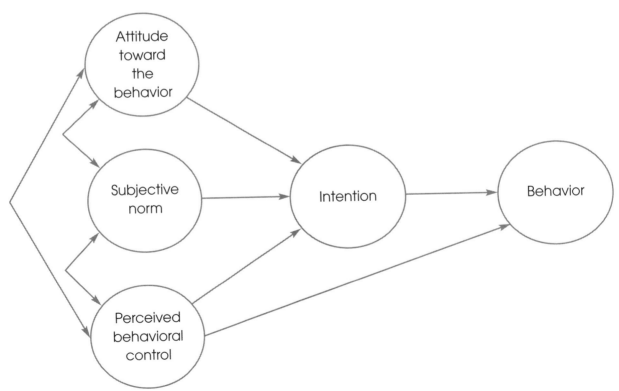

Figure 11.3. Adapted from Ajzen, I. & Madden, T. J. (1986). Prediction of goal-directed behavior: Attitudes intentions and perceived behavioral control. *Journal of Experimental Social Psychology, 22,* 453–474.

have and the fewer obstacles they anticipate, the greater their perceived control over the behavior. For example, if exercise were the behavior in question, we would assume that the more favorable the attitude and subjective norm toward exercise and the greater the person's perceived control over factors affecting exercise participation (e.g., distance from workout facility, injuries, time, partner to exercise with), the stronger the intent to exercise would be.

Relationship to exercise. Research testing the theory of planned behavior has been encouraging and provides at least partial support for the theory and the key variables within the theory. For example, two experiments designed to test the model demonstrated that the theory of planned behavior was superior to the theory of reasoned action with respect to predicting class attendance and receiving an "A" grade. There was specific support for the notion of perceived behavioral control (the new critical variable) as a predictor of behavioral intentions as well as motivation.

Studies have also examined the relevance of the theory of planned behavior on exercise adherence. The key point to most of these studies was to determine if perceived behavioral control could predict some aspect of exercise intention or behavior. In general, results were positive as perceived behavioral control contributed to the prediction of the intention to do aerobics regularly (Gatch & Kendzierski, 1990). Dzewaltowski, Noble, and Shaw (1990) found similar results for the prediction of intention to participate in physical activity where the degree of perceived behavioral control increased, so did physical activity participation. Moreover, in two studies, Godin, Valois, and Lepage (1993) found that for adult males and nonpregnant females as well as for pregnant women, perceived behavioral control contributed to the prediction of intention to exercise, although it did not predict actual exercise behavior. Thus, although perceived behavioral control helped predict intentions to exercise, it did not always predict actual exercise behavior. One explanation for perceived behavioral control's lack of influence on exercise behavior is that exercising is a behavior under volitional control. Thus, the theory of planned behavior should be most useful in helping researchers understand the formation of intentions to exercise and thus help develop interventions aimed at modifying exercise behavior.

Furthermore, a study by Mummery and Wankel (1999) investigated how well the theory of planned behavior would predict the adherence to training and practice behaviors of adolescent swimmers who were drawn from 19 different swimming clubs across Canada. Although this is a sport setting, the focus was on adherence to practice and training behaviors and not on performance, which makes this study more applicable to exercise. Results revealed that training

intention was significantly related to training behavior and that the direct measures of the theory of planned behavior (i.e., attitude, subjective norm, and perceived behavioral control) were good predictors of training intention. In essence, the components of the theory of planned behavior helped predict intention to adhere to the training regimen, and this in turn helped predict actual adherence of the swimmers. That is, swimmers holding positive attitudes toward training, believing that other individuals important to them thought they should complete the training as assigned, and holding positive perceptions of their ability to complete the training as required formed stronger intentions to train (and actually adhered to training) than did those who did not hold such beliefs.

Along these lines a recent study (Courneya, Vallance, Jones, & Reiman, 2005) found that the TPB was a very good predictor (predicting 55% of the variance) of exercise intentions in a group of cancer survivors. The key variable in helping to predict intentions to exercise was perceived behavioral control (followed by attitude and subjective norms), thus underscoring the notion that the perceived ease or difficulty of performing a behavior is a good predictor of whether that behavior will actually be performed. Courneya et al. found that only about 50% of cancer survivors actually intended to exercise despite their conditions. The development of a positive mental attitude was the most important belief, whereas lack of energy and fatigue was seen as the major barrier.

Finally, there have been a number of reviews that have systematically investigated the effectiveness of the TPB (e.g., Godin & Kok, 1996; Sutton, 1998). One such review (Hausenblas, Carron, & Mack, 1997) found that the TPB constructs have considerable utility in explaining and predicting exercise behavior. In fact, the authors recommend that knowledge of these constructs could help exercise leaders as well as exercisers better understand the critical elements regarding starting and adhering to a physical activity program.

Self-Efficacy Theory

The theories that have been presented illustrate some of the ways social cognitive scientists have sought to explain individual differences in the propensity to adopt a behavior such as exercising. Although the health belief model puts health-related behaviors and their understanding at the center of protecting against disease or improving health, the theory of reasoned action and the theory of planned behavior focus more on the decision-making process involving intentions and perceived behavioral control. In the self-efficacy approach (Bandura, 1977, 1986, 1997), it is hypothesized that all behavioral changes are mediated by a common cognitive mechanism termed *self-efficacy*. In short, efficacy expectations are the individual's beliefs in his or her capabilities to execute necessary courses of action to satisfy situational demands. It should be noted that more recently, Bandura (1995, 1997) has refined the definition of self-efficacy (now termed *self-regulatory* efficacy) to encompass those beliefs regarding individuals' capabilities to produce performances that will lead to anticipated outcomes. In a strong statement, Bandura (1997) argues that "unless people believe they can produce desired effects by their actions, they have little incentive to act. Efficacy belief, therefore, is a major basis for action" (pp. 2–3).

It is then theorized that these efficacy expectations influence (a) the activities that individuals choose to approach, (b) the effort expended on such activities, and (c) the degree of persistence demonstrated in the face of failure or aversive consequences (Bandura, 1986). For example, people who are efficacious in their running ability will likely choose to engage in running and exert greater effort and persistence when running, compared to individuals who lack efficacy in running. In addition to influencing behavior, efficacy beliefs are hypothesized to influence individuals' affect, thought patterns, and motivation. Thus, to use the above example, those with high running efficacy will likely experience more positive affect, set higher goals, and have higher motivation regarding running compared to individuals lacking efficacy.

Self-efficacy theory is a social cognitive approach to behavioral causation in which cognitive, physiological, behavioral, and environmental factors operate as reciprocal interacting determinants of each other. This interactional model is known as *reciprocal determinism* (see Figure 11.4). In essence, this interacting process states that behavior and human functioning are determined by the interrelated influences of individuals' physiological states, behavior, cognitions, and the environment. Moreover, self-efficacy theory focuses on the role of self-referent thought and provides a common mechanism through which people demonstrate control over their own motivation and behavior. As a demonstration of its usefulness in predicting health-related behaviors, self-efficacy has been shown to be a good predictor of behavior in a variety of health settings, such as smoking cessation, weight management, and recovery from heart attacks.

It is interesting to note that self-efficacy theory distinguishes between efficacy expectations and outcome expectations. The expectation of outcome is the individual's estimate that a given behavior will lead to certain results. For example, individuals may, as a result of exercising, expect outcomes such as loss of weight or increased cardiovascular fitness.

Relationship to exercise. In the past 15 years or so, self-efficacy theory has been used extensively to help predict exercise behaviors. Although self-efficacy can affect exercise behavior, in a true reciprocally determining fashion, exercise can also act as a source of efficacy. We will first focus on how efficacy expectations can influence exercise behavior and then on the impact of exercise on self-efficacy. But to set the stage for the discussion of specific studies, some overall summary reviews will be noted. For example, three reviews report that self-efficacy influences exercise adherence in various populations (Bandura, 1997; McAuley & Courneya, 1993; McAuley & Mihalko, 1998). In fact, results provided support for the notion that self-efficacy can act as both a determinant and outcome of exercise behavior. Furthermore, it was

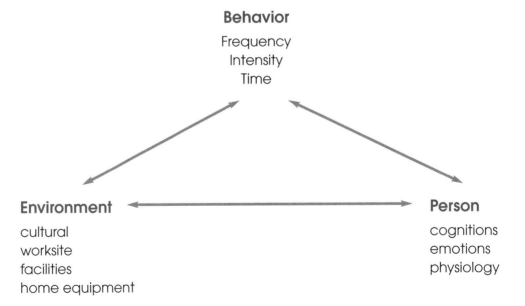

Figure 11.4. Theoretical model of exercise behaviors.

found that self-efficacy exerts the greatest impact on adherence when individuals are initiating a regular exercise program or attempting long-term maintenance of regular exercise. Finally, besides influencing exercise behavior, self-efficacy was found to influence exercise intention, effort expenditure, and attributions. Specifically, high-efficacy individuals exerted more effort, attributed outcomes to internal, stable factors, and intended to exercise significantly more than low-efficacy individuals.

Along these lines, Sallis and his colleagues (Sallis, Haskell, Fortmann, Vranizan & Solomon, 1986; Sallis, Hovell, Hofstetter, & Barrington, 1992; Sallis et al., 1989) provide evidence that self-efficacy can play an important role in the etiology of exercise theories. Specifically, when data from the Stanford Community Health Survey were used, it was reported that self-efficacy was significantly related to exercise theories at different stages of the natural history of the exercise process. Moreover, self-efficacy was the most consistent predictor of changes in exercise behavior over time despite the fact that many variables were used to predict exercise changes.

Research by McAuley and colleagues (McAuley, 1993a, b; McAuley & Courneya, 1992, 1994; McAuley, Courneya, Rudolph, & Lox, 1994) has indicated that exercise-related self-efficacy plays different roles at different stages in the exercise process and that employing efficacy-based strategies in training studies seems to enhance adherence to exercise behavior. In fact, the transtheoretical model presented next will discuss these different stages in more detail. This is especially true in sedentary older adults. For example, in investigating exercise adherence of older adults in an exercise program lasting 6 months, with follow-ups by telephone and mail 4 months after program termination, results revealed that only self-efficacy was a significant predictor of exercise behavior (e.g., Bock et al., 1997).

It is interesting to note that the role of self-efficacy expectations has also been investigated within the context of other theoretical models of exercise adherence. For example, in some studies, self-efficacy was defined similarly to the concept of perceived behavioral control, which is a critical concept in the theory of planned behavior (although self-efficacy has not been universally accepted as a theoretical equivalent to perceived behavioral control; e.g., Biddle, Goudas, & Page, 1994). However, in these studies, where self-efficacy has been seen as equivalent to perceived behavioral control (e.g., DuCharme & Brawley, 1995; Rodgers & Brawley, 1996), results have revealed that self-efficacy was predictive of exercise intentions and exercise behavior in novice exercisers. Although some researchers have viewed self-efficacy and perceived behavioral control as equivalent, Bandura (1997) has argued that self-efficacy expectations are unique from

different components of the theory of reasoned action and theory of planned behavior. He thus argues that these concepts should be investigated separately. Moreover, in research emanating from the transtheoretical model, efficacy has typically been viewed as confidence to participate in exercise in the face of difficult situations. Furthermore, from an empirical point of view, research has generally found a linear increase in self-efficacy across exercise participation (e.g., Cardinal, 1997; Gorley & Gordon, 1995; Marcus, Pinto, Simkin, Audrain, & Taylor, 1994).

Exercise effects on self-efficacy. Finally, as noted previously, considerable research has focused on the effects of exercise on self-efficacy. In essence, exercise can act as a source of information for feelings of efficacy, and the exercise bouts can take both chronic and acute forms (e.g., McAuley & Blissmer, 2000; McAuley & Courneya, 1992). In the case of acute exercise effects on self-efficacy, exposure to a bout of activity serves as a mastery experience, and self-efficacy expectations can thus be enhanced. For example, studies have indicated that acute changes in such physical activities as walking, cycling, and sit-ups can produce positive changes in perceived self-efficacy (e.g., McAuley, Bane, & Mihalko, 1995). At the chronic level, it has also been shown that longer-term exercise interventions (especially with clinical samples, such as individuals suffering from coronary heart disease or chronic obstructive pulmonary disease) have produced increases in feelings of self-efficacy (Kaplan, Ries, Prewitt, & Eakin, 1994; McAuley & Katula, 1998). In summary, a fairly large literature strongly suggests that the effects of exercise on perceptions of personal efficacy are consistent and robust for clinical and asymptomatic populations as well as for acute (e.g., graded exercise tests) and long-term (fitness class programs). In addition, a variety of exercise behaviors influenced self-efficacy, including walking, strength training, volleyball, aerobic dance, and exercise as part of a cardiac rehabilitation program. Therefore, practitioners should try to implement programs in which changes in self-efficacy are a central component to changes in exercise behavior

Transtheoretical Model

For many years, models and programs to change behavior have focused predominantly on the extinction or control of negative behaviors such as smoking, substance abuse, and obesity rather than on positive behaviors such as exercise. In much of that early research, it was found that it was extremely difficult to change behaviors that had become habitual over a long period. In fact, it was discovered that people in behavior-change programs passed through specific changes as they struggled to change their longtime behaviors. In essence, in the past, behavior change was often construed as an event such as quitting smoking, drinking, or overeating, but repeated observations showed behavior change as a process that occurs over time. From these observations came the development of the transtheoretical model (Prochaska & DiClemente, 1983; see Figure 11.5) of behavior change.

Although the previous models are useful in attempting to understand why people do or do not exercise, they tend to focus on a given moment in time. However, as noted above, the transtheoretical model argues that individuals progress through a series of stages of change, and movement through the stages is thought to be cyclic, not linear, because many do not succeed in their efforts at establishing and maintaining lifestyle changes. In addition, change is seen as a lengthy process involving stages where the cognitions and behaviors of individuals are different. Thus, a "one size fits all" approach does not work as noted by one of the top researchers in this area (Marcus et al., 2000). This notion of rejecting the "one size fits all" approach was seconded in a recent study (Lippe, Zioegelmann, & Schwarzer, 2005) using a stage-specific model that made a distinction between non-intenders, intenders, and actors in terms of physical activity. Like Prochaska and DiClemente (1983) earlier, they found that understanding the different stages that individuals are in (and then matching interventions to stages) helped predict the intended and actual exercise behavior.

Along these lines, it is important to note that the concept of stages falls somewhere between those of traits and states. Specifically, traits are typically viewed as stable and not open to change. States, on the other hand, are readily changed and typically lack stability. Second, stages are both dynamic and stable. That is, although stages can last for a considerable period of time, they are susceptible to change. For example, a sedentary woman may think about exercising but enjoys watching her favorite programs on TV and thus stays sedentary for months. Then, someone buys her a pair of walking shoes and volunteers to walk with her. After a year of walking, she gets an injury, stops walking entirely, and doesn't pick it back up even after the injury is healed. The cyclical pattern of the stages-of-change model can be seen in Figure 11.5

In developing this model, six stages were hypothesized:

Precontemplation. In this stage, individuals do not intend to change their high-risk behaviors in the foreseeable future. Regarding exercise, this usually means the person is not anticipating starting exercising in the next 6 months. In essence, these people are "couch potatoes." People may be at this stage for a variety of reasons. For example, they may be uninformed or underinformed about the consequences (especially long-term) of their behavior, or they may have tried to change their behavior a number of times and have become demoralized about their ability to change. Finally, they may be defensive due to social pressures to change. They may even dislike the exercise experience itself. In any of the above cases, these people tend to avoid reading, talking, or thinking about the behavior that needs to be changed (Prochaska & Velicer, 1997a). In other theories, these people are typically classified as resistant or unmotivated, not really ready to make any positive changes. In reality, many of today's traditional health-promotion programs are not really ready for such individuals, and these programs are therefore not motivated to match the specific needs of these special people. In essence, programs tend to be interested in people who are exercising regularly or will begin to exercise soon.

Contemplation. In this stage, people seriously intend to exercise within the next 6 months or at least are contemplating exercising within the next 6 months. They are typically more aware of the pros of changing behavior (here the positive effects of exercise) but are also acutely aware of the cons of this behavior change (e.g., more time away from the family). This delicate balance between the costs and benefits of

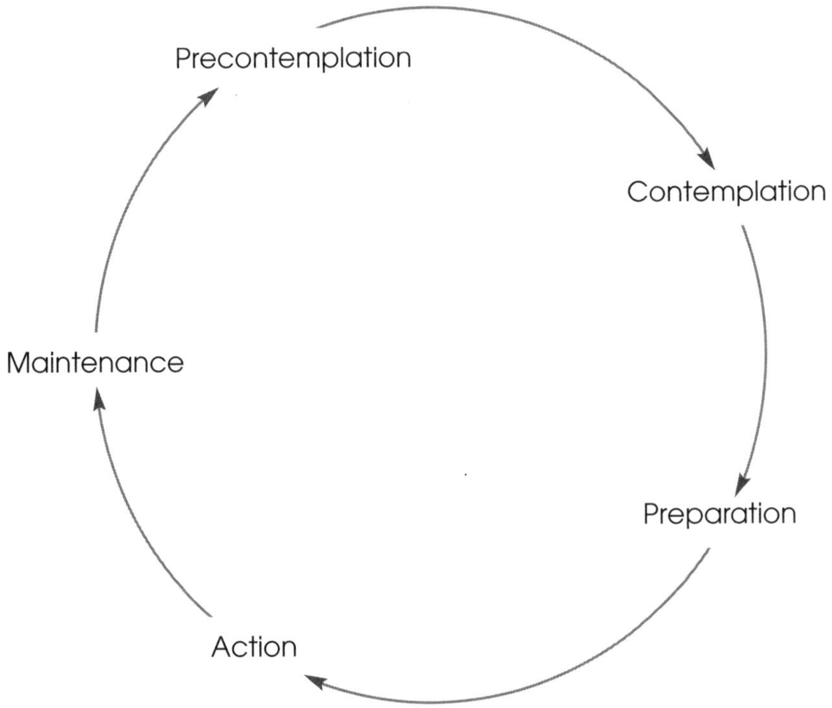

Figure 11.5. Cyclic pattern of stages of change.

changing behavior can produce profound ambivalence that can keep people "stuck" in this stage for long periods. This has often been characterized as *chronic contemplation* or *behavioral procrastination*. Therefore, despite their intentions, research has revealed that these individuals usually stay in this stage for about 2 years. So the couch potato has a fleeting thought about starting to exercise but is unlikely to act on that thought. In essence, these people are not really ready for traditional action-oriented programs.

Preparation. People in this stage are usually intending to take action in the near future, usually within the next month (e.g., "I plan on exercising three or more times a week for 20 minutes or longer"). In addition, these individuals usually have taken some significant action in the past year such as joining a health club, contacting a physician, doing a little exercise, or buying a piece of exercise equipment. In essence, these people have some sort of a plan of action. Hence, our couch potato may actually exercise, but not regularly enough to gain major benefits. Finally, preparation is not a stable stage, and people in it are more likely than precontemplators or contemplators to progress over the next 6 months.

Action. This is the stage in which people have made specific overt modifications in their lifestyle within the past 6 months. In essence, individuals in this stage may exercise regularly but have been doing so for less than 6 months. This tends to be the busiest stage in which the most processes of change are being used. (These processes will be discussed in the upcoming section.) This is also the least stable change and tends to correspond with the highest risk for relapse. Because action is observable, behavior change often has been equated with action. The difficulty is coming to a consensus on what really represents action. Generally speaking, individuals must attain a criterion that health professionals agree is sufficient to reduce risks for disease. Unfortunately, this is not always an easy task. Take smoking, for example. In the past, reducing the number of cigarettes was seen as action, but today, only total abstinence counts. In terms of exercise, what are the minimum frequency, duration, and intensity of exercise necessary for a person to be considered in the action stage? Some health professionals would argue that 3 days a week for 20 minutes at 50–70% of maximum heart rate is necessary. What if someone is walking 3 days a week for 20 minutes, but the intensity level is below 50% of maximum heart rate? Would this person be considered in the action phase? A research rule of thumb is, when in doubt, use a stricter criterion in order to obtain clearer results about how people change. So our couch

potato is now an active potato, but could easily fall back into his or her old couch-potato ways.

Maintenance. Maintenance is the period from 6 months after the criterion has been reached until such time as the risk of returning to the old behavior has been terminated. For example, individuals in this stage have been exercising regularly and have done so for more than 6 months. Once they stay in this stage for 5 years, it is likely that they will continue to maintain regular exercise throughout the life span except for injury or other health-related problems. In this stage, people are working to prevent relapse, but they do not apply change processes as frequently as people do in the action stage. Although relapse (the return from action or maintenance to an earlier stage) is always a problem when talking about behavior change, in exercise, only about 15% of the people regress all the way

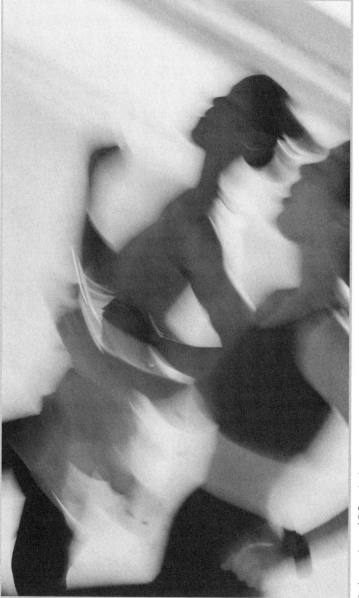

back to the precontemplation stage (and most of these will return to the contemplation or preparation stage for another serious attempt at action). At this stage, one is truly an active potato—probably for a lifetime.

Termination. Termination is the stage in which individuals have zero temptation to engage in the old behavior and 100% self-efficacy in all previously tempting situations. No matter whether they are depressed, anxious, bored, lonely, or angry, they are sure they will not return to their old unhealthy habit as a way of coping. In areas like smoking and alcoholism, it has been shown that approximately 20% of people in these groups had reached the criteria of zero temptation. In the area of exercise, it might be an ideal goal to expect a lifetime of maintenance without ever really reaching termination because there always may be temptations. So our couch potato may never reach this stage of termination, but if he stays on maintenance, then that might be sufficient.

Applications to Physical Activity

The early research on the stages-of-change model has come predominantly from work with smokers. For example, research has demonstrated that approximately 40% of smokers are in the precontemplative stage and another 40% in the contemplative stage, with approximately 20% in the preparation stage (Prochaska & Velicer, 1997a). These results indicate that action-oriented cessation programs will not match the needs of the vast majority of smokers (nor do they match people who are currently not exercising). In applying the model to exercise, one strength would appear to be its dynamic nature because exercise researchers have recommended dynamic models that focus on the transitions that occur in adoption and maintenance of a behavior (Sallis & Hovell, 1990; Sonstroem, 1988).

The initial application of the transtheoretical model to exercise was conducted at the University of Rhode Island (Sonstroem, 1988). However, the majority of work done with this model as applied to exercise has been conducted by Marcus and her colleagues. For example, in a large (over 1,000 participants) work-site exercise-promotion project (Marcus, Rossi, Selby, Niaura, & Abrams, 1992), participants were classified into the following categories: (a) 24% in precontemplation, (b) 33% in contemplation, (c) 10% in preparation, (d) 11% in action, and (e) 22% in maintenance. This pattern of distribution of stages of change is similar to the distribution of stages of change for other behaviors such as smoking cessation and weight control. It is interesting to note that participants in different stages used different processes of behavior change (which will be discussed shortly). For example, participants in the preparation stage used more behavioral

processes, such as putting things around the house to remind them to exercise, than did people in other stages. In addition, although there were many similarities between the findings in this study and those for smoking cessation, there were important differences. Specifically, the use of behavioral processes declines from the action to maintenance stage in smoking cessation, but there is no such decline in exercise.

Research has demonstrated that when there is a mismatch between stage of change and intervention strategy, attrition is high. For example, if an individual is in the contemplation stage and the intervention focuses on maintenance strategies (e.g., refining specific types of exercise behavior) instead of motivational strategies for the contemplators, dropouts will increase. In essence, we simply cannot treat people with a precontemplation profile as if they were ready for action intervention and expect them to stay with the program. Therefore, matching treatment strategies to an individual's stage of change is one strategy to improve adherence and reduce attrition. For example, initial research using smokers (and later on using exercisers) has indicated that the best strategy to promote retention is matching interventions to the stage of change (Prochaska & Velicer, 1997a). Results from these studies indicate that a reasonable goal for any therapeutic intervention is to help people progress one stage, which makes them about two-thirds more successful than people not progressing any stages. If perchance they progress two stages, then they are about two and two-thirds more successful at longer-term follow-ups.

The underlying theme of the transtheoretical model is that people are at different levels of readiness to change their behavior; therefore, different strategies or interventions are needed to bring about the desired change (Prochaska, DiClemente, & Norcross, 1992). This matching approach was taken by Marcus and her colleagues (Marcus, Banspach, Lefebvre, Rossi, Carelton, & Abrams, 1992). Participants for this program (called Imagine Action) started at different points, with 39% classified in the contemplation stage, 37% in the preparation stage, and 24% in the action stage. There was a 6-week intervention that consisted of matching self-help materials and activity to the particular stage of development of the participants. For example, the manual for contemplators was called *What's In It For You* and focused on increasing lifestyle activity such as taking the stairs instead of the elevator as well as the perceived barriers such as exercise taking up too much time. For individuals in the preparation stage, the manual was called *Ready for Action* with the goal to get people into action, which meant regular exercise in this case. The manual focused on helping people to overcome the barriers and experience the benefits of physical activity through the use of goal setting, rewarding themselves

Matching the Exercise to the Individual's Stage of Development

It appears that matching people based on their stage of development to specific interventions and strategies enhances the effectiveness of behavioral interventions. As described in the text, this approach has been successfully used in exercise interventions. Some of these studies have lacked proper controls; thus, a more controlled study was conducted by Marcus and colleagues (Marcus, Emmons, Simkin, Taylor, Linnan, Rossi, & Abrams, 1994). In this follow-up study, employees from a work-site promotion situation were randomized to a stage-matched self-help intervention or standard-care self-help intervention. This particular intervention consisted of printed materials that were distributed to participants at baseline and one month after baseline.

Individuals in the stage-matched group received manuals specifically tailored to their stage of readiness to exercise at the start (i.e., baseline) of the program. One month after the program began, individuals also received a second manual in the series. For people in the precontemplation stage, a manual entitled *Do I Need This?* was developed that focused on increasing the awareness of the positive effects of physical activity and encouraging individuals to think about the barriers that prevented them from exercising in the first place. Because they were not really ready to exercise, this manual did not have specific suggestions for starting an exercise program. For individuals in the contemplation stage, a manual entitled *Try It, You'll Like It* was developed. This manual focused on describing reasons to stay inactive but spent more time on the reasons to become active such as health and well-being. Aids to becoming more active such as setting specific, realistic goals and rewarding one-

self after successful completion of tasks (e.g., keeping to a low-fat diet, having successful exercise bouts) were also included.

For individuals in the preparation stage, a manual entitled *I'm On My Way* was developed. The information in this manual not only focused on the benefits of physical activity and goal setting but also included tips on performing safe and enjoyable activities as well as common obstacles to regular involvement in physical activity (e.g., perceived lack of time). For those in the action stage, the pamphlet called *Keep It Going* was developed. This manual provided information on such topics as staying motivated, enhancing confidence, benefiting from physical activity, active planning, and overcoming obstacles. For those people who had reached maintenance, materials entitled *I Won't Stop Now* were developed. These emphasized the benefits of physical activity, injury avoidance, proper goal setting, planning, rewards for oneself after success, and variation in activities to reduce boredom. People in the standard-care control group received standard materials from the American Heart Association because these are excellent materials readily available for use.

Results from this controlled-intervention study revealed that 3 months after the program concluded (compared to baseline information), more participants in the stage-matched group demonstrated stage progression whereas participants in the standard-care group displayed stage stability or stage regression. In essence, the matched-stage approach seemed more effective in producing positive changes in exercise intentions and behavior.

for the activity, or applying time-management skills to fit the activity into a busy schedule. For example, an individual was encouraged to watch the news on television while exercising on the stationary bicycle or to go dancing with a significant other rather than sit in a movie theater. Finally, for individuals in the action stage, a manual called *Keeping It Going* was developed, which focused on keeping up a regular program of physical activity for individuals who had been exercising for only a short period. These individuals were at great risk of slipping back into the preparation stage, which meant not exercising at all or exercising only

occasionally. Therefore, the manual focused on providing hints to troubleshoot situations that might lead to a relapse such as a vacation, illness, or injury. In addition, the manual tried to provide guidelines and hints for using goal setting and gaining social support to keep exercise going on regularly.

Results of this matching approach revealed that the intervention was successful in getting people to actually exercise or at least closer to exercise. That is, 30% of those in contemplation and 61% of those in preparation at baseline progressed to the action stage, with an additional 31% of the contemplators progressing to

---

Table 11.1
Exercise Processes of Change

Processes	Example
Cognitive Processes	
Consciousness raising	I recall information people have personally given me on the benefits of exercise.
Dramatic relief	Warnings about health hazards of inactivity move me emotionally.
Environmental reevaluation	I feel I would be a better role model for others if I exercised regularly.
Self-reevaluation	I am considering the idea that regular physical activity would make me a happier person.
Social liberation	I find society changing in ways that make it easier for the exerciser.
Behavioral Processes	
Counter-conditioning	Instead of remaining inactive, I engage in some physical activity.
Helping relationships	I can rely on my friend to help me exercise.
Reinforcement management	When I exercise regularly, I reward myself.
Self-liberation	I convince myself that I can keep exercising.
Stimulus control	To increase the probability of exercise, I put different reminders around the house.

Adapted from "The Stages and Processes of Exercise Adoption and Maintenance in a Worksite Sample," by B. H. Marcus, J. S. Rossi, V. C. Selby, R. S. Niaura, and D. B. Abrams, 1992, *Human Psychology, 11*, p. 390.

---

the preparation stage. Additionally, there was little regression to an earlier stage of development, with only 4% of those individuals in preparation and 9% of those in action actually regressing. These findings demonstrate that a low-cost, relatively low-intensity intervention can produce significant improvements in stage of exercise adoption. A similar study using a randomized design is presented in the accompanying box

Although these theories have been presented individually, they often bear a relationship to one another. For example, one study (Gorley & Gordon, 1995) found a relationship between self-efficacy and the transtheoretical model. Specifically, they found that self-efficacy to overcome barriers to exercise increased systematically throughout the stages of change. In addition, Sullum, Clark, and King (2000), tracking the exercise behavior of college students, found that students who became inactive over an eight-week period had lower self-efficacy at baseline

than did those who maintained their exercise level. Finally, investigating the virtual opposite of self-efficacy (temptation), researchers have found that although temptation (the urge to engage in a behavior during difficult situations) and self-efficacy function inversely across the stages of change, temptation is typically a better predictor of relapses (Hausenblas et al., 2001; Redding & Rossi, 1999). To demonstrate the change over stages, results of one study found that maintainers reported the lowest temptation to not exercise and the highest confidence to engage in exercise compared to individuals in other stages.

In conclusion, the popularity of the transtheoretical model in the health community, exercise literature, and its use by practitioners appears to outweigh the objective research evidence. The popularity could be attributed to a number of factors, although the most intuitively appealing feature is that it offers the potential to match an intervention to the state of readiness for change. This

Using Theory to Help Inform Practice

Much of this chapter has been aimed at trying to provide you with an understanding of the some of the major theories that have been developed to help explain and predict exercise behavior. So, from a practical point of view, let us take a look at how understanding these theories might help us predict the exercise behavior of an individual. You should understand that each theory has its own specific variables that its theorists see as most predictive of exercise behavior, and these were explained in detail in the chapter. This example will focus on taking bits and pieces from the different theories to help the practitioner make more informed decisions about promoting exercise behavior.

Your friend Kira (age 27) has not exercised for several years. She is already becoming overweight, and her blood pressure and cholesterol are on the high side. Besides changing her diet, you feel that a program of regular exercise would be beneficial to Kira from both a physical and a psychological standpoint. You are familiar with the theories of exercise behavior, and you plan to use this information to help your friend start and continue to exercise.

You first need to know what stage (from the transtheoretical model) Kira is in so you can devise a program to match that stage. You find out that she is in the contemplation stage and that she is seriously thinking about exercising due to her condition, but has not really done anything proactive thus far. Based on this, you start by informing her of the benefits of regular physical activity as well as some of the typical barriers that she will need to overcome (as well as strategies for overcoming these barriers such as time management and goal-setting skills).

You also know from the health belief model that people's likelihood of engaging in preventive health behaviors such as exercise depends on the person's perception of the severity of the potential illness as well as her appraisal of the costs and benefits of taking action. Therefore, it is your job to convince Kira of the severity of her potential problems (e.g., obesity and high blood pressure can lead to such things as heart attacks and strokes) as well as all the psychological and physiological benefits of exercise (e.g., greater self-esteem, reduced risk of cardiovascular disease, weight control, and reduction of stress and depression). You can do this by provid-

ing her written information or simply by talking to her about these pros and cons of exercising. In addition, because the health belief model also argues that "cues to action" are important variables predicting exercise behavior, you can provide Kira with an exercise machine, a newspaper article detailing the positive effects of exercise, or perhaps a guest pass or membership into a fitness club near her house.

You also know from the theories of reasoned action and planned behavior that subjective norms and perceived behavioral control are critical determinants of Kira's intention to exercise, which in turn should influence her actual exercise behavior. Along these lines, because subjective norms refer to the person's beliefs about others' opinions about the importance of exercise, you (as well as enlisting significant others) can try to convince Kira that exercising is positive and that all these important people in her life believe that exercise is a good thing. This positive social pressure to exercise will, it is hoped, cause Kira to want to exercise, in part, because the significant people in her life believe that exercise will produce positive benefits for her. In addition, it is important that Kira feel that changing her exercise behavior is under her control (perceived behavioral control). In this regard, changing a person's beliefs about her ability to exercise can directly affect behavior without influencing intentions and thus is a very powerful variable in predicting exercise behavior. Therefore, helping Kira build up her belief of control (maybe you can volunteer to do something for her while she is exercising) and convincing her that she does have the opportunity to exercise are important ways that you can influence her exercise behavior.

Finally, from self-efficacy theory, you know that a key determinant in exercise behavior is a person's belief that she can execute the necessary behaviors to produce a desired response. Up to this point, Kira has not really believed in herself, and she is not sure that she has the ability or motivation to exercise on a consistent basis. You know that the strongest source of self-efficacy is performance accomplishments, so you can try to convince Kira that she can, in fact, exercise

Continued on next page

Using Theory to Help Inform Practice (cont.)

on a regular basis. One of the best ways to do this is for Kira to actually start exercising so that she can believe that she can, in fact, exercise regularly. So you agree to be Kira's partner (see next chapter) and set a specific time to meet to exercise 3–4 days per week for 30 minutes each time. You also have Kira's family and friends encourage and support her exercise behavior and do whatever is necessary to allow her to exercise. Once Kira starts to exercise, we know from research that exercise can positively affect self-efficacy, so her belief in herself should grow with each exercise bout.

Therefore, we are taking the major concepts from each of the theories to try to help Kira increase her exercise. In essence, knowing the explanations each theory proposes regarding exercise behavior helps inform us about the factors to focus on in trying to have people start or continue an exercise program. It has been said that nothing is more practical than a good theory, and this example illustrates that knowing the theories of exercise behaviors can help inform practice to enhance the probability of engaging in exercise and adhering to an exercise program over time.

type of research has been proven successful by Marcus and her colleagues (1992; 1998), although more research is necessary before more firm conclusions can be made regarding the efficacy of the transtheoretical model. But until that time, it appears that its appeal to practitioners will result in continued use in exercise settings as the whole notion of different stages makes intuitive sense to professionals in the exercise area.

Processes of Behavioral Change

The stages of change described above document when people change, but the processes of change describe how people change (Prochaska, Velicer, DiClemente, & Fava, 1988). Processes of change are covert or overt activities that individuals use to modify their experiences and environments in order to modify behavior. To help exercisers progress through the stages, we need to understand the processes and principles of change. A number of retrospective, cross-sectional, longitudinal, and intervention studies have found that different change processes are emphasized at the various stages of change. In fact, one of the fundamental principles for progress is that different processes of change need to be applied at different stages of change. Traditional conditioning processes like counter-conditioning, stimulus control, and contingency control can be highly successful for participants taking action, but can produce resistance with individuals in precontemplation. With these individuals, more experiential processes like consciousness raising and dramatic relief might prove more effective in reaching people. Along these lines, research has revealed that people use a range of strategies and techniques to change behaviors and these strategies are the processes of change. Processes can be divided into two categories: cognitive and behavioral. These processes

are listed in Table 11.1, and these are just samples from the Processes of Change Questionnaire developed by Marcus and colleagues (Marcus et al., 1992). Use of the cognitive processes tends to peak in the preparation stage, and use of the behavioral processes tends to peak in the action stage.

In making exercise decisions, individuals also do a kind of cost-benefit analysis called decisional balance. Specifically, when people are considering a lifestyle change, they weigh the pros and cons of a given behavior (e.g., Should I begin exercising?). In one study, researchers found that usually in the precontemplation and contemplation stages, the cons are greater than the pros. However, a crossover usually occurs in the preparation stage, and then the pros outweigh the cons in the action and maintenance stages (Prochaska et al., 1998). Therefore, it's important for exercise specialists to help individuals contemplating exercise realize all of the benefits of exercise to help them move from contemplation to preparation.

Summary

In this chapter, we have learned that despite the positive information being conveyed about exercise, we still have a large majority of the population (both youth and adults) who do not exercise regularly enough to gain these positive benefits both physiologically and psychologically. The question remains, why are so many people not exercising despite all the positive benefits that can accrue from regular exercise?

One way in which to understand this phenomenon and eventually help people begin exercising and stay exercising is through an understanding of the models that have been developed to predict exercise behavior. Many models have been developed, but we have focused on those that have generated the most research support in the literature and/or have practical applications to enhancing exercise behavior. The models reviewed included the health belief model, the theory of reasoned action, the theory of planned behavior, self-efficacy theory, and the transtheoretical model. Although all of them have implications for increasing physical activity, the chapter focused more on the transtheoretical model as a way of changing exercise behavior. This is because several other theories have been tested using a stage-of-change approach, there is good preliminary research support for the model, and it makes good intuitive sense. Matching treatment to the stage an individual happens to be in at a given moment in time maximizes the individual nature of an intervention and thus increases the probability for success.

Can You Define These Terms?

attitude toward exercise

cues to action

intention to exercise

matching hypothesis

perceived behavioral control

processes of behavioral change

reciprocal determinism

self-efficacy

stages of change

subjective norms

Can You Answer These Questions?

1. Why is it important to understand the reasons people start and adhere to exercise programs? Use data from the Department of Health and Human Services to discuss your answer.

2. Discuss the major points regarding the health belief model as they relate to exercise behavior. Devise a scenario that uses the health belief model to predict exercise behavior.

3. Discuss the major components of the theory of reasoned action and the theory of planned behavior. How are these two theories similar and different?

4. If you had a friend who was not exercising, how would you use the theory of planned behavior to help this person start and continue to exercise?

5. Discuss the major predictions and key variables in self-efficacy theory as they relate to behavior change.

6. Provide specific examples of how self-efficacy can affect exercise behavior as well as how exercise behavior can influence feelings of self-efficacy.

7. Discuss the transtheoretical model of behavior change, including the different stages of change for an exerciser.

8. How does the transtheoretical model support the notion of treatment-client matching?

9. Give three examples of cognitive processes and three examples of behavior processes of exercise-behavior change.

CHAPTER 12

Motivational Determinants of Exercise Behavior

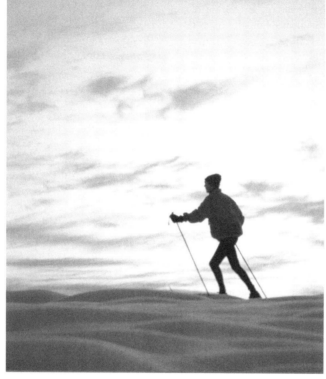

Photo courtesy of © Eyewire Images

After reading this chapter, you should be able to

- Identify the benefits of exercise,

- Identify the costs of exercise,

- Explain the problem of exercise adherence,

- Discuss the demographic determinants of physical activity,

- Explain the personal/cognitive determinants of physical activity,

- Explain the programmatic determinants of physical activity,

- Explain the environmental determinants of physical activity, and

- Discuss the characteristics of physical activity.

Introduction

Chapter 11 discussed a number of theories that help us determine and predict exercise behavior. We suggested that all potential exercisers know and evaluate the reasons for exercising as well as potential barriers or costs of exercising. However, we did not discuss those topics in detail, so we will do so now. In addition to considering why people simply might start an exercise program, we will discuss issues related to exercise maintenance, because maintenance of physical activity over a period of time has most certainly been problematic, as evidenced by the great dropout rate in exercise programs.

Reasons to Exercise

With the prevalence of people either not exercising at all (usually in the precontemplative or contemplative stage) or not exercising enough to gain physiological or psychological benefits, the initial problem we typically have to tackle is getting these people exercising in the first place. People are motivated for different reasons, but a good starting place to get people to initiate or stay with an exercise program is to emphasize the several diverse benefits of exercise (U.S. Department of Health and Human Services [USDHHS], 1996, 2000). The issue of maintenance as well as initiation is a critical one because individuals must continue to be physically active to sustain the full health benefits of regular physical activity (Marcus et al., 2000).

Weight Control

We know that the share of adults who are overweight is on the rise nationally and internationally. For example, in the United States, it is estimated that 70 to 80 million adults and 15 to 20 million American teenagers are overweight. By 1995, the percentage of adults over age 20 who were overweight climbed to approximately 35% (Dortch, 1997), and the prevalence of obesity increased from 12% in 1991 to 18% in 1998, making the United States arguably the most overweight nation on earth (Mokdad et al., 1999). Recent statistics for 2004 indicate that the U.S. population has become even more overweight and more obese. For example, statistics for 2004 indicate that 65% of the adult population is overweight and 30–35% is obese. Moreover, for ages 6–18 the rate of kids overweight has tripled since 1980. In addition, recent research has revealed a similar level of obesity for a number of other countries around the world, thus demonstrating that this is a worldwide epidemic.

For most people, when they think about losing weight, they think about dieting because many people's typical diets are filled with fast foods, high cholesterol, and poor nutrition. Although dieting certainly helps people to lose weight, exercise plays an impor-

tant role that is often underrated. For example, running three miles five times a week can produce a weight loss of 20 to 25 pounds in a year if caloric intake remains the same. The key thing is to make exercise part of the daily regimen and not an add-on after the day is almost over. Keeping weight down not only can help reduce risk for coronary heart disease (see below), but many people also feel that their appearance is greatly enhanced if they are looking trim and in shape. Maybe the most important point is that exercise can be fun and enjoyable, something to look forward to, not something that makes the participant cringe.

Reduced Risk of Chronic Diseases

There has been a good deal of research investigating the role of regular physical activity in the reduction of chronic disease states (see Berger & Motl, 2001; Biddle & Mutrie, 2001; Landers & Arent, 2001, for reviews). Results generally reveal that regular exercise can help reduce the probability of such diseases as hypertension, coronary heart disease, osteoporosis, diabetes, and strokes. This, in turn, will reduce the overall mortality rate as well as increase longevity. Although we still do not know the exact amount of exercise required to achieve these desired effects, it is clear that exercise exerts a positive influence on reducing the probability or severity of these diseases.

As noted by the USDHHS (1996), the relationship between physical inactivity and cardiovascular illness is approximately equivalent to that between smoking and coronary heart disease. In fact, the 1996 Surgeon General's report (USDHHS, 1996) noted three consistent conclusions from the studies on the relationship between physical activity and physical health. First, people of all ages can benefit from regular moderately intense physical activity several days a week for 30–60 minutes per day. Second, regular physical activity not only reduces the risk of premature mortality and acquiring the diseases noted above, it also is important for maintaining the health of people's bones, muscles and joints, as well as being a useful aid in the prevention of osteoporosis. Third, activities that develop muscular strength via resistance training should be performed at least twice per week to yield significant fitness benefits.

Reduction in Stress and Depression

Regular exercise also has been associated with increased psychological well-being. In particular, as noted in Chapters 3 and 5, research has shown that regular physical activity is associated with decreases in anxiety and depression (many times induced by increases in stress) as well as improving overall mental health (Landers & Arendt, 2001.; USDHHS, 1996, 2000). Our society has seen recently a tremendous increase in the number of people suffering from anxiety disorders and depression, and exercise is one way to cope more effectively with the world around us. (See Chapter 5 for a detailed review of the relationship between exercise and mood states such as anxiety and depression.)

Enjoyment

Although many programs will focus on providing information about the benefits of physical activity, we know that many people still do not exercise on a regular basis to receive these benefits. This is particularly important when looking at reasons for initiation of exercise programs versus adherence to these programs. Specifically, although many people start exercise programs to improve their health and lose weight, they rarely continue these programs unless they find the experience enjoyable. In general, people continue an exercise program because of the fun, happiness, and satisfaction it brings (Kimiecik, 1998), as well as simply "feeling good" after exercising (see Chapter 5). So in trying to get people to adhere to programs, it is especially important that these programs tap the participants' enjoyment of the activity. In essence, exercise should be intrinsically motivating if we are to adhere to it over a long period. This strategy is highlighted in more detail in Chapters 13 and 15.

Enhanced Self-Esteem/ Self-Concept

As noted in Chapter 4, one of the major psychological benefits of exercise is an increase in self-esteem (Sonstroem, 1997). In fact, from a public health perspective, the strongest evidence for the positive effects of exercise on mental health is for self-esteem. Enhanced self-esteem and self-concept have significance for mental health because they provide a feeling of value or worth, and they are generalized indicators of psychological adjustment. Furthermore, when increases in fitness or ability occur, there is a similar change in body image or self-perceptions (Fox, 2000). The great thing is that even walking around the block or working out at the club for a half hour can give people a sense of satisfaction from accomplishing something they couldn't or didn't do before. Furthermore, many people who exercise regularly start to feel more confident about the way they look, and this can be a big part of developing self-esteem. Specifically, one's weight appears to tie into self-esteem (especially physical self-esteem); thus, staying in shape by exercising can help build confidence to exercise (e.g., to be seen in

public), which, in turn, can eventually have a positive impact on self-perceptions.

Socializing

One of the reasons often cited for exercising or joining an exercise program is the chance to socialize and be with others. Exercise can provide an outlet to meet new people, which can often lead to camaraderie and friendship. With the fast pace of our society and people spending more time alone on the Internet and with other types of communication devices, there is a perception that there is less time to spend with friends and family. Exercising is a potential way to get with and meet people, and almost 90% of exercise program participants prefer to exercise with a partner or group rather than alone. Along these lines, although it is usually more enjoyable to exercise with somebody else, social support is also derived from others who are exercising, and this can also enhance personal commitment to exercise (Willis & Campbell, 1992). In fact, a review by Carron, Hausenblas, and Mack (1996) found that social support consistently was related to increased exercise behavior. The notion of social support is further developed in Chapter 13 because it is one of the major strategies to enhance exercise adherence.

Excuses to Not Exercise

Despite recent national and international reports regarding the variety of psychological, physiological, and social benefits of exercising, we know from the statistics that many people still choose not to exercise. Although these individuals put forth a variety of reasons for not exercising, a study out of Canada found that people usually cite lack of time, lack of energy, and lack of motivation as their primary reasons for inactivity (Canadian Fitness and Lifestyle Research Institute, 1996). It is interesting to note that these are all factors that fall under an individual's control as opposed to environmental factors, which are often out of our control (see Table 12.1). This is consistent with previous research, which has found that the major reasons for attrition from an exercise program were under a person's control (e.g., lack of motivation, time management). These results strongly suggest that participation in physical activity is modifiable if people have the desire to change their sedentary behavior (this is consistent with the stages-of-change model presented in the previous chapter). Therefore, it is incumbent on fitness professionals to develop strategies to counteract these amendable barriers to maximize exercise participation (see Chapter 13). Some of the most persistent given reasons for not exercising are discussed below.

Table 12.1		
Barriers to Physical Activity		
Barrier	**Individuals who cite this as a barrier to participation (%)**	**Type of barrier**
MAJOR BARRIERS		
Lack of time	69	Individual
Lack of energy	59	Individual
Lack of motivation	52	Individual
MODERATE BARRIERS		
Excessive cost	37	Individual
Illness/Injury	36	Individual
Lack of facilities nearby	30	Environmental
Feeling uncomfortable	29	Individual
Lack of skill	29	Individual
Fear of injury	26	Individual
MINOR BARRIERS		
Lack of safe places	24	Environmental
Lack of child care	23	Environmental
Lack of a partner	21	Environmental
Insufficient programs	19	Environmental
Lack of support	18	Environmental
Lack of transportation	17	Environmental

Note: Adapted from Progress in Prevention, by Canadian Fitness and Lifestyle Research Institute, 1996.

Perceived Lack of Time

The most frequent reason typically given for inactivity is lack of time. In fact, in the Canadian study, 69% of those surveyed cited lack of time as a major barrier to physical activity (Canadian Fitness and Lifestyle Research Institute, 1996). Are we talking about a real lack of time, or is "lack of time" just a simple and convenient excuse for not exercising? Research has revealed that it appears to be a perception of lack of time because a close look at schedules usually reveals that this lack of time is more in someone's head rather than being a reality. The problem appears to be one of priorities, as people simply don't put exercise high enough on their list. They seem to have time to watch TV, hang out, talk on the telephone, or read the newspaper, but not enough time to exercise. Only when fitness professionals make programs enjoyable, satisfy-

ing, meaningful, and convenient can exercising compete well against other leisure activities. In devising programs of physical activity therefore, fitness professionals need to look at the reasons why people exercise and why they adhere to exercise over time.

Lack of Energy

For many people (59%, in fact), lack of energy is a major barrier to physical activity (Canadian Fitness and Lifestyle Research Institute, 1996). In today's society, everyone seems to be on the go all the time, and these busy schedules provide a nice excuse for feeling fatigued and thus not exercising. Because our busy schedules are often related to our jobs or careers, this fatigue typically is more mental than physical and is, in fact, often stress-related. In Chapters 5 and 6, we discussed that exercise could help produce positive mood-enhancing effects and actually increase perceptions of energy (Thayer, 1996; Thayer, Newman, & McClain, 1994). In essence, individuals can change their perceived levels of energy through exercise as simple as brisk walking. Therefore, fitness professionals should emphasize that a brisk walk, bicycle ride, or tennis game can relieve tension and stress and at the same time be more energizing. Physical activity therefore can help reduce the stress occurring from daily hassles (e.g., walking can increase one's energy level), especially if these activities are structured to be fun and enjoyable.

Lack of Motivation

Another reason typically given for not exercising is lack of motivation. There is no doubt that it takes commitment and dedication to maintain regular physical activity when our lives are already busy with work, family, and friends. It is easy to lose our motivation to exercise, especially if other aspects of life take up a lot of energy and motivation. Therefore, it is important to remember the physiological and psychological benefits of being physically active and to make these activities enjoyable and part of our daily regimen. In addition, making the activity enjoyable is critical to keeping motivation high. For example, setting specific, attainable goals can help enhance motivation.

The use of goal setting (as well as other strategies) aimed at improving adherence to exercise is detailed in Chapter 13.

The Problem of Exercise Adherence

As noted in Chapter 11, once sedentary people have overcome inertia and start exercising, the next barrier is to keep on exercising. This is harder than it seems, as research has consistently found that approximately 50% of participants drop out of exercise programs within the first 6 months (see Figure 12.1). Even among the habitually active, unexpected disruptions in activity routines or settings can interrupt or end a previously continuous exercise program. Relocation, medical events, and travel can impede the continuity of activity reinforcement and create new activity barriers. Along these lines, Sallis and colleagues (1990) found that from a sample of over 500 current exercisers, 40% had experienced an exercise relapse (stopped exercising for at least 3 months) and 20% had experienced three or more relapses. The most frequent reason for relapse was injury, which was followed by work demands, lack of interest, lack of time, family demands, end of sport season, bad weather, and stress. Dishman and Buckworth (1997) note that these events may have a more limited impact if the individual antic-

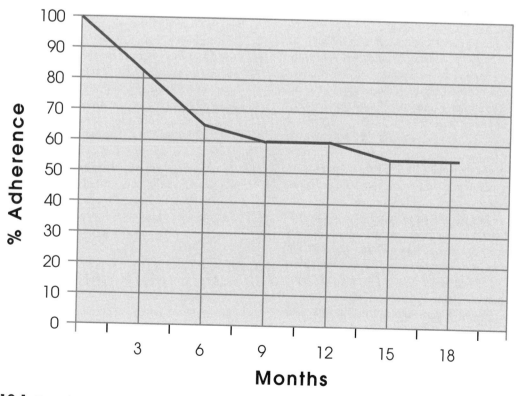

Figure 12.1. Drop in adherence rates for individuals trying to maintain regular exercise.

ipates and plans their occurrence, recognizes them as temporary impediments, and develops self-regulatory skills for preventing relapses to inactivity. For example, what contingency plans might you have if you injured your shoulder (or other upper body part)? Stationary bikes, for instance, might be employed in the interim until the upper body injury is healed.

Along these lines, Prochaska and Velicer (1997b) note that, in the sense that there is a high relapse rate in exercise programs, exercise is like dieting, quitting smoking, or cutting down on drinking alcohol. Specifically, as reported in the previous chapter, it was shown that people typically intend to change a habit that affects their health and well-being negatively, and they typically want to start exercising again after relapsing. In the stages-of-change model reviewed in the last chapter, these people would be in the contemplative stage. To get people who are thinking about exercise to actually exercise, a heavy media advertising campaign from sportswear companies and fitness clubs is typically mounted before the beginning of the year to feed on people's New Year resolutions to start exercising next year. These companies are usually successful in getting people to start exercising again. However, these newcomers typically drop out in 6 to 12 months. So, when people start an exercise program, why don't they stick with it?

Determinants of Exercise Adherence

As noted in the previous chapter, one way to help understand this dropout phenomenon is through the models of exercise adherence. Another way is to gain a better understanding of the determinants of exercise behavior, and this will be the focus of the rest of the chapter. Determinants have been used to denote a reproducible association or predictive relationship, rather than imply cause and effect, because many or most of the studies in this area have been correlational (Buckworth & Dishman, 1999). These determinants fall into a number of different categories, and we examine each category, highlighting the most consistent specific factors related to adherence and dropout rates. Table 12.2 summarizes the positive and negative influences on adherence along with the variables having no or mixed influence on exercise adherence (Dishman & Buckworth, 1997; Dishman & Sallis, 1994; Heaney & Goetzel, 1997). Like Dishman and Buckworth, we will focus on studies in which the sample size was relatively large (i.e., weighted sample size) because this approach typically yields a better estimate of the true effect of how these determinants actually affect the population under study. A final note of caution is warranted here. Specifically, determinants of physical activity are not isolated variables, but

they influence and are influenced by each other as they contribute to the behavioral outcome. Therefore, although presented separately, these determinants do not act in a vacuum, and they are affected by environmental and personal factors.

Personal Factors

The first set of factors potentially related to exercise adherence that we will present is termed personal characteristics. These can be further divided into the three categories, including demographics, cognitive variables, and behaviors.

Demographics

As seen in Table 12.2, demographic variables traditionally have had a strong association with physical activity.

Socioeconomic status. Research has indicated that people with higher income and more education are more likely to be physically active than are those with lower income and less education. Specifically, for individuals earning less than $15,000 annually, 65% are inactive as compared to 48% of those earning more than $50,000. In addition, of those with less than a high school education, 72% are sedentary as compared to 50% of college-educated individuals (U.S. Centers for Disease Control and Prevention, 1993). Thus, having more education is associated with higher levels of adherence although the effect of participating in exercise among healthy people has been contrasted with all groups of patients. However, there have not been many studies investigating exercise behavior for people who had coronary heart disease (CHD) or were at high risk for CHD, nor were there many for people who had other chronic diseases or had physically or developmentally disabling conditions. This type of analysis would be important when investigating the impact of disease on exercise adherence.

Age. Using age as a variable, physical activity typically declines as one gets older, with a 50% decrease from ages 6 to 16. This result contributes to the increased childhood obesity documented by the USDHHS (2000), which has shown that this decrease in moderate-vigorous physical activity (at least 3 days per week) from grades 9 through 12 occurs both for males (80% to 67%) and for females (65% to 45%). This decline in physical activity continues throughout adulthood (Leslie, Fotheringham, Owen, & Bauman, 2001) and appears to continue to age 80 with progressively fewer people exercising on a regular basis. In fact, Ruuskanen and Puoppila (1995), using over 1,200 participants, found a significant decline in physical activity between ages 65 and 80 due to such things as impaired health and reduced cardiovascular functioning, as well as social isolation due to poor health. In addition, the Norwegian Confederation of Sports

Table 12.2
Known Determinants of Exercise Adherence

Determinant	Positive	Negative	Neutral
PERSONAL FACTORS			
Demographics			
Age		✓	
Blue-collar occupation		✓	
Level of education	✓		
Gender (male)	✓		
High risk for heart disease		✓	
Socioeconomic status	✓		
Overweight			✓
Cognitive/personality factors			
Attitudes			✓
Barriers to exercise		✓	
Enjoyment of exercise	✓		
Expectation of health benefits	✓		
Intention to exercise	✓		
Knowledge of health and exercise			✓
Lack of time		✓	
Mood disturbance		✓	
Perceived health or fitness	✓		
Self-efficacy for exercise	✓		
Self-motivation	✓		
Behaviors			
Diet			✓
Past childhood unstructured physical activity			✓
Past adult unstructured physical activity	✓		
Past program participation	✓		
School sports			✓
Smoking		✓	
Type A behavior pattern		✓	
ENVIRONMENTAL FACTORS			
Social environment			
Class size			✓
Group cohesion	✓		
Physician influence			✓
Past family influences	✓		
Social support friends/peers	✓		
Social support spouse/family	✓		
Social support staff/instructor	✓		
Physical environment			
Climate/season		✓	
Cost			✓
Disruptions in routine		✓	
Access to facilities: actual	✓		
Access to facilities: perceived	✓		
Home equipment			✓
Physical activity characteristics			
Intensity		✓	
Perceived effort		✓	
Group program	✓		
Leader qualities	✓		

Note: Adapted from Weinberg, R. S., & Gould, D. (2003)
Foundations of sport and exercise psychology, Champaign, IL: Human Kinetics, pp. 409–410.

(1984) observed an increasing appreciation of the contribution of exercise to health and a diminished valuation of the fun and enjoyment of exercise among older adults. Thus, it would make sense that the health and enjoyment aspects of exercise should be emphasized when working with older populations. In essence, it is always important to know with whom we are working in order to maximize the effectiveness of any intervention

Gender. Regarding male-female comparisons, no consistent significant differences (in reduction of physical activity) have been observed, although differences do appear occasionally in some particular studies. In essence, individual differences should always be noted. Finally, as noted earlier, it has consistently been found that males have higher levels of physical activity than females (although decreases do not differ), which, in part, can be attributed to sociocultural influences.

Ethnicity. In a study conducted by the Centers for Disease Control and Prevention (USDHHS, 2000), ethnic differences were found to affect physical activity. Specifically, 36% of White Americans were sedentary followed by 42% of Asians or Pacific Islanders, 46% of American Indians, 52% of Black or African Americans, and 54% of Hispanic Americans. These discrepancies are apparent even at the high school level, with 67% of White students engaging in vigorous physical activity compared to only 60% of Hispanics and 54% of African Americans. Along these lines, a study by King and colleagues (2000) included a large percentage of nonwhite participants. These women have been underrepresented in previous studies or had been virtually absent from the literature (Taylor, Baranowski, & Young, 1998). Yet it is believed from the little data that are available that these individuals might be especially at risk for low levels of physical activity (Eyler et al., 1998). Specifically, using a large population of African-American, Hispanic, American Indian, and Alaskan Native women, it was found that the barriers to exercise were similar to (although not the same as) those of a comparable group of White females.

For example, for all ethic subgroups, caregiving duties and lack of energy to exercise ranked among the top four most frequently reported barriers. Caregiving was also identified as an important barrier to physical activity participation among women in a larger population-based study (over 15,000 respondents) that included 15 European Union member states (Zunfl et al., 1999), as well as in a community-based physical-activity intervention targeting rural Latino families (Grassi, Gonzales, Tello, & He, 1999). However, frequently observing others exercising in their neighborhood increased physical activity participation for African-American women, and not being in good health was associated with less physical activity for

American Indian and Alaskan Native women. Interestingly, discouragement from others about exercise was associated with more exercise in Hispanic women, and being self-conscious about one's own appearance increased physical activity in American Indians-Pacific Islanders. With respect to self-consciousness, it is possible that appearance motives might increase interest and participation in physical activity. On one hand, it is possible that greater levels of physical activity, which often occur in public venues or settings, lead to increased awareness that others may be noticing one's appearance. On the other hand, in the case of discouragement from others, more criticism from others might be related to choosing to spend more time exercising. More research is definitely needed in this area before firm conclusions can be made. Nevertheless, to maximize the effectiveness of any intervention aimed at increasing levels of physical activity, it is important to note the population subgroup with which one is working.

Education. Research clearly indicates that level of education is positively associated with leisure time physical activity (Ross, 2000). For example, only 6% of adults older than 25 with less than a 9th grade education engage in vigorous physical activity compared to 32% who have a college degree or greater (USDHHS, 2000). It appears that even the level of parents' education is important as 68% of high school students who reported engaging in vigorous exercise had parents with at least some college education, whereas only 54% of high school students reported engaging in vigorous exercise if their parents had no college education. Interestingly, even the level of education of other members in the community has an impact on physical activity levels. Specifically, Ross (2000) found that people exercised more if their neighbors had college degrees. In fact, the level of education of one's neighbors was a better predictor of physical activity than was one's own education level. In a sense there seems to be a social facilitation effect of others, on one's own level of physical activity.

Other demographic variables. Staying with the theme of individual differences (based on demographics), consistent findings have been observed for smokers and blue-collar workers, with these individuals more likely to drop out of exercise programs or exercise regularly than are either nonsmokers or white-collar workers (Dishman & Buckworth, 1997). Also, blue-collar workers and smokers are less likely to use work-site exercise facilities. This may be due to the fact that many blue-collar workers may carry with them the perception that on-job activity is adequate for health and fitness despite low actual exertion. Regarding obesity (another individual difference factor), early results indicated that obese individuals were generally less active than those of normal weight and were less likely to adhere to exercise programs. Due to the difficulty in actually exercising, it was felt that obese people might respond better to alternative routines of moderate activity such as walking than to more vigorous fitness regimens. However, more recent research has revealed no association between obesity and physical activity, and obese individuals do not react more favorably to lower metabolic activities such as walking. Therefore, exercise professionals need not alter activities just based on the notion of a client's weight, although this should be factored into the total exercise picture.

Cognitive/Personality Variables

A number of cognitive and personality variables have been investigated in the past 20 years to determine if they help predict and are related to patterns of physical activity.

Self-motivation. If we take a look at personality variables first (these trait variables tend to be relatively stable over time), a trait measure of self-motivation has been a relatively consistent correlate of physical activity, with people high in self-motivation generally being more physically active. Self-motivation has been conceived as a personality variable in which an individual continues to persist at an activity without any external inducements. For example, an individual who continues to exercise regularly without any assistance from significant others might be considered to be high on self-motivation if this is a typical kind of behavior. In essence, does the person exhibit this type of persistence across different situations?

Empirical evidence suggests that self-motivation may reflect self-regulatory skills such as effective goal setting, self-monitoring of progress, and self-reinforcement that are believed to be important for maintaining physical activity (Dishman & Buckworth, 1997). For example, successful endurance athletes consistently have scored high in self-motivation, and self-motivation has discriminated between people adhering to versus dropping out of a variety of physical activity-related programs across different programs, such as corporate fitness, preventive medicine, cardiac rehabilitation, commercial spa, and athletic conditioning.

Combined with other measures, self-motivation can predict adherence even more accurately. For example, when self-motivation scores were combined with percent body fat, about 80% of subjects were correctly predicted to be either adherents or dropouts (Dishman, 1981). However, it is important to note that some studies do not find self-motivation differing between adherers and dropouts, and, thus, it is always useful to understand adherence based on the person and the situation in which the person is placed (e.g., interactional model). For example, a person might be high in self-motivation but be low in social support

and have a high exercise intensity that might negate self-motivation effects.

Self-efficacy. Another important personality variable that has been a consistent predictor of exercise behavior is self-efficacy. In fact, self-efficacy has received the most support of any personal variable in predicting adherence, accounting for 25% to 35% of the variation in physical activity in most studies. Self-efficacy was discussed in detail in the previous chapter under social cognitive models and can simply be defined as the belief than an individual can successfully perform a desired behavior. It has been found that self-efficacy beliefs about one's ability to exercise have predicted compliance with an exercise prescription in both heart and lung disease patients as well in

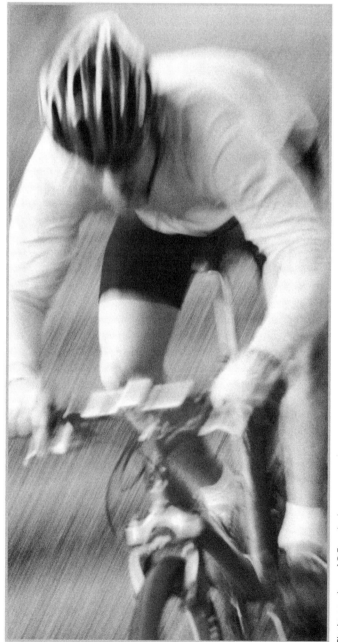

Photo courtesy of © Eyewire Images

normal adults (McAuley & Blissmer, 2002). Getting started in an exercise program, for example, is likely affected by the confidence one has in being able to perform the desired behavior (e.g., walking, swimming, running, cycling, aerobic dance) and keeping the behavior up over time (i.e., maintenance). Many people who haven't been exercising regularly may feel awkward and self-conscious about their bodies. Therefore, it is important to help people feel confident about their bodies through offering social support encouragement and tailoring activities to meet their needs and abilities. These all help to enhance feelings of self-efficacy, which will, in turn, enhance the likelihood that people will initiate and adhere to an exercise program or regimen.

Knowledge of physical activity. In addition to self-efficacy and self-motivation, the cumulative body of evidence also supports the conclusion that knowledge, attitudes, values, and beliefs regarding physical activity are associated with increased physical activity levels among adults as well as with adherence to structured physical activity programs (e.g., Marcus et al., 2000). In fact, research has revealed that knowledge, attitudes, values, and beliefs regarding physical activity can be modified in population-based educational campaigns, and these changes then influence individuals' intention to be active and finally their actual physical activity. Along these lines, research has indicated that intentions have accounted for about 50% of the variation in self-reported physical activity. More specifically, Courneya, Friedenreich, Arthur, and Bobick (1999) found that intention to exercise was a positive determinant of cancer patients' actual exercise after surgery. In essence, if you can change people's intention to exercise, then you have a good chance of changing their actual exercise behavior.

It is therefore important that individuals receive information regarding the benefits of regular physical activity (such as is done in many of the programs testing the stage model of exercise adherence discussed in the previous chapter) along with ways to overcome perceived barriers as a way to change their attitudes and beliefs regarding regular exercise. This type of information delivery also helps get people to actually act on this information. As alluded to above, an example of how to provide this type of information was discussed in the previous chapter when presenting research on the stages-of-change model (Marcus, Rossi, Selby, Niaura, & Abrams, 1992) with the distribution of exercise-specific manuals to participants based on their current stage of physical activity.

As you will learn in the next chapter, however, simply changing attitudes may not always be enough to change actual exercise behavior. For example, changing attitudes might be enough to get people started in an exercise program, but these changes alone will typically not be enough to make people adhere to an exercise program. Estimates from several countries indicate that more than half of the public is aware of fitness-promotion programs (in essence, they have the knowledge to change behavior), but less than 20% felt themselves influenced by such programs. Educational campaigns (i.e., increased information) may more effectively increase physical activity if they dispel misinformation that might impede activity for some groups. This is especially the case if knowledge about effective goal setting and other behavioral skills is reinforced by successful experience or peer models that demonstrate the skills and desirable outcomes (Dishman, 1993).

For these education campaigns to be very effective, they should tie into people's personal meaning of exercise, which will be discussed in Chapter 14. More specifically, one person might relate more to the health benefits of exercise whereas another might be more "turned on" by the recreational aspect of exercise. Furthermore, exercise can provide an avenue for increasing self-awareness and exploration and an opportunity for self-reflection; it can facilitate self-responsibility, or it can help bring body and mind together. So it is very important that these messages are in concert with the personal meaning people attach to their exercise to increase the probability that the messages will be meaningful and thus acted upon.

As noted above, it is extremely important that we also make the activity enjoyable and fun for the person involved if we expect this person to maintain this exercise behavior over time. The importance of the concept of enjoyment along with a focus on play is highlighted in Chapters 2, 13, and 15. In essence, as noted earlier, enjoyment has been a consistent determinant of increased physical activity, and we will discuss ways to enhance enjoyment of physical activity and exercise in the next chapter.

Behaviors

The previous discussion centered on demographic and cognitive/personality variables related to exercise. What are the actual behaviors of people that are related to exercise participation?

Past participation in physical activity. Of the many behaviors studied in relation to predicting physical activity patterns in adulthood, previous physical activity and sport participation have produced some of the most consistent findings. In fact, in supervised programs where activity can be directly observed, past participation in an exercise program has been shown to be the most reliable predictor of current participation (Dishman & Sallis, 1994). However, it does seem to matter whether one's participation was in childhood or early adulthood. Specifically, research with a wide range of participants has revealed that past (recent past) program participation and adulthood physical activity are more predictive of current levels of exercise than early childhood physical activity.

Along these lines, it is important to note that most studies that track physical activity participation across ages are based on correlations from an earlier age to a later age in a longitudinal fashion. In general, researchers have found moderate correlations tracking physical activity from childhood to adolescence, lower correlations from adolescence to young adulthood, and relatively weak correlations from childhood and adolescence to older adulthood (Janz, Dawson, & Mahoney, 2000; Malina, 2001). In essence, when trying to predict from a younger age to an older age, physical activity prediction is not very strong.

However, if people have participated in and adhered to an exercise program in the recent past, then they are more likely to adhere in the near future. Evidently, the key behavior is that an individual has developed a fairly recent habit of being physically active in his or her adult years regardless of the activity pattern in childhood. In fact, research has revealed that habit is often as strong a predictor of physical activity as attitudes, self-efficacy about exercise, and intentions to exercise (Godin, 1994). As one exerciser put it, "Once I was in a program, I knew what it took to stay active and learned the importance of exercise, so it was just a matter of time before I was going to start another program." Therefore, we can seemingly overcome a childhood that was lacking in physical activity by developing an adult habit of physical activity. This prediction of increased involvement following recent participation in physical activity holds for adult men and women in supervised fitness programs, and it is consistent with observations in treatment programs for patients with coronary heart disease and obesity. So it's important then to get initial exercisers into programs.

Conversely, little evidence indicates that mere participation in school sports in one's youth in and of itself will predict adult physical activity. Similarly, there continues to be little support for the notion that activity patterns in childhood are predictive of later physical activity. In fact, prospective studies have not shown a relationship for adherence to cardiac rehabilitation exercise programs or for physical activity in the community at large with participation in interscholastic or intercollegiate athletics. However, active children who receive parental encouragement for physical activity were more active as adults than were children who were sedentary and did not receive parental support. Along these lines, an extensive survey of 10 European countries and approximately 40,000 schoolchildren revealed that children whose parents, best friends, and siblings took part in sport and physical activity were very likely to take part themselves and continue to exercise into adulthood (Wold & Anderssen, 1992). In addition, other research from the Netherlands revealed that there was a 10% decline in physical activity from ages 12 to 18 except in the most active 10% of the children, whose participation remained stable over time. These results underscore the importance of encouraging and getting youngsters involved in regular physical activity and sport participation early in life, especially at a high and regular level of physical activity, as well as providing lots of adult support and encouragement for this participation.

Environmental Factors

The environment would seem to offer the potential to impact on physical activity. Let's take the differences in travel activity among people in the Netherlands, Canada, and the United States. Specifically, people in the Netherlands use their bicycles much more and walk much more than do their Canadian and American counterparts. In fact, people in the Netherlands use a car for only 44% of all trips in urban areas, whereas in Canada 74% of all trips are taken by car and this number rises to 84% in America. One factor that has been mentioned as a possible explanation is the physical environment of the roadways. For example, in the Netherlands, roads and paths are constructed to facilitate cycling and walking with separate paths and right of way for cyclists. However, in North America, many roadways are developed without bicycle paths, or even sidewalks. With attached garages, many North Americans don't even have to step out of the house to make a trip. Some people would argue that this can, in part, be explained by cultural difference. Although cultural norms undoubtedly have an impact on travel patterns, studies have revealed that in the U.S. and Canada, 46% and 70% of respondents, respectively, said they would cycle to work more often if safe bicycle lanes were provided (Puchjer & Lefevre, 1996).

As a result, environmental factors have been shown to be a critical ingredient in adhering to exercise programs. At times, the environment can help regular participation in physical activity, but at other times, it can hinder participation. Environmental factors can include a whole host of variables including the social environment, such as family and peers, the physical environment, such as weather, time pressures, and distance from facilities, as well as the characteristics of the physical activity itself (e.g., intensity, duration, frequency). Environments that promote increased activity, while offering easily accessible facilities and removing real and perceived barriers to an exercise routine, are likely prerequisites for successful maintenance of exercise behavior change. For example, adherence to physical activity is higher when individuals perceive that they have time to be active, are supported by their family and close friends (social environment), and have more opportunity to exercise due to better access to an exercise or fitness facility (physical environment). Unfortunately, most of the determinants that have been studied in the past have focused on psychological, demographic, behavioral, and programmatic factors rather than on environmental variables (Sallis & Owen, 1999). However, some recent studies (as reported below) have started to provide information on environmental factors affecting physical activity. Ecological models of physical activity emphasize the expected interplay of demographic, psychological, social, and environmental variables in influencing physical activity patterns. Some of the more prominent environmental factors, both physical and social, affecting physical activity are discussed below.

Physical Environment

As noted above, the physical environment itself can have an important impact on exercise adherence. We will now review some of the important physical determinants of exercise.

Physical location. In terms of the physical environment, one of the central factors appears to be whether or not the person has a convenient location to participate in physical activity either near the home or at the workplace. Interestingly, both the perceived convenience and actual proximity to home or work site are fairly consistent factors as to whether someone chooses to exercise and adheres to a supervised exercise program (King, Blair, & Bild, 1992). The closer to home or work the exercise setting is to the individual, the greater the likelihood of his or her beginning and staying with a program. However, individual differences, of course, need to be considered. The importance of the environment is consistent with some theories (e.g., Bandura, 1997) that have suggested the potential importance of the immediate environment in influencing physical activity levels.

As a result of the possible importance of location in relation to adoption and maintenance of physical activity, a number of potential settings for exercise programs have been explored in addition to the more traditional home and work-site settings. These have included such places as primary and secondary schools, senior centers, places of worship, and recreation centers. In documenting these changes, results from research have revealed the potential effectiveness of community-based physical activity programs, especially if they are convenient to the participants (Smith & Biddle, 1995). The importance of convenience to exercise facilities is supported in a different way by the results of King et al.'s (2000) study. Specifically, they found that approximately two-thirds of women from different ethnic groups expressed a preference for undertaking physical activity on their own with some instruction, as opposed to going to an exercise group at a workout facility. The authors hypothesize

that the preference for activities one can undertake on one's own probably reflects the roles that convenience and flexibility play in influencing people's physical activity choices as well as subsequent participation levels. These results underscore the importance of continuing to fashion effective physical activity programs that are appealing to the large number of people who prefer to "go it alone" rather than join a community class or group.

Besides the actual physical location itself, the geographic location has an impact on physical activity, as it is affected by the climate or season. For example, physical activity levels are lowest in the winter and highest in the summer, with summer being lighter longer and having temperatures more conducive to outdoor activity. Along these lines, from observational studies, the time spent outdoors is one of the best correlates of physical activity in preschool children (Kohl & Hobbs, 1998).

Neighborhood design. It has been hypothesized that one's own physical environment (i.e., neighborhood) would have an important influence on levels of physical activity. In fact, Sallis (2000b) has noted that one of the major reasons for the current epidemic of inactive lifestyles is the design of modern built environments. The best supporting evidence comes from transportation research showing that urban environments in the United States are designed with formidable barriers to walking and biking as part as everyday life. Similarly, many "established" neighborhoods were built with little thought in mind to the physical activity and recreational needs of the people living there. In fact, people often give this reason for not getting into an exercise program in the first place. Unfortunately, to date, little research has investigated these neighborhood and transportation variables as they may relate to physical activity levels, but it seems logical that creating environments that encourage (rather than discourage) physical activity via walking, cycling, and other types of exercise would be an important factor in encouraging more active lifestyles. Hence, this seems a fertile area for applied research for those interested in increasing physical activity levels.

Along these lines, Booth, Owen, Bauman, Cavisi, and Leslie (2000) examined the perceptions of the environment and physical activity in Australians older than 60 years of age. Results revealed that participants who were more active perceived that they had greater access to a recreation center bicycle track, gymnasium, and parks, as well as perceiving footpaths to be safer. Furthermore, footpath safety and access to a local park provided the best predictors of physical activity. In another study using over 2,000 Australian college students (over 40% of which were not regularly or consistently active), Leslie et al. (1999) found that people who stayed active continued participating regardless of their physical location. So there is something to be said about developing a habit of physical activity.

Time constraints. Although not classically seen as an environmental variable, one could include perceived lack of time in this group, as it is often related to one's perception of his or her physical environment. As noted at the outset of the chapter, a perceived lack of time has been found to be the most prevalent and principal reason given for dropping out of supervised clinical and community exercise programs (Dishman & Buckworth, 1997). In essence, when time seems short, people typically drop exercise because it is not a priority in their lives. How many times have you heard someone say, "I'd like to exercise but I just don't have the time"? What we have found is that people really have a perceived lack of time, and this often simply reflects a lack of interest or commitment to exercise. This notion is supported by research, indicating that regular exercisers are at least as likely as the sedentary to view time as a barrier to exercise (Dishman, 1997). For example, women employed outside the home are more likely than full-time homemakers to exercise regularly, and single parents are more physically active than families with two parents. So it is not clear that time constraints truly predict or determine exercise participation. Rather, physical inactivity might have more to do with poor time-management skills than lack of time. To illustrate, for some individuals, a lack of appreciation of the benefits of exercise may result in a low task priority in their busy day, and, thus, they perceive no time to exercise.

Along these lines, it is interesting to note that although lack of time was cited as a major reason for physical inactivity, home exercise equipment has not solved the inactivity problem. Specifically, Americans spent nearly three times as much on home exercise equipment from 1986 to 1996 ($1.2 billion to $3 billion). However, during that period, moderate to vigorous physical activity only increased 2%, as a lot of that equipment ended up in people's garages and closets.

If sedentary people lack motivation, rationalizing that they do not have enough time to exercise (even with exercise equipment in the house) represents an easy excuse for not exercising in the first place. Despite this fact, exercise leaders should try to schedule programs at optimal times for busy people. Regardless of a leader's best efforts and intentions, this may still result in exercising on one's own, rather than with a group or formal exercise program, if a convenient time cannot be scheduled. Before and after the workday seem to be more popular than during lunch for both formal and informal exercise programs. However, other times might also work (especially for informal individualized exercise), and these individual differences should be accounted for whenever possible. Studies have shown that trying to squeeze an exercise class in during the lunch hour causes people to drop out. Therefore, helping new exercisers deal more effectively with time management might be especially beneficial as well as helping them find ways and places to exercise on their own.

Social Environment

Besides one's physical environment, an individual's social environment can be just as, if not more, important in facilitating physical activity. Along these lines, one of the key aspects of the social environment is social support. Social support from family, friends, and significant others has been consistently related to adult physical activity and adherence to structured exercise programs (USDHHS, 1996). To illustrate, when dealing with youth, findings from developmental psychology suggest that peers would have the most influence on adolescent physical activity. In the sport/physical activity realm, however, parents have also been shown to be critical providers of social support and encouragement for sport and physical activity. This social support could take the form of parents' providing information on physical activity, viewing a child's play or practice, discussing physical activity with the child, offering to exercise with the child, and assisting the child (e.g., providing transportation to practice) in physical activity interests. Along these lines, research (Taylor, Baranowski, & Sallis, 1994) has revealed consistently positive associations between parental encouragement of activity and young children's immediate physical activity. In essence, more active parents tend to have more active children, and parental prompts for children to play outdoors, rather than watch television or play video games, increase children's level of physical activity. A meta-analysis by Carron and Hausenblas (1996) found that support from the family and support from important others had a consistently moderate effect on one's intention to exercise.

Of all the social influence variables studied, social support of one's spouse or significant other has received the most attention and most support in enhancing physical activity. In particular, a spouse has great influence on exercise adherence, and a spouse's attitude can exert even more influence than one's own attitude (Dishman, 1994). An example of the tremendous influence spouses can have on exercise adherence comes from the Ontario Exercise-Heart Collaborative Study (Oldridge et al., 1983). Specifically, the dropout rate among patients whose spouses were indifferent or negative toward the program was three times greater than among patients with spousal support. In this study and in most other studies, spousal support is generally defined as the demonstration of a positive attitude toward an exercise program and the encouragement of involvement in it. Expressing interest in program activities, enthusiasm for the spouse's progress, and willingness to juggle schedules to facilitate exercise participation are examples of this type of support.

Although the notion of spousal support will be discussed in the next chapter when we explore characteristics of successful intervention programs, a few points are noteworthy here. First of all, exercise professionals can possibly use spousal support in different ways, such as by arranging an orientation session for family members, offering a parallel exercise program for them, or educating spouses on all aspects of the exercise program to foster an understanding of the goals. In one study on cardiac rehabilitation, the dropout rate, which had been 56% before initiation of the spouse program, reduced to only 10% for patients with a spouse in the support program (Erling & Oldridge, 1985). The nice thing is that the social support could be as simple as a few encouraging words, such as saying, "Way to go" or "I'm proud of you" as someone is trying to stay physically active. Such personalized social reinforcement can exert a positive influence on exercise adherence and does not cost anything to the provider of this reinforcement.

Physical Activity/Program Characteristics

Both practitioners and researchers have realized that the actual characteristics of the physical activity itself can have a great impact on an individual's continued participation in that activity. This observation is supported by the quantitative research of Dishman and Buckworth (1997), which demonstrates that such physical activity characteristics as exercise intensity, type of physical activity, and exercise measures utilized affect the maintenance of physical activity programs. Some of the more important factors influencing exercise participation are reviewed below.

Exercise Intensity/Duration

There is no doubt that the intensity of one's physical activity is an important factor related to adherence and maintenance of exercise programs. It makes sense that high-intensity exercise is more stressful on the system than low-intensity exercise, especially for people who have been sedentary. In essence, individuals generally find higher-intensity activities more physically painful and more demanding in effort expenditure. This, in turn, can make the activity seem less enjoyable. As a result, there are more dropouts from exercise programs where the intensity levels are higher. In fact, it is noted in Chapter 6 that high-intensity exercise can sometimes be related to negative or undesirable mood change, which would also make exercise a less enjoyable activity. Although early research showed little

relationship between exercise intensity and adherence in supervised programs, there was a negative relationship (i.e., higher intensity, lower adherence) between intensity and adherence in unsupervised programs (Dishman, 1997).

Research (Dishman & Buckworth, 1997) has also indicated that the highest levels of adherence occurred when exercise was done at a lower intensity (i.e., less than 50% of maximum heart rate—usually walking programs) than at a higher intensity (i.e., 50%–70% of maximum heart rate—usually jogging/aerobic programs). An interesting gender difference was found in a study of California adults where more men (11%) than women (5%) adopted vigorous exercise such as running during a year's time, but a comparatively higher proportion of women (33%) than men (26%) took up moderate activities such as walking, stair climbing, and gardening. Probably the key point was that both men and women were more likely to adopt regular activities of a moderate intensity than of higher intensity. Furthermore, adoption of moderate activities was associated with a dropout rate of 25% to 35%, which was roughly half (50%) of that seen for vigorous exercise (Sallis et al., 1986). However, recent research (Anton et al., 2005) has revealed that previous exercise participation might moderate the intensity-adherence relationship. Specifically, results revealed that participants with higher levels of past exercise showed better adherence to higher intensity exercise but tended to have poorer adherence to moderate exercise intensity. Thus, in prescribing an exercise regimen, the intensity of previous exercise needs to be considered to maximize the effects of the program since not everyone adheres more to moderate intensity levels of physical activity.

In addition to the above findings, research has found that adherence rates in exercise programs were best when individuals were exercising at 50% or below their aerobic capacity (USDHHS, 1996). By lowering the intensity level and extending the duration of the workout, a person can achieve nearly the same benefits as from a high-intensity workout. Best results seem to be obtained when the duration of the exercise program is between 20 and 30 minutes. However, for people who are unable to set aside 20–30 minutes to exercise, accumulation of shorter bouts of exercise (e.g., taking the stairs) throughout the day is recommended. In fact, recent findings have indicated that people can gain benefits (e.g., reduction of weight, lowered blood pressure) by doing some physical activity rather than no physical activity. So building in short durations of exercise throughout the day such as parking the car farther from the office, taking the stairs whenever possible, or taking short walking breaks during the workday would be helpful and provide some health-related benefits. This is consistent with current

American College of Sports Medicine Guidelines recommending that people should exercise on most days (30–60 minutes in total) at a moderate level of intensity. Furthermore, it is suggested that an intensity similar to brisk walking would provide the needed level of intensity. Thus, the previous research demonstrating that adherence to exercise is higher with walking, as opposed to running programs, is consistent with providing individuals a high enough intensity to derive health-related benefits.

Although most research has focused on the intensity of exercise, there is some research investigating the duration of the exercise bout. Specifically, Jakicic, Wing, Butler, and Robertson (1995) varied exercise bouts from 20 minutes to 30 minutes to 40 minutes per day. Results revealed that participants in the shorter exercise group exercised for more days and for a longer total duration compared to individuals in the longer exercise bout. Thus, as noted above, it appears that exercise can be accumulated more effectively (as recommended by the American College of Sports Medicine) by performing a number of short bouts of exercise.

An important part of any physical activity program relates to the propensity of injury resulting from that program (or, more particularly, the intensity of exercise characterizing the program). Research has consistently revealed that there is a strong relationship between physical activity and orthopedic injuries with rates running as high as 50% per year for those who regularly engage in high-intensity physical activities such as running. In fact, injury is the most common reason given for the most recent relapse from exercise, and participants who report temporary injuries are less likely than healthy individuals to report vigorous exercise (Dishman, 1997). It has also been found that people reporting injury also report significantly more walking for exercise. These results suggest that many injured people can still engage in regular walking and that injury appears to have a strong influence on maintenance or dropout from regular physical activity. In essence, injury appears to cause people to change the intensity of their exercise program, but if exercise has been established as a lifestyle pattern, exercise is continued despite the injury (Hofstetter et al., 1990).

Unfortunately, in starting an exercise program, many people try to do too much the first couple of times out and wind up with sore muscles, injuries to soft tissues, or orthopedic problems. Of course, for some individuals, such an injury is just the excuse they need to quit exercising. The message is that a person is much better off doing some moderate exercise like walking or light aerobics than trying to shape up in a few weeks by doing too much too soon.

Exercise Leader

If you talk to anyone who has been involved in a supervised exercise program, it quickly becomes apparent that the qualities of the exercise leader are paramount in determining the success of the program and the perceived enjoyment that people have in the program. In essence, anecdotal reports and other related research tell us that program leadership is an important factor in determining the success of an exercise program. Along these lines, Peter-

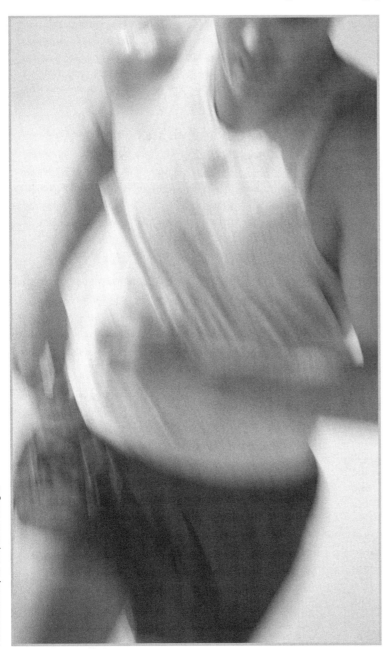

Photo courtesy of © Eyewire Images

son (1993) identified 24 qualities that were reduced to three general categories of good exercise leaders, including

(a) behavioral (the ability to instruct with proper technical execution, stay focused, and be energetic),
(b) communicative (the ability to express themselves clearly and listen to class members), and
(c) motivation (ability to motivate both the participants and themselves, be decisive, and use group processes effectively).

By doing these things, a good leader can compensate to some extent for certain deficiencies in a program, such as lack of space or equipment, whereas weak leadership can result in a breakdown in the program, regardless of how elaborate the facility.

This underscores the importance of evaluating not only a program's activities and facilities but also the expertise and personality of the program leader(s). Most people starting a program need extra motivation, and the leader's encouragement, enthusiasm, and knowledge are critical. Good leaders also show concern for safety and psychological comfort, expertise in answering questions about exercise, and personal qualities with which participants can identify (Weinberg & Gould, 2003). Remember, though, that program participants should find a good match in style with a leader who fits their individual needs, interests, and abilities. Not everyone needs an outspoken, effusive exercise leader like Jane Fonda or Richard Simmons, but everyone does need to connect with the exercise leader at some level and in some way, so all exercisers should try to find the person and the program that best matches their needs. In fact, research has revealed a positive relationship between instructor efficacy and adherence, indicating that participants who perceived their exercise leader more positively had higher levels of adherence (Gyurcsik, Culos, Bray, & DuCharme, 1998).

Some interesting research has investigated the interaction of the qualities of a leader and the type of group environment that is created (Fox, Rejeski, & Gauvin, 2000). Specifically, the type of leadership style (socially-enriched versus bland) and the type of class/group environment (socially-enriched versus bland) were systematically varied. For example, in the socially-enriched leadership style, participants' first names were used, specific positive reinforcement was given, participants were engaged in conversation before and after class, and encouragement was provided before and after a mistake. This contrasted to the bland leader, who did not use participants' names, engage in general conversation, give reinforcement, or provide encouragement after a mistake. Results revealed that participants enjoyed the class more when both the group environment and leader were enriched. However, only the group environment mattered when

participants were asked whether they intended to return to a similar class. Similarly, in a recent extension of the above study (Bray, Millen, Eidsness, & Leuzinger, 2005), it was found that both leadership style (instructionally and motivationally enriched) and exercise program choreography (variable choreography) produced the most enjoyment in participants. Since enjoyment is typically related to increased adherence, then it is likely that this type of leader behavior and environment would lead to greater adherence, although this needs to be empirically tested.

To get the best exercise leader possible, Smith and Biddle (1995) note that certain programs in Europe have developed special training programs to empower these leaders to promote physical activity with their client groups. These training courses focus on behavioral change strategies rather than a repertoire of physical movement skills. In essence, the role is to promote physical activity in the community rather than simply teach exercise classes. These programs are in their infancy and should be evaluated by outcome research in the near future.

Group vs. Individual Programs

Research has been very consistent in indicating that group programs lead to better exercise adherence than do programs that are more individual in nature (Dishman & Buckworth, 1996). The benefits of group programs are numerous and can include enhanced enjoyment, higher levels of social support, increased sense of personal commitment to continue, and opportunity to compare progress and fitness levels with others. In part, belonging to a group fulfills a basic need for affiliation with others and tends to be a greater commitment to exercise when others are counting on us. For example, if you and a friend agree to meet at 8:00 in the morning five times a week to run/walk for 20 minutes, you are likely to keep each appointment so you don't disappoint your friend. So even if you don't feel like getting up and exercising that morning, chances are you will because you know your friend is up and out waiting for you. It should be noted that although group programs are generally more effective than individual programs, certain people prefer to exercise alone for convenience as was noted earlier in this chapter. In fact, approximately 25% of regular exercisers almost always exercise alone. Consequently, it is important for exercise leaders to understand the advantages and disadvantages of exercising alone or in a group so programs can be tailored to meet the needs of each individual.

Settings for Exercise Interventions

In their extensive review of the literature, Dishman and Buckworth (1996) were among the first researchers to

CASE STUDY 12.1

Increasing Exercise Adherence: A Case Study Based on the Determinants of Exercise

Manny, who is 42 years old, was thinking about getting into an exercise program. He had not been exercising for the past 6 or 7 years and was told by his doctor that he should start exercising because his blood pressure and cholesterol were both on the high side. He was also 15–20 pounds overweight. Manny used to play sports in high school, but since he got married, had a family (two children, ages 12 and 7), and spent a lot of hours trying to get his own computer networking business off the ground, exercise just seemed like the last thing left in his day. Based on the reasons to exercise, barriers to exercise, and the determinants of exercise adherence, what would you do with Manny to increase the probability that he will start an exercise program and continue one for a long time to come?

Because Manny already has some of the physical signs related to increased probability of cardiovascular disease, the first strategy would be to reinforce the physical benefits of regular exercise in reducing cardiovascular and other diseases. The critical role that regular exercise plays in this regard should be emphasized, and anecdotes about people with conditions similar to Manny being helped by physical activity, which might "hit close to home," should be enumerated. Manny should also be made aware that, in addition to the physical benefits, physical activity has many psychological benefits such as reductions in anxiety and depression, as well as increased levels of confidence and self-esteem. Moreover, it can be fun and enjoyable at the same time. Along these lines, like many others, Manny seems to give perceived lack of time as the primary reason for his decreased physical activity levels over the past few years. In reality, it is

the low priority that exercise receives that makes it appear that he has little time left to exercise. Especially with the doctor's instructions, exercise should now be placed as one of the top priorities, and behavioral steps should be taken to make exercise a part of Manny's daily regimen. For example, exercise should be one of the first things that Manny does during his day as opposed to one of the last. This will help ensure that exercise happens regularly and at the outset of his day.

Based on the available data, make sure that Manny gets lots of social support, especially from his family and spouse, because this is a consistent predictor of adherence. You should also let Manny choose whether he wants a formal exercise program or a program that he does on his own to match his schedule. If he chooses a formal program, try to make this community based because this appears to enhance exercise maintenance. In terms of the types of activities in his program, they should include low- to moderate-intensity activities and possibly some ball sports because he seems to continue to enjoy "playing games" rather than simply exercising. You should also encourage a buddy system, especially if he chooses to exercise on his own, because exercising and working out with somebody appear to be critical to program success and maintenance. Work with Manny on setting realistic, specific, and short-term goals to enhance his self-motivation and to help him see continued progress toward achieving his goals. Finally, make his physical environment as conducive to exercising as possible. This might mean pointing out some convenient running, walking, or cycling paths in or near his neighborhood.

systematically investigate the role that the setting has on the effectiveness of exercise interventions. Although the setting is not technically a characteristic of the physical activity itself, the program must take place somewhere, and the place of the physical activity seems to be a determinant of adherence (King, 1994). The main settings for exercise interventions include (a) school, (b) work site, (c) home, (d) community, and (e) health care facility. Although successful interventions can be found in all sites, research reveals that community-based exercise interventions produce the most positive effects (Buckworth & Dishman, 2002; USD-

HHS, 1996). However, examples of successful interventions can be found at all sites.

For example, Stone, McKenzie, Welk, and Booth (1998) reviewed 14 different studies conducted at school sites and summarized the results using three specific categories. First, school-based interventions appeared to improve knowledge and attitudes about physical activity. Second, interventions conducted at schools increased the amount of physical activity in the physical education classes. Third, these school-based interventions generally did not help increase the amount of time spent in physical activity outside of the school setting. Similarly, Dishman and colleagues (1998) examined 26 studies investigating physical activity interventions conducted on the work site itself. Results revealed only a small positive effect was seen between these worksite studies and increases in physical activity. Finally, Simons-Morton, Calfas, Oldernbuurg, and Burton (1998) summarized 12 studies conducted to test the effects of physical activity interventions in health care settings. Although the review found generally positive findings in the short-term, the effects seem to decrease over time.

Despite the occasional success at other sites, the literature strongly indicates that community-based approaches offer the best way of reaching large amounts of people through exercise programs (Dishman & Buckworth, 1997). A number of community organizations provide attractive settings for physical activity programs. An example of such a community-based program was adopted by the Institute for Aerobics Research, where a Campbell Soup Company-sponsored program called FITNESSGRAM was implemented (Blair, Clark, Cureton, & Powell, 1989). FITNESSGRAM is a physical fitness assessment and feedback program for youth that is designed to enhance awareness of and encourage greater participation in physical activity. It incorporates exercise logging with feedback and participation rewards and has been implemented in a number of community settings throughout the country, such as YMCAs and recreation centers. Preliminary results reveal that this type of community program provides a useful standardized method for assessing children's fitness levels and for encouraging continued improvement.

More recently, Blissmer, Marquez, Jerome, and Kimiecik (2005) noted that some of the largest community-level campaigns, such as the Standford Five City Project, the Minnesota Heart Health Program, and the Pawtucket Heart Program, included exercise as a component but also involved multiple behavioral targets. These education-based interventions have had some success in increasing knowledge about exercise but only modest effects of actually increasing exercise behaviors. Community-based programs that involve more than educational messages, such as teaching specific exercises, have been more effective in increasing levels of physical activity.

Examples of Successful Community-Based Programs

As noted in the text, community-based exercise programs seem to produce the highest rates of exercise participation and adherence. Let's take a closer look at a few successful community-based programs and some of the characteristics that have made them successful.

Places of worship seem to offer a means of targeting the family and have been suggested as particularly appropriate settings for reaching population segments that have been traditionally underserved in health promotion. For example, programs such as the Fitness Through Churches project, which targets African-American residents in North Carolina, and the Health and Religion Project in Rhode Island use both personal-interpersonal strategies such as exercise classes and organizational strategies such as training church volunteers to disseminate information to other church members. Early results support the feasibility of these approaches, but achieving sustained physical activity participation awaits future follow-up research from these and other studies.

The use of competition has also been employed in community-based programs to facilitate exercise participation. Specifically, the Stanford Coming Alive Program, Team Health Program, and the Minnesota Shape Up Challenge Program (see King, 1994) used competition as well as goal setting, regular tracking of physical activity, feedback, and incentives to promote increases in exercise participation. The Minnesota and California programs involved a competition among a number of work sites in the community regarding the number of stairs climbed, which was a central (although routine) measure of physical activity. The Team Health Program focused on one work site in Dallas, and their contest occurred within members of this group. Results have indicated significant increases in physical activity participation during the contest period. In addition, an effort to extend such contests to a traditionally hard-to-reach segment of the employee population (in this case, blue-collar workers) resulted in a 25% increase in the number of employees engaged in physical activity vigorous enough to improve fitness during the 4-month contest period (King, Carl, Birkel, & Haskell, 1988). These contest periods have been more recently used successfully, so it seems that they are a good way to get individuals involved with exercise programs and to continue to exercise over time.

In closing, it should be noted that although the different determinants of exercise adherence have been looked at separately in the present chapter (as is the case in many of the empirical studies), in real-life situations, one must consider the interaction and interplay among these variables. A good example of this approach comes from the research of King et al. (1997). This study focused on approximately 270 healthy, sedentary adults who were followed over a 2-year period so that exercise adherence could truly be observed. A number of factors were entered into the equation to help in achieving the maximum prediction possible. Results revealed that less-educated individuals who were assigned to supervised home-based exercise and who were less stressed and less fit at baseline than other individuals had the greatest probability of successful adherence by the second year. Overweight individuals assigned to a group-based exercise program were the least successful 2 years later, with only 7.7% adhering to their exercise program. These results demonstrate the importance of taking a close look at both person and situational variables in determining the best program to enhance adherence to exercise programs.

Summary

In this chapter, we have provided an overview of the basic determinants of regular physical activity based on the empirical literature. The chapter started by discussing the benefits (e.g., reduction of cardiovascular disease, decreased anxiety and depression, and enhanced self-esteem) and barriers (perceived lack of time, low motivation, and lack of energy) related to physical activity. The problem of exercise adherence was noted because approximately 50% of individuals starting an exercise program will drop out within 6 months. As a result, there has been a history of empirical research in the past 20 years investigating determinants of physical activity. These determinants can be classified as follows: (a) demographic factors, (b) cognitive/personality factors, (c) behavioral factors, (d) environmental (social and physical) factors, and (e) characteristics of the physical activity. Much of the research on these factors has produced inconsistent findings, or there is insufficient research investigating certain factors. The factors that have been consistently related to increased levels of physical activity include the following: (a) higher self-motivation, (b) more social support, (c) immediate past adult participation in physical activity, (d) perceived time, (e) access to facilities, (f) nonsmoking, (g) higher education levels, (h) lower intensity of physical activity, and (i) community settings. This kind of information should help health-fitness professionals in devising programs that maximize participation in regular physical activity and maintain these levels over time.

Can You Define These Terms?

attitudes and beliefs about physical activity

barriers to regular physical activity

benefits of regular physical activity

characteristics of exercise leaders

demographic variables

exercise intensity

past participation in physical activity

perceived lack of time

physical environment

self-motivation

social environment

social support

Can You Answer These Questions?

1. Why is it important to understand the reasons people start and adhere to exercise programs? Use data from the Department of Health and Human Services to discuss your answer.

2. Your friend is sedentary and needs to start a regular exercise program but doesn't consider it important. What are three reasons you would cite to convince your friend?

3. Why is exercise adherence so difficult to maintain?

4. What are the relationships among body fat, risk of cardiovascular disease, and adherence? What implications do these have for the practitioner?

5. Discuss three environmental (physical and social) factors as they relate to exercise adherence and the structuring of exercise programs.

6. If you were setting up an exercise program, would you try to target group programs or individual programs related to exercise adherence? (Use research to support your conclusion.)

7. Social support appears to be related to exercise adherence. Devise an exercise program based on research that enhances the social support of the participant.

   (a) Discuss three personality/cognitive factors that have shown to be consistent determinants of exercise adherence.

   (b) Discuss the efficacy of using different settings (e.g., school, worksite, health-care, community) to enhance physical activity. Which is the best one? Provide an example.

CHAPTER 13

Motivational Strategies to Enhance Exercise Adherence

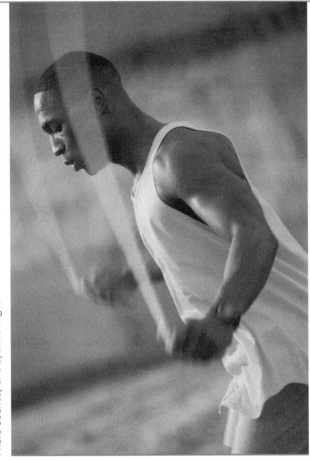

Photo courtesy of © Eyewire Imges

After reading this chapter, you should be able to

- Identify behavior modification strategies for increasing exercise adherence,
- Identify reward strategies for increasing exercise adherence,
- Identify goal-setting strategies for increasing exercise adherence,
- Identify cognitive strategies for increasing exercise adherence,
- Identify decision-balance strategies for increasing exercise adherence, and
- Identify intrinsic strategies for increasing exercise adherence.

Introduction

In the previous two chapters, the models of exercise behavior and determinants of exercise adherence were discussed at length. A key reason for bringing these issues to light is that they help inform the practitioner of the factors to consider when designing and implementing exercise-change programs. As a result, presumably you now know numerous factors that influence individuals to stay in or drop out of exercise programs. Unfortunately, these reasons and factors are typically correlational, telling us little about the cause-effect relation between specific strategies and actual behavior. In addition, no single theoretical approach to exercise behavior has proven comprehensive enough to satisfy all areas of application. Therefore, sport and exercise psychologists have used the information regarding the determinants of physical activity along with the behavior-change theories to develop and test the effectiveness of different strategies to enhance exercise adherence.

It is important to note that any intervention should always attempt to match the individuals in the program and the situational/environmental factors surrounding the program. In this regard, the matching hypothesis and interactional model discussed in the previous two chapters should always be kept in the forefront of any program decision. In essence, consistent with the transtheoretical model, practitioners should always be sensitive to the stage of their participants and individualize as much as possible a program that matches this stage. It should be noted that a quantitative review of 127 studies examining the efficacy of interventions for increasing physical activity among 130,000 people in community, school, work, home, and health-care settings (Dishman & Buckworth, 1996) found that interventions, on the average, increased adherence from the typical rate of 50% to approximately 85%. In addition, it is important to keep in mind that there is a wide range of effectiveness in the interventions studied based on a number of individual and environmental factors. For example, generally larger effects are found for interventions increasing low-to-moderate intensity activities than for strength training activities, and effects are greater when supported or delivered through audio or visual media (Gauvin, Levesque, & Richard, 2001). In addition, emphasizing leisure physical activity, community approaches, group approaches, and unsupervised physical activity appears to enhance the effects of various interventions. Thus, interventions to enhance exercise adherence can work; the key is to find the best intervention for the particular setting and people in that setting. Although these techniques can be classified in different ways, in this chapter the categories and approaches will be (a) behavior modification approaches, (b) cognitive/behavioral approaches, (c) decision-making approaches, (d) social support approaches, and (e) intrinsic approaches.

Behavior Modification Approaches

From the exhaustive review by Dishman and Buckworth (1996), it was found that behavior modification approaches to improving exercise adherence consistently produced extremely positive results. These approaches might affect an element of the physical environment that acts as a cue for behavior change. For example, the sight and smell of food might be a cue to eat, and the sight of a television after work, a cue to sit down and relax. If you want to promote exercise, one technique is to provide cues that will eventually become associated with exercise. Similarly, the type of reinforcement, either positive or negative, provided for exercising or not exercising can also be a powerful determinant of future action. For example, to increase exercise adherence, incentives or rewards have been given for staying with the program. Below, we will discuss in more detail some of the specific behavior modification interventions that have been employed to enhance exercise adherence. Because these have proved most effective in enhancing adherence behaviors (and have been used most often from an applied perspective), we will spend the most time discussing these strategies.

Prompting

One technique for establishing a behavior is the use of *prompts*. A prompt is a cue that initiates a behavior, and these can be verbal, physical, or symbolic. For example, a verbal prompt may be a simple statement such as "Okay, let's get going" or a slogan that is meaningful to the individual such as "You can hang in there." A physical prompt might be helping someone get over a "sticking point" in a particular weight-lifting activity. A symbolic prompt generally reminds a person to begin or continue a behavior, such as leaving out one's workout gear the night before to promote physical activity or placing a Post-it note on the refrigerator. The goal is to increase cues for the desired behavior and decrease cues for competing behaviors.

Although prompts are helpful in beginning new behaviors or in getting past difficult points, they should not be continued indefinitely because people can start to rely on these prompts too much. Moreover, because prompts are usually discontinued at some point, people need to find other sources of motivation (hopefully internal) to continue participation. Although prompts such as signs and posters can be helpful, eventually prompts can be gradually eliminated through a process called *fading*, which means less and less use over time. This gradual withdrawal of the prompt allows an individual to gain increasing independence without the sudden withdrawal of support.

A good example of the use (and withdrawal) of a prompt occurred in a study that used cartoon posters (symbolic prompt) placed near elevators in a public building to encourage stair climbing (Brownell, Stunkard, & Albaum, 1980). Results revealed that the percentage of people using the stairs rather than the escalators increased from 6% to 14% after posters were put in place. Unfortunately, 3 months after the posters were removed, stair use returned to 6%. In a similar study (Blamey, Mutrie, & Aitchison, 1995), a motivational sign that read "Stay healthy, save time, use the stairs" was posted in an underground station where commuters could take the stairs (30 steps) or an escalator. Stair use went from 8% to 17% while the sign was posted, but declined after the sign was removed, with a downward trend suggesting an eventual return to baseline. Finally, in a more recent extension (Vande Auweele, Boen, Schapendonk, & Dornez, 2005), a health sign linking stair use to health and fitness was placed at a junction between the staircase and

elevator, increasing stair use significantly from baseline (69%) to intervention (77%). A second intervention involved an additional e-mail sent a week later by the worksite's doctor, pointing out the health benefits of regular stair use. Results revealed an increase in stair use from 77% to 85%, although once the sign was removed stair use declined to around baseline levels at 67%. This is a good demonstration of how effective just a sign can be, but yet it also shows that people easily go back to their old behavior (if the new behavior has not been internalized) if the sign is removed.

Prompts can also be helpful when combined with other techniques. For example, in one study, self-monitoring was combined with different schedules of calling participants to prompt them to walk. Frequent calls or prompts (once a week) resulted in three times the number of reported episodes of physical activity than resulted from calling every 3 weeks (Lombard, Lombard, & Winett, 1995). Combining self-monitoring with additional external prompts appears to maximize adherence to exercise programs.

Verbal prompts are a different example of prompting used to encourage exercise participation. These prompts can come from an exercise leader who is try-

CASE STUDY 13.1 — *Basic Elements of Contracting*

The basic elements of a contract were described by Kanfer and Gaelick (1986). A hypothetical example of a contract will be provided here. We will use the case of Sally, whose main goal is to lose weight because she has been sedentary for several years and wants to get back into shape.

1. First, a clear description of the target behavior should be stated. Although there are several things that Sally hopes to accomplish, such as reducing cholesterol and increasing cardiovascular function, her main goal is to lose weight. Along these lines, in consultation with her doctor, it is decided that Sally should aim to lose 20 pounds. This forms the basis for the contract.

2. The next step is to set the exact timeframe in which to lose this 20 pounds. Because it is deemed realistic that Sally should lose 2 pounds per week, the contract reads that she will lose 20 pounds in 10 weeks.

3. The behaviors that need to occur to make this happen are now elaborated upon. Spe-

cifically, Sally contracts to attend an exercise class four times a week for one hour each time. She will also attempt to change her eating habits to consume no more than 1,800 calories per day.

4. Specific positive reinforcements for achieving certain aspects of the contract or moving towards the right direction are identified, as are aversive consequences for not fulfilling contract behaviors. For example, with the help of the fitness instructor, Sally identifies the purchase of an expensive piece of clothing as a reward and some unwanted housework as an aversive consequence.

5. A bonus clause might be put into the contract if Sally achieves her goal. If she does reach her goal, then she would be able to purchase something extravagant, such as a new television.

6. To keep a clear track of the behaviors related to the contract, Sally states that she will keep a weekly journal of her exercise, diet, and weight, and the instructor will review the journal weekly.

ing to encourage participants to exercise harder or more vigorously, saying such things as "Keep up the good work," "You can do i," "Hang in there," and "Just a little longer." In addition, verbal prompts can come from the participant in the form of self-talk, which is similar to the verbal cues provided by an instructor, except that it comes from the participant herself and is more personalized.

Contracting

Another way to change exercise behavior is to have participants enter into a *contract* with the exercise practitioner. Written statements that outline specific behaviors and establish consequences for fulfillment are known as contracts. In essence, contracts typically specify expectations, responsibilities, and contingencies for behavioral change. Usually, the purpose of these contracts is to maintain or enhance an individual's motivation to continue exercising. More specifically, Kanfer and Gaelick (1986) identified the purposes of contracts as helping the client take action, establishing criteria for meeting goals, and providing a means for clarifying consequences.

The literature on exercise change cites a number of advantages for setting up contracts. First, contracting involves the client in the behavioral change strategy, which typically increases the individual's commitment because a more collaborative approach is perceived. Second, a written contract enables there to be verification of a person's intentions, and this is usually clearer than merely an oral contract, which can be unclear and easily forgotten. Third, by establishing a contract, a public commitment (rather than a private commitment) is conveyed, and this, in turn, should foster an increased sense of self-control. If the client monitors the contract, the likelihood of treatment adherence increases. This was the case in a study in which participants signed a statement of intent to comply with the exercise (Oldridge & Jones, 1983). Research has found that people who sign such a statement have significantly better attendance than do those who refuse to sign. Thus, individuals choosing not to sign a statement of intent to comply can be signaling that they need special measures to enhance their motivation.

Charting Attendance and Participation

Public reporting of attendance and performance is another way to increase the motivation of participants in exercise programs. Performance feedback can be made even more effective by converting information to a graph or chart (e.g., Franklin, 1984). A performance or attendance graph usually represents data in a form easily understood by everyone involved. The chart is helpful and motivational in that it can tell a person at a glance what changes are taking place and if he or she is on target for the behavior involved. The visual representation of progress by a chart is extremely helpful because a person can even note small changes in behavior and performance. This may be important to maintain interest, especially later in a program when the individual reaches the point where improvements are often small and occur less frequently. In addition, recording and charting keep individuals constantly informed, and often the increased cognitive awareness is all that is necessary to bring about changes in the target behavior. Furthermore, if people know that their workout record is available for everyone to see, they are much more likely to strive to keep up the positive behavior (or improve upon some poor behavior) to reach their goals than if the information is kept private. This public information also allows exercise leaders as well as other program participants to offer praise and encouragement to the participant.

An example of public charting improving performance and behavior comes from a classic study of youth swimmers by McKenzie and Rushall (1974). In this study, practice behaviors were publicly recorded with a check for first simply attending practice, then for attending practice on time, and finally for attending practice on time and swimming the required amount. Results revealed that absenteeism and tardiness were significantly reduced and the number of yards swum daily by each swimmer was increased significantly due to the public display of target behaviors.

A similar finding was achieved in a program focusing on increasing physical activity but also offering some rewards for goal attainment. Specifically, in a program called the Miles Club (Henning, 1987), runners and walkers recorded their weekly mileage on a public chart. As they reached certain designated intervals, they were rewarded with engraved paperweights and gift certificates, which enhanced the desired behavior. In addition, a competition was set up among different teams of people within the program. A team challenge board posted in a prominent location generated interest and enthusiasm for the contest. This competition also improved the overall participation, and group morale also increased. It should be noted, however, that the public nature of these programs can pose a threat to confidentiality. If this is the case, then that person should not be required to participate, and an alternative record system that is accessible only to that person (and possibly the exercise leader) should be implemented.

Although not classically a charting approach (but a participation approach), including top managers into corporate fitness programs has also been successful. In one program, top managers got involved in a fitness program, and this greatly helped the success of the program (Hobson, Hoffman, Corso, & Freismuth, 1987). When employees see the company president running around in the gymnasium or fitness facility, they oftentimes see that person in a different light and may be challenged to match his or her commitment. In addition, observing one's supervisor struggling like everyone else conveys the message that exercise and fitness are important. Certainly, if top managers, CEOs, and the like have the time for fitness activities, then these activities must be important to the company. Finally, with the informal "give and take" that exercise often provides, there is typically an increase in the "team spirit" of the employees. As a cautionary note, not all managers feel comfortable exercising with their employees, and their needs must also be taken into consideration when devising corporate physical activity programs.

Rewarding Attendance and Participation

Besides simply charting attendance and participation records, some studies and programs focused on the use of rewards in enhancing exercise adherence. Using the reward approach, one study employed two rewards for attendance during a 5-week jogging program. First, there was a $1 weekly deposit return contingent on participation. Second, all participants contributed $3 each and were required to attend exercise four out of five sessions per week to qualify for the lottery (in essence, this was an attendance lottery). At the end of the study, a winner was chosen randomly from among the qualifiers. The two interventions resulted in 64% attendance, whereas participants in a control group attended only 40% of the classes (Epstein, Wing, Thompson, & Griffiths, 1980).

Most researchers agree that if people are to benefit from a fitness program, they should have some financial investment in it. If individuals have little or no financial interest in their program, they will probably sign up for it, but chances are they will drop out in a fairly short time. With this in mind, an approach that has proved effective in corporate programs is for the company to pay most (but not all) of the program cost. Researchers compared four methods of payment and found that program attendance was better when participants were either reimbursed based on attendance or split the fee with their employer. Interestingly, the lowest attendance was found when the company paid the entire fee (Pollack, Foster, Salisbury, & Smith, 1982). Following this model, the Campbell Soup Company required employees to pay $50 the first year. If they exercised 3 times a week or more during the second year, they paid only $25. If employees continued to exercise at this rate, they paid nothing the third year (Legwold, 1987). In general, results were encouraging for initial attendance or adherence but less so for long-term improvement. Additional incentives or rein-

forcement must be provided throughout the program to encourage adherence over longer periods.

Providing Feedback on Progress

An important motivational technique that capitalizes on individuals' inherent interest to reach certain outcomes is to provide periodic feedback on how individuals are progressing. Providing feedback regarding various fitness tests such as submaximal exercise tests, resting/recovery pulse rate, and body composition measures can be very motivational to people in exercise programs. An aerobic instructor praising a participant for finishing an especially hard routine would be an example of positive reinforcement or feedback that is meant to increase motivation and eventual participation. In one study, Scherf and Franklin (1987) developed a data documentation system for use in a cardiac rehabilitation setting in which participants' number of laps walked and run, body weight, resting heart rate, and exercise heart rate were recorded on individual forms after each exercise session. These records were easily accessible and were reviewed monthly with the participants by staff members. From these records, report cards were generated, and they were then returned to the participants with appropriate comments. Individuals who met certain performance goals were then recognized in a monthly awards ceremony. This program resulted in better exercise participation and adherence as well as higher levels of motivation and enthusiasm.

In another study, giving feedback to individuals during a program session was found to be more effective than praising the whole group at the end (Martin et al., 1984). Specifically, giving feedback to runners individually produced higher levels of program attendance and adherence three months after program termination than did group feedback. These results underscore the notion of individualizing feedback as much as possible.

Cognitive/Behavioral Approaches

Cognitive/behavioral approaches evolved out of the operant conditioning behavior modification theories that dominated psychology in the 1940s, '50s and '60s. In one form or another, these approaches all assume that private or internal events, or thinking, have an important role in behavior change. Two techniques that will be discussed below are goal setting and association/dissociation.

Goal Setting

One technique that can be considered both cognitive and behavioral is goal setting. Goal-setting research emanated from the industrial/organizational literature where this technique has been used extensively to enhance motivation and increase employee output. The acceptance and use of goal setting has come in response to overwhelming evidence for its motivational and performance-enhancing effects in the organizational and industrial literature. Specifically, in a review of over 400 studies, using over 40,000 participants, Locke and Latham (1990) found that setting specific, difficult goals significantly enhanced performance when compared to setting easy goals, "do your best" goals, or no goals.

As noted above, such consistent findings from the industrial and organizational literature have led many individuals involved in sport and exercise to employ goal-setting techniques to improve performance, enhance adherence, and increase motivation. Although not quite as impressive, in a meta-analytic review of the literature, Kyllo and Landers (1995) found that goal setting can help improve performance and enhance motivation in sport and exercise settings. In fact, many of the original studies investigating goal setting were conducted using fitness activities such as sit-ups, push-ups, weight lifting, and aerobics. It should be noted, however, that certain factors need to be in place to enhance the probability that goal setting will be effective. These factors are highlighted in the accompanying box.

Although goal setting has been investigated in both sport and exercise settings, in one study focusing on exercise, it was found that 99% of participants enrolled in an intermediate fitness class set multiple, personally motivating goals for their exercise participation (Poag-DuCharme, & Brawley, 1994). Clearly, individuals do set personal goals for their exercise participation, and they perceive these goals as being able to influence actual exercise behavior. In addition, participants appear knowledgeable about what exercise behavior is needed to meet their goals, information that is a requirement for effective goal setting. In essence, it seems that most people involved in exercise programs set goals to help them maintain their exercise regimen and to keep up their motivation to maintain their level of activity. Therefore, it is important that the goals people set maximize their effectiveness in helping them reach their physical activity and exercise objectives.

The above study found that not only did people set goals, but most exercise participants also appear to set multiple, personally motivating goals for exercise participation. These goals appear to be a combination of outcome-based goals (e.g., I want to lose 20 pounds) and behavior-based goals (I want to walk/run for 30 minutes, 5 times per week). The exercise goals that were most often reported included increasing cardiovascular fitness (28%), toning or strengthening muscles (18%), losing weight (13%), and exercising regularly (5%). Along with these multiple goals, were

multiple action plans to reach these goals. The most commonly identified action plans (which remained consistent from program onset to mid-program) were to bring fitness clothes to school (25%), attend fitness classes regularly (16%), and organize time/work around fitness (9%). On the average, most participants reported only two behavioral strategies to employ for goal attainment, and such a small number of plans might be related to why so many people drop out of exercise programs.

In investigating the types of goals that are most effective in an exercise setting, Martin and his colleagues (1984) found that flexible goals that participants set themselves resulted in better attendance and 3-month maintenance of exercise behavior than did fixed, instructor-set goals. Specifically, attendance rates were 83% when participants set their own goals, compared to 67% when instructors set the goals. Furthermore, 47% of those who set their own goals were still exercising 3 months after the program ended (compared to 28% of the people for whom the instructor set goals). These results underscore the importance of getting participant input when goals are set for exercise participants, because such involvement helps commitment to the goals and eventual adherence.

In addition to getting input from the participants, results revealed that time-based goals resulted in better attendance (69%) than did distance-based goals (47%). Longer-term, or distal (6-week), goal setting produced better attendance (83% vs. 71%) and better 3-month exercise maintenance (67% vs. 33%) than did proximal (weekly) goal setting (Martin et al., 1984). The best thing to do with goals is to combine short-term and long-term goals so the final outcome and the process of reaching that outcome are both specified.

Association/Dissociation

Although goal setting involves both some cognitions (thoughts) and some behaviors, association and dissociation strategies involve predominantly thoughts (which eventually will affect behavior). In essence, what people think about and focus their attention on while exercising is also important. When the focus is on internal body feedback (e.g., how their muscles feel or their breathing feels), it is called *association*; when the focus is on the external environment (e.g., noticing how pretty the scenery is or listening to music on an iPod while exercising), it is called *dissociation*. This dissociation usually acts as a distraction from focusing on the pain and fatigue that often accompany vigorous physical activity. When someone exercises with an iPod on, playing music, this is a great example of using a dissociative technique to get the mind off what the person is doing, and this usually makes the time appear to pass more quickly.

Principles of Effective Goal Setting

Goals Should Be Specific, Rather Than General.

It has been clearly shown in the literature that general goals such as "do your best" are not as effective as specific goals. Specific goals are usually quantifiable, and they inform a person of exactly what needs to be done. For example, a specific goal would be for a person to exercise (either running or fast walking) four times a week for 30 minutes each time.

Goals Should Be Realistic and Challenging, but Attainable.

Another consistent finding in the literature is that goals should be challenging (moderately difficult) because they produce better results than do easy goals. In research with college athletes and Olympians, Weinberg, Burton, Yukelson, and Weigand (1993, 2000) found that these individuals preferred moderately difficult, challenging goals that they felt were difficult, yet attainable. Exercisers also prefer realistic goals because they help keep motivation high to continue working toward achieving their specific goals.

Goals Should Be Both Short Term and Long Term.

A long-term goal provides information about where one is going. Short-term goals, on the other hand, provide information regarding progress toward the long-term goal. By setting intermediate, short-term goals, people can see if their progress toward reaching their long-term goal is on track. Also, short-term goals are more manageable than long-term goals, which, at times, can appear daunting. For example, an individual may want to lose 50 pounds in the next year, and this might very well seem like an impossible task. If the person breaks that down to short-term goals of losing about one pound a week, then this seems much more realistic and attainable.

Goals Should Be Written.

Goals are much more effective when they are written down, especially in a place that the participant can see every day. This is why many exercise programs have bulletin boards with participants' daily/weekly progress prominently displayed. Writing goals down increases com-

mitment to reaching those goals and is an important part of successful goal-setting practices (Weinberg, Butt, & Knight, in press).

Goals Should Be Accepted by the Participant.

Goals that are meaningful and important to the participant are more likely to result in commitment to their attainment. Research has consistently demonstrated that participants should "own" their goals. One way to accomplish this is to have fitness participants actively participate in the formation of these goals. Their input is critical to their acceptance of the goals, and this enhances motivation and commitment.

Goal Strategies Should Be Explicitly Defined.

One of the areas in which exercisers fall down is that they do not specify how they are going to reach their goals. It is all well and good to have a goal to lose 50 pounds in a year, but how are you going to reach this goal? Are you going to exercise for 4 days a week, 30 minutes each time? Are you going to change your eating habits and patterns and reduce caloric intake? These questions need to be explicitly answered, and action steps specified that describe behaviors to reach these goals.

Goals Should Have a Feedback Mechanism Built In.

Goals need to be periodically evaluated to determine if the participant is on track to meeting his or her objectives. For example, measurement of percent body fat and flexibility are examples of periodic assessments that inform participants of their progress toward meeting their goals. This type of feedback can also serve a motivational function to keep people going. A number of fitness activities have built-in feedback because we always know how much weight we lifted, how many sit-ups we did, or how long our run was. Sometimes, however, we need additional feedback, and this could come from the instructor in a supervised program, or individuals can provide feedback to themselves in the form of checking on weight loss or dress/pants size.

Research has revealed that people who dissociate have significantly better attendance (77%) than do those who associate (58%). In a study of a 12-week exercise program (Martin et al., 1984), the dissociative subjects were also superior to the associative subjects in long-term maintenance of exercise after 3 months (87% vs. 37%) and 6 months (67% vs. 43%). Focusing on the environment instead of on how one feels is apparently helpful for exercise adherence rates, perhaps because thinking about other things reduces boredom and fatigue. Although associative techniques typically help elite athletes, exercisers also can use these techniques effectively. When the activity is over, associative techniques such as taking your resting heart rate or getting in touch with your musculature during a relaxation exercise while "cooling down" can become more important, but as you will see later in the chapter, association can be important when trying to achieve flow states, and these states appear critical for exercise maintenance.

Decision-Making Approaches

Deciding whether to start an exercise program can often be a difficult decision. As noted in Chapter 11, these undecideds are typically in either the precontemplation or contemplation stage. They are thinking about exercising but have not really started to exercise. People can stay in this stage for a long time (up to 2 years); thus, it is necessary to develop techniques that will help people make the decision to exercise. One technique that has been demonstrated to be effective in helping people make exercise decisions is the decision balance sheet.

Decision Balance Sheet

To help people in the decision to start exercising (as well as start other positive behaviors such as stopping smoking and quitting alcohol), a technique known as a decision balance sheet was developed (Hoyt & Janis, 1975), and this was later applied to exercise (Wankel, 1984) to make people aware of potential benefits and costs of an exercise program. In devising a decision balance sheet, individuals write down the anticipated consequences of exercise participation in terms of the following categories: (a) gains to self, (b) losses to self, (c) gains to important others, (d) losses to important others, (e) approval to others, (f) disapproval to others, (g) self-approval, and (h) self-disapproval. However, more recently, it appeared more efficacious to simply label things as the "pros" and "cons" of changing behavior. It is expected that after reviewing these positive and negative consequences, people will see that there are many more positives than negatives to exercise and will then make a decision to exercise. Although they may know this in their mind, writing

these ideas down in a systematic fashion helps people focus on the reasons for their decision.

In one study (Hoyt & Janis, 1975), participants who completed a decision balance sheet attended 84% of the classes over a 7-week period, whereas controls attended only 40% of the classes. In a variant of this study applied specifically to increasing exercise participation and adherence, Wankel and Thompson (1977) compared using a full balance sheet (where both positive and negative consequences of exercise are enumerated) to using a positive-only balance sheet, which deleted reference to any anticipated negative outcomes. Results revealed that both types of balance sheets produced higher attendance rates than did a control condition. Collectively, the evidence available demonstrates the effectiveness of involving participants in decisions before initiating an exercise program. Using a decision balance sheet appears to be a good way to get people involved in the decision-making process.

As a practical example, let's look at some typical statements regarding engaging in regular physical activity. These would get a "pro" or "con" designation and then rated from "1" (not important at all) to "5" (extremely important).

- I would feel better about myself if I exercised regularly.
- I would feel that I am wasting my time if I exercised regularly.
- I would be healthier and more fit if I exercised regularly.
- I would feel more tired if I exercised regularly.
- Other people would respect me more if I exercised regularly.
- I would spend less time with significant others if I exercised regularly.

Social Support Approaches

In the previous chapter on determinants of physical activity, it was noted that social support was one of the consistent factors related to elevated levels of participation and adherence to exercise programs. In an exercise context, social support refers to an individual's favorable attitude toward another individual's involvement in an exercise program. Most of the time, people think of social support as coming from significant others in the environment such as spouses, family members, and close friends. This type of social support may influence physical activity in many ways. For example, spouses, significant others, family members, and friends can cue exercise through verbal reminders such as "Hang in there" or "You're really looking good with all that exercise you are doing."

In addition, significant others who exercise may model and cue physical activity by their behavior and

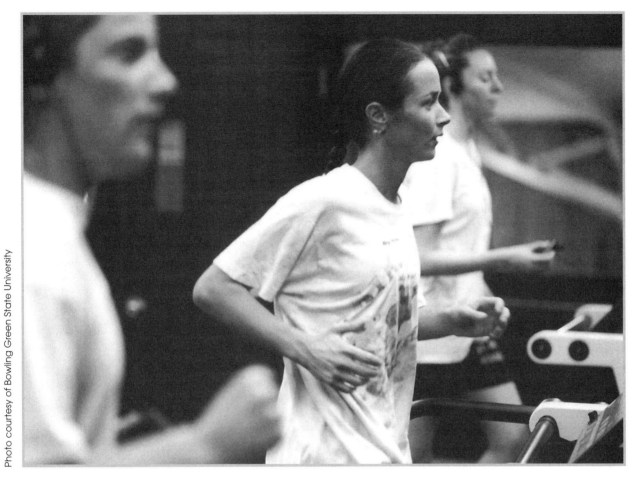

reinforce it by their companionship during exercise. Sometimes family routine is adjusted to allow exercise time. Often, people give practical assistance, providing transportation, measuring exercise routes, or lending exercise clothing or equipment. In a summary of the studies investigating the relationship of social support and adherence to exercise, research has revealed family and friends exert a strong influence on compliance with exercise programs (Carron, Hausenblas, & Mack, 1996). This positive influence of social support goes across a variety of different exercise behaviors. For example, social support was positively related to

(a) compliance with an exercise program after a heart transplant,
(b) adherence to a voluntary exercise program,
(c) children's physical activity levels, and
(d) school-based physical activity.

Furthermore, positive parental, family, and friend influence has been shown to increase the satisfaction the participants get from exercising, the participant's intention to exercise, and the participant's degree of self-efficacy. In addition, social support from family and friends has been consistently and positively related to adult physical activity and adherence to

structured exercise programs (U.S. Department of Health and Human Services, 1996). So it is therefore important to include the spouse or significant others when planning and implementing an exercise program, as this will not only enhance adherence, but also improve enjoyment of the activity itself.

In addition to the social support offered by significant others in the environment, the support that occurs inside a fitness class, especially the behavior of the fitness leader, is crucial for the adherence to exercise. By establishing a warm and nonthreatening relationship with the exerciser, the exercise leader may influence the individual's level of motivation. It appears important that the exercise leader create an expectation of participation that is challenging yet attainable to the exerciser. Then, the leader should reward these positive behaviors (and these rewards could simply be social reinforcement—e.g., "You're looking good" or "It's great to see you come here regularly"). For example, Martin et al. (1984) found that when a leader gives personalized, immediate feedback and praises attendance and maintenance of exercise, adherence improves. So exercise leaders can, and do, make a difference in exercise adherence, depending on the type and amount of social support provided. Of course, different people need different types and amounts of social support. Therefore, it is incumbent on the exercise leader to try to match the social support to the person as best as possible.

Another example of a social support program that focused on the behaviors of the leader was developed by Wankel (1984). This program included the leader, the class, a buddy (partner), and family members. Specifically, the leader regularly encouraged the participants to establish and maintain their home and buddy support systems, attempted to develop a positive class atmosphere, and ensured that class attendance and social support charts were systematically marked. Results showed that participants receiving social support had better attendance than did members of a control group.

The relationship among program members can also serve as a great source of social support. As relationships are formed within the exercise group, members begin to feel a greater sense of commitment and personal involvement and a greater reluctance to let the other members down through poor attendance or lack of effort. Along these lines, establishing a buddy system has been shown to be an effective way to help participants overcome the initial anxiety of beginning a program, as well as encouraging continued participation (Hobson et al., 1987).

An additional example of a program using social support was developed by King and Frederiksen (1984). In their program, they set up three- or four-member groups and instructed them to jog with at least one group member throughout the study. In addition, the groups took part in team-building exercises to promote group cohesiveness. These small social support groups increased attendance and improved exercise behavior. These studies all show the important role that social support plays in promoting adherence to exercise programs.

Although not directly related to exercise, the importance of social support is again seen in a meta-analysis conducted by Schwartzer and Leppin (1989). Specifically, they found that both for mortality and morbidity there was a relationship between social support and death and illness. That is, married people tended to live longer than single/divorced people (although individuals are at greater risk for passing away in the first six months of losing a spouse). In addition, married people are less likely to suffer health problems than are single/divorced people. So once again, having social support (in this case a spouse) is extremely important in promoting good health.

Ecological/Social Approaches

Most of the approaches to enhance physical activity studied thus far have been generally individualized in nature, focusing on specific kinds of person and indi-

vidualizing efforts to produce maximum benefit. In essence, the focus has been on intrapersonal factors (e.g., self-efficacy, intentions to exercise, self-esteem) and interpersonal factors (e.g., social support, social influence). However, more recently, the focus has somewhat shifted to a variety of targets emphasizing institutional factors, community factors, and public policy (McLeroy, Bibeau, Steckler, & Glanz, 1988). More specifically, an ecological program is one that included interventions aimed at both environmental and individual targets and that delivers these interventions in a variety of settings.

Examples of organizations that would be targeted are sports clubs, fitness centers, community centers, schools, and public health facilities. Similarly, entire communities (e.g., neighborhoods, towns, villages, small cities) might be targeted for a specific intervention. An example of some of the different types of interventions that might occur include

- open use of exercise facilities for families, couples, or small groups;
- discussion groups to promote maintenance of physical activity;
- support groups among families for remaining more active;
- services to link up clients to perform activities together (e.g., find a partner to play racquetball);
- personal training services to help get people to start exercising;
- influencing political representatives to legislate for the promotion of physical activity;
- increasing the accessibility of facilities in a community;
- meeting with the head of an organization to encourage employees to become more active;
- providing a toll-free number for community members looking to access physical activity resources in their community; and
- providing incentives to organizations (e.g., tax breaks) whose employees meet certain physical activity standards.

Let's look at a couple of specific examples of research that highlights this approach. A school-based intervention known as the Child and Adolescent Trial for Cardiovascular Health (CATCH) used 96 elementary schools in an attempt to change physical activity in physical education classes and outside school time (Luepker, Perry, & McKinlay, 1996). The intervention included classroom sessions targeting social cognitive variables like expectations and self-efficacy, as well as policy changes such as the provision of space, equipment, and supervision during non-school hours. Results revealed that physical activity increased during the three years of the study in both physical education classes and out-of-school activities. Most impressively, the out-of-school increase in physical activity was still present three years later.

One of the initial community-wide interventions that included policy and environmental approaches was the Naval Community Project in California (Lineger, Chesson, & Nice, 1991). Policy strategies included extending the hours that the community recreation center was open and communications between superiors and subordinates stressed the expectation that all members of the base should be involved in regular exercise. In addition, fruits and vegetables were included at all snack shops on the Naval base. Finally, environmental changes included the construction of bicycle paths, creation of jogging clubs, the opening of a women-only fitness center, and the purchasing of new exercise equipment for the gymnasium. Results revealed faster times for the 1.5 mole run, a reduced failure rate in physical fitness testing, smaller increases in sedentary individuals, and no increase in body fat (compared to controls who gained body fat). Impressively, these changes occurred across males and females, officers and enlisted personnel, and all age categories.

Intrinsic Approaches

Most of the previous approaches relied on some sort of "gimmick," knowledge, feedback, or reward system for enhancing exercise behavior. In addition, most of the practices fitness professionals presently employ to encourage people to exercise are based on the notion that knowledge about the disease risks of a sedentary lifestyle and the long-term health benefits of exercise is sufficient to get people exercising regularly. Although these helpful cues, knowledge, and rewards can certainly help improve exercise adherence, we all know that the best and most long-lasting motivation comes from within. In fact, the research is all too plain, finding that simply emphasizing the relationship between disease reduction and regular exercise is not sufficient to keep most people physically active over time. In addition, the external rewards for exercising must at some point diminish greatly or be totally removed from the environment. When this occurs, what is left to keep the person exercising for life? In essence, if this approach worked we would not have so many sedentary people and we would not have an obesity epidemic on our hands. Thus, despite the emphasis on health and fitness, eating properly and maintaining an active lifestyle, the large majority of people still fall short in achieving regular physical activity.

In essence, we have learned the hard way (with research from attempted cessation from smoking, alcohol, and other negative behaviors) that most people do not change their exercise behavior based on extrinsic long-term consequences. Of course, many people start an exercise program with an eye toward positive health gains such as improving physical fitness, losing weight, or decreasing the probability of certain disease states. For example, we probably all know people who have started a weight-loss program with some fancy diet (which may or may not include exercise as part of the program). Research and anecdotal reports have shown that many of these people were initially very successful in losing weight, but the key is that they were usually extremely motivated to do so and were willing to do almost anything to achieve this goal. Follow-up studies conducted several years later have typically indicated that these people have not only gained back the weight they had lost, but they also are even heavier now than when they started their weight-loss program. This is because most of these people never really changed their lifestyle or found a way to eat and exercise that was fun and enjoyable and that they could keep up for a lifetime.

In essence, Kimiecik (2002) argues that most exercise programs take an outside-in approach. That is, people are constantly told about the benefits of exercise and typically start to exercise because of some external reason, like losing weight or reducing the probability of cardiovascular disease. And as noted above, with lots of drive, determination, and motivation, people can be successful in maintaining an exercise program for a period of time. However, it is extremely rare for an individual to continue participating over a long period of time for these extrinsic reasons. Think of the kind of exercise behaviors that you do on a regular basis. You will probably realize that these activities are enjoyable to you. Thus, exercising with a friend, playing racquetball or tennis, or being part of a fitness class all emphasize the fun aspect of exercising. For this reason, Kimiecik argues that people should take an inside-out approach to exercise, emphasizing the enjoyment and fun of exercising and making it something to look forward to, not some dreadful means to an external goal (e.g., weight loss)

In addition, in the long run, overemphasizing the positive (extrinsic) outcomes of exercise can actually undermine an individual's motivation to exercise. Specifically, individuals can become so focused on obtaining these outcomes (*extrinsic motivation*) that they ignore the process of developing positive inner experiences with movement and exercise (*intrinsic motivation*). It is this intrinsic motivation that becomes a critical factor in maintaining exercise over a long period.

Intrinsic vs. Extrinsic Motivation

One way to look at the different types of methods and techniques used to motivate people to exercise is to view exercise motivation on a continuum from extrinsic to intrinsic motivation. Early research on intrinsic

Kimiecik (2002) offers a little self-assessment to help individuals determine where they currently are relating to being an intrinsic or extrinsic exerciser. The scoring (after the self-assessment) just offers some broad guidelines to help you assess where you currently are regarding intrinsic motivation and exercise.

1. The main point to moving my body is to experience it in the here and now.
   Agree _____ Disagree _____

2. Moving my body is not about long-term outcomes, but about the experience.
   Agree _____ Disagree _____

3. When I move my body, I feel free.
   Agree _____ Disagree _____

4. I experience my movement without judging my body.
   Agree _____ Disagree _____

5. When I move my body, I forget about thinking and let my senses (feel, touch, taste, hearing, smell) take over.
   Agree _____ Disagree _____

6. I allow my movement to embrace my whole being—mind, body, and spirit.
   Agree _____ Disagree _____

7. I am aware of my basic bodily signals and my bodily tension hot points.
   Agree _____ Disagree _____

8. I am aware of my breathing and how it varies through different movements.
   Agree _____ Disagree _____

9. I regularly distract my mind from my body during movement experiences.
   Agree _____ Disagree _____

10. I can focus on one thought or one feeling for at least five minutes during a movement activity.
    Agree _____ Disagree _____

11. I perform exercise as a mindful experience rather than as a mindless habit.
    Agree _____ Disagree _____

12. I often worry that others are evaluating my body when I am moving.
    Agree _____ Disagree _____

13. I sometimes connect exercise with my need to interact with others (social).
    Agree _____ Disagree _____

14. I sometimes connect exercise with my need to learn (mental).
    Agree _____ Disagree _____

15. I sometimes connect exercise with my need for meaning and purpose (spiritual).
    Agree _____ Disagree _____

Scoring:
Give yourself 1 point for "Agree" responses except for numbers 9 and 12. For those numbers give yourself 1 point if you responded "disagree."

Totals:

12–15: You are well on your way to becoming an Intrinsic Exerciser.

8–11: You have the makings of an Intrinsic Exerciser.

4–7: The Intrinsic Exerciser is there somewhere.

0–3: Your inner exercise tank is on empty. Start filling it up.

and extrinsic motivation emphasized the dichotomy between the two concepts. However, later research has found that this dichotomy is insufficient to adequately depict human behavior. Along these lines, the empirical and conceptual work on intrinsic motivation and external rewards by Deci and Ryan (1991) is particularly salient to the establishment of this continuum. In their development of *self-determination theory*, Deci and Ryan (1985, 1991) suggest that three psychological needs are especially crucial in energizing human action: autonomy, competence, and relatedness. The need for autonomy refers to the desire to be self-initiating in the regulation of one's actions. The need for competence implies that individuals want to interact effectively with their environment. Finally, the need

for relatedness pertains to the desire to feel connected with significant others.

With these needs in mind, Deci and Ryan (1991) view motivation in terms of varying degrees of self-determination, thereby leading to a continuum of different types of motives (see Figure 13.1). The proposed continuum is suggested to run from high to low levels of self-determination as an individual moves from intrinsic motivation to extrinsic motivation to amotivation (no motivation). Briefly describing this continuum will help us better understand the motives for exercise initiation and maintenance.

Self-determination theory predicts that both intrinsic and extrinsic motivations are multidimensional in nature (Vallerand & Losier, 1999). For example,

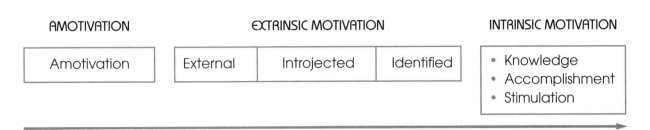

Figure 13.1. Adapted from Vallerand, R. J., & Losier, G. F. (1999). An integrative analysis of internal and external motivation in sport. *Journal of Applied Sport Psychology, 11,* p.153.

intrinsic motivation can have three forms: intrinsic motivation toward knowledge, toward accomplishment, and toward experiencing stimulation. Intrinsic motivation toward knowledge involves engaging in exercise for the pleasure of learning something new (like a new step in an aerobics class) or of knowing more about the activity. Intrinsic motivation toward accomplishment occurs as one derives pleasure from reaching personal goals such as walking for 60 minutes without stopping. Intrinsic motivation toward experiencing stimulation refers to engaging in exercise for the pleasant sensations derived from the activity itself, such as those described later in this chapter by Maddux (1997).

Extrinsic motivation also is conceived as being multidimensional, but without going into detail, the different types of extrinsic motivation are known as external regulation, introjected regulation, identified regulation, and integrated regulation. In general, when an individual is motivated extrinsically, then he or she is performing an activity in order to receive some reward. There are degrees of extrinsic motivation, with external regulation being the most extrinsic (e.g., exercising in order to win a participation contest) and identified regulation being the least extrinsic (exercising to lose weight because looking good is important). The key point, however, is that intrinsic motivation forms the basis for long-lasting adherence to exercise. Extrinsic motivation can be successful, but usually it is relatively short-lived. That is why people tend to start to exercise for extrinsic reasons (e.g., to lose weight), but they stay with exercise for more intrinsic reasons (to enjoy the experience). As Kimiecik (2002) has noted "to become a regular exerciser over a long period of time, you must learn to love to move your body" (p. 4). So here are some ways in which to enhance our love and intrinsic motivation to exercise.

Focus on the Experience Itself

It appears that if we are to really help sedentary people develop positive exercise habits that will last a long, long time, we need to focus more on making the exercise experience a positive one, rather than simply attempting to change behavior. If people change their behavior (and they can certainly do this), this usually results in a short-term solution for a long-term problem. Rather, the focus needs to be on changing the quality of the exercise experience. Most individuals are well aware of the desired outcomes of exercise. However, far fewer understand and then obtain the inner skills that are critical for motivating themselves to be physically active on a regular basis (Kimiecik, 1998).

A similar point is made by Maddux (1997) in his thoughtful article on the relationship of healthy behaviors, habit, and happiness. He persuasively argues that thinking about the future may be a good way to get people to begin to exercise, but as the statistics reveal, it appears not to be a good way to get them to adhere to exercise over time. People drop out of exercise programs (as well as smoking, drug, and diet programs) at very high rates in part because they expect such activities to become easy, habitual, and mindless, when, in fact, they are very difficult and mindful. When people find it hard to continue, they think something must be wrong, they become discouraged, and then they eventually quit. Furthermore, Maddux argues that we inadvertently tie exercise with a struggle with death. In essence, if people exercise, they will live a longer, happier life, and if they do not, they will die early.

One way to get people to continue exercising and adhering to exercise programs, perhaps, is to teach them to do it mindfully (not mindlessly via a habit). People should be in the present moment while exercising, and exercise should be something done for its own sake, instead of for some future gain. In essence, we should be telling people, "When you run, only run. When you lift weights, only lift weights, and when you are doing aerobics, only do aerobics." Maddux (1997) suggests that when individuals run, we should tell them the following:

> "Do not run thinking anything at all. Just run. Just breathe. Just take one step at a time. Just be in the present moment. If you experience discomfort or even pain, notice that. If you have thoughts about stopping, notice that too." (p. 343)

What this really is about is the ability to be in the present moment, to be fully focused and concentrated on the activity, not the goal. It is this ability that will make the activity enjoyable over the long haul.

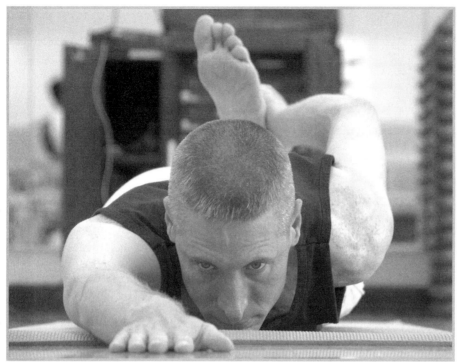

Photo by Jason M. Webb, courtesy of US Air Force

Process Orientation

So, how do we make an activity enjoyable so that we can stick with it for a long time? One way is to focus on the process instead of the product of these movement activities. For example, many exercise programs focus on the product of the exercise, which might be weight control, reduction in risk for certain diseases, or high levels of physical fitness. As noted above, these are the primary reasons that people exercise in the first place. Research and experience have consistently shown that maintenance of exercise is related more to the process of the movement, which emphasizes intrinsic motives.

Certainly, for many people who exercise regularly, it is natural to focus both on the process and product of the activity at different times in order to remain physically active. For example, at times, a product orientation would be appropriate because on some days, the notion of weight control might prompt the activity. More often, however, a process orientation is related to maintaining exercise over time.

Moving toward the intrinsic side of the continuum is a critical step that people must take if they are to move from little or no exercise to regular exercise day after day. Without this transformation, as demonstrated time and time again, many people will drop out of exercise programs or try unsuccessfully to stay motivated by bouncing from one exercise program to the next (Kimiecik, 1998). What happens to many people is that they stay focused on the outcome of the exercise such as losing weight and never really learn to enjoy the experience of exercise. That is, people never really focus on the process of the exercise. Research has revealed that the focus on process, as opposed to outcome, is related to long-term maintenance of exercise (Field & Steinhart, 1992). People who focus solely or predominantly on the outcome usually run into the various societal and physical barriers discussed in Chapter 11, which eventually lead to a termination of exercise. So people who want to become lifelong exercisers need to make the shift from being more outcome oriented to being more process oriented. One way to this is through a focus on flow.

Flow States

If exercisers are to move from a product to a process orientation, then a focus on flow states is one way to achieve this transformation. From a definitional point of view, *flow* has been conceived as an optimal psychological state of mind that usually occurs when the challenge of a situation or an activity matches the skills the individual brings to the situation. The concept of flow has been popularized by over 30 years of investigation by Csikszentmihalyi (1997b). His original work focused on understanding what makes a task intrinsically motivating. To accomplish this, he studied and interviewed people who performed activities with high intensity and effort (and sometimes great physical risk), yet few external rewards. These included rock climbers, dancers, amateur athletes, chess players, and musicians. His lifelong research program has revealed that flow states seem to be the result of several factors including (a) setting clear goals, (b) losing one's self-consciousness, (c) immersing oneself totally in the activity, merging action and awareness, (d) feeling a sense of control, (e) focusing on the activity itself, and (f) balancing skills and challenges (Csikszentmihalyi, 1997b). These factors underscore the importance that a process orientation has on ultimately experiencing a flow state.

Although some of the recent research has focused on elite athletes and their search for flow, much has also been written about flow states from an exercise point of view. For example, research on the "runner's high" would be one example in which the focus has been on the quality of the experience and not on the outcome of some performance. Although some elite athletes train to achieve these flow states, research has shown anyone

Achieving Flow States

As noted in the text, achieving flow can significantly help individuals maintain and adhere to an exercise program. In essence, the focus should be on the positive aspects of the experience itself rather than merely on the outcome. How do we achieve these flow states? Below are a few helpful hints that might increase the probability of getting into flow with our exercise (Kimiecik, 1998).

Balance Challenge and Skill.

A key part to the definition of flow is that the individual's skill level should match the challenge that is presented. Doing something that is extremely easy or very hard will usually not keep someone in a flow state. For many beginning exercisers, after exercising for a couple of months or so, boredom oftentimes sets in because the novelty of the experience wears off. So, if the activity becomes too easy, more difficult goals should be set, or the activity itself could be changed to increase the challenge. Conversely, if the challenge is greater than the skill level, people typically become anxious, and they avoid the exercise environment. Either more modest goals might be set (for example, exercising 3–4 days a week instead of 5–6), or the environment could be changed (e.g., exercising with someone you feel comfortable with if you are uncomfortable with your body).

Enhance Concentration and Awareness.

Focusing on the "here and now" is another critical aspect of achieving the flow experience. It is essential that people try to stay in the moment while exercising because this keeps the focus on the process of movement, not the end result. Focusing on one's breathing or being aware of the movement itself are two strategies to enhance focus and concentration on the task. For example, Kimiecik (1998) describes a technique that he uses to enhance his concentration. Specifically, he tries to repeat the word "left" when his left foot strikes the ground while running as he simultaneously exhales. This process is repeated when the right foot hits the ground. He offers that this has helped improve his concentration, and time seems to pass very quickly.

Become Aware of Internal Feedback.

Another important aspect of the flow experience is learning how to gauge and process the feedback that is provided by the mind and body during exercise. The kind of feedback received is not important. Instead, becoming aware of the feedback and knowing how to process it are of much greater importance. An exercise professional can help this process by asking the exerciser questions such as "How did your body feel today? or "What were you thinking during your exercise bout?" The exerciser can ask himself or herself these same questions.

It should be noted that some people like to dissociate from the exercise experience by listening to headphones or watching TV while riding the stationary bicycle. Although these techniques can help beginners with attendance and adherence to exercise programs, in the long run, these exercisers become less and less able to develop a keen awareness of their physical experience. To maximize the exercise experience, at some point people have to start associating with their bodies and "getting into the exercise" instead of trying to tune out.

Set Clear Goals.

It is important that every exerciser know what he or she wants to accomplish. Although this may seem easy, many people, in fact, are not very clear on their specific goals (at least for an individual exercise session). It may seem that setting clear goals goes against the whole notion of getting in touch with the exercise experience, but nothing could be further from the truth. Remember that the purpose of goal setting is to focus the exerciser's attention on the task at hand. It is likely that when exercisers become bored, it's because they are not clear about their goals and they are not concentrating on the task at hand. Then, too, goals might change from session to session. For example, some days a runner might just want to be with friends and emphasize the social nature of the exercise experience. Other times, the goal might be to focus on the beautiful surroundings and physical environment, and on other days, the goal might be simply to keep up good form. In any case, exercisers should clearly be aware of what they want to accomplish when they go out and exercise.

can achieve them, regardless of skill level. In essence, although flow states might vary in intensity, anyone can increase the chances of experiencing flow in a given situation by developing the appropriate mindset and mental strategies. Of course, flow is not the only source of motivation for regular exercisers, but it can be an important part of developing an intrinsic orientation and a process approach to exercise. That is, when we exercise in a flow state, it is usually such a positive experience that we want to repeat it again and again. According to Csikszentmihalyi (1997b), the important thing is to enjoy the activity for its own sake and to know that what matters is not the result, but the control one is acquiring over one's attention. The accompanying box provides some strategies on how to achieve different aspects of the flow experience.

Guidelines for Improving Exercise Adherence

Several elements have emerged in this chapter (as well as in Chapters 11 and 12) as keys to enhancing adherence to exercise. We will now consolidate these elements into guidelines for the aspiring fitness professionals as well as for people considering starting an exercise program or for those who want to make exercise a lifelong pursuit. These have been discussed at length in the chapters, so we will only list them at this point. They should help focus you on some of the major points in helping make exercise programs more successful. These are provided in no special order, and they are not prioritized in any way. They are just meant as tips for maximizing the effectiveness of exercise programs.

- Obtain social support from spouse, family members, and peers. (Support from significant others has consistently been shown to enhance exercise adherence.)
- Provide rewards for attendance and participation. (Rewards should be used judiciously, but they have been shown to be effective, especially in the short run.)
- Provide cues for exercise such as signs, posters, and cartoons. (Cues help remind people to exercise, but their removal typically means people return to their old habits.)
- Have participants complete a decision balance sheet before starting the exercise program. (Noting the pluses and minuses of exercising has been shown to help people make the decision to exercise.)
- Match the intervention to the stage of change of the participant. (The matching hypothesis is one of the central tenets of effective exercise programs.)

- Make exercise an enjoyable experience. (The research on intrinsic motivation and flow consistently points to the fact that people need to become intrinsic exercisers to adhere for the long haul.)
- Find a convenient place to exercise. (People are more likely to exercise if they perceive it is convenient for them to do so.)
- Practice time management skills. (Many people view lack of time as a barrier to exercise, but research has clearly shown it is simply a perceived lack of time. So making exercise a priority and managing time more effectively are critical in this regard.)
- Promote exercising with a group or friend. (Group programs have consistently been shown to be more effective than individual programs. However, do remember that some people need to exercise by themselves due to time constraints so individual differences are always important to keep in mind.)
- Have participants sign a contract or statement of intent to comply with the exercise program. (This helps enhance commitment to the program and eventual adherence to exercise.)
- Have participants reward themselves for achieving certain goals. (These rewards can help sustain motivation and keep people interested in the exercise program.)
- Tailor the intensity, duration, and frequency of the exercise. (People need to feel comfortable in their exercise program.) The program should be challenging, but it must meet the individual needs of each participant. Trying to exercise 30 minutes per day (although not 30 minutes at once) will help build flexibility and make goal setting more realistic.
- Give positive feedback. (All exercisers need some positive reinforcement, especially at the beginning stage, so exercise leaders and others should be free with praise.)
- Encourage goals to be self-set, flexible, and time based, not distance based. (Flexible goals that are set by the individual offer the greatest amount of commitment and allow for a wider range of behaviors, which is especially important in the early stages of an exercise program.)
- Participants should focus on internal (associative) cues (e.g., breathing, feeling of muscles) when exercising rather than on external (dissociative) cues. Although external distractions are helpful, for long-term adherence, exercisers need to focus more on the process and experience of the movement to maximize enjoyment.

Enhancing Lifelong Physical Activity for School and Community Programs

The Centers for Disease Control (1997) authored a report that highlighted the potential of community-based interventions aimed at promoting physical activity throughout the lifespan. Although the recommendations are focused on school and community programs, they can readily be generalized to any type of community-based physical activity intervention.

Recommendations	Description
Parental Involvement	Encourage parents to take part in physical activity programs as well as to support their children's participation.
Community Programs	Encourage participation in and provide for a variety of community-based physical activities for a wide range of ages and abilities.
Health Education	Make sure that the principles and benefits of regular physical activity are incorporated into school-based health education programs.
Personnel Training	Make sure that individuals are properly trained in school, coaching, recreation, and health-related jobs so that they can promote and encourage participation in regular physical activity.
Policy	Develop and implement policies that encourage and promote lifelong regular physical activity.
Health Services	Assess the participation levels of youngsters in regular physical activity, counsel them about the benefits of physical activity, and promote participation in different activities.
Environment	Provide and develop safe and enjoyable environments that encourage physical activity.
Physical Education	Encourage the regular offering of physical education in the schools and develop a curriculum that encourages enjoyment of physical activity, and helps students develop the knowledge, skills, and attitudes to lead physically active lifestyles.
Extracurricular Activities	Offer out-of-school physical activity programs that are enjoyable and meet the needs of students.
Evaluation	Make sure to regularly evaluate school and community physical activity programs as well as the viability of the facilities.

Summary

In Chapters 11 and 12, we discussed the models and determinants of exercise adherence because they provided us with information about the approaches and strategies that might be most effective in sustaining exercise programs. This is especially important because, at this point, only a small percentage of people exercise regularly enough to gain physiological and psychological benefits. In the current chapter, specific strategies were identified from the literature in the hope of enumerating what appears to work best in fostering exercise adherence. A wide variety of strategies were discussed including those involving behavior modification approaches such as prompting, setting up contracts based on attendance and participation, charting attendance and participation, and prompting exercise behavior. Other effective approaches were also discussed including the use of rewards, goal setting, cognitive strategies, decision balance sheets, feedback, and social support.

The last of the strategies discussed revolved around enhancing intrinsic motivation by focusing on the process of movement instead of the end product. Ample evidence indicates that for long-term maintenance of exercise to occur, people have to become intrinsic exercisers. In essence, they must come to enjoy participating in the activity itself, a condition that can be achieved by embracing the concept of flow. In essence, exercisers have to learn to enjoy the activity for its own sake, and not rely on external inducements to continue exercising. These external rewards certainly can be effective, but long-term maintenance of exercise usually means that the person finds fun, enjoyment, and fulfillment in the act of exercising itself. This state of mind is what exercise professionals need to foster when attempting to enhance exercise participation. The chapter ended with some tips and guidelines for maximizing the effectiveness of an exercise intervention.

Can You Define These Terms?

association

behavior modification

charting

contracting

decision balance sheet

dissociation

flow

intrinsic motivation

prompts

social support

Can You Answer These Questions?

1. Discuss the research using prompts to facilitate exercise adherence.

2. If you were going to use contracting as a method to enhance adherence, as an exercise professional, describe the type of contract you would draw up to facilitate adherence.

3. Based on research about the effects of goal setting on adherence, how would you use goals in setting up an exercise program? What goals are most effective?

4. How is a decision balance sheet used to help people stick with an exercise program? What research studies demonstrate its effectiveness?

5. Discuss two studies of using social support for enhancing adherence.

6. Discuss the research on using charting of attendance and participation to enhance adherence.

7. You want to get your exercise group intrinsically motivated to exercise. What practical steps would you take to accomplish this task?

8. What is a flow state, and how might it be related to exercise adherence?

9. Discuss three ways to enhance flow states that might produce longer-term adherence to exercise programs.

10. Using the guidelines for enhancing exercise adherence, design a program that would maximize adherence rates.

11. How would you use associative and dissociative strategies to maximize exercise adherence?

12. Briefly describe the empirical research relating to the effectiveness of goal setting.

CHAPTER 14

Personal Meaning in Physical Activity

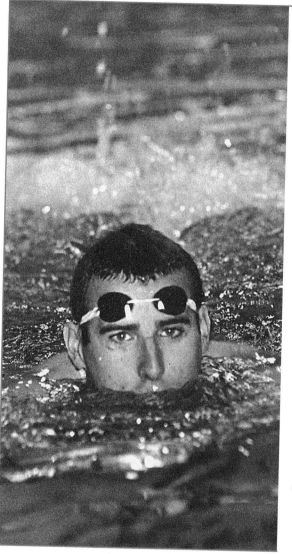

After reading this chapter, you should be able to

- Explain why both qualitative and experimental research is needed to study personal meaning in physical activity,

- Discuss the value of critical pedagogy in the training of physical educators and sport scientists,

- Identify some of the paradoxical meanings of exercise,

- Highlight cultural views of exercise that preclude understanding personal meaning in physical exercise,

- Illustrate the roles of fun and enjoyment throughout a lifetime of exercise,

- Describe the importance of freedom as a meaning of exercise,

- Reflect on the personal meanings of exercise for yourself at the different stages of your life thus far, and

- Discuss the transformational powers of exercise.

Introduction: Personal Meaning in Physical Activity

There are times when I am not sure whether I am a runner who writes or a writer who runs. Mostly it appears that the two are inseparable . . . .

Writing is the final form of the truth that comes from my running. *For when I run, I am a hunter and the prey is my self, my own truth* [italics added] . . . .

To reach these recesses, these hiding places below the conscious, *I must first create a solitude* [italics added]. I must achieve the *aloneness that is necessary for the creative act* [italics added] whether one is a master or a common man like myself. Because nothing creative, great or small, has been done by committee. (Sheehan, 1978, p. 13)

My fitness program was never a fitness program. It was a campaign, a revolution, a conversion. *I was determined to find myself. And, in the process, found my body and the soul that went with it* [italics added]. (Sheehan, 1978, p. 62)

I ask these students to reexamine that idea and choose the *body* [italics added]. Not to the exclusion of the *mind and soul but in conjunction with them* [italics added]. To see themselves as evolving wholes. Body and mind expressing the personality that is the self. (Sheehan, 1992a, p. 129)

Your body reveals you within and without. It tells the perceptive observer your philosophy, your view of the universe. (Sheehan, 1992a, p. 129)

Personal meaning in exercise captures the very *heart* of exercise. The quotations from George Sheehan depict a few personal meanings—at least the meanings of physical activity to Sheehan. In this chapter, you will examine personal meanings associated with exercise in an attempt to understand the actual lived experience of exercise, or how exercise is perceived by the individual. See Table 14.1 for the diverse personal meanings of exercise explored throughout this chapter. Personal meaning in exercise is interactive, which emphasizes that meaning is closely aligned with factors such as the

- Exercise setting,
- Goals of the exerciser,
- Type and intensity of exercise,
- Exercise partners, and
- Participant's previous experiences.

Table 14.1
Meanings of Exercise Explored in This Chapter

- A means to an end
- Absorption in the moment
- Appearance enhancement
- Become stronger—physically and psychologically
- Communion with nature
- Competition
- Defying death and the aging process
- Drudgery
- Empowerment and self-responsibility
- Escape from anxiety and depression
- Escape from tedium of daily existence
- Establish psychological endurance
- Freedom
- Health
- Inspiration, or disillusion
- Integration of body-mind-heart-spirit
- Liberation, or oppression
- Moving for the sake of moving
- Obligation (obligatory exercise)
- Opportunity for fun and enjoyment
- Opportunity to look within
- Persistence and a sense of continuity
- Physical attractiveness
- Potential for accomplishment for oneself, or failure
- Rapturous, peak moments
- Search for spirituality
- Self-awareness, self-exploration, and self-reflection
- Social interaction
- Solitude
- Something to be avoided
- Time alone

Because of these influences, personal meaning is larger than the exercise behavior itself, and it depends on that person's conscious awareness and interpretation of the experience.

Meaning of Exercise: A Relative Lack of Information and Impediments to Looking Within

When exploring the psychological effects of exercise, both desirable and undesirable, creation of personal meaning often is omitted. Thus, there is a relative lack of knowledge within exercise psychology about what exercise means to the participant. This lack is surprising because personal meaning, as previously observed, reflects the heart of the exercise experience. The running philosopher Sheehan recognized the lack of knowledge about meaning and devoted a chapter to it in *Dr. George Sheehan on Getting Fit & Feeling Great* (1992a). Despite Sheehan's initial analysis, there is a need for a greater understanding of meaning within physical activity. This chapter introduces you to some of the diverse meanings. First, though, you will explore three impediments to examining meaning in exercise: (a) emphases on accomplishment and an outward focus, (b) quantitative research approaches, and (c) the difficulty of looking within.

Emphasis on Utilitarian Accomplishment and an Outward Focus

Why is it that exercise and sport scientists seem to have neglected the personal meanings of physical activity? One reason may be that modern Western society tends to be utilitarian and heavily focused on technology. Thus, endorsement of the biomedical model of health with its utilitarian focus on disease treatment and prevention may preclude a focus on the meaning of health and exercise. As a result, our society values the tangible outcomes of exercise such as decreased heart rate and percent of body fat, and distance run or other performance indices that are assumed to represent reality, a reality that is out there in the world (Stelter, 1998). Many of us give little attention to inward, subjective experiences that occur during exercise.

The whole of exercise tends to remain compartmentalized because of the focus on its parts such as skill development, enhanced physical fitness, and the health benefits such as weight loss. As aptly noted by the psychologist and philosopher Ken Wilber (1996), you can take a watch apart to better understand its components; however, the parts will not tell you what

time it is. The whole (such as exercise) often is more than the sum of its parts. Thus, personal meaning of exercise is much more than improving our moods and decreasing body fat. Participants generate their own personal meanings of exercise from environmental signals such as light, sound, and touch (Stelter, 1998). "In this theoretical approach 'information' generates *meaning* [italics added] from signals" (Stelter, p. 10).

Research Approaches: Quantitative and Qualitative

Another possible reason for the neglect of the personal meaning of exercise is that quantitative research—a key means of establishing knowledge—emphasizes measurable, objective data that are necessary for statistical analyses. In contrast to traditional, utilitarian, medical models of exercise and the associated quantitative approach, personal meaning is a subjective experience that is difficult to measure. Too often, factors that are difficult to measure are considered to be unreal, unimportant, or not worth the effort needed to investigate them.

Our knowledge about exercise includes obvious parts: physiological training principles; biomechanical analyses; historical, cultural, and social contexts; and psychological techniques for performance enhancement. However, the exercise experience also includes less obvious feeling states, many of which are nearly impossible to capture: unity of body and mind, valuation of personal effort and struggle, pleasant fatigue of exertion, ecstasy, and peak moments. To gain knowledge about the multiple and unique personal meanings and interpretations of physical activity experiences, reflective research methods known as *qualitative research* are needed, as well as the more traditional quantitative research methods.

Qualitative research, which relies heavily on description, can be used in conjunction with quantitative or positivist research to reflect the wholeness of the human movement experience. Bob Brustad (1997), a noted specialist in the social psychology of exercise and sport, has emphasized that the positivist experimental model of research is fine as far as it goes. However, the positivist model, which accentuates objectivity and reductionism, is limited if it is the *only* model used to investigate the dynamic psycho-social-physical world of exercise. Qualitative research permits the capturing of "reality" from the perspective of an individual who exercises and emphasizes diversity of expression. In qualitative research, the researcher is an observer rather than a data gatherer. A goal within qualitative research methodology is to describe the many exercise events and interactions that influence the meaning of physical activity.

The Difficulty of Looking Within

An additional factor contributing to a lack of information about the personal meaning in exercise is that many of us lack the skill or inclination for turning our focus inward and engaging in self-analysis. This inward focus is a prerequisite for understanding the meaning of physical activity. Like most individuals, each of us occasionally may overlook the personal side of our lives and discount its importance (Wilber, 1996). Perhaps we are afraid of what we might find. We often go through our days priding ourselves on being efficient and focusing on school, work, and our list of "things to do." It almost is as though the personal-meaning aspects of our beings do not exist, or do not matter. This view is surprising because idiosyncratic, personal meanings have a large influence on our behavior, mood states and psychological well-being, and overall quality of life (Berger & Tobar, in press).

As a result of the historical valuation of quantitative research and a general lack of looking inward, chapters focusing on personal meaning are difficult to write. Little information is available, and discussion of personal meaning is vulnerable to criticism by proponents of the positivist model of research. For many of these reasons, chapters on the topic often are not included in textbooks. This is a serious omission because it limits our understanding of the exercise experience. In this chapter, you will begin to explore a sampling of diverse aspects of personal meaning. Personal meanings are context specific and may vary from one person to another. More specifically, meanings of exercise are influenced by the following:

- *Exercisers' characteristics* such as motivation, goals, personality, and physical conditioning;
- *Exercisers' previous exercise experiences*;
- *Contextual factors* of exercise such as competition, surrounding scenery, physical appearance of other exercisers in the area, and exercise leader;
- *Cultural factors* such as gender, race, and age;
- *Social factors* such as the valuation of exercise by immediate family, spouse or partner, and close friends; and
- Exercisers' personal interpretations of the whole exercise experience.

The Meaning of One Exercise Experience: A Physical Education Class

To illustrate the diverse meanings of exercise, take a moment to explore one aspect of physical activity with which most people are familiar: a physical education class, commonly referred to as a "gym" class. What is the meaning of gym to you? Gym might mean a time for fun; a time for exercise; a time to yell, to be boisterous, and to express yourself. Gym might mean an opportunity to play. If these were your answers, then it is likely that you are physically talented and/or feel secure in your movement capabilities. To others, the word *gym* might mean something to avoid. This negative meaning might result from a teacher who loudly pointed out mistakes or errors in moving, your personal feeling of being physically inept or awkward, from the need not to embarrass yourself around your friends, from bullying or taunting by classmates, or a host of other things.

In addition to personal responses and meanings of physical education, school physical education programs are in crisis throughout the United States, as concluded by Mary McElroy (2002) in her text examining general resistance to exercise. The ethos of competition and individual achievement, community funding resources for schools, and the limited time for academic classes within the school day create a complex interplay of competing factors. These factors and others detract from offering quality physical education classes, the establishment of physical skillfulness, and development of personal meanings that are conducive to lifetime exercise participation. Capturing part of the crisis in physical education programs, George Sheehan (1978) has described how he watched with envy when children answered the call "Come and play," and he asked an important question:

> What happens to our play on our way to becoming adults? Downgraded by the intellectuals, dismissed by the economists, put aside by the psychologists, it was left to the teachers to deliver the *coup de grace*. "*Physical education*" was born and turned what was joy into boredom, fun into drudgery, pleasure into work [italics added]. (pp. 72–73)

There are numerous meanings associated with the word *gym*, just as there are for *exercise*. *Physical education* has positive meanings for some people, neutral ones for others, and negative meanings for some others. Partly as a result of their exercise experiences in physical education classes, in school playgrounds, and in neighborhood ballgames, a large segment of the population, as much as 88%, tends to exercise less than required for enhancing their health (U.S. Department of Health and Human Services, 1996).

To correct the negative view and events within physical education classes, Fernandez-Balboa (1997) suggests that the training of physical education teachers be based on a critical pedagogy. Critical pedagogy encourages open communication and reflection in the gymnasium. This pedagogy enables teachers and students to share their goals, needs, fears, and other things that facilitate discovering the meaning of exercise by becoming thinking, feeling, imaginative, and intuitive beings. The relatively new critical pedagogy approach is a quest for the highly desirable qualities of social justice, freedom, equity, and institutional change. A goal of critical pedagogy is to go beyond criticism and argumentation and to focus on reflection and viable ways of teaching. Critical pedagogy includes consideration of many topics of importance in exercise psychology:

- Active change from *burning* bridges between various subspecializations within physical education to *building* bridges across academic specializations to provide a holistic understanding of human movement,
- Discrimination issues in physical education and sport, especially in regard to access to facilities and quality coaching,
- Ethics of health promotion that presently focus more on treating the symptom (i.e., heart disease, high blood pressure, etc.) than on the cause,
- Negative as well as desirable health effects of exercise,
- Personal meanings in physical activity,
- "Scientization" of physical education, or the rejection of everything in physical education that is not scientific, and
- Valuing of high-performance exercise and sport.

Paradoxical Meanings in Exercise

This chapter on personal meaning explores only some of the connotations of exercise to help you assist your students and clients in discovering some of the many meanings for themselves. It is important to recognize and acknowledge that there are diverse meanings—both positive and negative—within physical activity. As observed by Wankel and Berger (1990) in their examination of the psychological and social benefits of sport, "sport, like most activities, is not 'a priori' good or bad but has the potential for producing both positive and negative outcomes" (p. 167). The same is true for exercise.

Exercise can liberate or oppress, encourage or alienate, inspire or disillusion, and it can also be a source of satisfaction and achievement or a source of disappointment and failure (Tinning, 1997). In addition, exercise can enslave or free the participant, prevent or encourage psychological development, and be a source of body-mind integration or disassociation (Fahlberg & Fahlberg, 1990). These paradoxical meanings of physical activity reflect a diversity of movement forms and our own movement capabilities, as well as our age and gender (DeSensi, 1996). If you are familiar with some of the personal meanings of exercise, you might be able to use them to assist individuals who wish to exercise, or exercise more than they currently do, and to find their own personal meaning in exercise activities.

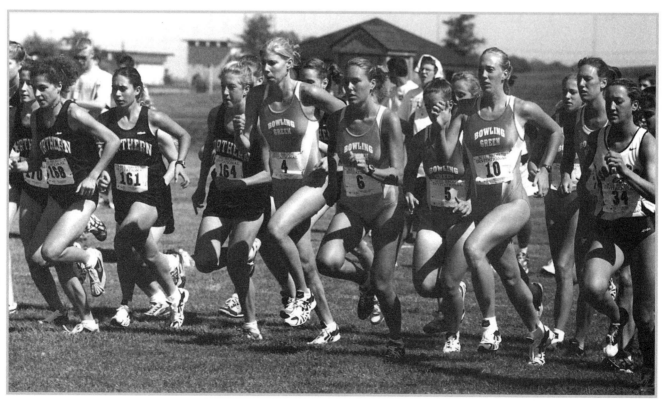

Meanings of Exercise in Specific Cultural Groups

The meanings of physical activity examined in this chapter tend to reflect the values, experiences, and perspectives of Americans of Anglo-Saxon descent and habitual exercisers, rather than athletes. Thus, these meanings and perspectives are culturally biased. This bias is due in part to the participants tested, the perspectives of authors of the available literature, and the focus of this textbook on *exercise* psychology. Highlighting the need to investigate the cultural implications of exercise and other forms of physical activity, Duncan and Robinson (2004) concluded,

> We cannot assume that White-American culture is representative of all cultures; this kind of totalizing practice stands in the way of knowledge . . . Yet in practice, White researchers ignore this principle all of the time . . . As we have seen, the bodily ideals discussed in this paper differed from those assumed to be universally embraced. (p. 98)

There is a great need for an examination of the meaning of physical activity in specific ethnic and racial groups, athletes and exercisers, different social classes, crosscultural populations, different age-groups, and people with specific health concerns such as cancer, heart disease, and AIDS. This process has just begun, and two groups, African Americans and athletes, are described below as examples of the needed research on the meaning of exercise in specific cultural groups.

African-Americans

In one of the few examinations of the meaning of exercise to African-Americans, Airhihenbuwa, Kumanyika, Agurs, and Lowe (1995) reported the results of their focus group interviews examining perceptions and beliefs about exercise. The study participants did not consider recreational exercise to be an important or necessary component of their lives. Despite the apparent lack of interest in recreational exercise, 64.5% of African-American adult women are overweight and/or obese in comparison to 46.6% of all American women (National Center for Health Statistics, December 5, 2005). Further support of the need for physical activity in the African-American population is the relatively high prevalence of coronary heart disease and Type 2 diabetes that can be controlled or prevented by increased physical activity (Duncan & Robinson, 2004; American Diabetes Association, 2005).

Key meanings of exercising for this sample of African-Americans were (1) to become more physically attractive to the opposite sex and (2) to become physically stronger in order to survive in their environ-

ment (Airhihenbuwa et al., 1995). African-American women, in particular, seem to have no single, ideal physical shape that dominates their preferred body ideal(s) and/or resulting participation in exercise activities (Duncan & Robinson, 2004). Emphasizing the need to focus on the meaning of exercise as a way to encourage broader exercise participation, Duncan and Robinson (2004) concluded,

> In fact, it may be that the biomedical model of health/fitness is not appropriate to all groups of White-American women either. The first author of this paper, a White woman, agrees with the focus group's argument that *health/fitness should be approached holistically as a lifestyle change affecting mind, body, and spirit, rather than merely as a diet or an exercise program* [italics added]. Our studies of socio-cultural groups different from our own reveal an important truth: We have much to learn. (p. 99)

These studies by Airhihenbuwa and colleagues (1995) and Duncan and Robinson (2004) are only a beginning of the quest to understand the meanings of exercise for specific segments of the population. Considerable research is needed to understand exercise meanings for men and women of diverse ages from various exercise and sport backgrounds, racial and ethnic groups, social classes, and nationalities.

Former Competitive Athletes

Another cultural group in regard to examination of the meaning of exercise is composed of former athletes. Investigating the meaning of movement to former competitive athletes, Jill Tracey and Tim Elcombe (2004) examined three hypotheses related to a relative lack continued lifetime exercise participation of this cultural group. Their hypotheses reflect the counterintuitive data emerging that indicates that former athletes *fail* to live healthier, more productive, or longer lives once they conclude the competitive sport phase of their lives. It seems that the personal meaning of physical activity, rather than knowledge about its health benefits, influence participation in exercise activities.

Tracey and Elcombe (2004) suggest throughout their analysis of the complex dynamics of meaningful movement that the sport experience itself may serve as a deterrent to lifetime exercise participation. The following hypothesized meanings of physical activity in general to competitive athletes may serve to deter their lifetime participation in physical activity (Tracey & Elcombe, 2004).

- *Hypothesis #1: Atypical physical behaviors.* This first hypothesis is that the sport culture is antithetical to lifelong exercise participation, because of its emphasis that suffering, pain, and injury during competition are necessary components of physical activity. The "no pain, no gain" sport mantra reflects the emphasis on suffering as a necessity in the training and competition process. Since pain and injury are *atypical* aspects of everyday living, are not enjoyable, and serve as deterrents to exercise participation, they are counterproductive to creating patterns of lifelong exercise participation.

- **Hypothesis #2: The utilitarian uses of physical activity.** The second hypothesized meaning is that physical activity is *a means to the end of winning* within the culture of competitive sport. This emphasis on winning and intense athletic training regimes often begins in youth sport and continues to the professional level. With physical activity being viewed as a duty or mechanized routine controlled by coaches or conditioning professions, sport and exercise tend to lose their appeal, enjoyment, and fun. This second meaning focusing on the utilitarian purpose of physical activity also deters athletes' lifetime exercise participation.

- **Hypothesis #3: The consequences of an athletic identity.** The third hypothesis is that *athletic identity*, or the extent to which participants see themselves as athletes, may deter exercise participation upon completion of their competitive sport careers. Sport means high performance; exercise means drudgery and relative lack of skill. Former athletes who have a strong athletic identity may struggle with and become embarrassed by their post-career diminished physical abilities or fitness levels. As a result, former athletes may avoid physical activity, since they no longer are as highly skilled as before (Tracey & Elcombe, 2004).

Fortunately, Lance Armstrong, the world class cyclist who was struggling with chemotherapy to treat his testicular cancer, was able to change the meaning of physical activity (1) from a focus on fitness and competition to (2) the pure enjoyment of exercise as Armstrong describes in the following quotation.

It became an increasing struggle to ride my bike between the chemotherapy sessions, and I had to accept that *it was no longer about fitness* [italics added]. Now I rode purely for the sake of riding—and that was new for me. To ride for only half an hour. I had never gone out for such a trivial amount of time on a bike.

I didn't love the bike before I got sick. It was simple for me: it was my job and I was successful at it. *It was a means to an end* [italics added] . . . a potential source of wealth and recognition. But it was not something I did for pleasure, or poetry; it was my profession and my livelihood, and my reason for being, but I would not have said that I loved it.

I'd never ridden just to ride in the past—there had to be a purpose behind it, a race or a training regimen. Before, I wouldn't even consider riding for just thirty minutes or an hour. Real cyclists don't even take the bike out of the garage if it's only going to be an hour-long ride.

Bart would call up and say, "Let's go hang out and ride bikes." "What for?" I'd say.

But now I not only loved the bike, I needed it. I needed to get away from my problems for a little while, and to make a point to myself and to my friends [italics added]. I had a reason for those rides: I wanted everyone to see that I was okay and still able to ride—and maybe I was trying to prove it to myself, too. (Armstrong & Jenkins, 2000, pp. 148–149)

Commonly Expressed Meanings in Exercise

For many participants, exercise provides a concrete activity—namely, movement—for taking care of our needs and, in a broader sense, for taking care of ourselves. Whether exercise provides these important opportunities to each of us depends partially on our own personal construction of the meaning of exercise (Berger & Tobar, in press). Some commonly expressed meanings of exercise include the following:

- Exercise can be fun and enjoyable because it gives us an opportunity to be lighthearted and joyful while moving.
- Exercise provides an avenue for increasing our exploration and awareness of our selves.
- Exercise can be freeing as exercisers learn to examine, set, and change their personal goals.
- Exercise also provides an opportunity for self-reflection. Spending time alone and relishing the experience are other possible meanings of exercise.
- For some participants, exercise facilitates empowerment and self-responsibility.
- Other participants note the importance of communing with nature, of being outdoors and experiencing the elements, of feeling close to the earth.
- Defying death and the aging process is an additional conscious or unconscious meaning of exercise.
- More esoteric meanings of exercise include a search for spirituality and a feeling of body-mind-heart-and-spirit integration.

In the following sections, you will examine these meanings in more detail.

Fun and Enjoyment

Fun and enjoyment are highly related meanings of exercise, and their presence greatly enhances our quality of life. However, it is difficult to distinguish between fun and enjoyment as illustrated by the first and third definitions of *fun* in the *Merriam-Webster's Collegiate Dictionary* (2003):

> **1 :** what provides amusement or *enjoyment* [italics added]; *specif*: playful often boisterous action or speech <full of ~> **2 :** a mood for finding or making amusement <all in ~> **3 a :** AMUSEMENT, ENJOYMENT <sickness takes all the ~ out of life **b** : derisive jest : SPORT, RIDICULE <a figure of ~>. (p. 507)

From these definitions, it would seem that fun and enjoyment are nearly synonymous because the word *enjoyment* is used to define the word *fun*. However, the difference between the two words is captured by the first definition which emphasizes boisterousness.

In contrast to the excitement and boisterousness of fun, enjoyment is a quieter, more peaceful, and less intense experience. A dictionary definition of *enjoyment* is

> **1 a :** the action or state of enjoying **b :** possession and use <the ~ of civic rights> **2 :** something that gives keen satisfaction <the poorest life has its ~s and pleasures>. (*Merriam-Webster's Collegiate Dictionary*, 2003, p. 414)

Further defining enjoyment, Kimiecik and Harris (1996) described enjoyment as "an optimal psychological state that leads to performing an activity for its own sake and is associated with positive feeling states" (p. 256).

In real life, exercisers might *enjoy* swimming laps, jogging, or playing basketball. However, rock climbing, downhill skiing, and other exciting activities may be *fun*. A single activity also may change from being fun to being enjoyable, depending on environmental conditions. Mountain biking over rugged terrain may be *fun* on a beautiful, spring day that is 60 degrees Fahrenheit; the same mountain biking might be considered *enjoyable*, but not fun, on days that the temperature dips to a chilly 30 degrees. Of course, determining which physical activities are fun and enjoyable remains in the eye of the beholder. Different types of exercise have different meanings for different individuals (Berger & Tobar, in press). Take a moment to list the types of exercise that are fun and the ones that are enjoyable to you. How did you arrive at your decisions? The frequent mentioning of fun and enjoyment as primary reasons for participating in physical activity supports including both of them as major meanings of physical activity (e.g., Berger & Motl, 2001; Douillard, 1994; Fine & Sachs, 1997).

Fun and enjoyment: Often-missing components. Most children seem to find physical activity fun. Games of tag, hide-and-go-seek, and simply twirling around until dizzy can occupy large blocks of time. As we grow older, however, we tend to forget this wonderful aspect of exercise. As we pass from childhood to adolescence, we tend to become more conscious of an evaluative aspect of moving and may become preoccupied with moving "properly." We begin to compare our movement abilities with peers and with athletes we see in the media. When we compare ourselves to our well-coordinated peers and major sports figures, some of us conclude that we just are "no good" when it comes to movement. The incentive to avoid failure or negative comparisons with others can become *more important* than expressing ourselves through movement. This thought could cause us to stop exercising altogether.

As adults, we become purposeful, practical, and utilitarian. We focus on accomplishing our daily tasks, which often are not fun. Fun and enjoyment are not items on our daily list of "things to do." Our list may or may not include exercise. If it does, the exercise probably is not for fun and enjoyment, but for health, fitness, and appearance benefits. Emphasis on health and appearance may provide fertile ground for exercise serving to impair our health. This is evident in disordered eating syndromes such as bulimia and anorexia, social physique anxiety (unfavorable comparison of our bodies to media images of the ideal physique), and identity issues characterized by low self-esteem (Brustad, 1997). Therefore, regardless of our age, we each need to include fun and enjoyment in each day—ideally, some of it is in the form of exercise.

The Fahlberg Exercise Plan emphasizing fun and playfulness. The 7-Part Wellness Exercise Plan of Larry and Laurie Fahlberg (1990) emphasizes the importance of fun and enjoyment in physical activity. This exercise plan is designed for the long-term promotion of exercise and focus on fun, enjoyment, personal growth, and health. The exercise plan is in direct contrast to the standard three-part exercise prescription of intensity, duration, and frequency. According to Fahlberg and Fahlberg, only compulsive individuals adhere to an exercise program that is not enjoyable. Their exercise plan emphasizes the need to consider the participant's needs and preferences and includes seven components (see Table 14.2). These components emphasize the importance of exercise enjoyment, a positive supportive environment, and valued personal meanings. The combined components emphasize personal well-being and the health-enhancement journey rather than the fitness outcome. Note that Fahlberg and Fahlberg (1990) designed the exercise components in Table 14.2 for movement specialists in diverse specialty areas to use as possibilities, not as formulas. All

Table 14.2
Seven-Part Exercise Plan for Health and Wellness
(Fahlberg & Fahlberg, 1990)

Components in the Exercise Plan	Description
Psychosocial considerations	**Focus** on personal meaning and enjoyment in a positive, supportive atmosphere.
A rate of progression that prevents exercise dismfort and injury	**Accept** a slower rate of progress than sport and competition to encourage enjoyment. Slower progression encourages lifetime participation.
Environmental and contextual	**View** the exerciser in a broad context of supports and constraints. **Create** an empowerment approach to exercise to avoid designing exercise interventions in lives of "deficient" individuals. **Establish** a goal of engendering feelings of self-responsibility and enjoyment.
Exercise mode or type	**Include** variety and fun to facilitate long-term health rather than short-term fitness.
Duration	**Suggest** (rather than prescribe) how many minutes per day for exercising. **Aim** for a lifetime duration.
Intensity	**Recognize** that high intensity is less important for enjoyment and personal development, than for fitness and athletic purposes.
Frequency	**Be Open** to participants' preferences and choices.

exercise programs, regardless of their specific components, need to facilitate empowerment, joyful self-expression, and freedom of choice for the participants.

Freedom and Its Relationship to Personal Goals and Meaning

Freedom can be another meaning found in exercise. When we exercise, we are free to exercise in any way that we wish. Within minimal constraints such as our financial resources and the amount of time we have available, we are free to choose the type of exercise, the location of our exercise sessions, the people with whom we exercise, our exercise intensity, the length of an exercise session, and the frequency of our exercise sessions.

Freedom is a recurring theme throughout Western civilization and is an important element in exercise.

Freedom is theorized to have three levels, any of which we can include within our exercise sessions (Fahlberg & Fahlberg, 1997). The first level is the freedom to make personal choices and the freedom to act on them. Many of us find that reaching this first level is difficult due to a pattern of repressing our true thoughts and feelings, and also to subtle forms of oppression. The second level of freedom is to transcend socially conditioned values and wants and to become an authentic form of ourselves. This level of freedom is more difficult than the first to attain, because it requires us to be attuned to socially and culturally constructed constraints, and then to separate ourselves from these values and viewpoints as we make truly independent choices. The third level represents the freedom from body and mind. Body and mind are only temporary phenomena that eventually will die. Freedom on this third level reflects who we are rather than what we get.

Freedom and exercise. Maintaining a sense of freedom while exercising is a difficult goal. Too often, we base our exercise goals on the socially prescribed values of a lean body, firm muscles, and youthful appearance, as well as the exercise leader's "prescription" of exercise intensity and duration. The term *fitness prescription* certainly has an impressive aura of science. However, the word *prescription* negates free choice, and results in disempowerment. Exercise prescription is the antithesis of freedom.

Freedom of choice is a much less verbalized meaning of exercise than is physical fitness. However, freedom is an important human value, and encourages movement from biomedical, technological, and utilitarian exercise goals to *emancipatory exercise goals* that foster body-mind integration. As noted by Fahlberg and Fahlberg (1997), the shift from utilitarian to body-mind integration is not new, but the portion of people who exercise for emancipation is increasing. The technological goal of attaining a "perfect body" is an obsession that tends to limit both health and freedom. Exercise can be enslaving and prevent development, or it can be freeing and facilitate personal growth. Fahlberg and Fahlberg (1997) emphasize three basic premises in their exploration of freedom, health, and human movement in the postmodern era:

- Human freedom is possible by means of emancipatory reason;
- Lifelong human development beyond socially acceptable behavior is possible; and
- Human movement that embodies body-mind integration can be a facilitator of personal freedom and human development.

Within a particular exercise session, there can be a huge freedom of choice. As noted by Sheehan (1978),

> Then I discovered running and began the long road back [to his true self]. *Running made me free* [italics added]. It rid me of concern for the opinion of others. Dispensed me from rules and regulations imposed from outside. Running let me start from scratch.
>
> It stripped off those layers of programmed activity and thinking. Developed new priorities about eating and sleeping and what to do with leisure time. Running changed my attitude about work and play. (p. 27)

Unfortunately, many people are not aware of their freedom to choose whether they want to exercise on a given day, how they might want to exercise, or what they might actually choose to do during a particular exercise session. Some exercise leaders adopt an autocratic stance regarding how intensely and for how long a person "should" exercise and offer the opposite of freedom: exercise prescriptions, the need for rigid exercise adherence, and an almost blind compliance to exercise guidelines. These exercise "shoulds" need careful scrutiny as possible limitations on freedom, self-exploration, and personal empowerment. As movement specialists, we need to facilitate and enhance conditions in which exercisers can experience freedom for themselves. Fahlberg and Fahlberg (1997) observed that

> Many of us live imprisoned much of the time in a variety of ways. At least two of the jail house bars are cast by psychological and social forces. Typically, we have various degrees of awareness of some of these bars; whereas other bars escape our awareness and, therefore, limit our possibilities to free ourselves. For example, psychologically, we are imprisoned and influenced by unconscious forces, whereas, socially, we operate with unexamined assumptions that limit our freedom (Fromm, 1969; McCarthy, 1981). But it is not necessary to remain so confined; a new, more exalting vision can include the path leading beyond social oppression and psychological repression. We will define *health as the freedom to travel this path*, [italics provided] in accord with developmental potential. (p. 69)

Freedom of choice: To not exercise. Choosing not to exercise also is an important aspect of choice. Freedom of choice within the sometimes-coercive exercise environment is a crucial element within exercise (Fahlberg & Fahlberg, 1997). We need to protect freedom and maintain the element of choice within our clients' and students' exercise programs. Maintaining freedom within many exercise settings, however, is more difficult than it initially seems. As exercise experts, it is important that we avoid telling our clients and students what they "should" do in regard to their exercise programs. Many exercisers tend to compete with themselves and constantly strive to do "more" at a faster pace. In regard to exercise, "enough is enough" does not appear to apply.

A constant focus on self-improvement does not provide exercisers with opportunities for true self-reflection. Are exercisers free to do what they want when they exercise? Alayne Yates (1991), a professor of psychiatry at the University of Arizona, has emphasized the lack of self-reflection that characterizes many runners. In a classic book, *Compulsive Exercise and the Eating Disorders: Toward an Integrated Theory of Activity,* Yates investigates obligatory runners who do not have the freedom to choose the type of exercise in which they want to participate or how long and far they want to run. She also compares obligatory runners to people with eating disorders and examines the psychological, sociocultural, and biological similarities between the two groups. Obligatory runners are not free to make choices about whether they will exercise. However, obligatory runners do report some positive meanings in exercise that are available to all exercisers. Yates reports that

> Obligatory runners continue to run in part because they *derive substantial benefit from the sport* [italics added]. This is the case even when the running is painful and driven. They are *soothed and invigorated* [italics added] when they run; they *feel proud of the body and in command of their future* [italics added]. Max describes the runner's high as *enormously satisfying, a sensation of floating through space* [italics added]. Dick describes running as providing *a sense of power, control, and well-being. His body seems alive with grace and vigor* [italics added]. (p. 41)

Health and Appearance

Health and improved appearance are two common meanings of exercise. Health has multiple components as illustrated in Figure 14.1. Maintaining a regular exercise program enables each exerciser to reach a variety of personal health goals. Common exercise goals include losing a few pounds, toning our bodies, enhancing our cardiorespiratory health, as well as socializing or "catching up" with our friends while exercising. These goals tend to be reflected in New Year's resolutions and often are based on societal values, rather than the exerciser's own. Because these goals reflect "shoulds" based on technological ration-

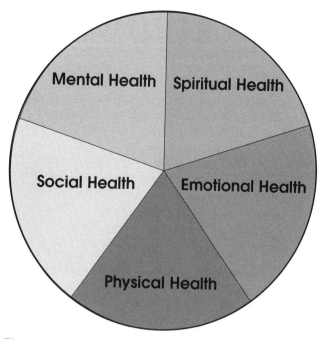

Figure 14.1. Balanced components within the holistic concept of health (Greenberg, 1998).

ality rather than "wants" that might reflect self-emancipatory goals, many individuals abandon their New Year's resolutions within a few months.

The general lack of success in adopting and adhering to exercise programs for enhanced health and appearance makes it important to examine a host of exercise goals to understand the meanings of exercise and what enables some people to be successful exercisers. Exercise means more than following a scientific prescription of what and how to move. Exercise can be a celebration of life.

Health includes physical, social, spiritual, emotional, and mental components as depicted by the circle in Figure 14.1 (Greenberg, 1985, 1998). According to Greenberg's (1998) holistic model of health, each component is of equal value and is represented by an equal portion of a circle. Many individuals exercise either too little or too much for optimal health, and thus they represent the common imbalances depicted in Figure 14.2. If an individual devotes too much time and energy to one component such as exercise, the physical component of health grows out of proportion, and the imbalance has undesirable effects on the other health components. For example, with an overemphasis on the physical component, the excessive exerciser's health is "out of round" or imbalanced, as illustrated in Figure 14.2. Health is a paradoxical meaning of exercise. Exercise is a highly desirable activity. Yet beyond a certain amount, more exercise does not necessarily result in greater health.

When too much exercise detracts from health and appearance, the participant may not be aware of the

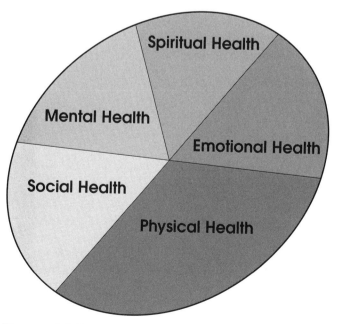

Figure 14.2. Unbalanced, lower levels of health (Greenberg, 1998).

CASE STUDY 14.1 — *Exercise and Health: Jim's Lack of Balance*

I could not help wondering if Jim was healthy. Several years had passed—five to be exact—since we last saw each other, and I was looking forward to catching up on old times. When I asked the standard, "How've ya been?" Jim replied that he never felt better. He took up jogging and now was up to 50 miles a week. As a result, he gave up cigarettes, became a vegetarian, and had more confidence than ever.

In spite of Jim's reply, I need (*sic*) further assurance. Jim look (*sic*) like "death warmed over." His face was gaunt, his body emaciated. His clothes were baggy, creating a sloppy appearance. He had an aura of tiredness about him.

"How's Betty?" I asked.

"Fine," Jim replied. "But we're no longer together. Betty just couldn't accept the time I devoted to running, and her disregard for her health was getting on my nerves. She's still somewhat overweight, you know, and I started viewing her differently when I became healthier myself."

(Greenberg, 1985, p. 403)

---

undesirable effects, although the people around that individual may be. The negative aspects of exercise are not as visible as the positive and include cases of exercise addiction, overcommitment to exercise, overuse injuries, and eating disorders as examined in Chapter 16 on exercise concerns. This darker side of exercise illustrates that health consists of far more than physical health and high fitness levels. The comments in Case Study 14.1 about a runner named Jim illustrate the negative influence of exercise on health:

Jim was pleased that he was jogging, stopped smoking, became a vegetarian, and felt more confident. By overemphasizing his physical health, however, he damaged his overall health. He neglected his social health by spending too little time and energy on his marriage and other relationships. He also may have harmed his mental health if he was exercising so much that he experienced undesirable mood changes as commonly occurs in overtraining with increased fatigue and depression and decreased vigor (O'Connor, 1997). Exercise could damage Jim's health even more if Jim develops an overuse injury.

The question remains, is Jim healthier with this particular exercise routine than before he started his exercise program? Only Jim can answer this question because he alone knows the status of his social, spiritual, emotional, and mental health. In conclusion, we often equate habitual exercise and physical factors with health. Health, however, is multifaceted, and includes a balance of physical, social, spiritual, emotional, and mental components.

Time Alone

Another meaning of exercise is time—time to be alone with one's self. Time alone often includes peace, quiet, and contemplation, which are important components of a well-lived life. Carving out a bit of quiet time in our day is a central message in a variety of religious faiths, stress management techniques, and theories that focus on creating inner wisdom, strength, and creativity (e.g., Cameron, 1992; Cunningham, 1997). Exercise can create a break in our daily routines, *and* we can experience time alone by participating in a solitary form of exercise such as jogging, swimming, weight training, rock climbing, or scuba diving. The running philosopher George Sheehan (1984) captured the importance of time spent alone while exercising and the accompanying peace, quiet, and contemplation that occur while jogging:

I am surprised to find that I have been contemplating while out on the roads. I engage in what Aquinas called the highest human activity: contemplating while out on the roads . . . One need not be a trained philosopher to do this. It is human nature to look inward and examine oneself and the world. Fortunately for me, running frees me to do that—it allows me to become absorbed in my thought . . .

In using my body, I become disembodied. I become pure intellect. My life becomes thought. Motion makes time stand still, and I am completely in the present . . . For the moment, reasoning, evaluating, and judging are suspended—the person is getting to the soul's center.

Josef Pieper, the German theologian, claims that ultimate happiness consists in contemplation. (p. 37)

Being alone provides the exercise participants with time: time to reflect, time to contemplate and learn from the reflection, and even time to be silent without the emanation or bubbling up of any thoughts. Many runners, including the one obligatory runner described in Case Study 14.2, prefer to run alone. It is likely that exercisers in many other activities also prefer to exercise alone for the following reasons aptly described by runners such as Marilyn, who was a participant in a study by Yates (1991).

CASE STUDY 14.2 *Exercise and the Importance of Time Alone for Marilyn*

. . . Yet, like Marilyn who meditates as she runs, obligatory runners prefer to be alone. If they happen to run with another, they may run silently. When they are by themselves, *they think special thoughts, make unique calculations and comparisons, and immerse themselves in the sensations of the body and mind.* Solitary activity provides them with *the chance to reflect, to problem solve, to savor the run, to visualize themselves in action, and regroup for the challenge ahead.* Running alone is one method of *resolving the resentments which stem from being misunderstood by the boss or being taken advantage of by the spouse or children* (italics added).

(Yates, 1991, pp. 41-42)

Self-Exploration, Self-Awareness, and Self-Reflection

In addition to providing opportunities for fun and enjoyment, freedom, health, improved appearance, and time alone, physical activity can facilitate self-exploration, self-awareness, and self-reflection. Exercisers can become aware of thought processes that occur before, during, and after exercising. For example, by honestly exploring the role of exercise in their lives, participants can examine what is important and then reflect on its meaning. For example, they might ask, "Do I choose to find time for exercise in my busy day? Is exercise important to me in my life? What is my value system? Do I choose to exercise today? Do my beliefs and values match my actual behavior?" The priorities of your exercise clients and students may or may not include exercise. Recognizing the priorities and meanings of exercise to your clients is a foundation for your professional interactions with them.

Specific types of exercise such as jogging, lap swimming, and other solitary forms are conducive to self-exploration and introspection, to thinking in general, and to gaining self-understanding. Reflecting on the self-exploration and introspective opportunities in some types of exercise, a woman jogger reports,

> When I'm running, it seems like I'm dreaming and a lot of thoughts go through my mind very, very quickly. And you can get in touch with things quickly if you are aware of what you're doing and what the day has been like. (Berger & MacKenzie, 1981, p. 104)

Supporting the self-exploration and the self-awareness that are available through habitual participation in physical activity while running, Sheehan (1978) reflected,

> When I was young, I knew who I was and tried to become someone else. I was born a loner. I came into this world with an instinct for privacy, a desire for solitude and an aversion to loud voices, to slamming doors and to my fellow man. I was born with the dread that someone would punch me in the nose or, even worse, put his arm around me.
>
> But I refused to be that person. I wanted to belong. (p. 26)

Creating time within each day for exercise provides participants with an opportunity for reflection and self-exploration. Including exercise in a busy day could mean that exercisers like themselves enough to do something that is important to them. Exercisers recognize that they are physical beings who benefit in a multitude of ways by exerting themselves physically. Through exercise, participants have opportunities to experience body-mind unity, have time for themselves, and especially have time for reflection. Physical exercise can provide participants more energy, vigor, and desirable mood changes as suggested in Chapter 6, and exercise can moderate our stress levels as reviewed in Chapter 8. However, some of the health goals of exercise can be enslaving rather than emancipatory as discussed in Chapter 16 as evidenced by people in quest of the "perfect" body, by those who use exercise as an obsessive form of weight control, and by compulsive and/or addicted exercisers (Fahlberg & Fahlberg, 1997). As exercise psychologists, exercise physiologists, athletic trainers, and teachers, we need to contemplate the importance of exercise and its meaning in our clients' and students' lives. With this information, we can assist them in balancing personal freedom with their health and other goals.

Empowerment and Self-Responsibility

The concepts of empowerment and self-responsibility in exercise are closely interwoven with the meanings of freedom, self-exploration, and increased personal awareness. *Empowerment* is defined as the individual's ability to direct his or her own life by making wise choices and maintaining them (Rappaport, 1981).

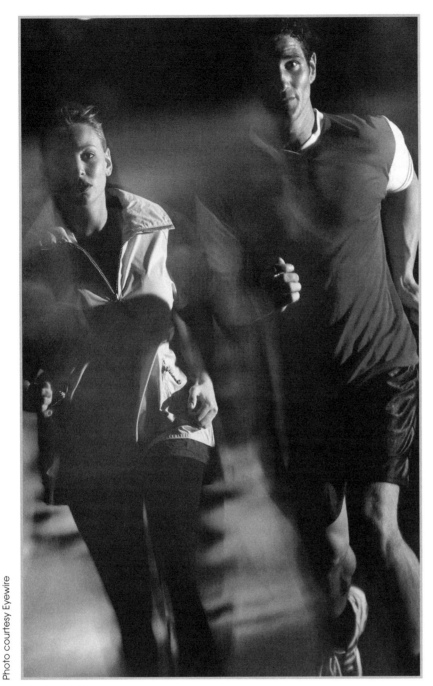

an exercise class leader or fitness facility. As suggested by Fahlberg and Fahlberg (1990), program staff in exercise centers, personal exercise trainers, and other movement specialists who do not recognize the problems associated with an overemphasis on the physical component of health unwittingly may be encouraging exercisers to become dependent on exercise.

Making responsible personal choices means that exercise participants have the freedom to avoid an overemphasis or dependence on exercise to the exclusion of the other health dimensions of intellectual, emotional, social, occupational, and spiritual activities depicted in Figure 14.1. Dependence (or addiction) to exercise is an effective means of repression and avoidance of self-responsibility, as long as the person is able to exercise. Unfortunately, an inability to exercise for someone who is dependent on exercise can lead to a personal crisis as illustrated by the following vignette:

> I got injured in a motorcycle accident and it was really hard. I was burned out too, and I got sick and had a virus. But I just never quite got it back together, so I ended up in the hospital with this virus, and, boy, it seems like my life just fell apart. Couldn't exercise, couldn't do anything, just lethargic and it was like my life had come to an end.... (Fahlberg & Fahlberg, 1994, p. 106)

Communion With Nature

Another meaning of exercise is associated with increased opportunities to be outdoors in nature. Exercising outside presents opportunities for participants to observe and be a part of nature, as well as to be close to the earth. Regardless of whether exercisers are walking, jogging, playing a game of tennis or golf, rock climbing, skiing, or whitewater rafting, they have an opportunity to be outdoors and a part of nature. Price (1983) captures the meaning of communing with nature while skiing:

winter beauty surrounds me here
    alone among the hills
        I soar in rhythm to the falling snow
            and feel its gentle touch upon my soul

today I feel as if God planned
    all urgencies should fall away

Empowerment is both individualized and contextually dependent upon environmental conditions and perceived options (Fahlberg & Fahlberg, 1990; Rappaport, 1981). *Self-responsibility* is an individual's recognition that she or he has choices (Fahlberg & Fahlberg, 1990). With choice, exercisers also use their cognitive capacities to better understand their bodies' needs and the meanings in exercise. This mental challenge may contribute to exercisers' mental well-being and health.

Empowerment and self-responsibility are central concepts in being a physically educated person, one who is able to choose among a host of exercise parameters and health outcomes rather than being dependent upon

and only winds

　　that whirl the snow

　　　　should give motion to my day

that I should sense

　　the rhythm of the downhill run

　　the rise and fall of slopes beneath my skis

　　the long

　　　　slow

　　　　　　sweeping

　　　　　　　　turns

　　　　　　　　　　through silent pines

that I should see my signature of wholeness

　　undersigned

　　　　in space

　　　　　　and time

and know this rhythmic design

　　transforms discordant motions

　　　　of the

　　　　　　body

　　　　　　　　soul

　　　　　　　　　　and

　　　　　　　　　　　　mind.

(p. 75)

Being outside provides exercisers with an opportunity to notice the air temperature, the color of the sky, cloud formations, occasional rainbows, the majesty of trees, and the shape and color of leaves and flowers, the strength of the sun, the color of the sky, the movement of the breeze, and a host of other characteristics. Being surrounded by nature gives exercisers a wonderful opportunity to practice mindful meditation while increasing their awareness of the here and now as they exercise. Participants can be totally caught up in the experience and fully in the present moment as they complete various movements and feel their bodies responding while being surrounded by nature. In capturing the importance of nature for some exercisers, Wilber (1996) has described some of the related meanings:

> At the psychic level, a person might temporarily dissolve the separate-self sense (the ego or centaur) and find an identity with the entire gross or sensorimotor world—so called *nature mysticism*. You're on a nice nature walk, relaxed and expansive in your awareness, and you look at a beautiful mountain, and wham!—suddenly there is no looker, just the mountain—and you are the mountain. You are not in here looking at the mountain out there. There is just the mountain, and it seems to see itself, or

you seem to be seeing it from within. The mountain is closer to you than your own skin. (p. 202)

> A spontaneous environmental ethics surges forth from your heart, and you will never again look at a river, a leaf, a deer, a robin, in the same way. (p. 204)

In conclusion, exercisers experience nature in their own individual ways. However, the term *communing with nature* seems to capture a hard-to-describe meaning that some exercise participants value. As Stelter (1998) notes in his discussion of the theory of meaning and understanding, "There is a co-dependency between the subject and the environment" (p. 19). Communing with nature seems to be particularly important when attempting to capture the meaning of outdoor exercise for participants.

Delaying the Aging Process

For some participants, delaying the aging process is another conscious or unconscious meaning associated with exercise. Exercisers delay the aging process in numerous ways. By exercising, participants can maintain or even increase muscle mass, establish cardiorespiratory fitness and reservoirs of endurance and vitality, and maintain strong bones.

To understand the multiple roles of exercise in the aging process, it is helpful to examine what aging actually entails. Aging is a group of universal processes that occur with the passage of time as described in Chapter 19, "Exercise for Older Individuals." Emphasizing the

Table 14.3
Commonly Employed Age Categories (Spirduso, 1995, p. 8)

Description	Age in years
Infant	0–2
Child	3–12
Adolescent	13–17
Adult categories	18–64
Young adult	18–24
Adult	25–44
Middle-aged adult	45–64
Old categories	65–120
Young-old	65–74
Old	75–84
Old-old	85–99
Oldest-old	100+

centrality of time in the aging process, people often are separated into the different age categories illustrated in Table 14.3. The term *old* refers to people who are older than the "middle-age" category in the table. In general, society considers people who are 65 years of age or older as old. The four age ranges within the "old" category illustrate large differences in physical abilities of the young-old, old, old-old, and oldest-old. The "old" category spans 55 years based on the assumption that the maximum human life span is around 120 years. Reference to the period of life beyond 65 as "the third age" emphasizes the possibilities for a meaningful, healthy, and vital life during this third portion of our years on earth.

Postponing the aging process is a reoccurring meaning of exercise for some participants. Exercise can serve as a vehicle to slow the aging process and even to increase the length of life. Thus, exercise affects both the quality and quantity of life. Truths about aging that Waneen Spirduso and her colleagues (2005) observed at the beginning of their encyclopedic book on the physical aspects of aging include the following:

- Everyone does it, and
- Everyone does it differently. (p. 3)

Despite individual differences in the aging process, the research evidence is clear. As illustrated in a classic book, *Inside Running*, written by Dave Costill (1986), a respected exercise physiologist, highly trained exercisers have the maximum oxygen uptake of sedentary individuals who are 20 years younger. In addition, most habitual exercisers have lower blood pressure and pulse rates, greater muscle mass, increased joint flexibility, less fat tissue, and greater respiratory capabilities and oxygen uptake than do their younger, sedentary peers (Spirduso, Francis, & MacRae, 2005). Exercise's physiological benefits help to reduce mortality and morbidity (being physically and mentally incapacitated).

Research evidence supports the likelihood that habitual exercisers who expend over 2,000 calories per week in moderate or intense physical activity live two years longer than sedentary individuals who expend fewer than 500 calories a week (Lee & Paffenbarger, 1996). In their review of the relationship between exercise and mortality, Lee and Paffenbarger concluded that exercise helps participants to avert premature mortality rather than actually extend the life span. In age-groups from 45–54 to 75–84, the greater the amount of intense exercise, the lower the mortality rate.

Table 14.4

D.A.R.E. Guidelines for Reaching 100 Years of Age: Areas in Need of Attention (Bortz, 1996, pp. 90-92)

Diet	**A**ttitude	**R**enewal	**E**xercise
Eat to reach 100	Believe in 110	Recharge yourself	Take the first step
Read well to eat well	Find meaning	Stay in flow	Make time for exercise
Know when to eat	Be necessary	Think travel	Keep strong
Be fat alert	Be an optimist	Keep in rhythm	Stay loose
Don't dry up	Be a good loser	Afford retirement	Work dem bones
Count cholesterol	Have guts	Keep working	Respect your back
Keep your fiber up	Stay in touch	Sleep enough	Know that aging is incurable
Take a coffee break	Learn to learn	Cherish your world	Keep your oxygen tanks full
Beware of free radicals	Get high on helping	Relearn, rethink, reeducate	You don't have to win
Examine the pros and cons of protein	Maintain the creative spark	Think when, where, and why retire	Know how hard, how long, and how often to exercise

Note: From Dare to Be 100 (pp. 90-92), by W. M Bortz II, 1996, New York: Fireside.

Postponement of Death With Immortality Projects

Postponing death is another conscious or unconscious meaning of exercise. In fact, exercise has been described as an "immortality project" (Fahlberg & Fahlberg, 1997; Wilber, 1983, 1996). Viewing exercise as an immortality project emphasizes the biomedical, mechanistic model of physical activity. Exercise that is strenuous enough to produce desirable changes in body fat, bone density, and heart rate enables participants to postpone death, as long as it does not exacerbate existing medical conditions.

Emphasizing the value of exercise—along with other factors of diet, attitude, and renewal—in postponing death and in preventing premature aging, Walter Bortz (1996) has published the book, *DARE to be 100*. Bortz is a well-respected researcher in the area of aging who has written more than 100 studies, a faculty member at Stanford University Medical School, a practicing physician, and a past president of the American Geriatric Society. Based on his years of research and interest in the area of aging, Bortz lists 99 active strategies or steps in the quest for living well to the age of 100. Groupings of the 99 DARE steps are represented in Table 14.4. These include 18 **D**iet-related steps, 35 **A**ttitude-related steps, 20 steps for **R**enewal, and 25 **E**xercise-related steps. The first letters of each of these categories fit together to spell the word *DARE*, which is part of the book title. Following all of Bortz's 99 steps on a daily basis would be a major immortality project.

Staying too busy to think about death. Habitual physical activity serves to postpone death by helping the participant avoid consideration of the inevitability of death. If people exercise long enough and hard enough, they have little time or energy to ponder their demise. By keeping busy through activities such as exercise, careers and work, and service to the community, the inevitability of death can be ignored or successfully repressed. This meaning of exercise was noted by Yates (1991) throughout *Compulsive Exercise and the Eating Disorders: Toward an Integrated Theory of Activity* and initially by Yates, Leehey, and Shisslak (1983) in their classic study of individuals who are unable to "not run" and who build their lives around running. The following quotation illustrates the relationship between exercise, business, and death:

> Obligatory runners and anorexic women must continue to prove themselves by running or dieting . . . They are satisfied by moving toward a goal, not by achieving it; in fact the goal itself is entirely secondary and is reset at will to rationalize the continuation of the process . . . The *endless quest . . . is perpetuated by the fear that if one stops, one will cease to exist* [italics added]. (Yates et al., 1983, p. 225)

Enriching the present with acceptance of mortality. The use of exercise to avoid contemplating our eventual death is counterproductive to self-development. Psychologists and philosophers (Fahlberg & Fahlberg, 1997) suggest that we do not begin to live fully until we confront the inevitability of death. Accepting death as a valuable part of life can be freeing and contributes to the overall quality of life. As conceptualized by Fahlberg and Fahlberg (1997), the realization of death is accompanied by existential angst characterized by personal discomfort and anxiety. However, acknowledging death as part of life and accepting the unavoidability of our physical death enable a more aware, more intense participation in the present movement.

The existentialist view of death is that many of our daily activities are in service of postponing or hiding from the inevitability of death:

> We lie about our mortality and finitude by constructing immortality symbols—vain attempts to beat time and exist everlastingly in some mythic heaven, some rational project, some great artwork, through which we project our incapacity to face death . . . We lie about the richness of the present by projecting ourselves backward in guilt and forward in anxiety . . . In place of the authentic or actual self, we live as the inauthentic self, the false self, fashioning its projects of deception to hide itself from the shocking truth of existence. (Wilber, 1996, p. 194)

Rather than remain in this angst-ridden existential state, Wilber (1996) proposes that individuals move into a transpersonal stage characterized by a superconsciousness where the observing self transcends the mind.

Search for Spirituality

> I express myself with and through my body. I am called to be the body I become. My profession is how my body plays, what becomes my body's sport. So my physical education is no less important than any other part of my education. And the physical manifestation of myself deserves, indeed *requires*, equal time with my other functions.
>
> I will be fit because I must. I will find my sport because without it I will be incomplete. If I am fortunate I will find an area where movement of body joins movement of the mind and movement of the *spirit* [italics added]—and discover that activity in which the subsequent repose coincides with heightened states of being, and affirmation of myself and all creation. (Sheehan, 1992a, pp. 33–34)

Another meaning found in exercise and in the wellness concept of health (see Figure 14.1) is a sense of spirituality. Spirituality is defined as experiencing the presence of a higher power, a unifying force, or an energy often referred to as "God" (Gorsch, Baumeister, Cameron et al., 1998; Miller & Thoreson, 1999). Spirituality reflects individual experience and includes personal transcendence and meaningfulness. It is a multidimensional construct that includes discovering the "truth" about who we are, why we are here on earth, whether there is a God, and what our relationship to Him or Her is (Gorsch et al., 1998). During exercise, this presence or Godly awareness can be close to the individual. *Presence* and *energy* are additional words for describing spirituality. Either of these terms allows for bidirectional interaction between the individual and the spirit.

Spirituality may or may not have religious connotations. A person may be spiritual but not identify with any religion such as Christianity, Judaism, or Buddhism. The terms *spirituality* and *religion* are not synonymous. Religion is characterized by the organized activities of a church group, sect, or cult. The term *religion* is used to reflect formally structured religious institutions (Gorsch et al., 1998). As noted by Miller and Thoresen (1999), spirituality can reflect an individualistic perspective:

> . . . spirituality, which might center on material experiences such as mountain biking at dusk [italics added], quiet contemplation of nature, reflection on the direction of one's life, and a feeling of intimate connection with loved ones . . . Clearly, spirituality and religion are not the same. (Miller & Thoresen, 1999, p. 7)

Spirituality is a word closely tied to religion and pertains to the inner life. To acknowledge some people's lack of belief in religious doctrine, spirituality can be separated into secular spirituality, which is without religious overtones, and religious spirituality, which is for people who value faith in the divine (Ardell, 1996). Although it is hard to define, spirituality is an integral component in health and wellness (Miller & Thoresen, 1999; see Figure 14.1).

Spirituality is a commonly expressed meaning of exercise as captured by Eva Bednarowicz (2004) in her essay, *The Amen of Running*. As described in the essay, runners and perhaps participants in other types of exercise can converse with God and become aware of the presence of a deity in their lives during an exercise session. Exercisers can find presence or energy in nature, in the peace and quiet of solitary exercise, in religious references to taking care of the body, in awareness of the magnificence of the human body created according to some divine plan, and in a host of other situations and meanings.

Integration of Body, Mind, Heart, and Spirit in Personal Transformation

Closely associated with the search for spirituality is the opportunity to integrate body, mind, heart, and spirit while exercising. Exercise participants often express an appreciation of being a fully functioning, whole being as experienced during physical activity. This meaning of exercise is difficult to explain, but it is mentioned in diverse readings (e.g., Douillard, 1994; Leonard & Murphy, 1995). In a book guiding people in the realization of integrating body, mind, heart, and soul, George Leonard and Michael Murphy (1995) explore ways to unify and honor these components within ourselves. Emphasizing personal transformation as the "ultimate adventure," Leonard and Murphy report,

> Today another process is underway throughout much of the world, a grassroots understanding that *spirit* and *body* are joined, that *mind* can somehow influence matter, that lives can radically change, that the further evolution of humankind is possible. The evidence of this process is all around us, in books that come out of nowhere to top the national bestseller lists, in polls on spiritual matters, in sometimes sensational images in the popular media of angels among us, of contacts with alien civilizations. (p. 195)

Leonard and Murphy have been writing thought-provoking books about exercise for the past 25 years. Leonard, a writer who coined the phrase *human potential* in the early 1960s (Leonard & Murphy, 1995), has written a variety of books that focus on the exercise experience. These books include *The Ultimate Athlete: Re-visioning Sports, Physical Education, and the Body* (1975), and *Walking on the Edge of the World* (1988). Murphy is a cofounder of the Esalen Institute, a center for the development of human potential. Murphy has written numerous books on exercise, including *Golf in the Kingdom* (1972), *The Future of the Body: Explorations into the Further Evolution of Human Nature* (1992), and *In the Zone: Transcendent Experience in Sports* (with White; 1995). Together, Leonard and Murphy (1995) wrote a workbook for integral transformative practice (ITP) entitled *The Life We Are Given: A Long-Term Program for Realizing the Potential of Body, Mind, Heart, and Soul.* This book reflects their lifetime quest to assist people in tapping their potential to learn, love, feel deeply, and create. The ITP program assists participants in transforming their lives through long-term commitment and through balanced, comprehensive practice of integrating spiritual, psychological, social, nutritional, and body techniques in already busy lives.

An underlying premise in *The Life We Are Given* is that human growth and personal transformation occur from practices that incorporate the whole person. The ITP program depicted in Table 14.5 includes the seven components listed. Several of these can be accomplished through exercise: plans or affirmations, integral transformation practice Kata, aerobic exercise, the body as a teacher, nutrition, and the social sense of community. Leonard and Murphy

(1995) recognize in their program that exercise can help human beings grow beyond our customary daily levels of functioning. Supporting the importance of freedom in movement, the ITP approach is *not* to view movement as a mechanical process that yields specific benefits but

> . . . as a fundamental expression of our embodiment, essential to our practice precisely because it is valuable *for its own sake* . . . But the real juice of life is to be found not so much in the products of our efforts as in the process of living itself in how it feels to be alive. (Leonard & Murphy, 1995, p. 117)

We can try to use exercise to circumvent our censorship of ourselves and to facilitate awareness of additional parts of ourselves that are not readily available to our consciousness. Transformative movement is effective because body and mind are integrated (Csikszentmihalyi, 1997a; Fahlberg & Fahlberg, 1997; Leonard & Murphy, 1995). When exercise is used for transformative purposes, there is no focus on performance or quality of movement. There is no right or wrong way to move. According to May (1974), "we learn that technique can be used as an intellectualizing defense against understanding of the self" (p. xi). Emphasis on exercise performance or skill can be absolutely detrimental to transformation (May). One possible way to address this issue "is to affirm to yourself: 'I am moving for myself, for my own pleasure. This is a gift to me!' When you understand this, there is no pressure to do it right to please the instructor or even your own inner critic" (Bonheim, 1992, p. 26).

Additional Meanings Within Exercise

Thus far, we have highlighted some of the common personal meanings within exercise. Undoubtedly, you can suggest other meanings. To broaden the scope of movement and its meanings, additional meanings are briefly identified in this section. Some of the meanings are interrelated and augment those elements that already have been discussed. The interrelationships and agreement among the various meanings reinforce the likelihood that they are experienced by multiple exercise participants.

Table 14.5
Integral Transformative Practice (ITP); Leonard & Murphy, 1995

Component	Description
Plans or Affirmations	• Changes that are in the realms of normal means such as the following: taking two inches off a waistline, exceptional achievements, meta-normal accomplishments, and overall good health. • Good health reflected by the affirmation, "My entire being is balanced, vital, and healthy" (Leonard & Murphy, 1995, p. 22).
Integral Transformative Practice (ITP) Kata	• 40 minutes of specified exercises: warm-ups, balances, stretches, deep and rhythmic breathing, progressive relaxation, transformational imaging and meditation.
Aerobic Exercise	• Minimum of 2 hours of aerobic exercise weekly—any type of exercise the participant chooses. • Sessions of at least 30 minutes each. • Three sessions of strength training recommended each week.
The Body as Teacher	• The body can show us how to live a balanced, natural life and can be a key teacher of human evolution.
Nutrition	• Consciously eating food for transformation: eating wisely; eating less; eating foods low in fat and high in fiber, • Instead of counting calories, eat fruits, vegetables, beans, and legumes.
Community	• The magic of community emphasizes oneness with others in a tightly knit group working and playing together.

Absorption in the Moment

Exercise gives us an opportunity to be totally in the here and now. We can be totally absorbed in the movement pattern, the immediate environment (nature, music, friends), regulation of our exertion, and just the use of our bodies. This meaning is closely associated with peak moments and being in the zone.

Meditation

Meditation emphasizes mind-body interactions. When we engage in meditation, we repeat a word or sound. When intrusive thoughts appear, they are passively disregarded, and there are specific bodily responses that are healthful. These responses include decreased metabolism, rate of breathing, and heart rate as well as distinctive slower brain waves. Many exercisers, particularly runners, have reported that exercising is a time for meditation. This may reflect the time for quiet that running affords and its repetitive motion. Each foot strike may be comparable to saying a mantra over and over. Solomon and Bumpus (1981) have suggested that the altered states of consciousness experienced by some exercisers are similar to the psychological changes reported in studies of those engaged in transcendental meditation. Meditating while exercising continues to be seen as a valuable approach to using exercise for personal transformation as suggested by Bonheim (1992) in *The Serpent and the Wave: A Guide to Movement Meditation.*

Moving for the Sake of Moving

Another meaning of movement is the opportunity it presents to be fully functioning physical beings. We have bodies. Perhaps as a result of relatedness to our evolutionary past and subsequent movement up the phylogenetic scale, we need to use our bodies even though we have no need to flee or catch prey (Fixx, 1977). Physical activity needs no justification for meaning. It just "is." The following quotation by Fahlberg and Fahlberg (1997) illustrates the experience of just "being" while exercising:

> Unlike socially conditioned behavior, the authentic being is constituted by intrinsic meaning. People at the existential level realize that they are worthy simply because they exist, rather than because they produce or conform to whatever it is that society happens to value at the time. For example, when we engage in movement for the sake of movement, not to achieve a socially dictated goal, its intrinsic value emerges. (p. 82)

Peak Moments

Peak moments create very special meanings in exercise and are temporary experiences of transcendence as described in Chapters 3 and 15. Peak experiences, flow, peak performances, and the exercise high are profound and life enhancing. They improve the overall quality of our lives. Peak moments are highly memorable, and contribute greatly to the meaning of exercise. These moments include

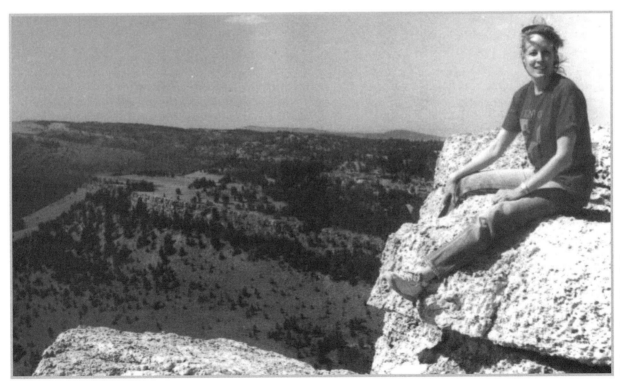

Photo courtesy of Bonnie Berger

- Total absorption and the centering of attention in the exercise,
- Loss of concern about performance and surroundings,
- Feelings of ecstasy and euphoria,
- A sense of power,
- Altered perceptions of time, and
- A sense of body-mind-heart-spirit unity (Berger & Motl, 2001; Csikszentmihalyi, 1997b).

Peak moments are very difficult to capture with words, yet many exercisers have reported experiencing them (Nelson, 2004). In his reflective essay, Steve Nelson attempts to describe the runner's high. As he describes it,

> The runner's high is an act of remembrance. And forgetting. It's a matter of opening up. And closing down. It's everything and nothing at once, the rapture of motion and falling mindlessly back into nature. (Nelson, 2004, p. 53)

Nelson continues to describe the peak moment of the runner's high by comparing his experiences when walking and running and the importance of his mind being free to wander.

> Why is it that the idea of a walk around the neighborhood bores me, while the notion of a run over the same streets enchants? If we can answer this, we're on our way to understanding the runner's high, or the runner's mind at least. A walk, you see, is easy, and though your mind is free to wander, the problem is that it doesn't wander far enough. We control the wandering, and it never gets too far. A run, on the other hand, requires concentration, and in an experienced runner the mind and body learn to work together, with a concentration that becomes second nature, and allows one's mind to wander in a different way, forgetting the thoughts at the top of the mind and going deeper, toward a more essential version of the self.
>
> The only thing I know for sure about the runner's high is that I can't describe it. (Nelson, 2004, pp. 53–54)

Persistence and a Sense of Continuity

By doing something over and over on a regular basis, we become better at what we are doing. Knowing that we will manage to exercise each day, no matter what happens to our schedule, provides us with a sense of continuity, predictability, and habitual return to the familiar. With exercise, we learn that the movements and physical exertion will become easier week by week, year by year. The Nike slogan "Just do it" captures this focus on the importance of persistence and continuity in an unpredictable world.

Strength and Endurance: Physical and Psychological

This meaning of exercise refers to a hard-to-describe personal experience. Building physical strength and endurance through any type of exercise can transform itself into a feeling of psychological strength and endurance that carry over to other aspects of life. Feelings of psychological strength may result from increased physical endurance and vigor, seeing positive results from our perseverance, and feelings of self-efficacy. Habitual exercise seems to result in a quiet, internalized feeling: "I can do it. I am a strong and capable person." More simply, strength is the feeling "I can!" Endurance is the feeling that one can complete an activity—a feeling that "I can persist" through to the completion of this activity.

Summary

Exercise has so many meanings, both positive and negative, that it is impossible to capture them all. Many of the meanings within the exercise experience are not necessarily independent of one another. They are interrelated and interdependent. Separately or in combination, the meanings of exercise can make our lives more fulfilling. Exercise has the potential to foster unity of body, mind, heart, and spirit. As noted by Martin Seligman (2002; Peterson & Seligman, 2004), former president of the American Psychological Association, there is a set of human strengths that serve as buffers against mental illness and that enhance our overall quality of life.

Exercise provides opportunities for participants to test and develop their perseverance, optimism, hope, and courage. These desirable psychological characteristics and others can be important factors in the exercise experience. They are related not only to mental illness but also to health, well-being, personal development, and creating personally fulfilling, productive, and meaningful lives.

Given all that we are learning about the *mind-body* relationship and the effects of behavior and mental well-being on the body, it is surprising that more is not known about the *body-mind* relationship. Exercise enables us to strengthen our bodies, increase our physical endurance, and create a reservoir of energy. The meanings of movement explored in this chapter include fun and enjoyment, self-exploration, freedom, health, self-reflection, time alone, empowerment, communing with nature, delay of the aging process, postponement of death, spirituality, meditation, movement for the sake of moving, peak moments, persistence, and strength.

Exercise has transformational powers by enabling participants to reach more of their potential with the integration of body, mind, heart, and spirit. As DeSensi (1996) aptly captured in the Fifth Delphine

Hanna Interdisciplinary Lecture sponsored by the American Alliance for Health, Physical Education, Recreation, and Dance, virtue, knowledge, and wisdom are personal meanings of movement:

> The meaning of movement is found certainly in reflection, but meaning is also available in the immediate present. Both reflective thinking and immediate experience are important. The analysis within reflection creates an objective means by which we create meaning, after the fact. But the meaning of movement experiences in the context of the present is as valuable and authentically subjective and valid . . . (p. 529)

> I do wish sometimes, though, that my unique meanings and experiences weren't so ineffable so that I could share them with others and have them know and feel what meaning I experienced. But that is *my* unique experience. So this is the body I am and that is the body you are—this is each of us, unique, alive, moving, learning, experiencing, knowing, and understanding meanings of movement. Let us celebrate it. (p. 529)

Can You Define These Terms?

athletic identity

body-mind integration

communing with nature

delaying the aging process

empowerment

freedom

freedom in exercise settings

freedom to not exercise

fun and enjoyment

health

immortality projects

integration of body, mind, heart, and spirit

paradoxical effects of exercise

paradoxical meanings in exercise

peak moments

personal transformation

qualitative research

religion

search for spirituality

self-exploration

transformation

utilitarian foci in exercise and physical activity

Can You Answer These Questions?

1. Is the whole of exercise larger than the sum of its parts? Explain the bases for your response.

2. How might the use of critical pedagogy change procedures for teaching physical education in schools?

3. What kinds of questions are best investigated by qualitative and quantitative research approaches? Give an example or question for each type of research investigation.

4. How and why do the meanings of exercise differ within specific cultural groups?

5. Why is it likely that the meanings of exercise differ in African Americans and Americans of Anglo-Saxon descent?

6. How would you identify and illustrate specific meanings of exercise to competitive athletes?

7. Can you give personal examples of paradoxical meanings in exercise; that is, how exercise can liberate or oppress, and also inspire or disillusion?

8. How might ethnicity, culture, and social class influence the meanings of physical activity?

9. How do exercise prescriptions reduce the element of freedom in exercise settings?

10. Do you think that the meanings of exercise may differ in diverse physical activities such as swimming, jogging, rock climbing, and squash? Explain your response.

11. What were the meanings of exercise you experienced when you were in elementary school or in high school?

12. Can you provide insights into the meanings of exercise for several different members of your family?

13. What is your personal concept of health? Do you think that Jim, as described in the chapter, is healthy?

14. Have you personally been aware of body-mind integration during any of your exercise sessions? If so, describe your experiences.

15. What aspects of your exercise sessions create fun and enjoyment?

CHAPTER 15

Peak Moments in Exercise

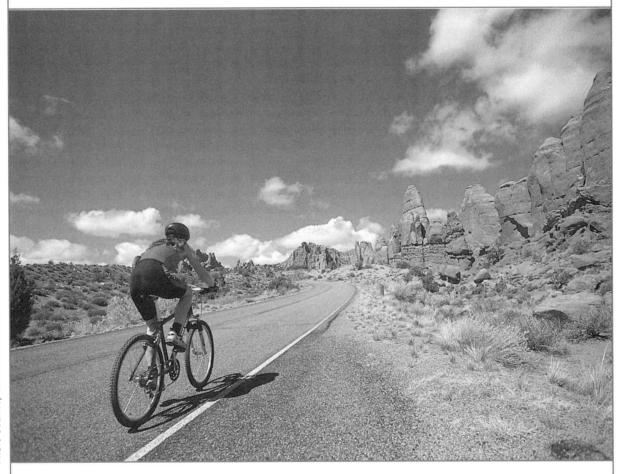

After reading this chapter, you should be able to

- Define and distinguish among three types of peak moments in exercise: peak experience, peak performance, and flow;

- Discuss a specific type of peak moment, the runner's high, and the required conditions for its occurrence;

- Explain ways by which peak moments may be facilitated; and

- Contrast the cognitive strategies known as association and dissociation as they relate to exercise.

Introduction and Definition of Terms

"Would anyone like to join me for a walk?"

"Yeah. I'll go. How far do you want to walk?"

"I'm not sure—let's just go and see how we feel. We'll take it easy and stop when we're tired. We'll play it by ear, but we have to be back in an hour for dinner. We don't want to hold everyone up."

"I'm leaving now for my power walk. I want to see if I can cut at least 30 seconds off my best time for three miles. I'm really going to bust it—hit it as hard as I can. If things go well I'll see you in about 27 minutes. Bye."

Each of us experiences exercise in different ways. In fact, the intensity, duration, and goals of our exercise are likely to vary though we may be engaged in the very same activity. As noted in Chapter 12, even motives for exercising are person-specific. Some of us exercise because we have been instructed to do so by a physician, coach, or physical therapist. Others exercise because the experience provides fun or enjoyment, as discussed in Chapter 14. Perceptions about the value of our exercise—its enjoyability and memorability—are related to our view of its meaningfulness, which, in turn, depends on our personal needs, interests, philosophy and attitude about life in general and health in particular. For some of us at certain times, physical activity assumes an unusual significance. Its

---

Table 15.1
Components of the Mindset During Flow: What's Happening Mentally During Flow

1. **Challenge-skills balance:** The exerciser is able to meet the challenge, and the challenge is formidable. She must extend herself to satisfy the task's requirements.

2. **Action-awareness merging:** An effortless fusion of mind and body occurs. The exerciser feels at one with his movements. If the exerciser is using skis, a bicycle, an oar, or any other equipment, there is the feeling of being part of it—being at one with the machinery or device. A fluidity and automaticity of action occur that meld with mental processes.

3. **Clear goals:** Goals clarify the behavior necessary to satisfy a task. When attentional focus is sharpened, there is reduced opportunity for distraction. A fully focused exerciser is confident of every step/move. She knows exactly what to do—what comes next.

4. **Unambiguous feedback:** Information about the movement's correctness or accuracy must somehow reach the exerciser. He must *know* that his goals are being met and that he indeed has what it takes to meet the challenge; that is, "I'm doing it." This information may come from internal or external sources, but it must be clear, definite, and immediate.

5. **Concentration on the task at hand:** During flow, no extraneous thoughts are present. Only what is presently being done is narrowly focused upon. Concentration is extended throughout the activity's duration.

6. **Sense of control:** A feeling of invincibility prevails. The specter of failure—of not completing the exercise or of slipping or falling—is totally absent. "Nothing can go wrong."

7. **Loss of self-consciousness:** There is no worrying about oneself. The exerciser does not think about or concentrate on himself. Therefore, issues that may inhibit performance such as self-doubt or worry that "I'll fall or crash" are excluded from thought. The question of "How am I doing?" never emerges, nor does concern about how others in the environment may see the exerciser.

8. **Transformation of time:** Time speeds up or slows down. This is exemplified in Case Study 15.1, which portrays the perceptions of Doug, the baseball batter, who claimed, "It was like everything was in slow motion." For Doug, the pitch came in slow motion. Sometimes the feeling persists that time moves forward with incredible speed. An experience that actually took place during the course of an hour appears to be complete in merely a few moments. In other words, during flow, the physical activity is timeless.

9. **Autotelic experience:** Jackson and Csikszentmihalyi (1999) refer to this dimension as the final or culminating experience of flow—"the result of the other eight components" (p. 30). The interpretation of the activity is "just a wonderful event"—"a real rush, something fabulous."

Adapted from *Flow in Sports: The Keys to Optimal Experiences and Performances* (pp. 16–31), by S. Jackson and M. Csikszentmihalyi, 1999, Champaign, IL: Human Kinetics. Copyright 1999. Adapted with permission.

quality is extraordinary, strange—even surreal. With reference to the quality of our exercise experience, three terms are currently in vogue: flow, peak experience, and peak performance. All three are used loosely to refer to special, sensational, enormously gratifying, and, in some cases, bizarre or extraordinary events involving physical activity. At least, these events are perceived as such by the individual experiencing them.

Jackson and Csikszentmihalyi (1999), two scholars who have written extensively about these phenomena, represent *flow* as an element of *peak experience* and *peak performance*. That is, flow is typically present when these unusual happenings and achievements take place, although they are more likely to occur during work rather than leisure endeavors (Csikszentmihalyi & LeFevre, 1984). However, Jackson and Csikszentmihalyi direct most of their analyses and discussion of flow to high-level sport behavior. But it is clear from their writing that casual participants in games, sport-like activities, and exercise also experience flow. Jackson and Csikszentmihalyi believe that "because flow is so enjoyable, we tend to seek out situations where we can experience it. This necessarily involves developing skills and taking on increasingly greater challenges" (p. 13). What exactly is flow and how is it different from peak experience and peak performance?

Flow

Flow, as described by Csikszentmihalyi (1975b, 1997b), is associated with play and similar pleasurable conditions. Flow equates with enjoyment, and people therefore participate in certain activities because they are fun or intrinsically rewarding. But flow is not just fun—it's a state of total involvement in an activity that requires complete concentration (Csikszentmihalyi, 1999).

Flow may be encountered at different levels. Listening to a humorous story may not produce ecstasy, whereas achieving something challenging will generate a much higher degree of flow. Flow situations involve challenges that are compatible with an individual's skill levels and frequently occur in games and play. However, the challenge must be substantial, but not overwhelming. The skier who descends a difficult trail in full command may experience flow. The rock climber who scales a formidable face under remarkably clear and sunny skies may also report it. But Csikszentmihalyi cautions that you can't make flow happen. All you can do is learn to remove obstacles in its way.

Beginners in exercise or sport are not likely to get a sense of flow because the activity may be too demanding and therefore cause anxiety. And because of their assumed low level of fitness or skill they are not good candidates. Their thoughts tend to be focused on the demands of the activity rather than on stimuli conducive to flow. In order for flow to occur, self-consciousness

---

CASE STUDY 15.1

A Baseball Player Describes His Experience With Flow

Doug Mientkiewicz, a former Florida State University baseball star, played for the United States team at the 2000 Olympic Games in Sydney, Australia. Team USA won its first three games to stay in the winner's bracket and then came up against one of the strongest teams in the tournament, Korea. At the bottom of the eighth inning, with bases loaded, Mientkiewicz came to the plate to face a reputedly hard-throwing relief pitcher by the name of Pil-Jung Jin. Mientkiewicz recalls, "I was like, 'Wow.' But I was seeing the ball really well and all five pitches (the count went to 3 balls, 2 strikes) could have been strikes. Suddenly, everything became so clear it was spooky. It was like everything was in slow motion." Doug swung and drove the ball into the stands. The grand slam did it and Team USA won the game 4–0. Seven days later they beat Cuba by the same score and won an unprecedented gold medal for the United States.

---

must be eradicated. In other words, beginners, because of their insecurity about satisfying basic physical requirements of the activity, are not eligible for flow.

Table 15.1 lists nine fundamental dimensions of flow, as identified by Jackson and Csikszentmihalyi (1999). Notice how these dimensions emphasize freedom from awareness of self, the absence of evaluation of the performance, and feeling of exclusive involvement with the activity to the exclusion of everything else. Those who have experienced this mindset sometimes use some of the following expressions by way of referring to it: "in the zone," "in the groove," "in the bubble," "focused," and "everything clicks."

A measure of flow in sport and physical exercise settings has been constructed by Jackson and Marsh (1996). The Flow State Scale (FSS) has 36 items and 9 scales (4 items in each scale) and these are shown in Table 15.1.

In addition to *flow*, two other terms deserve attention in our discussion, namely, *peak experience* and *peak performance*. A clarification of the differences among these three experiences follows.

Peak Experience

A peak experience is intense in that it requires considerable effort and high levels of concentration. Involvement of others in the exercise may inhibit occurrence of the peak experience because the required narrowed and acute attentional focus may be disrupted. Therefore, cyclists riding in a pack, or "lunch bunch" swimmers getting in their laps in a crowded lane are not good candidates for peak experiences. But skydivers floating along above land (Privette & Bundrick, 1991) and English Channel swimmers virtually isolated in an aquatic environment are. A peak experience is also positive; that is, the participant views its consequences as beneficial, including high levels of happiness (Laski, 1962; Maslow, 1962, 1970, 1971). Peak experiences are perceived by persons to be among the most thrilling, exciting, and fulfilling events in their lives. Such experiences involve deep immersion in an activity that holds substantial value and appropriateness to life. However, award-winning or record-setting achievements are not necessarily involved. Maslow (1970) used this term to refer to moments of *self-actualization*, when individuals have attained complete satisfaction of lower-level physiological and social needs. When all is well and beautiful and basic needs have been met, the individual is "self-actualized" and encounters the extremely gratifying peak experience. Such experiences, according to Maslow, are unique, involuntary, and of brief duration. Maslow's insights were innovative and important in that they encourage focus upon and study of self-actualization and similar events as measurable and explainable physiological phenomena. He has thus relocated human experiences that were previously and exclusively understood only as mystical or religious happenings into the realm of science—notably the science of psychology.

Peak Performance

A second term, *peak performance*, describes an episode of superior functioning (Privette, 1964, 1965, 1968, 1981, 1982; Privette & Landsman, 1983), with an emphasis upon *superior*. It involves an optimal level of achievement by the individual and requires superb focus. Peak performances are typically perceived as unique and are not necessarily accompanied by feelings of enjoyment. Here, the emphasis is upon elements of the behavior such as accuracy, speed, or grace. In the peak performance, the participant perceives these aspects to have been present at unusually high levels. For example, the skier has the "absolutely,

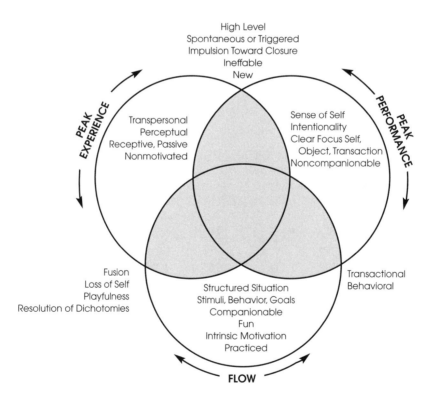

Figure 15.1. A representation of the overlapping elements of the three peak moments. Among components shared by all three are absorption, joy, and valuing. From "Peak experience, peak performance, and flow: A comparative analysis of positive human experiences,": by G. Privette, 1983, *Journal of Personality and Social Psychology*, 45, p. 1366. Reprinted with permission.

positively, best run" of her life—never before has she made her way down any trail with such control, maintenance of rhythm, and perfect form.

Distinguishing among types of peak moments. Exercise provides an excellent opportunity for any or all of the aforementioned experiences. Moreover, peak experience, peak performance, and flow may also account for the motivation to engage in exercise. One may exercise with the hope of achieving these states. Because the terms *peak experience*, *peak performance*, and *flow* are often, but incorrectly, used synonymously, the following clarification, provided by Privette and Bundrick (1991), is helpful:

> Peak experience is intense joy, a moment of highest happiness that stands out perceptually and cognitively among other experiences. Peak performance is superior functioning, releasing latent powers to behave effectively in athletic prowess, artistic expression, intellectual endeavors, interpersonal relationships, moral courage, or any activity. Flow is an intrinsically rewarding experience chosen for its own sake and often, but not necessarily, characterized by optimal performance or feeling responses. These events share many qualities: absorption, joy, spontaneity, a sense of power, and personal identity and involvement. (p. 171)

All three are transcendent, uplifting, absorbing, and memorable. Those who have experienced them delight in offering personal accounts of their occurrence, and typically express an eagerness to replicate them. Unfortunately, this is not easy to accomplish at will. What we can do, however, is attempt improvement of personal exercise-related or movement skills to the extent that future challenges are well within our range of competence. When compatibility exists between situational demands and task requirements and the degrees of preparedness to meet them, flow and peak achievements are most likely to occur. When we are secure in our assessment that the job before us is well within our ability, we are free to experience flow and peak experiences. Physical activity is a fertile opportunity for all three.

Additionally, as Privette (1983) suggests, peak experience and peak performance represent optimal levels of an experience, and both are subjective. In the peak experience, an individual encounters exceptionally high levels of happiness and fulfillment (Maslow, 1962) and unusually high levels of intensity and richness (Leach, 1963). The peak experience stands out from other experiences because it is meaningful or significant. It may also refer to a category of activities. An example of a peak experience might be figure skating, which provides a good deal of pleasure for participants. Merely lacing up one's skates, gliding out onto the ice, and spending a recreational hour in this playful

activity provides enormous gratification. But peak performance is different in that it refers to a singular event or behavior that an individual recognizes as unique because of its exceptionally high level of function. Peak performance therefore involves achievement of one's full potential. The competitive figure skater has had a peak performance when he flawlessly executes his routine— something he has never done before. When you are in the midst of a peak performance, you are completely focused and have a very clear insight into the process you are experiencing. There is also a sense of power and correctness of action, almost a feeling of invincibility. However, enjoyment is not necessarily a part of peak performance. A peak experience, on the other hand, may be a rare happening in your life and thus be noteworthy, or it may occur often or continuously (Privette, 1983). But it does not involve optimal or superior behavior.

Researching peak moments. Peak moments in exercise have not been studied as much as those in sport. However, McInman and Grove's (1991) review of the research literature relative to such experiences in sport does provide a basis for understanding these phenomena in the context of exercise. Among the pertinent issues they raise are:

1. What are the optimal conditions for facilitating peak experience, peak performance, and flow?
2. How can opportunities for the generation of these three be optimized?

Although these questions are appropriate and important, definitive answers are not yet available. To this end, factors that may facilitate peak moments in both sport and exercise are discussed in sections of this chapter that follow.

Exercisers and athletes may experience peak moments (peak experience, peak performance, and flow) more frequently than they report. Some individuals may have difficulty in articulating or conceptualizing the peak moment; that is, they may have trouble talking about or describing the experience (Murphy, 1977; Panzarella, 1980). Perhaps, as McInman and Grove (1991) suggest, the ambiguity concerning the frequency with which peak moments are reported has to do with the kinds of questions asked by researchers. Thus, tighter, more objectively conceived, and more standardized questions asked of exercisers and athletes might yield higher incidences of peak moments. Wuthnow (1978) has expressed the feeling that very large numbers of people have had such experiences.

An attempt to provide a series of structured questions that would generate information about situational factors preceding the peak moment has been made by Privette (1984). Privette's Experience Questionnaire (1984) provides 42 items to which subjects respond in accordance with a five-point Likert scale, enabling them to express an event's importance. Their answers are made relative to a personal incident that they are asked to recall about peak experience, peak performance, flow, failure, or an average event. Nine additional items probe circumstances occurring immediately prior to the target event.

Despite efforts to describe conditions that may precipitate peak moments, these experiences tend to occur spontaneously and thus are difficult to predict. Even an absolutely perfect performance may not result in the perception of a peak moment. Many exercisers cannot relate to *peak moments* on a personal experiential level. Despite years and years of swimming, jogging, cycling, skating, skiing, etc., they have yet to experience a peak moment. It does not happen to everyone.

A Specific Type of Peak Moment: The Runner's High

To be "high" is to be exultant—to suddenly have a realization of enormous power, ability, comfort, and control. When you are high, you are excited and "perfect," as is everything around you. You are in total harmony with the environment and all of its parts. Your sense of well-being is so profound and complete that you are euphoric. For some persons, being high involves "spinning out" or altering consciousness. In this state, your sensitivities to surrounding stimuli—awareness of what's going on around you—become altered. Common objects may suddenly be interpreted in strange ways, and insights occur that are so new and different that they may appear to be bizarre.

The material in Case Study 15.2, "An Account of the Runner's High," depicts perceptions about a 15-kilometer run of a most unusual nature. The "high" runner reports indefatigability and a conviction that he could run 100 miles with comfort. In a fascinating account of the psychology of long-distance runners, William P. Morgan (1978) exemplifies peculiar insights of runners while experiencing the "high." One runner felt that he was hovering above his body during the run and able to look down upon himself. Another became convinced that he could run through an oncoming truck and emerge unscathed from its other end. Obviously such remarkable perceptions during a run are potentially hazardous, to say the least. They may account for attitudes and behaviors that fly in the face of reality. If you truly believe you are capable of running through a truck, you are at risk.

Various synthetic chemicals and plant derivatives (e.g., opiates) have been known for centuries to produce many of the above effects. However, can physical exercise such as running cause alteration of consciousness? Is there such a thing as the runner's high, and if so, under what specific conditions may it be experienced? We now turn to these questions with a particular emphasis upon running, for there is some evidence that it is in this form of exercise that these phenomena actually occur.

Production of the Runner's High

In an effort to explain causality (in contrast to antecedents or conditions for the high), Pargman and Baker (1980) speculated that certain chemicals secreted by the body itself (endogenous products), for example, enkephalins and beta-endorphins, may be responsible for altering consciousness. These substances have been shown to be present in the blood in increased amounts during and after sustained, rhythmic, rigorous exercise such as running (Farrell, 1985; Steinberg & Sykes, 1985). Both chemicals are very close in molecular structure to opium derivatives (juice of the opium poppy), which have, for centuries, been known to produce mind-altering effects (Hughes et al., 1975; Viveros, Diliberto, Hazum, & Chang, 1979). Although the exact physiological roles of enkephalins and beta-endorphins are still unclear, these endogenous substances somehow produce an analgesic state (insensitivity to pain) and reduce responsiveness to external stimuli (Kirkcaldy & Shephard, 1990). They have also been shown to be responsible for other biochemical chains during or after exercise that may ultimately result in less fatigue and easier or more comfortable exercise (Grossman & Sutton, 1985), thus enabling the runner to experience the high. As Riggs (1981) concluded years ago, "Whether this describes the state encompassed by the term 'runner's high' is unclear" (p. 226). This absence of clarity still remains today. Additional research is necessary to explain the biochemical bases of this phenomenon, although the state described above is, indeed, attainable (Hawkes, 1992).

Conditions for Experiencing the Runner's High

The runner's high was described more than 25 years ago as an exercise-induced altered state of consciousness (Pargman & Baker, 1980). More recently, Arne Dietrich (2003) has proposed that this unusual experience may be due to *transient prefrontal deregulation*. Dietrich's hypothesis appears to be as attractive (and testable) as any others currently available and may eventually prove to be the most sustainable. In effect, he suggests that because activation of the frontal lobe of the brain's cortex is reduced or deregulated during exercise, high cognitive functions ascribed to this location are reduced. Exercise is indeed associated with increased activation of certain brain parts; notably, those affiliated with motor and several of the sensory systems. But this deregulation occurs at the expense of stimulation of the prefrontal lobes of the cortex, which are apparently not required for running (but needed for other exercise forms). Many of the alleged phenomena reported as part of the runner's high are, according to Deitrich, "consistent with a state of frontal hypofunction" (p. 10). Among these are the phenomena reported by Sachs (1980), such as time-lessness, living in the here and now, reduced awareness of one's surroundings, and diminished attentional capacities. Less prefrontal cortex function is required during an activity such as endurance running than, for example, basketball or chess. This frontal hypofunction may be the answer to the so-called "high" claimed by some runners.

Michael Sachs (1997) has tried to describe the conditions required for the "high" state. He maintains that they are twofold: (a) the quality of the run itself and (b) the physical environment.

Quality of the run. The run during which the high is usually experienced is gentle, rather than intense or painful. The participant must let go of the run and not be focused upon its distance or time. The runner should be able to run comfortably for 5 to 10 miles if the high is to occur. Another factor often reported in the Sachs (1997) interviews is the runner's perception of an absence of personal problems and little anxiety about day-to-day affairs. Participants who dwell on anxieties and problematic situations are therefore not good candidates for experiencing the runner's high.

Environmental and climatic conditions. A number of runners who have experienced the high indicated that certain environmental factors were precursors. Among these are cool, calm weather, low humidity, absence of hills, and running in familiar areas with few distractions such as traffic and bumps in the road. However, one observation surfaced repeatedly; that is, even in the above conditions, there is by far no guarantee that the phenomenon would necessarily occur. The high is evidently unpredictable and not available to all runners. One of the authors of this book has been running for more than 40 years, and, to date, has not experienced consciousness alteration during a run.

Research on the Runner's High

A good deal of what is known about the runner's high derives from interviews with runners. Sachs and colleagues (Sachs, 1980; Sachs & Buffone, 1984; Sacks & Sachs, 1981) were among the first to study the runner's high, and much of what is known about it results from their work. Sachs (1980) interviewed 60 runners and found that 77% of them had experienced the high. On

CASE STUDY 15.2 *An Account of the Runner's High*

I sat on the locker-room bench, elbows on my knees, watching the perspiration drop from the tip of my nose and puddle on the tiled floor. My drenched shorts clung to my thighs, and my toes itched in my damp socks. The trail I had run was too tough. The hills were formidable, and the loosely packed sand had battered my calves. The eight miles had consumed a large measure of my energy, and I was spent . . . exhausted. I sat and breathed heavily trying to recover—postponing for a few moments the challenge of untying my laces, removing wet socks and shorts, and making my way to the shower. The last mile and a half had been particularly difficult; I'd even contemplated walking. Disgraceful . . . even to think about. So, I sat, sweated, and sighed.

Then, this guy walked in. I'd seen him before and, on one or two occasions, had been in a group run with him. A tall, skinny guy, he seemed uplifted, somehow relaxed. He was smiling as he began to speak, and the smile never left him as he delivered his bizarre accounting:

"Man, I've just run the most incredible 15K ever. I didn't want to stop. I could have gone forever. I never felt so strong . . . so powerful. It's as if I was floating without effort . . . without pain. My body seemed to separate from me and my mind . . . as if my legs were churning without me. I felt as though my body was in perfect synch with whatever the trail was demanding. The hills meant nothing. I didn't seem to be aware of them. All I could think of was the energy at my command and that my pumping knees and arms were unstoppable pistons that would move me surely and easily through any kind of obstacle or terrain. No challenge would be insurmountable. I felt myself to be some sort of uncanny, unstoppable machine, surging and pumping rhythmically and ceaselessly. I was in some kind of high . . . some sort of unreal spinout. I could have gone 100 miles without stopping. The 15K was like a half-mile warm-up jog. The run was fun . . . just a beautiful experience. I was the wind, a giant wave, rolling and rolling over anything and everything."

I looked at this guy. Ah . . . Would something like this ever happen to me?

the other hand, Weinberg (1980) reported that only 9% of his sample of runners had ever experienced this state. Sachs (1997) concludes that "the runner's high does exist, though not everyone experiences it" (pp. 280–281). Perhaps variables such as age, gender, number of years of regular running, and level of attained running fitness determine the existence or absence of the high. In addition, care must be given when establishing an operational definition of the runner's high so that those being queried are all contemplating the same phenomenon. When the term *runner's high* is employed, simply "feeling good" or "having a pleasant run" is not of essence. It may be that the term has not been standardized adequately and therefore has been presented to subjects in ways that vary from study to study. This may account for distorted results from surveys that have attempted to investigate the evidence of the high.

Facilitation of Peak Moments in Exercise

Can exercisers be taught to experience peak moments? Can flow be facilitated? Not very much is available in the research literature that addresses these questions. However, Gallwey (1982) has suggested that essential to these experiences is avoidance of conscious thinking about them. McInman and Grove (1991) put it this way: "While centering your attention, you should not be trying harder to concentrate. As soon as you begin a struggle to concentrate, you lose the ability to flow" (p. 347). From the few studies that have been published, it appears that the exerciser/athlete should center attention on a narrowed attentional field—on the important elements of the task—in order to optimize performance and achieve a peak moment as a byproduct. In other words, it's not a good idea to raise questions about the quality of your exercise or to think about whether or not you are experiencing a peak moment.

Peak moments—be they peak experiences, peak performances, or flow—involve the focus of attention, or cognitive control or directionality. That is, for peak moments to occur, participants should strive to disengage cognitively from their exercise. In particular, they should subdue perceptions of discomfort or pain. How may this be accomplished? What follows is a brief discussion of some cognitive strategies employed by exercisers in search of peak moments.

Cognitive Strategies: Association and Dissociation

When done at high levels of intensity or for long periods, exercise may cause pain or discomfort. Indeed, this is often the case. To alleviate such consequences, exercisers often resort to mental strategies such as *association* and *dissociation* (Morgan & Pollack,

1977). Association emphasizes monitoring one's feelings or inner conditions during participation whereas dissociation uses distracting techniques that are intended to take the mind off the activity. During running, for example, is it best to think about task-related phenomena such as tightness in the legs, heaviness of breathing, and running pace (the answer is no, if a peak experience is desired); or, would using dissociation techniques such as thinking about the environment, work, personal problems, and in general, focusing thoughts towards external sensations help the runner to better manage pain and discomfort? Related questions, particularly with regard to competitive runners, concern which of these cognitive strategies yields better performance outcomes and whether beginning runners or exercisers differ from experienced (e.g., better trained, faster) participants in their use of associative or dissociative cognitive strategies. These questions have been the basis of numerous research endeavors.

Researching association and dissociation. Cognitive strategies have been studied in competitive runners wherein mental demands challenge the participant as much as physical demands do (Silva & Applebaum, 1989). There is definitely a mental side to running that contributes importantly to competitive outcomes. However, expert opinion varies as to the most preferred mental strategies, since they may be specific to level of skill (Morgan, 1978; Sachs, 1984a; Schomer, 1986, 1987).

Silva and Applebaum (1989) found that among elite marathon runners (Olympic trial contestants), top finishers employed associative as well as dissociative techniques. That is, at different points in the run, cognitive strategies varied. It seems that lower-level performers employed dissociative strategies much earlier in the run and maintained them, in contrast to the top competitors, who shifted their strategies in accordance with the demands of the race. Morgan and Pollack (1977) reported similar results; that is, more experienced masters track-and-field athletes used associative mental coping strategies more often than did less experienced athletes. Tammen (1996) found that as running pace increased in a sample of elite middle and distance runners, there was a tendency to associate more. This makes sense in that it is probably more difficult to dissociate from the discomfort of exercise when the "going gets tough," and easier when comfort prevails.

Clingman and Hilliard (1990) reported the same tendency in race walkers. A study by Morgan, Horstman, Cymerman, and Stokes (1983) examined cognitive strategies in endurance performance in treadmill running. Two groups of subjects ran to exhaustion on a motor-driven treadmill at 80% of maximal aerobic power (a high level of intensity). Subjects in the first group were assigned a dissociation strategy. Those in the second group comprised the placebo or control group and were permitted to think about whatever they wished. Dissociation group members were able to exercise for a significantly longer period of time before quitting. Apparently, the distraction from sensory discomfort enabled subjects in the experimental group (dissociation) to endure longer.

In another study of undergraduate volunteers from university-sponsored jogging-for-fitness classes, those who used dissociative cognitive strategies showed greater improvement in times over trials for a 1-mile run than did students who reported using more associative strategies (Okwumabua, Meyers, Schleser, & Cooke, 1983). Thus, the performance of novice, noncompetitive runners also seems to benefit from the use of dissociative cognitive strategies. Subjects in this

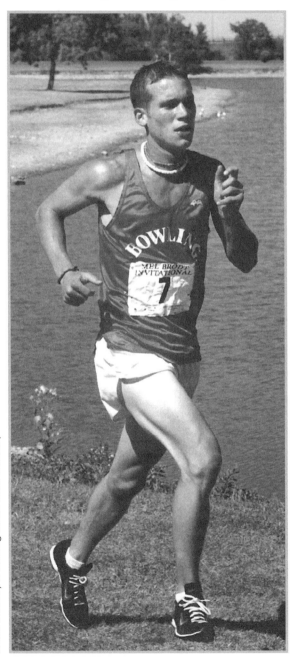

study were not assigned to associative or dissociative strategies but were queried periodically afterwards about the strategy they employed. Over time, while the semester progressed, the runners tended to increasingly use associative strategies. This suggests that as novice runners increase running fitness, they are better able (or prefer) to use associative cognitive strategies.

Similarly, Spink (1988) reported greater endurance on a leg-extension task in subjects receiving a dissociation/analgesic treatment including focus on something unrelated to the task plus the suggestion that they ". . . should feel a dramatic reduction in the amount of discomfort and pain experienced" (p. 101). Subjects in the dissociation-only group endured longer than did those in the control group, but not as long as the dissociation/analgesic group endured.

Unfortunately, cognitive strategy research in relation to the variables of endurance, pain, and discomfort (all considered to be perceptual cognitive phenomena) has been limited to a few exercise forms or sports. It has not incorporated many popular activities such as swimming, skating, and cycling. Pain or discomfort experienced during exercise is known as *performance pain*, in contrast to *injury pain* felt, for example, during injury rehabilitation. Both are capable of causing a variety of physical and emotional reactions. Performance pain may be interpreted as a controllable, short-lived perception that suggests to the exerciser that it is necessary to modify or halt the activity; injury pain is typically understood to be longer lasting, uncontrollable, and linked to negative emotions.

Gauron and Bowers (1984) showed that a cognitive-behavioral pain control technique was effective in managing pain in college athletes participating in a variety of sports; however, the implications for exercisers, per se, are limited. Nonetheless, some conclusions may be drawn from the aforementioned studies that bear upon the use of cognitive strategies during exercise:

1. Cognitive strategies such as dissociation can improve endurance.
2. Cognitive strategies such as dissociation may help manage pain when it is performance pain.
3. In endurance activities such as middle- and long-distance running, higher-level performers tend to use associative strategies. They apparently want information from their bodies, which they use to make decisions about their running mechanics, speed, and effort.

Exercisers who are unsure about whether to use associative or dissociative strategies should experiment with both in order to determine which is most helpful. Research findings typically involve the use of *inferences* that may or may not apply to individuals.

Rituals. Another approach to facilitating the peak moment is the use of rituals. Rituals, in this case, are behaviors or patterns of behaviors typically done knowingly before execution of a skilled movement. Apparently, less conscious effort is applied to irrelevant thoughts and stimuli when the performer is immersed in ritualized behavior (e.g., bouncing the basketball a prescribed number of times before the free throw or bouncing the tennis ball prior to the serve). In other words, distracting thoughts, particularly negative thoughts that emphasize failure or inadequacy, are less likely to emerge during ritualized behavior. Rituals, often referred to with the term *pre-shot behavior*, frequently help provide a comfort zone for the participant wherein positive thoughts are more likely to emerge. Sports with repetitious activity have been found by Csikszentmihalyi (1975b) to generate states of flow. This is also true of sports that provide fast and direct feedback (Furlong, 1976), probably because participants can learn quickly about the quality of their performance. Above all, the feedback must not result in conscious thinking about the activity. So, once again: to experience a peak moment, avoid focusing on the activity's quality. Don't make conscious thoughts to assess your performances.

Failure to Experience Peak Moments

Finally, those with meager exercise or sport experiences are not likely to have peak moments (Csikszentmihalyi, 1975b). Perhaps this is due to their personal resources being insufficient to satisfy task demands. Consequently, levels of anxiety or stress are too high, which results in inhibition of a clear focus, intrinsic motivation (fun), and spontaneity associated with peak moments. If a novice is attending closely to the activity (because he or she is insecure about its execution), the requisite disengagement is not likely to occur, and the peak experience, peak performance, or flow is, thus, inhibited. As Susan Jackson (1995) tells us, physical activity that does not emphasize the following salient factors is not likely to result in the occurrence of flow:

- high degree of preparation, both physical and mental;
- confidence;
- focus;
- how the activity felt and progressed; and
- optimal motivation and arousal level.

However, in a study by Stein, Kimiecik, Daniels, and Jackson (1995), certain hypothesized antecedents of flow in recreational sport participants, such as goals, perceived competence, and confidence, were not observed. Suffice it to say, not everyone who exercises regularly and rigorously is destined to personally have a peak moment.

Future Research Directions

Peak experiences are fascinating. Accounts of consciousness alteration, bizarre insights, and extraordinary achievements in sport are certainly intriguing. But research into such events should be extended to non-sport activities. Much of the work to date has focused upon running, to the exclusion of other activities such as rowing, cycling, and swimming.

Summary

The quality of exercise we experience may influence the intensity and duration of our exercise as well as the degree of motivation to exercise in the future. Exercise experiences perceived to be unsuccessful in some way may be avoided in the future, whereas experiences deemed meaningful and significant will likely be engaged in again. Peak moments such as peak experiences, peak performances, and flow may account for the continuation and enjoyment of exercise.

Peak experiences are associated with exceptionally high levels of happiness and fulfillment (irrespective of performance or outcome); peak performances are moments of superior functioning (irrespective of enjoyment); and flow is experienced during activities that are intrinsically rewarding and therefore enjoyable.

The runner's high is a specific type of peak moment during which the exerciser experiences euphoria and, at times, altered consciousness. Endogenous substances secreted by the body such as enkephalins and beta-endorphins play an important role in the production of the runner's high. When the quality of exercise is comfortable, the environment is familiar and free of distractions, and the weather is calm with low humidity, the runner's high is more likely to occur.

Peak moments may be facilitated through the use of cognitive strategies such as association and dissociation. Association involves recognition and regulation of internal states during exercise, whereas dissociation involves distraction from internal states during activity. Research findings indicate that higher-level performers employ associative strategies frequently, whereas lower-level performers rely upon dissociative techniques. However, when exercisers using dissociative strategies are compared to a control group, the former group is capable of sustaining exercise for longer periods of time than is the control group.

Individuals who perceive their personal resources as insufficient to fulfill the demands of exercise tasks are not likely to experience peak moments. The high levels of stress and anxiety that may accompany these perceptions interfere with their focus, diminish their motivation, and result in the failure to achieve peak experiences, peak performances, or flow.

Can You Define These Terms?

association

cognitive strategies

dissociation

flow

injury pain

peak experience

peak performance

performance pain

pre-shot routine

Can You Answer These Questions?

1. Why might inconsistencies be found in research concerning peak moments?
2. What physiological role does the body play in the production of the proposed phenomenon known as the runner's high?
3. Describe the quality of the run and the environmental and climatic conditions necessary for the occurrence of the runner's high.
4. Provide reasons why the incidence of the runner's high experience may vary across research studies.
5. How do the uses of associative and dissociative strategies contrast among athletes of differing skill level? How can these techniques affect exercise or sport performance?
6. How may rituals help facilitate peak moments?

CHAPTER 16

Exercise Concerns: Eating Disorders, Substance Abuse, and Exercise Dependence

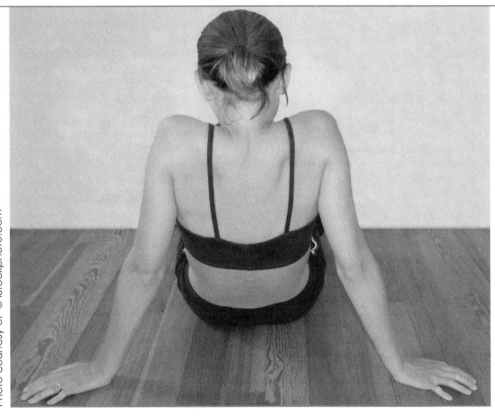

Photo courtesy of © iStockphoto.com

After reading this chapter, you should be able to

- Discuss the prevalence of eating disorders in sport/exercise,
- Explain the predisposing factors for developing eating disorders,
- Understand methods for recognizing disordered eating,
- Discuss the prevalence of substance abuse in sport/exercise,
- List the reasons that exercisers take drugs,
- Explain how to detect and prevent substance abuse,
- Understand methods for recognizing exercise addiction/dependence, and
- Discuss ethical considerations in eating disorders and substance abuse.

Introduction

In 1999, for the first time in 20 years, Willy Voet was not at the Tour de France, cycling's premier race. After Voet was caught transporting recreational and performance-enhancing drugs into France, he admitted that he had been giving drugs to cyclists over the past 20 years, creating quite a controversy in the cycling world. Of course, more recently has been the Bay Area Laboratory Cooperative (BALCO) scandal which has led to a congressional investigation into steroids in baseball. Star players such as Mark McGuire, Barry Bonds and Sammy Sosa (just to name a few) have been implicated in possibly taking steroids and a black cloud hovers over many players. In addition, there have been many anecdotal reports about exercisers and athletes of all ages—especially teenagers—using steroids, wanting to look good, strong, and "buff" for themselves or the opposite sex. University of Maryland basketball star Len Bias did not use steroids. He tried cocaine only once—and died of cocaine-induced heart failure just before embarking on his NBA career. He died not because he was a drug addict but because he decided to celebrate with a recreational drug, as some exercisers might do after reaching some milestone in their exercise program.

Although eating disorders have been found in a number of elite athletes such as ex-tennis player Zina Garrison (who suffered from bulimia, an eating disorder that involves food binges and self-induced vomiting), such disorders have also surfaced in exercisers. For example, one runner, who was a recovering bulimic, reported that during her worst period of self-abuse, she was visiting the bathroom five or six times a day and vomiting simply by flexing her stomach muscles. Of course, disordered eating patterns can be seen in people who are not athletes or regular exercisers. For example, Oprah Winfrey is a great example of a highly visible, high-achieving person who has lost weight, regained it, lost it again, and regained it again, etc., in a very public manner. This "yo-yo" effect of losing and gaining weight is typical of many people who diet off and on and do the same with exercise regimens. Many young people, similarly to those who take steroids, are influenced by societal expectations of the "thin body," and this starts them down the long path of disordered eating.

There is no doubt that although exercise is a healthy habit, it can occasionally have adverse consequences, such as a greater risk for injury (especially in competitive sports). And for certain vulnerable people (especially young women) exercise is associated with specific psychopathologies arising from eating disorders and distortions of body image (Buckworth & Dishman, 2002). Furthermore, a variety of physiological health hazards have been found to be associated with habitual physical activity and/or sport. These hazards include metabolic abnormalities (e.g., hypothermia in swimmers or dehydration in marathon runners), blood disorders (e.g., anemia in endurance athletes), and cardiac problems (e.g., arrhythmia as a result of prolonged vigorous physical activity). This chapter will focus more on the psychological issues related to physical activity and competition.

At first glance (despite some of the above anecdotal examples), the topic of psychopathology is not typically associated with sport and exercise participation. However, a number of case studies have revealed a wide variety of mental disorders in exercise and sport participants. Some of these disorders include clinical depression, panic disorder, schizophrenic disorder, seasonal affective disorder, obsessive-compulsive disorder, bipolar disorder, and Tourette's syndrome (Brewer & Petrie, 2002). Clearly, exercisers and athletes can experience a wide range of psychopathological conditions. For those interested in working with these populations, psychopathological behaviors should at least be considered as possible when certain symptoms are presented, but as noted above, addictive and unhealthy behaviors certainly are not limited to elite athletes. Drugs, steroids, alcohol, and smokeless tobacco are used even by youth who are not sport participants. However, descriptive and other data on these addictive and unhealthy behaviors have tended to be collected on athletes, so this will be highlighted in the data presented in this chapter. Like it or not, physical education, sport, and exercise science professionals must be prepared to deal with these issues. It should be noted that substance abuse, eating disorders, and addictive exercise behaviors are clinical issues requiring treatment by specialists. Still, non-specialists must learn to detect signs of these conditions and refer afflicted exercisers, students, and athletes to specialists for the treatment they need. Let us start with a discussion of eating disorders.

Eating Disorders

Due to the increased prevalence of both anorexia nervosa and bulimia in the general population, as well as the exercise/sport population, both these eating disorders have received more attention in the last 10 years or so. The findings relative to the increase in the obese and overweight throughout the world are consistent (see Chapter 12 for some of these statistics). In the United States alone, approximately 55% of the adult population (approximately 97 million) is now considered overweight (National Heart, Lung, and Blood Institute [NHLBI], 1998). This undoubtedly accounts for the widespread concern in our nation and has spawned considerable interest in weight-loss programs and strategies. Unfortunately, many of the popular diets are unsafe and can lead to disordered eating habits and patterns, but before we discuss some of these diet-related problems in more detail, let us establish clear definitions of these disorders

Anorexia Nervosa

According to the *Diagnostic and Statistical Manual of Mental Disorders*, also known as the DSM IV (American Psychiatric Association, 1994), the diagnostic criteria for *anorexia nervosa* include

- Refusal to maintain a minimal body weight normal for a particular age and height. This is typically defined as weight 15% below that expected.
- Intense fear of gaining weight or becoming fat, even though underweight.
- Disturbance in the way in which one's body weight, size, or shape is experienced (e.g., feeling fat even when obviously emaciated, feeling that one area of the body is too fat even when obviously underweight).
- In females, absence of at least three consecutive menstrual cycles when otherwise expected to occur (primary or secondary amenorrhea). (pp. 544–545)

Anorexia can lead to starvation, as well as other medical complications such as heart disease and death. In addition, it may be made worse because it involves denial of "abnormality." Anorexia nervosa is clearly a multidimensional disorder (not simply psychological, as many people believe). Specifically, familial, perceptual, cognitive, and possibly biological factors all interact in varying combinations in different individuals to produce slightly different types of disorders (Bordo, 1993). This realization is important, as we will see later in this chapter, in that the treatment of anorexia should also be multidimensional in nature. However, it is important to keep in mind that the primary criterion or essence of anorexia nervosa is a refusal to maintain a normal body weight.

Bulimia Nervosa

With regard to the other major category of eating disorders, bulimia nervosa, its diagnostic criteria include the following (American Psychiatric Association, 1994):

- Recurrent episodes of binge eating (rapid consumption of large quantities of food in a discrete period of time)
- A feeling of lack of control over eating behavior during the eating binges
- Engaging in regular self-induced vomiting, use of laxatives or diuretics, strict dieting or fasting, or

vigorous exercise in order to prevent weight gain
- A minimum average of two binge-eating episodes a week for at least 3 months
- Persistent over-concern with body shape and weight. (pp. 549–550)

The primary criterion for bulimia nervosa involves eating binges followed by inappropriate compensatory methods to prevent weight gain. The binge typical of bulimics usually progresses through four stages. First, there is often stress or a negative event, which acts as a trigger. Second, the person starts to eat avidly but privately, which continues until the binge seems complete. Third is the ending when the person is full, nauseated, or in pain, and therefore stops. Fourth, there are the consequences of one's actions, which at first may bring relief from stress but are soon replaced by shame, guilt, disgust, and feeling of loss of control (G. Fairburn & Wilson, 1993).

Although not considered strictly a part of the DSM-IV definition of anorexia or bulimia, the accompanying box briefly discusses some of the more common mental and physical complications associated with anorexia or bulimia.

One of the common contributing factors of bulimia is low self-esteem (Burckes-Miller & Black, 1988), and individuals often become depressed because of this feeling. This often leads to excessive eating in an effort to feel better, but then people feel guilty about eating, which, in turn, induces vomiting (because they feel they are eating too much and getting "fat") or causes people to take laxatives to purge the food. Although a severe problem, as we will see, bulimia is usually less dangerous than anorexia. The person with bulimia is aware he or she has a problem. In contrast, the anorexic often is not aware of his or her problems and believes that the problem simply rests with the distorted perceptions of others. In some cases, bulimia can lead to anorexia, and some individuals are characterized as *bulimarexic* (they have characteristics of both kinds of eating disorders). Within each disorder are progressive stages of involvement so behaviors can be seen as parts of a continuum rather than as an all-or-none phenomenon.

Binge Eating Disorder

Binge eating, without accompanying methods to prevent weight gain, has been suggested as a third separate major category for eating disorders. Along these lines, provisional criteria for the condition were established by the American Psychiatric Association (1994). The provisional criteria from DSM-IV include the following:

- Recurrent episodes of binge eating
- Rapid consumption of a large amount of food in a short time

Mental and Physical Complications of Eating Disorders

Many of the mental and emotional symptoms common to anorexia are directly related to the physical effects of starvation. However, other symptoms are related to the attitudes and behavior related to eating and weight.

Anorexia Nervosa—Mental Complications

- Reduced Energy Level. This is typically seen in fatigue, lethargy, persistent tiredness, apathy, dizziness, and lightheadedness.

- Social Isolation. The person isolates him- or herself from significant others and becomes increasingly aloof and withdrawn. Family relationships typically decline, and the individual starts to avoid peers.

- Lowered Mental Ability. People are usually not able to concentrate and have a decrease in alertness. There could be memory loss and diminished capacity to think.

- Mood and Attitude Problems. The person is often moody, depressed, irritable, anxious, and intolerant of others. The person's self-esteem is low; he or she has a distorted body image and "feels fat" despite an emaciated appearance.

- Food, Eating, and Hunger Issues. The person has a great fear of gaining weight, often eats alone, has unusual food-related behaviors (e.g., time of eating, size of bites), and needs to vicariously enjoy food (e.g., collect recipes, dream of food).

Anorexia Nervosa—Physical Complications

- Bone Problems. Decreased bone density may lead to fractures. There can be a retardation of growth and development of osteoporosis.

- Metabolic Issues. There is a good chance of abnormal temperature regulation and cold intolerance. This can be accompanied by abnormal glucose tolerance and high free fatty acids.

- Cardiovascular Problems. Commonly present are chest pain, arrhythmias, hypotension, edema, and changes in the electrocardiogram. Heart rates lower than 40 beats per minute are common.

- Gastrointestinal Problems. Constipation is likely, and this may promote laxative use. There are oftentimes vomiting and a feeling of fullness along with abdominal discomfort.

- Electrolyte Imbalance. The individual may be low in potassium, sodium, chloride, calcium, magnesium, and bicarbonate.

Bulimia Nervosa—Mental Complications

- Decreased Mental Ability. There is typically a loss of ordinary willpower, poor impulse control, and self-indulgent behavior.

- Mood Disturbances. There are usually increases in anxiety and depression along with mood swings, low self-esteem, and self-depreciating thoughts. In addition, there may be paranoid feelings, unreasonable resentments, excuse making, and impulsiveness.

- Food, Eating, and Hunger Issues. The person usually eats alone, eats when not hungry, fears binges and eating out of control, and has an increased dependency on bingeing.

- Purging. The individual feels the need to rid the body of calories consumed during binge (through vomiting, laxatives, diuretics, fasting, or excessive exercise).

- Weight. The person usually feels that self-worth is dependent on low weight. There is a constant concern with weight and body image.

Bulimia Nervosa—Physical Complications

- Neurological Problems. EEG changes are common, and people may even have epileptic seizures if there is an electrolyte imbalance.

- Metabolic Issues. Having too many high free fatty acids and too much B-hydroxbutyric.

- Electrolyte Imbalance. Bulimics are usually low in potassium and chloride. There might also be dehydration leading to cardiac arrest, renal failure, and muscle cramps.

- Gastrointestinal Problems. Typically there is increased likelihood of constipation.

- A sense of lack of control of eating during the episode
- Episodes associated with three or more of the following:
  — Eating faster than usual
  — Eating until feeling uncomfortably full
  — Eating large amounts when not hungry
  — Eating alone because embarrassed about how much one is eating
  — Guilt, depression, or disgust following overeating
  — Marked distress about binge eating
  — Episodes occurring on average 2 days per week for 6 months
  — Binges are not associated with the regular use of inappropriate compensatory behaviors. (p. 731)

It should be noted that because clinical cases often present themselves in diverse ways, diagnostic nomenclature rarely covers every possible presentation of an eating disorder (O'Connor & Smith, 1999). Therefore, the DSM-IV also contains another category called "eating disorders not otherwise specified" (NOS). For example, someone who meets all the criteria for anorexia nervosa yet has normal current weight would fit under this classification. Similarly, someone who meets all the criteria for bulimia except that the episodes are less frequent than twice per week or of a duration of less than 3 months would be classified as having an eating disorder "not otherwise specified."

Disordered Eating

As indicated above, anorexia and bulimia are not simply yes or no conditions, but rather each disorder has degrees. Thus, another category, termed *disordered eating*, refers to an entire spectrum of exaggerated eating patterns involving increased health risks. For example, an exerciser might not fit the classic definitions of either anorexia nervosa or bulimia nervosa. Yet he or she obviously has eating problems and is still at increased risk of developing serious endocrine, skeletal, and psychiatric disorders. Such an exerciser might meet all the criteria for anorexia except that body weight is in the normal range. Likewise, an exerciser might meet all the criteria for bulimia except the frequency of binges is less than twice a week for a duration of less than 3 months. Thus, at the extremes, disordered eating includes anorexia and bulimia. However, there is a great deal of middle ground (in fact, this might be the largest category of eating disorders) where there are still eating problems, but not quite severe enough to meet the criteria of the DSM-IV for either anorexia or bulimia. Therefore, it is important to understand and recognize the variety of different disordered eating patterns that might fit along this continuum.

Prevalence of Eating Disorders in Sport /Exercise

It has traditionally been difficult to get an accurate assessment of eating disorders in any population for a variety of reasons. First, these types of disorders are usually very secretive, and people are not always willing to share information on their disorder. For example, even the roommates and parents of those who have a problem often don't know what's going on. Sometimes they don't find out until it becomes almost catastrophic and professional help is necessary. So we may be seeing just the tip of the iceber. (Thornton, 1990, p. 118). Second, a number of different definitions have been used to identify eating disorders. (Some use a strict DSM-IV interpretation, and some are more liberal and

Are You a Dysfunctional Eater?

1. Do you regularly restrict your food intake?
2. Do you skip meals regularly?
3. Do you often go on diets?
4. Do you count calories or fat grams, weigh or measure your food?
5. Are you "afraid" of certain foods?
6. Do you turn to food to reduce stress or anxiety?
7. Do you deny being hungry or claim to feel full after eating very little?
8. Do you avoid eating with others?
9. Do you feel worse (anxious, guilty, etc.) after eating?
10. Do you think about food, eating, and weight more than you'd like?

A "yes" answer to more than three of these questions can indicate a pattern of dysfunctional eating (Berg, 2000). Dysfunctional eating typically includes three general categories. *Chaotic eating* refers to irregular eating such as fasting, bingeing, and skipping meals. *Consistent undereating* usually means not paying attention to hunger signals and regularly eating less food than meets one's daily needs. *Consistent overeating* means a person is overriding normal satiety signals and eating more on a daily basis than the body wants or needs.

look at any sort of disordered eating.) Third, in the competitive sport environment, an athlete may risk being dropped from a program or team if an eating problem is discovered. Fourth, the accuracy of assessment techniques used for identifying eating disorders has sometimes been questionable. In this regard, issues of instrument validity are obvious.

For example, one study investigating eating disorders in female college gymnasts (O'Connor, Lewis, & Kirchner, 1995) found (using more reliable and valid instrumentation) that although these athletes did have concerns about their weight and being thin, they did not exhibit extreme scores on standardized measures of psychological constructs with relevance to eating disorders.

In a follow-up study, O'Connor, Lewis, Kirchner, and Cook (1996) found that retired gymnasts no longer competing (average age of approximately 36 years) did not display any more eating disorders than did a matched control group. So, figures on the prevalence of eating disorders should be examined carefully before any firm conclusions are drawn. For instance, the prevalence of various eating problems such as eating only one meal a day in order to stay slim should not be automatically construed as disordered eating. Because of these assessment problems, descriptive data should be viewed with caution.

Given some of the limitations noted above, a summary of the prevalence of eating disorders in general, and in exercise/sport in particular, has recently been provided by various researchers (e.g., Berg, 2000; Brewer & Petrie, 2002; Goss, Cooper, Stevens, Croxon, & Dryden, 2005; Sanford-Martens, et al., 2005; Swoap & Murphy, 1995). Remember again that many of these data have been collected on athletes and not exercisers. However, the more similar the activity from sport to exercise (e.g., gymnastics, long-distance running), the more the findings probably generalize to exercisers. Some of the general conclusions are as follows:

1. An estimated 10% of high school and college students (most of them female) suffer from some sort of clinical eating disorder.
2. Death rates for anorexia nervosa and bulimia nervosa are estimated at 10 to 20%.
3. For girls in late adolescence and women in early adulthood, approximately 1.0% and 3.0% meet the diagnostic criteria for anorexia nervosa and bulimia nervosa, respectively. Men and boys tend to have a substantially lower rate than females.
4. Athletes and regular exercisers appear to have a greater occurrence of eating-related problems than do members of the general population.
5. A significant percentage of athletes engage in disordered-eating or weight-loss behaviors (e.g., binge eating, rigorous dieting, fasting, vomiting, use of diuretics), which, although sub-clinical, are important to examine.
6. Eating disorders and the use of pathogenic weight-loss techniques tend to have a sport-specific prevalence (e.g., they occur in sports such as gymnastics and wrestling rather than in archery and basketball).
7. Although anorexia and bulimia are special concerns in sports and physical activities emphasizing form (e.g., gymnastics, diving, and figure skating) or weight (e.g., wrestling), eating disorders have been found in a wide array of athletes as well as in exercisers.
8. In their meta-analysis, Hausenblaus and Carron (1999) found that males involved in sport and physical activity had higher scores (small but significant) on bulimic, anorexic, and drive for thinness indices than did non-participants. Female participants reported more anorexic and bulimic symptoms (small but significant) than did non-participants. Furthermore, males and females who competed in aesthetic sports (e.g., figure skating) consistently had the highest scores on the disordered-eating indices. Related to this finding, male athletes in aesthetic and weight-dependent sports self-reported more bulimic and drive for thinness symptomatology than did male non-athletes. Relative to females in the general population, females in aesthetic sports self-reported more anorexic and drive for thinness on various indices.
9. Although no firm prevalence data are available, up to 66% of female athletes may be amenorrheic as compared to just 2% to 5% of female nonathletes. Thus, many females who are very active in sport and exercise at an early age may eventually develop osteoporosis, which can result in increased bone fractures, increased skeletal fragility, and permanent bone loss (Sanborn, Horea, Siemers, & Dieringer, 2000).
10. Research has estimated that approximately 63% of all female athletes develop symptoms of an eating disorder between 9th and 12th grades. This does not mean that such a large percentage of athletes develop full-blown eating disorders, but it is an indication of the serious impact of weight, body image and shape, and performance pressures on athletes.

It is apparent from these data that disordered eating is most definitely a problem in our society and in certain athletic endeavors, but it is important to note that there is no compelling evidence that mere participation in sport or physical activity can directly cause an eating disorder. Interestingly, most studies, like those reported above, have focused on individuals in competitive sports. However, to a lesser extent, eating disorders have been studied in relation to physical activity behavior. A common misperception is that excessive exercise leads to the development of anorexia nervosa (O'Connor & Smith, 1999). In their review of literature, they came to the conclusion that "logic and empirical evidence dictates that excessive exercise cannot be a sole cause of anorexia nervosa" (p.1010). For example, despite the thousands of people who exercise regularly, only a very, very small proportion of those ever develop an eating disorder. In addition, increased physical activity with anorexia is paradoxical because very small amounts of food intake will typically result in reduced physical activity and fatigue. This is illustrated in a study (Bouten, Van Msarken Lichenbelt, & Westerderp, 1996), which found no differences between anorexics vs. controls in terms of physical activity, although anorexic women with a very low body mass index in fact exercised less than did a comparable normal-weight control group.

Although physical activity is not automatically associated with eating disorders, certain competitive sports appear to have more eating disorders associated with it. As we will see, certain behaviors by coaches or rules and regulations within specific sports might in fact contribute to the onset of an eating disorder. A first step in solving this problem is to identify and understand some of its causes and predisposing factors.

Predisposing and Contributory Factors

As professionals in the sport and exercise fields, physical education teachers, coaches, exercise leaders, and athletic trainers should understand the factors that might predispose an individual to develop an eating disorder. The assumption is that if you know the elements that are more likely to contribute to, or be related to, the development of an eating disorder, then you might possibly be able to alter them or at least prepare the individual for them. Although some of these factors include genetics, personality, and family background, which are largely stable and unchangeable, other factors relate to the sociocultural environment. Because the latter tend to be less stable, they are more amenable to intervention. Thus, knowledge about these factors might help prevent or reduce the probability of eating disorders developing in the first place, because behavior might be changed to avoid these situations (e.g., avoid sports where weight/appearances are

critical). Some of these factors are more related to the general population, and some are more specific to those individuals who are involved in exercise or competitive sport on a regular basis.

Sociocultural factors. The cause of eating disorders is certainly a complex question and may be even an unanswerable one, but some identified factors have been consistently related to the development of eating disorders. Traditionally, it was believed that the roots of eating disorders rested with pathological traits of patients and their dysfunctional families. However, recent research has focused more on the cultural emphasis on thinness, which has led to widespread body dissatisfaction (especially in women). Furthermore, many of the psychological traits once thought to cause eating disorders may instead be the result of starvation. According to anecdotal reports of weight-control specialists, for example, more and more clients are coming from wholesome, functional families. In essence, family attitudes that have been observed over the past 10–20 years are not consistently associated with the increases in eating disorders. Rather, it is a culture that values thinness that puts increased pressure on people (especially adolescents and young adults) to have a thin body. Of course, not all people develop disordered eating, and it is this argument that attempts to diffuse the role that culture plays. While other personal and biological factors should be considered (in a classic interactional research design approach), this does not diminish the importance of culture as a causal element in the development of eating disorders.

There is strong evidence, for example, of the major role that media (which oftentimes impart cultural

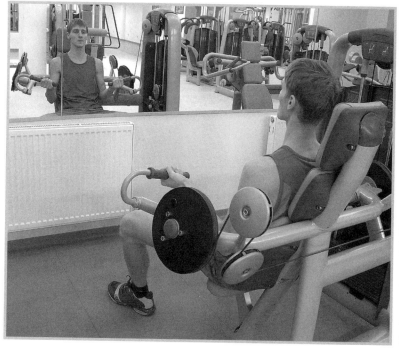

Photo courtesy of © iStockphoto.com

norms and values) can play in the development of eating disorders. In one study conducted in Fiji, within 38 months from the time satellite television came to the island in 1995 and began beaming images of thin actors and actresses, the number of teens at risk for eating disorders more than doubled to 29%. Furthermore, the number who vomited for weight control went up five-fold (Goodman, 1999). Cultural norms regarding the optimal body size and shape have had a great effect on both men and women (but especially women). For example, in one study of women free from eating-disorder symptoms, more than 95% overestimated their body size (on the average by 25%) as larger than it really was (Swoap & Murphy, 1995). This perception of feeling oversized or overweight is fairly typical, because the message we constantly receive from society is that thinness is highly valued and we should all strive to match the beautiful thin models we see on billboards and television.

Using in-depth interviews, C. G. Fairburn, Welch, and Doll (1997) conducted an interesting study that targeted social factors affecting the development of bulimia nervosa. Their results generally revealed that those who developed bulimia reported significantly worse social relationships than did those who belonged to a matched control group. Some of the major factors that appeared related to the development of bulimia included being sexually or physically abused, the pres-

ence of parental psychiatric disorder (e.g., depression, alcoholism, substance abuse), and other problems with parents such as minimal affection or frequent teasing and criticism. Thus, the quality of the environment in which one is raised appears to be an important consideration in the development of an eating disorder.

Weight restrictions and standards. A number of physical activities such as weight lifting, wrestling, and boxing commonly rely on weight classifications to subdivide competitors. In and of itself, this is not a problem. However, weight classification can become an issue when individuals feel that they have to perform below a weight that is appropriate for them, so that they can excel over lighter opponents. In essence, these people are often encouraged (either implicitly or explicitly) to try to "make weight" so they can compete at a lower weight classification, which presumably would give them an advantage against a lighter opponent. This practice of "cutting weight" may result in dropping up to 10 or 15 pounds immediately before weigh-ins, usually resulting in rapid dehydration. Crash dieting, use of diet pills, fasting, use of diuretics, laxatives, purging, and fluid restriction are all techniques to achieve this rapid weight loss (see Figure 16.1 for common weight-loss techniques used by athletes and exercisers).

Dieting is particularly prevalent among youngsters as research investigating over 11,000 high school stu-

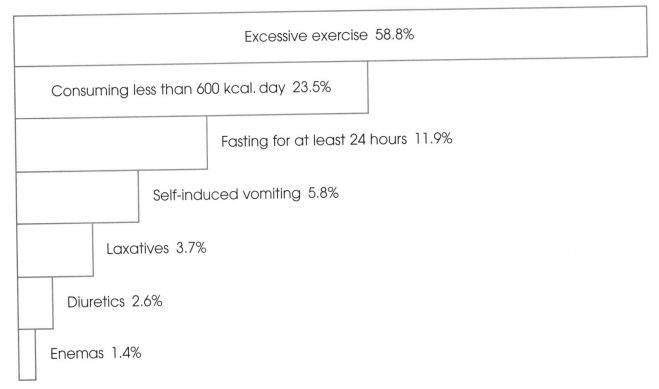

Figure 16.1. Common weight-loss techniques used by athletes.

dents found that more than 40% of the females were attempting to lose weight through some type of diet (Sedula, Collins, & Williamson, 1993). For these high school students, losing weight and looking thin made them fit in more and be better liked by their peers (at least this was their perception).

These techniques and resulting rapid dehydration can have both short- and long-term negative health consequences, especially if experienced repeatedly. For example, the rapid loss of body weight increases vulnerability to an overall weakened state, and as the medical literature shows, rapid dehydration is generally a dangerous behavior in terms of impact on the body (Webster, Rutt, & Weltman, 1990). As noted earlier, women are particularly prone to develop long-term health problems due to disordered eating to "make weight" or maintain a very low body weight, which can lead to osteoporosis and chronic amenorrhea. Everyone involved should discourage these methods of weight loss and dieting, even if they are imbedded in our culture.

Pressure from peers, coaches, and significant others. This pressure to lose weight or maintain a low body weight (or low percent body fat) might be considered part of the sociocultural environment discussed earlier. In this regard, coaches, significant others, and peers can play an important role in shaping the attitude and behaviors of individuals involved in sport and exercise. Unfortunately, these people sometimes knowingly or unknowingly encourage weight loss in exercisers either for enhanced performance or physical appearance. The greatest danger to an athlete's or exerciser's health exists when pressure is applied to lose weight in the absence of knowledge concerning safe and effective weight-management procedures. For example, in one study (Harris & Greco, 1990), 56% of gymnasts experienced pressure from their coaches to lose weight as there were, on the average, 6 team weigh-ins and 14 individual weigh-ins a month. The following account from the *Austin [Texas] American- Statesman* illustrates the role that a coach can play in promoting unhealthy attitudes toward weight and weight reduction as well as the pressure some athletes therefore feel to stay thin:

According to current and former swimmers, the pressure to meet weight guidelines was so intense that many routinely fasted, induced vomiting, used laxatives and diuretics, or exercised in addition to workouts. They did not want to be relegated to the group they called "The Fat Club." Primarily, the pressure came from the coach, until swimmers started to internalize it. Then it became self-inflicted torture, almost where some swimmers would weigh themselves three or four times a day . . . Weighing was a constant reminder of their weight, and former swimmers remember being at the swim center at 5:30 in the morning, looking at that stupid freight scale. The swimmers became obsessive with it, worrying about each pound— that's how fanatical it made them. (Halliburton & Sanford, 1989 a,b, pp. D1, D7, D8)

In addition to the pressure coaches can place on athletes, research has also revealed that many individuals involved in sport and exercise demonstrate relatively negative attitudes toward, and limited knowledge about, obesity (Griffin & Harris, 1996). Along these lines, exercisers tend to make decisions about the need for weight control on the basis of appearance rather than on objective indicators such as body-fat assessments.

There is additional pressure other than simply from coaches. For example, peer modeling can also be very important in the development of eating disorders. For example, one study (Chiodo & Latimer, 1983) found that most bulimic patients could identify specific incidents associated with the onset of vomiting and that many developed the problem after learning from someone else or the media about the behavior. Learning disordered-eating behaviors from others (or feeling pressured to use these behaviors to stay thin) can be a very powerful source of influence, especially for young people where approval from peers is so important in their lives. For instance, if two college students jog together and one finds out that the other purges to keep her weight down, then this might be incorporated into the friend's eating patterns because it might be seen as a relatively easy way to manage weight. Again, because thinness is so highly valued in our culture, this behavior from friends and peers can exert tremendous motivation to conform. Other people might take even offhand comments about weight gain and loss very seriously. This emphasis on thinness has also caused body-image disturbances that have been shown to be related to the development of eating disorders (O'Connor & Smith, 1999). Therefore, exercise professionals should be careful about irresponsible comments regarding weight gain or weight loss when interacting with students, athletes, and clients. You never know when a casual comment meant in jest might be interpreted in a way that contributes to disordered eating.

Performance demands. Our society has increasingly become interested in optimal performance, especially when it comes to exercise and sport. Along these lines, over the last 20 years, there has been an increased focus on the relationship between body weight or body fat and performance. First, it is important to note that body fat, not body weight, is the most critical factor for achieving high levels of personal performance (although weight alone can sometimes present limitations). For instance, an exerciser might have some difficulty participating in aerobic activities

Table 16.1

Body Fat Suggested Ranges for Men and Women Athletes in Different Sports

SPORT	MEN	WOMEN
Baseball, softball	8–16	12–18
Basketball	8–14	12–16
Bodybuilding	6–12	8–14
Canoeing and kayaking	8–14	10–18
Cycling	6–12	8–16
Fencing	8–14	10–16
Football	8–20	—
Golf	10–16	12–20
Gymnastics	7–14	10–18
Horse racing	8–14	10–18
Ice and field hockey	8–16	12–18
Orienteering	7–14	10–18
Pentathlon	—	8–18
Racquetball	8–16	10–18
Rowing	8–16	10–16
Rugby	6–16	—
Skating	5–12	10–18
Skiing	8–16	10–18
Ski jumping	8–16	10–20
Soccer	6–14	10–20
Swimming	6–12	10–18
Synchronized swimming	—	10–18
Tennis	8–14	10–20
Track-and-field		
Running events	7–14	10–17
Field events	8–18	12–20
Triathlon	6–12	10–17
Volleyball	7–15	10–18
Weightlifting	6–14	10–18
Wrestling	7–16	—

Adapted from Wilmore, J. H. (1992) Body weight standards and athletic performance. In Brownwell, K. D., Rodin, J., & Wilmore, J. H. (1992) *Eating: Body weight and performance in athletics* (pp. 315-329). Philadelphia: Lea & Febiger.

if he or she is overweight (despite not being over fat) due to the excess pounding on the body required in many aerobic activities. This observation is supported by research, which has indicated a correlation between low percent body fat and high levels of performance in a number of activities (Wilmore, 1992). Such findings have led many coaches, athletes, and exercisers to focus on weight control in an attempt to reach their optimal weight. However, at times this type of information has been inappropriately applied to athletes and exercisers, often pushing them well below their optimal body weight. In fact, some exercisers use excess exercise (to be discussed later in the chapter) as a primary way to control weight. Lower body fat, however, does not always mean better performance. Individual differences are critical here, and strict weight standards are therefore inappropriate.

As Wilmore (1992) suggests, there is typically a range of values for body fat related to optimal performance, and these differ between males and females (see Table 16.1). Specifically, females, on the average, have a higher percent body fat than men do; nevertheless, women are typically under more pressure and scrutiny to keep a very low percentage of body fat. This is especially true of athletes, even though the data indicate great individual differences among athletes and exercisers in relative body fat.

Judging criteria. This factor is directly related to sport competition. In sports and physical activities where physical attractiveness, especially for females, is considered important for success (gymnastics, figure skating, diving), it is often perceived that judges tend to be biased toward certain body types. In particular, very slender body builds are often seen as desirable. Anecdotal reports reveal that comments about losing a few pounds to look better are unfortunately communicated from judges to athletes. For example, an athlete might hear the comment "If you lost 5–10 pounds, you would probably do much better in competition next year." This type of comment can have a tremendous impact on an adolescent who fiercely desires success in sport and whose parents probably have spent tens of thousands of dollars on their child's training. It could eventually lead to disordered eating to obtain the desired look and body type. However, little evidence suggests that this weight loss will eventually lead to enhanced performance because the weight loss may, in fact, reflect loss of muscle mass, a loss that can be deleterious to performance. The following quote by a national champion figure skater describes how appearances are perceived as being tied to judging criteria:

"Skating is such an appearance sport. You have to go up there with barely anything on . . . I'm definitely aware of my weight. I mean I have dreams about it sometimes. So it's hard having people look at my thigh and saying 'oops, she's an eighth of an inch bigger' or something. It's hard . . . Weight is continually on my mind. I am never, never allowed to be on vacation." (Gould, Jackson, & Finch, 1993, p. 364)

Recognition and Referral of Disordered Eating

As alluded to above, although many exercisers and athletes might use pathogenic weight-loss methods frequently and experience eating disorders occasionally, these problems are not always obvious, and many cases go unrecognized and untreated. How then does one recognize and identify such a problem? This is definitely not an easy task, but physical education instructors, exercise leaders, athletic trainers, and coaches are in an excellent position to spot individuals with eating disorders. In addition, roommates, parents, and close friends should also have some knowledge of disordered eating because they might actually be the people closest to the individual with the problem. At times, immediate treatment might be appropriate, and at other times, the problem might be very difficult to diagnose.

Standardized Assessment

The major physical and psychological symptoms related to the recognition of eating disorders are presented in Table 16.2. Often, however, simply unusual

Table 16.2
Physical and Psychological-Behavioral Signs of Eating Disorders

Physical Signs and Symptoms	Psychological-Behavioral Signs and Symptoms
Weight well below normal range	Dieting very excessive
Considerable weight loss	Excessive eating—little or no weight gain
Extreme weight fluctuations	Excessive exercise that is not part of normal training program
Bloating	Excessive guilt about eating
Swollen salivary glands	Claims of feeling fat at objectively normal weight
Amenorrhea	Constant preoccupation with food
Carotinemia (yellowish palms or soles of feet)	Avoidance of eating in public and denial of hunger
Sores or calluses on hands from inducing vomiting	Hoarding food
Hypoglycemia (low blood sugar)	Disappearing after meals
Muscle cramps	Frequent weighing
Stomach complaints	Binge eating
Headaches, dizziness, or weakness from electrolyte disturbances	Evidence of self-induced vomiting
Numbness and tingling in limbs due to electrolyte disturbances	Use of drugs such as diet pills, laxatives, or diuretics to control weight
Propensity for stress fractures	
Bad teeth from gastric acid	

Note: Adapted from Garner, D. M., & Rosen, L. W. (1991) Eating disorders among athletes: Research and recommendations, *Journal of Applied Sport Science Research, 5*(2), 100-107.

eating patterns are among the best indicators of problems. For example, anorexics often pick at their food, push it around their plates, eat predominantly low-calorie foods, and then lie about their eating. On the other hand, bulimics often hide food and disappear after eating (so they can purge the food just eaten). Whenever possible, one should observe the eating patterns of students and athletes, looking for abnormalities.

There are also standardized self-report inventories to diagnose eating disorders, but these should be administered and interpreted only by trained professionals, such as a licensed psychologist. These might include the Eating Disorders Inventory-2, which measures individual eating attitudes and behavior (Garner, 1991); the revised Diagnostic Survey for Eating Disorders, which can be used as a self-report inventory or in a semi-structured interview (Johnson & Pure, 1986); or the Eating Attitudes Test (Garner & Garfinkel, 1979), which is a test of disordered-eating symptoms associated with anorexia nervosa. It is important to note that the context in which these tests are taken should be factored into any judgment regarding the individual involved. For example, a gymnast might get high scores on the Eating Disorders Inventory and thus be considered at risk for an eating disorder. However, because doing well in gymnastics, in part, is due to staying in shape and keeping weight down, it might be reasonable (and indeed necessary) for gymnasts to be concerned about their body composition and leanness. Therefore, "being preoccupied with being thinner" as a response may not really indicate anything psychopathological about the gymnast; rather, it may very well be a rational response in light of the requirements of the sport.

Assessment of Behavior and Personality

Besides the standardized assessments, one of the best ways to evaluate an eating disorder, especially for the non-expert or nonprofessional, is through observation. The use of behavioral observation often validates self-report or test data and can help clarify the nature of the problem. Table 16.2 displays many of the typical signs and symptoms of eating-behavior problems. Some of the more visual and possibly easily recognized ones include significant weight loss, especially for anorexics (or frequent fluctuations in weight); solitary eating; wide mood swings; and preoccupation with eating, food preparation, and caloric content of food. For example, bulimics might eat alone, making it easier to engage in purging after the meal, but because many bulimics tend to be near their normal or recommended weight, they are often more difficult to detect. They more typically have inconsistent eating patterns, either eating very little or much too much. Anorexics are often involved in

compulsive, ritualistic, or unusual eating. These might include cutting food into tiny morsels, eating only a very limited number of bland, low-calorie foods, creating unusual mixtures of food, or removing the breaded parts from foods. For example, one anorexic used to break off the ends of her french fries and eat only the middle portion. She explained this by saying, "The ends contained too much fat."

Regarding mood swings, self-worth issues are often a center point, but wide swings in depression and irritability are also common. Finally, it should be noted that an eating-disordered individual might have only some or none of the behaviors just described. For example, although perfectionist tendencies are typical of anorexics, they are also common in many other high-achieving individuals. Unfortunately, the emerging consensus is that no single personality structure is characteristic of eating-disordered individuals. Rather, eating disorders appear to be more multidimensional, developing in different people, at different times, for different reasons (Swoap & Murphy, 1995).

Referral of Eating Disorders

Knowing how and when to refer an individual suspected of an eating disorder for treatment is crucial. Therefore, judgments must be made, fairly early on, regarding when and if to refer. If there is severe pathology, then this typically does not present a referral dilemma. Cases that are mildly abnormal, however, present more of a problem (e.g., maybe the person has a very restrictive diet and thus is vomiting occasionally). Even in these cases, the person should be at least referred to a trained professional for an assessment.

The earlier the referral, the better chance there is of helping the individual. In many cases, however, because many athletes and exercisers have perfectionist tendencies and desire to please others, they often have difficulty admitting that a problem even exists. Therefore, these people should be approached very carefully with an emphasis on their feelings rather than a direct focus on their eating behaviors (Thompson, 1987). Focusing on eating behaviors and attempting to exert control in this area can often be counterproductive because eating is often the only thing the individual really feels that he or she can control. Along these lines, it's important not to exacerbate the problem (often done with bulimics, in particular) by being overly vigilant and trying to catch the person in the act (e.g., vomiting). All this usually does is create more pressure for the bulimic, which can oftentimes simply make the symptoms even worse.

If an eating disorder is suspected, the person (whether it is a fitness professional or a friend) who has the best rapport with the individual should schedule a private meeting to discuss his or her concerns

(Garner & Rosen, 1991). As noted above, the emphasis here should be on the person's feelings rather than directly focusing on eating behaviors. Be supportive in such instances and keep all information confidential. Referrals should then be made to a specific clinic or person rather than a vague recommendation such as

"You should seek some help." If an individual is still hesitant, then suggest that he or she see the referral person simply for an assessment to determine if there is a problem. The individual is often more amenable to a referral for assessment than for "therapy." Always try to make sure an appointment is made (or even you can

Reducing the Probability of Disordered Eating in Athletes and Exercisers

Perhaps one of the most important services we can provide as health care professionals is promoting the prevention of a problem. This is definitely the case with disordered eating in sport and exercise. Along these lines, we list some suggestions for effectively reducing the probability of eating disorders or disordered eating in exercise and sport environments. It would be a great contribution if we could help prevent, or at least reduce the probability of, these disorders from occurring in the first place. For a more detailed discussion of this issue, interested readers are encouraged to read Thompson and Sherman's (1993) guide to helping individuals in sport and exercise contexts.

Promote Proper Nutrition.

Accurate and usable nutritional information is critical and integral to anyone dealing with weight issues. Unfortunately, research indicates that many exercise and sport participants have limited or incorrect views on proper nutrition (Brewer & Petrie, in press). Therefore, exercise professionals (in particular) should become educated (or better educated) regarding proper nutrition and weight control so they can pass this information on to the athletes and exercisers. Modeling of good nutritional practices by family members, coaches, and exercise leaders is one positive step in promoting healthy nutritional practices.

De-emphasize Body Weight.

Unfortunately, the focus in our society has been on body weight, and ideal body weight for different body sizes. This only causes people to become more obsessed with achieving this desired weight or look. We, as exercise professionals, must move the focus away from the obsession with weight to a focus on fitness. Research has clearly shown that there is no ideal body composition or weight for an athlete or exerciser because such attributes can fluctuate

greatly due to such elements as type of sport, body build, metabolic rate, and natural variations in body composition (Davis, 2000). Rather, as seen in Table 16.1, perhaps some ranges can be developed for different activities, and these can provide exercisers and athletes with much more leeway in achieving their goals.

Promote Sensitivity to Weight Issues.

In working with sport and exercise personnel in the prevention of pathogenic weight-loss practices, we must all be sensitive to the weight-control and dieting issues that exercise and sport participants typically face. Fitness leaders, athletic trainers, coaches, and good friends can have powerful effects on individuals, so be careful when making remarks regarding weight control. Practices such as emphasizing the importance of thinness, repeatedly weighing-in, associating weight loss with enhanced performance, minimizing the detrimental and unhealthy effect of rapid weight gain or loss, and making unfeeling remarks can all help encourage disordered-eating patterns, and such practices need to be avoided at all costs.

Facilitate Healthy Management of Weight.

One positive outcome of the increase in weight-control problems over the past 10 years is that we have learned a great deal about behavioral approaches to the management of weight and the effectiveness of a variety of weight-management strategies. Perhaps, most important for education efforts aimed at changing attitudes, much has been learned about the effects of unhealthy weight-loss methods on performance and health concerns. Health care and exercise professionals must take the lead in emphasizing the relationship between body type and weight, the realities of optimal body composition, and weight for optimal health and performance. Only through such efforts will important strides be made to reduce the incidence of disordered eating in our population.

make the appointment) because often the person will not follow through. The accompanying box provides suggestions for helping eating-disordered individuals in exercise programs.

Substance Abuse

It was not surprising when it was made known to the public that many of the East German and Soviet athletes (especially women) were taking performance-enhancing drugs in preparation for the Olympic Games before the Iron Curtain disintegrated in approximately 1990. In fact, team doctors, under orders from the highest political powers, routinely prescribed drugs for athletes and then kept careful records regarding the effects of different dosages on performance and the length of time needed in order to test clean. Athletes have been taking steroids and other performance-enhancing drugs for decades to try to gain a competitive advantage over their opposition. Even the threat of death is evidently not a deterrent as long as victory is guaranteed. As one long-distance runner purportedly said, "You have guys who will go to the funeral of a friend who died from taking drugs and come home and inject it again." The seductive draw of taking drugs, no matter what the side effects or consequences, is highlighted in a 1995 poll of 198 athletes, most of them U.S. Olympians or aspiring Olympians. Athletes were given the following scenarios:

(a) You are offered a banned performance-enhancing substance with two guarantees: (1) you will not be caught, and (2) you will win. Would you take the substance?

(b) You are offered a banned performance-enhancing substance that comes with two guarantees: (1) you will not be caught, and (2) you will win every competition you enter for the next five years and then you will die from the side effects of the substance. Would you take it?

In answering the first question, 195 athletes said yes; three said no—a stunning 98%. In answering the second question, 120 of the athletes said yes (approximately 60%), and 75 said no. In essence, despite the fact that they would die in 5 years, the importance of winning and being number one was evidently more critical than even living.

What is surprising is that despite the dire warnings of the negative psychological and physiological effects of steroids and other performance-enhancing and recreational drugs, their use appears on the upswing (Swoap & Murphy, 1995). Moreover, a person doesn't have to be an elite or professional athlete to use drugs. Although we often hear of some of the more high-profile cases of substance abuse in high-level sport (e.g., tennis player Jennifer Capriati, golfer John Daly, baseball player Daryl Strawberry, soccer player Diego Maradona), the abuses go far beyond elite sport. For example, many recreational athletes or exercisers have started to use drugs to help them look better to the opposite sex, to simply build more bulk or better looking muscles, to control weight, and to improve performance. Although a great deal of the initial research was conducted with high school, college, and elite athletes, more and more research is being conducted on drug use by people who might be termed exercisers or recreational athletes (Weinberg & Gould, 2003). Remember, though, that not all drug use is bad. For example, many drugs are developed and needed to offset intense pain and enhance healing. So, drugs per se are not the problem, as long as the drugs being used are legal, are prescribed by appropriate medical personnel, and do not have any known harmful short- or long-term consequences. In essence, it is the misuse of drugs and the use of illegal and harmful drugs that are the real problems in sport and exercise environments. In addition, abuse occurs, both with performance-enhancing drugs such as steroids and so-called recreational or social drugs such as cocaine or marijuana. So let us start by taking a closer look at what substance abuse really is.

The *Diagnostic and Statistical Manual of Mental Disorders* (American Psychiatric Association, 1994) lists the following criteria for psychoactive *substance abuse*:

A. A maladaptive pattern of psychoactive substance use indicated by at least one of the following:
(1) continued use despite knowledge of having a persistent or recurring social, occupational, psychological, or physical problem that is caused or exacerbated by use of the psychoactive substance.
(2) recurrent use in situations in which use is physically hazardous (e.g., driving while intoxicated).

B. Some symptoms of the disturbance have persisted for at least one month, or have occurred repeatedly over a longer period of time.

Any exercise professional should know these criteria, as they will be helpful in the identification and eventual treatment of the problem, but there is also a need to define not only drug abuse, but also drug use. For example, if an individual uses a drug to relieve physical pain from injury, does this amount to drug use? If an individual uses marijuana once to help cope with performance anxiety, would this be considered drug use? These are the sort of difficult questions that have made firm conclusions much more difficult in this area. Unfortunately, an in-depth examination of how substance abuse affects exercisers and athletes is beyond our scope here. For more detailed information, we recommend several excellent books or chapters on the subject (Anshel, 2001; Stainbeck, 1997; Swoap & Murphy, 1995 ; Voy & Deeter, 1991). Similar to the discussion of eating disorders, we will begin with an overview of the prevalence of drug use and abuse in sport and physical activity.

Prevalence of Substance Abuse in Sports

In a fashion parallel to the reporting of eating disorders, it is inherently difficult to get an accurate picture of substance use and abuse due to its sensitive and personal nature. This is especially true in exercise settings because the athletic settings have dominated the research landscape in most previous reports. In the athletic domain, athletes are often hesitant to say that they have used drugs (even in purportedly anonymous surveys) due to potentially negative repercussions (e.g., being cut from the team) or their own approach of wanting to look good in society's eyes. Thus, once again, these data should be viewed with caution.

Anecdotal reports of drug use in sport/exercise. To begin with, there is much anecdotal evidence regarding substance use and abuse. This starts as far back as the 3rd century B.C., when Greek athletes experimented with many types of psychoactive substances to improve performance (Chappel, 1987). In recent years, however, we are starting to hear many anecdotal reports of athletes using drugs in professional, Olympic, and college sports. As noted earlier, the scandal originating out of BALCO—involving mostly high visibility baseball players—resulted in a congressional hearing on steroid use in sport and exercise. A number of players were accused of using steroids either intentionally or inadvertently. For example, Barry Bonds (who has over 700 lifetime homers and broke the season single record of home runs at 72) stated that he was given rubdowns with a clear substance that was probably a steroid, but he insists he didn't know it was a steroid. In fact, many people are calling for an asterisk to be placed next to the name of players who reportedly used steroids during the time they set records or achieved particularly high levels of performance.

Of course it is difficult to document the use of steroids without tests to prove their actual usage. However, circumstantial evidence regarding changes in body type and size and musculature as they correlate with increases in performance can be very damaging to a player's credibility. In addition, statements like those given by Mark McGuire at a congressional hearing that "I only want to talk about the present" in addition to not denying (or confirming) drug use while playing casts a dark cloud over the performances of certain players. Rafael Palmero (who has over 500 homers and 3,000 hits), who testified that he never

took performance-enhancing drugs in front of a Senate subcommittee, tested positive for drugs and has since been released by the Baltimore Orioles. This close scrutiny has led baseball commissioner Bud Selig to suggest a penalty of a 50 game suspension for first time offenders. In fact, recently, a new substance abuse policy was passed for Major League Baseball indicating a 50 game suspension for the first failed drug test, a 100 game suspension for the second failed drug test, and permanent suspension for a third failed test. Only time will tell if these more stringent measures have an impact on baseball (or will players find a way around the drug testing?).

One particularly popular and misunderstood drug is androstenedione, which is better known as creatine (Anshel, 2003). Its popularity soared when Mark McGuire said he used it during his then-record 70 homer season. At the time, creatine was not banned from baseball (categorized as a nutritional supplement) although it was banned by the Olympic Committee. Ostensibly, creatine increases muscular power

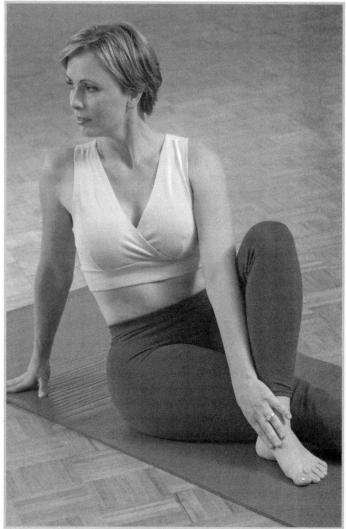

Photo courtesy of © iStockphoto.com

and speed in sport events. Its increased popularity is because it is not considered an anabolic steroid and is legally available over the counter. Whether or not it is effective as a performance enhancer appears to depend on the type of sport in question. In reviewing the literature regarding creatine, Anshel (2001) concludes that "even if creatine improves lean body mass and muscular strength, it may help performance only in sports that require repetitive, high-intensity, very short-term tasks with a brief recovery period" (p. 421). Given the uncertain long-term effects of prolonged creatine use, athletes should avoid this substance or take it under the close supervision of a physician.

Another popular drug is ephedra which is categorized as a stimulant and has mainly been used by dieters and athletes because it stimulates the heart and central nervous system to lose weight, increase metabolism, and burn fat. Ephedra can be very dangerous for athletes because it can deplete the body of water and cause stimulant-like effects (e.g., increased blood pressure and heart rate). The NCAA has banned ephedra since 1997, and in 2001 the National Football League became the first professional sports league to ban ephedra, stemming from the deaths of Rashidi Wheeler, a Northwestern University football player, and Korey Stringer, an offensive lineman for the Minnesota Vikings. In 2003, Baltimore Orioles pitcher Steve Bechler died of a heatstroke and was taking ephedra, causing Major League Baseball to ban the drug (Bacon, Lerner, Trembley, & Seestedt, 2005).

Although there has been a recent emphasis on steroids and amphetamines, the drug of choice was long been alcohol. This drug use was "brushed under the table" in years past (like many other scandals), but as the media and journalism have changed, it has reached front-page news in recent years. We probably are familiar with the long list of high-profile athletes such as Dexter Manley, Lawrence Taylor, Dwight Gooden, John Daly, and Chris Mullen, who have abused alcohol or have admitted to, or been caught, using illegal drugs. In some cases, their careers have been terminated, and they have served prison sentences due to repeated drug use and violations of league policy. In addition, unfortunately we have also seen some deaths due to drug use and abuse in sport such as those of Lyle Alzado and Len Bias. Furthermore, less lethal physical maladies such as sterility, kidney stones, irregular heartbeat, and hypertension, as well as psychological problems such as heightened anxiety, short attention spans, increased depression and aggression, and suicidal tendencies have been reported as being due to drug use (Anshel, 1997). Finally, the use of needles to inject drugs (especially anabolic steroids) may increase the probability of contracting HIV and hepatitis C infections, although little published research has addressed this potential problem.

Girls and Steroids

For a number of years researchers have noted the increase in steroid use among teenage boys both to perform better and look better. But an alarming number of young girls, some as young as nine, are using bodybuilding steroids—not necessarily to get an edge on the playing field, but to get the toned sculpted look of models and movie stars. Girls are getting their hands on the same dangerous testosterone pills, shots, and creams that created a scandal in Major League Baseball and other sports. In most cases, these illegal steroids are gotten from relatives, friends, or a gym. In fact, research has revealed that often these are the same girls who have an eating disorder.

Statistics reveal that overall, up to about 5 percent of high school girls and 7 percent of middle-school girls admit to trying anabolic steroids at least once, with the use of the drugs rising steadily since 1991. Researchers say most girls are using steroids to get bigger and stronger on the playing field and they attribute some of the increase in steroid use to girls' rising participation in sports. But plenty of other girls are using steroids to give themselves a slightly muscular look. With young women, they appear to use it more as a weight control and body fat reduction.

In teenage girls, the side effects from taking male sex hormones can include severe acne, smaller breasts, deeper voice, irregular periods, excess facial and body hair, depression, paranoia, and the fits of anger dubbed "roid rage." In addition, steroids also carry higher risks of heart attack, stroke, and some forms of cancer.

Lyle Alzado (1991), former National Football League star who subsequently died of massive brain tumors (which he attributed to the continued use of steroids during his playing career), candidly discussed the use of steroids in his sport. He contended that 90% of the athletes he knew were on steroids and that the coaches implicitly knew what was going on but conveniently looked the other way. He noted that he could easily pass drug tests by stopping his drug intake about a month before the test.

In another example of self-reported drug use, a story in *Sports Illustrated* (Chaiken & Telander, 1988) detailed the effects of prolonged steroid use on Tommy Chaiken, who played football for the University of South Carolina. This report provided significant insight into the numerous social and psychological pressures that foster drug use in sport (in this case, anabolic steroids) including the encouragement of coaches and the pressures to succeed. Chaiken and Telander noted that there were no team rules or other forms of communication that discouraged drug taking. From his abuse of steroids, Chaiken developed a variety of physical and psychological ailments, including chronic aggression, depression, testicular shrinkage, hair loss, insomnia, poor vision, chronic anxiety, hypertension, a heart murmur, and benign tumors.

As alluded to by Chaiken and Telander (1988) and Alzado (1991), coaches are often implicitly or explicitly involved in "their" athletes' use of drugs. For example, after having his gold medal taken away, sprinter Ben Johnson asserted that his coach knowingly gave him a banned substance: "Charlie Francis was my coach. . . . If Charlie gave me something to take, I took it" (*Time*, June 26, 1989, p. 57). In fact, in Francis' testimony in court, he stated that he told Johnson "that drugs marked the only route to international success and admitted that he provided such chemicals to his charges" (*Time*, June 26, 1989, p. 57).

Research evidence of drug use in exercise/sport. As we consider not only anecdotal evidence from athletes, but also data accruing from scientific studies, it becomes obvious that most of the latter have focused on alcohol and steroid use. For example, an early study has particular relevance to exercise because it focused on high school students in general, and not on athletes. Specifically, Taylor (1987) reported that over one million Americans had used or were using steroids for non-medical purposes. This use is typically designed to increase performance or improve physical appearance. In fact, steroid use among high school students was as common (unfortunately) as the use of crack cocaine. This early use of steroids by high school students was confirmed by a report in the Steroid Trafficking Act (1990), which found that up to 500,000 male high school students use, or have used, steroids, with more than one third starting by the age of 15 and two thirds by 16. More recently (National Institute of Drug Abuse, 2000), the use of anabolic steroids to increase muscular size and strength by high school seniors has been conservatively estimated at 3%. However, the prevalence is typically three to five times

Table 16.3
Common Recreational Drugs and Their Side Effects

Drug	Side Effects	
Alcohol	Feeling of confidence	Emotional outbursts
	Slowed reaction time	Lost inhibitions
	Distorted depth perception	Muscular weakness
	Difficulty staying alert	Decreased reaction time
	Reduced strength and speed	Dizziness
	Mood swings	Liver damage
		Reduced endurance
Marijuana	Decreased hand-eye coordination	Decreased alertness
	Increased blood pressure	Increased heart rate
	Distorted vision	Slowed reaction time
	Decreased physical performance	Decreased mental performance
Cocaine	Physical and psychological addiction	Death from circulatory problems
	Increased strength	Violent mood swings
	Dizziness	Decreased reaction time
	Anxiety	Vomiting
		Hallucination

higher in males than in females (Middleman & DuRant, 1996). However, female use is on the rise.

Along these same lines, research using almost 4,000 male high school students (Whitehead, Chillag, & Elliot, 1992) found that the most common use of drugs was to improve physical appearance, not to improve physical performance. Similarly, Melia, Pipe, and Greenberg (1996) surveyed over 16,000 Canadian students from grades 6–12. They found that approximately 3% of this sample ingested banned substances in attempts to enhance performance, but more important, to improve body build (however, the numbers of athletes reporting steroid use dramatically increases when elite Olympic-level athletes are surveyed, with usage rates sometimes approaching 50%). Therefore, we are not simply looking at steroids or other drugs as performance enhancers; rather, for the general population (at least high school age) exercising aerobically and lifting weights, the more typical reason for using drugs is simply to look better and appear more attractive. Essentially, many of the non-athletes (mostly males) took steroids to become more muscular, not to increase performance, but rather to increase self-esteem and peer approval.

But to be fair, there are other data that suggest that although physical appearance is an important use of steroids by high school students, it isn't the most important. Specifically, in a review of literature (Yesalis & Cowert, 1998), it was found that the main reasons high school students took steroids was to improve performance, enhance physical appearance, quicken injury recover, and fit in socially. However, performance enhancement and physical appearance were by far the two most prevalent reasons for taking steroids.

Because alcohol is the most widely used drug, several studies have focused on its use by athletes. One study found that 55% of high school athletes reported using alcohol in the past year (Green, Burke, Nix, Lambrecht, & Mason, 1996) whereas another study (Carr, Kennedy, & Dimick, 1990) found 92% of high school athletes reporting alcohol use. In college samples, alcohol use was consistent across studies, with reported use being 88% (College of Human Medicine, 1985) and 87% (Evans, Weinberg, & Jackson, 1992). In addition, in most studies, male athletes' use of alcohol was higher than that of non-athletes whereas no differences were found between female athletes and non-athletes in their use of alcohol. Although formal studies are hard to find, anecdotal reports indicate the prevalence of alcohol in exercisers to be similar to that found in athletes, but to reiterate, drug use is an area in which usage estimates must be viewed with extreme caution. Still, the widespread use of legal drugs such as alcohol and tobacco, as well as of illegal drugs such as cocaine and marijuana, has been linked to a host of negative health effects (see Table 16.3).

Likely Causes of Drug Use by Exercisers and Athletes

Exercisers and athletes use drugs for a variety of reasons, and it is important to understand these reasons, so that strategies can be devised to reduce, if not eliminate, the problem. Although a variety of categories of the causes of drug use have been developed, we will group them under three general categories: (a) physical, (b) psychological, and (c) social (see Anshel, 1997, for an extensive review of the causes of drug use).

Physical Reasons

The most common physical reasons for taking drugs are to enhance performance, to look more attractive by building bigger muscles, to cope with pain and injury rehabilitation, and to control weight. Regarding increasing performance, individuals take drugs with the expectation that they can increase their strength, endurance, alertness, and aggression or decrease fatigue, reaction time, and anxiety. However, taking drugs to enhance performance is clearly cheating. Those who take drugs and win must realize that winning is not a sole result of their training and performance, but is, in part, a result of cheating. Even if they are not caught, they'll always know the victory was not their own.

Rehabilitation from injury is another physical reason that individuals take drugs. Physical therapy and rehabilitation are usually not pleasant processes and typically involve a good deal of pain. Along these lines, drugs can attenuate pain and help an individual cope psychologically with the physical discomfort of the injury. In addition, fear of losing a starting position is often a reason that athletes want to rush back from an injury, and they feel drugs can sometimes speed that recovery process. As noted earlier, many exercisers take drugs (especially steroids) simply to look better and to be more attractive to the opposite sex. These individuals are not necessarily interested in performing better; rather, they are more concerned with simply having their bodies look good, strong, and firm. Finally, some individuals take drugs, especially, amphetamines and diuretics, to control appetite and to reduce fluid weight. For example, exercisers take diuretics to help themselves keep slim and trim as reducing fluid weight is much easier than following a strict dietary regimen.

Psychological Reasons

It is extremely common for athletes and exercisers (as well as others) to use recreational drugs for psychological and emotional reasons. These drugs often provide a convenient escape from unpleasant emotions when an individual has trouble dealing with sport, exercise, or personal environment. For example, one consistent finding is the use of drugs to help improve self-confidence. Many people doubt their own skills and abilities even when, from an objective point of view, they are indeed skilled. So resorting to drug use in order to feel more confident about performing optimally or simply looking good does definitely occur. Exercisers constantly seek confidence in the way that they look or in the image that they convey to others. Possibly related to feelings of low self-confidence is one side effect of taking anabolic steroids—increased feelings of aggressiveness (as noted by Chaiken's story above). This aggressive behavior often seen as a side effect of taking steroids can also provide a sense of invulnerability and thus enhance self-confidence (Anshel, 2001).

Another typical psychological use of drugs is related to coping with increased stress and anxiety. Of course, we all feel these emotions at some time or another. However, drug use can act as a means for coping with this stress, especially for exercisers who use exercise as a way to reduce stress (see Chapter 5). For example, some exercisers may have difficulty balancing being away from their family, staying in shape, and still functioning at a high level at home and at work. Sometimes it seems easy to just take a drug to escape temporarily from such anxieties and unpleasant emotions. This might especially be the case if the individual feels that he or she does not have a strong social support system to help talk through the problems they are experiencing.

Related to low self-confidence and increased feeling of stress is a fear of failure that is tied to both exercisers' and athletes' typically strong affiliation between sport/exercise success and self-esteem. Expectations for success from friends, parents, and coaches can often be too high, and drugs are sometimes viewed as a way to combat this source of stress as well as to protect self-esteem. Thus, one of the most important roles of fitness and sport professionals is to enhance participants' self-esteem. By doing so, they can provide an important barrier to substance abuse. Fortunately, sport and physical activities themselves appear to be excellent vehicles for improving self-esteem.

Social Reasons

Social pressures are also important causes for turning to drug use. For exercisers (especially younger exercisers), pressure from peers and the need to gain group acceptance are especially apparent because adolescents usually just want to fit in with their peers. They may drink, smoke, or take performance-enhancing drugs not so much because they want to, but to be accepted by their peers. From a variety of anecdotal reports, it appears that the lure of steroids is often too strong for many adolescents to resist due to the extreme demands on conformity in this age-group. In addition, Martin and Anshel (1991) found that individuals involved in sport were more inclined to choose a peer-prevention assistance strategy to deal with a drug problem of a friend or teammate than to ask parents or coaches to cope with the problem. So finding good friends who accept you for who you are (not what drug you choose) is especially important for adolescents instead of going along with the crowd. This is especially problematic for males who seem to be more prone to "macho behavior" in the desire to fit in with the group. Thus, it is important for teachers, coaches, and athletic trainers to repeatedly communicate the importance of being oneself and not giving in to pressure from so-called friends.

One of the strongest social ways in which behaviors are transmitted from adults to children and adolescents is through modeling. Accordingly, the development of appropriate and inappropriate behaviors in exercisers is often derived from the modeling of their older, more experienced counterparts. Psychologists regard adolescence as a time when young people explore their identity and experiment with drugs, particularly alcohol and tobacco, often developing behavioral patterns that affect the rest of their life (Wragg, 1990).

Athletes, in particular, have become highly visible through television and other media, and many youngsters use these professional, Olympic, and college athletes as role models. Therefore, the development of appropriate as well as inappropriate behaviors in young participants is often derived from watching and reading about their sport heroes. One does not need to be a star athlete to influence the attitudes of adolescents. If someone is working out to stay in shape (even if using drugs to do so), this person still can be seen by the adolescent as a positive role model due to his or her physical stature. Unfortunately, perceptions that exercisers and highly skilled athletes ingest drugs and the mindset that "if it doesn't hurt so-and-so, it won't hurt me" provide an attractive rationale for adolescents to take drugs (Anshel, 2001).

The bottom line is that drug use is often implicitly sanctioned for young people using the professional athlete or regular exerciser as a role model. This modeling effect is particularly influential during adolescence when many youngsters are exploring their identities while being exposed to drugs. Thus, health/exercise professionals and peers, as well as parents and coaches, need to provide appropriate models for youngsters with a focus on personal growth and responsibility.

Sometimes, exercisers and athletes simply engage in the use of drugs (usually recreational) for the purposes of fun or experimentation. Oftentimes, these people do not see the long-term potential negative consequences of their drug use. Attempts at "just one hit" (which is purportedly what Len Bias did with cocaine and he died of an overdose) and denial of any possible addiction to the drug help contribute to the individual's comfort with drug experimentation. This notion of fun and simple experimentation is consistent with the widespread use of drugs (especially those perceived as not really harmful, such as alcohol) in adolescents. Therefore, strong education programs need to be given to youngsters as they consider occasional recreational drug use in their teenage years.

Here are a few quotes which highlight some of the different uses of drugs:

(a) Pain/injury: "The drugs help me recover faster."
(b) Fear of failure: What if the other team takes them and I don't? Who do you think will have the advantage?"
(c) Improve performance: "Drugs help me play more aggressive."
(d) Peer pressure: "It's the 'in' things to do at a party. All the guys do it."
(e) Modeling: "All the pros do it and it doesn't hurt them."
(f) Weight control: "I take pills so I can 'make' (not put on) weight."
(g) Improve strength: "Steroids help me bulk up."

Drugs and Their Effects

Thus far, we have discussed the prevalence of drug use and the reasons for drug use, as well as provided a definition of substance abuse. We have not, however, really discussed the different types of drugs and their effects, both physically and psychologically. Of course, many different classifications have been employed in the past, but for our purposes in the sport and exercise realm, drugs can be classified as (a) *performance-enhancing drugs* and (b) *recreational drugs*. Performance-enhancing drugs include anabolic steroids, beta-blockers, peptide hormones, and stimulants used by athletes or exercisers to increase strength and endurance, reduce fatigue, calm nerves, and increase alertness. In addition, narcotic analgesics (anti-inflammatory drugs) have been used to reduce or block pain, and diuretics have been used to temporarily lose weight. Table 16.4 lists six general categories of performance-enhancing drugs, their potential performance-enhancing effects, and psychological and medical side effects associated with their use.

Recreational drugs (also known as street drugs) are substances that alter the perceptions of incoming stimuli. In general, people seek out and use these drugs for personal pleasure. In addition, they may be trying to escape pressures, to fit in with friends who use drugs, or to look for thrills and excitement that seem to escape them in everyday life. Because these typically inhibit response, decision making, and attentional focus, these drugs generally inhibit rather than

enhance performance. As noted earlier, Table 16.3 lists three common recreational drugs—alcohol, cocaine, and marijuana—and their side effects. Tobacco is another widely used recreational drug associated with negative health effects. Most people know the negative effects of cigarettes and cigars, but smokeless tobacco should not be forgotten, as its use has recently increased in teenage athletic populations. Snuff and chewing tobacco are associated with lip, gum, and other oral cancers.

Prevention/Control of Substance Abuse

The effectiveness of strategies to reduce the probability of drug use in sport and exercise settings is often a function of factors such as the individual's perceived needs for using drugs, the type of drug usage, and the demands of the sport or exercise program, as well as situational factors such as the expectation of others, boredom, and stress. However, it is important to realize that substance abuse is a clinical matter. Therefore, unless we have specific training in this area, sport and fitness personnel are unlikely to be involved in drug treatment programs. As a result, the focus of this section will be on trying to prevent drug use and abuse. Along these lines, some suggestions for helping prevent or at least reduce the probability of drug use are presented below. Before we begin, it should be pointed out that some of the traditional approaches to preventing or reducing drug use have not delivered consistently positive results. For example, a comprehensive study by Tricker, Cook, and McGuire (1989) using almost 10,000 sport/exercise participants found that drug education deterred only about 5% of the regular users from experimenting with drugs, and drug testing and knowledge of punishment deterred 5% of the social users. So it appears that we need more than mere deterrence strategies, and educational strategies should be carefully thought out if they are to be effective. As pointed out in a thorough review of literature by Nicholson (1989), "while distribution of information plays an important consciousness-raising function, it should not be considered as a strategy to reduce the drug use of athletes and exercisers" (pp. 50–51)

Teach Coping Skills

As noted earlier, increased anxiety and stress along with decreased levels of self-confidence and self-esteem can contribute to drug use. One of the techniques that sport and exercise psychologists have employed to help cope with stress and self-confidence issues is the learning of coping strategies. These strategies might include changing negative to positive self-talk; learning relaxation strategies such as progressive

Table 16.4
Major Categories of Performance-Enhancing Drugs in Sport

Stimulants	Various types of drugs that increase alertness, reduce fatigue, and may increase competitiveness	Reduced fatigue, increased alertness, endurance, and aggression	Anxiety, insomnia, increased heart rate and blood pressure, dehydration, stroke, heart irregularities, psychological problems
Narcotic analgesics	Various types of drugs that kill pain through psychological stimulation	Reduced pain	Constricted pupil size, dry mouth, heaviness of limbs, skin itchiness, suppression of hunger, constipation, inability to concentrate, drowsiness, anxiety, physical and psychological dependence
Anabolic steroids	Derivatives of the male hormone testosterone	Increased strength and endurance, improved mental attitude, faster training and recovery rates	Increased risk of liver disease and premature heart disease, increased aggression, a variety of gender-related effects (e.g., infertility in males and development of male secondary sex characteristics in females)
Beta-blockers	Drugs used to lower blood pressure, decrease heart rate, and block stimulatory responses	Steadied nerves in sports such as shooting	Excessively slowed heart rate, heart failure, low blood pressure, light-headedness, depression, insomnia, weakness, nausea, vomiting, cramps, diarrhea, tingling
Diuretics	Used to help eliminate fluids from the tissues (increase secretion of urine)	Temporary weight loss	Increased cholesterol levels, stomach distress, dizziness, blood disorders, muscle spasms, weakness, impaired cardiovascular functioning, decreased aerobic endurance
Peptide hormones and analogues	Chemically produced drugs designed to be chemically similar to existing drugs	Increases strength and endurance and muscle growth	Increased growth of organs, heart disease, thyroid disease, menstrual disorders, decreased sexual drive

relaxation, the relaxation response, and biofeedback; attentional control training; and thought stopping. If sport and exercise participants can learn these techniques, then they will be better equipped to deal with issues of anxiety and self-confidence when they arise.

Help Structure Free Time

Anecdotal and empirical literature has consistently linked excessive and unstructured free time with increased drug use. In this regard, research has revealed that a person's peer group is the single most important source for determining recreational activities, including drug use (Wragg, 1990). Therefore, the peer group is especially important in adolescence, and should be used to help develop healthy alternatives for athletes and exercisers to help them overcome the boredom often associated with taking drugs.

Educate Participants About the Effects of Drug Use

Although, as noted above, mere education is not always the answer to reducing the use of drugs, it can help if this information is delivered effectively. The key here is to be informative and accurate regarding both the negative and positive (performance-enhancing) effects of various drugs. Using examples of high-visibility athletes who have successfully coped with drugs or have managed to stay away from drug use, as well as actually bringing in high-visibility people (especially athletes), can be very helpful and influential. In addition, people who see and hear of drug abuse on a regular basis such as athletic trainers, physicians, and psychologists can also serve as effective speakers.

Set a Good Example

Actions speak louder than words, so coaches and exercise leaders should monitor their own actions and not smoke, chew tobacco, or drink excessively. Such behavior sends a powerful message against the use of drugs. In addition, we should keep winning in perspective and reduce the pressure to win at all costs. The individual who allows performance outcome to supersede the concern for the player's health and welfare is as dishonest and unethical in performing his or her job, as is the individual taking the drugs.

Develop Programs That Have More Severe Sanctions Against Drug Use

At the professional level, besides all the above, policies need to be developed that inhibit the use of drugs Most major sports leagues have some sort of drug pol-

icy that has consequences for athletes using drugs. These policies are listed in the accompanying box. You can see that they vary in terms of severity and as noted earlier, Major League Baseball is proposing stronger sanctions. There is usually a battle with the various players' associations in terms of the severity of these penalties with some people arguing that athletes need to be helped, not punished, for potential drug use. But as one professional baseball player said in regards to the proposed 50 game suspension for first time steroid users, "this will surely eliminate steroids in baseball." Only time will tell if more severe sanctions actually reduced steroid use or if athletes simply find another was to beast the system.

Detection of Substance Abuse

Of course, if we are to help reduce the probability or likelihood of substance use and abuse, then we need to know how to detect the signs and symptoms. Although you have been given some of the effects of the major drug categories, it is useful to list the consistent signs and symptoms of substance use. With these in our arsenal, we might be able to detect a problem before it gets too serious and out of hand. Here are several signs and symptoms that characterize people who are substance abusers:

- Change in behavior (lack of motivation, tardiness, and absenteeism)
- Change in peer group
- Major change in personality
- Major change in athletic or academic performance
- Apathetic or listless behavior
- Impaired judgment
- Poor coordination
- Poor hygiene and grooming
- Profuse sweating
- Muscular twitches or tremors

It is important to note that the presence of these symptoms in athletes and exercisers does not necessarily mean they are substance users or abusers because these symptoms could also reflect other emotional problems. Thus, a fitness professional who observes these symptoms should first talk to the concerned party to validate his or her suspicions. In fact, careful listening is a simple but excellent way to obtain information about substance use and abuse, though it should be noted that hard-core substance abusers are notorious for lying and denying the problem. So, if doubts remain after the initial talk with the individual, confidential advice should be solicited from a substance abuse specialist. A referral process similar to the one described earlier regarding eating disorders should also be followed when dealing with an individual with substance abuse problems.

Exercise Addiction

In Chapter 15, we discussed the notion of the runner's high and the positive feelings that can accompany regular exercise. These positive feelings associated with a desirable activity like running or other aerobic physical activity were originally termed *positive addiction* by Glasser (1976) in his landmark book. In more current terms, this may be seen as more of a "compulsion to exercise" rather than as an "addiction to exercise." In general terms, being positively addicted to exercise means that a variety of psychological and physiological benefits will typically occur as a person continues to participate in regular physical activity, which is seen as important in these people's lives. This involvement represents for them a "healthy habit." However, this "healthy habit" may turn into a dependence on exercise as first seen by the work of Bakeland (1970). Specifically, he had difficulty recruiting regular/habitual exercisers (5–6 days per week) who were willing to abstain from exercise for one month despite being offered substantial amounts of money to do so. So, after having to

settle for 3–4 days a week exercisers, Bakeland found that these participants reported decreased psychological well-being (e.g., increased anxiety, nocturnal awakenings, decreased sexual drive) during the one-month they were deprived of exercise. This was the beginning of the notion that exercise could turn from a positive to a negative addiction.

Definitional Considerations

There is no doubt that the subject of "overexercising" has generated increasing research interest over the past two decades. Much of this interest has emanated from the area of eating disorders discussed earlier, because hyperactivity is a pronounced clinical feature of many patients with this disorder (Davis, 2000). More specifically, studies have consistently found that about 80% of female patients with anorexia nervosa and 50% of those with bulimia nervosa exercise excessively during an acute phase of their disorder (Davis, 1997).

Habitual and excessive exercise is not simply a female phenomenon. Rather, it has been suggested that habitual running is the male analogue of an eating disorder (Yates, Leehey, & Shisslak, 1983). Essentially, motivation for exercising is largely focused on body image and weight concerns, and this is especially seen in people who engage in bodybuilding (Pierce & Morris, 1998). Indeed, a subgroup of bodybuilders has been identified who display a type of body-image disturbance in which there is a pathological fear of being too small and a perception of oneself as weak although actually strong and muscular. In addition, these weight-lifting activities consume huge amounts of time and thus interfere with normal life activities (Pope, Katz, & Hudson, 1993).

Although some excessive exercising might be seen as pathological, exercising with great regularity does not necessarily mean that a person is negatively addicted to the exercise. Unfortunately, much of the research investigating the area of over-exercising has focused on being addicted to exercise, and thus, anyone for whom exercise is a regular habit is often seen as being addicted to exercise. In fact, a recent study revealed that individuals classified as "obligatory runners" scored within the normal range on a series of psychopathological paper-and-pencil measures (Powers, Schocken, & Boyd, 1998). High-level exercising, in fact, may be accompanied by very different levels of functioning. This point was highlighted in the clinical work of de la Torre (1995), who notes that intense exercising can range from a very healthy behavior to one that is seen as pathological and addictive. De la Torre describes three different profiles of exercisers to highlight this continuum. More specifically, there is the "healthy neurotic," whose regular exercising is accompanied by a sense of accomplishment and achievement.

There is the "compulsive exerciser," whose exercising ties into compulsivity needs by providing a strict sense of routine, while providing a sense of control over his or her life. Finally, there is the "exercise addict," whose exercise itself controls and dominates the individual's life, and the exercise is critical to controlling the exerciser's mood and affect. Only in the last case would we really consider it exercise abuse, but classifying these approaches is a difficult task.

To make matters even more complex, a number of terms have been used in the literature to describe various aspects of exercise dependence. In fact, Hausenblas and Downs (2002a) located more than 130 research, review, and popular articles on exercise dependence. In their review they found that exercise dependence research is characterized by three general approaches: (a) comparing exercisers to eating disorder patients, (b) comparing excessive to less excessive exercisers, and (c) comparing exercisers to non-exercisers. Much of the research is inconsistent due to a lack of a clear definition of exercise dependence. As de la Torre (1995) has noted above, these range from terms that would be seen as more pathological, to those that would appear to be more positive in nature. As noted by Carron, Hausenblas and Estabrooks (2003) these include terms such as exercise addiction, obligatory exercise, excessive exercise, chronic joggers, obsessive exercise, fitness fanaticism, habitual runners, negative addiction, and compulsive runners.

In an effort to provide some direction for future research, Hausenblas and Downs (2002b) stated that exercise dependence (addiction) should be defined as

Exercise Dependence Scale

Directions: The questions refer to current exercise beliefs and behaviors that have occurred in the past 3 months.

1	2	3	4	5	6	7
Never						Always

1. I exercise to avoid feeling irritable _____
2. I exercise despite recurring physical problems _____
3. I continually increase my exercise intensity to achieve the desired effects _____
4. I am unable to reduce how long I exercise _____
5. I would rather exercise than spend time with family/friends _____
6. I spend a lot of time exercising _____
7. I exercise longer than I intend _____
8. I exercise to avoid feeling anxious _____
9. I exercise when injured _____
10. I continually increase my exercise frequency to achieve the desired effect _____
11. I am unable to reduce how often I exercise _____
12. I think about exercise when I should be concentrating on school/work _____
13. I spend most of my free time exercising
14. I exercise longer than I expect _____
15. I exercise to avoid feeling tense _____
16. I exercise despite persistent physical problems _____

17. I continually increase my exercise duration to achieve the desired effects _____
18. I am unable to reduce how intensely I exercise _____
19. I choose to exercise so that I can get out of spending time with family/ friends _____
20. A great deal of my time is spent exercising _____
21. I exercise longer than I plan _____

Scoring:

Component	Item Numbers
Withdrawal	1, 8, 15
Continuance	2, 9, 16
Tolerance	3, 10, 17
Lack of Control	4, 11, 18
Reduction in Other Activities	5, 12, 19
Time	6, 13, 20
Intention Effects	7, 14, 21

Categorizing participants into either at-risk for exercise dependence, non-dependent symptomatic, or non-dependent-asymptomatic groups

Individuals who are classified into the dependent range on 3 or more of the DSM IV criteria are classified as exercise dependent

The dependent range is operationalized by a score of 5–6 on that item

The symptomatic range is operationalized by a score of 3–4 on that item

The asymptomatic range is operationalized by a score of 1–2 on that item

a multidimensional pattern of physical activity that leads to significant impairment or distress as manifested by three or more criteria from a list of seven (DSMIV, 1994). These seven criteria are as follows:

(a) Tolerance—Increased physical activity is needed to achieve the desired effect.
(b) Withdrawal—The cessation of exercise produces negative symptoms or exercise is used to prevent these symptoms from occurring.
(c) Intensity—Exercise is undertaken with greater intensity, duration, or frequency than intended.
(d) Lack of control—Physical activity is maintained despite a consistent desire to cut down or control it.
(e) Time—Considerable time is spent in activities essential to physical activity maintenance.
(f) Reduction in other activities—Social, occupational or recreational pursuits are reduced or dropped because of physical activity.
(g) Continuance—Physical activity is maintained despite the awareness of a persistent physical problem (e.g., injury).

In fact, Hausenblas and Downs (2002) developed an Exercise Dependence Scale (see accompanying box) using the DMS IV criteria noted above which provides a reliable and valid measure of the different components of exercise dependence

Negative Addiction to Exercise

As noted above, although there have certainly been numerous reports of positive addiction to exercise, there are, of course, some people for whom exercise starts to control their lives (Benyo, 1990; Davis, 2000). These people develop a psychological or physiological dependence on a regular regimen of exercise that is characterized by withdrawal after 24 to 36 hours without exercise. The withdrawal that accompanies the cessation of exercise might include physiological and psychological symptoms (discussed in more detail later). However, in the long term, cessation of regular exercise can cause personality changes that might remain with the individual until he or she resumes a normal or typical exercise activity.

As Morgan (1979) originally noted, exercise can thus become a negative addiction that eliminates other choices in people's lives. What typically happens to people who become negatively addicted to exercise is that their lives tend to become structured around exercise. For example, home and work responsibilities often take a back seat and suffer due to exercise commitments. It has been noted that negative exercise addiction represents personal and social maladjustment. These symptoms also parallel other addictive behaviors, which are usually characterized by increasing dose dependence and withdrawal symptoms under deprivation.

So how do people originally become addicted to exercise? Typically, the person may start to exercise (usually in adulthood) to derive some health benefits (as noted in Chapter12) such as losing weight or improving physical fitness. In the meantime, due in part to the exercise, the individual starts to feel better about him- or herself, and self-esteem often improves in a dramatic sense. These exercisers develop a sense of control over their bodies that they were not able to gain simply by dieting. This feeling of control over their bodies often generalizes to a sense of control over other parts of their lives. This eventually leads to enhanced feelings of self-confidence and belief in their abilities.

Symptoms of Negative Addiction to Exercise

When people addicted to exercise are asked why they exercise, their answer is not, for example, because exercise is good for them or they enjoy the experience. Rather, they indicate that they participate in exercise because they "have to." Interviews with these people have revealed that they are totally consumed by the need to exercise, as this becomes the main driving point in their lives. In fact, research has also revealed that the person who is addicted to exercise will continue to exercise despite medical, social, or vocational information to the contrary (Adams & Kirkby, 1998; Benyo, 1990; Davis, 2000).

In addition, when individuals addicted to exercise are deprived from regular exercise, they tend to develop a variety of symptoms and these can start as quickly as missing just one day of exercise (Aidman & Wollard, 2003). These symptoms can be categorized as follows:

(a) Affective Symptoms—hostility, anger, guilt, anxiety, decreased self-esteem, depression, sexual tension, frustration
(b) Cognitive Symptoms—confusion, impaired concentration
(c) Social Symptoms—withdrawal from social interactions
(d) Physiological Symptoms—lethargy, decreased vigor, disturbed sleep, tics, muscle soreness, fatigue, gastrointestinal problems

An example of how a regular exerciser might differ from an addicted exerciser is the way to cope with an injury. So, for example, a runner who injures her lower leg might still swim or ride a stationary bicycle. For a true exercise addict, however, a mere substitution is sometimes not enough. As one dedicated runner (who might be considered negatively addicted) said when having to substitute cycling for running due to a tear in the Achilles tendon, "It was like methadone maintenance for a heroin addict." In essence, nothing really substitutes for the desired activity, and if an alternative is found, it sometimes simply continues to promote the negatively addicted behavior. However, work by Morrow (1988) has produced a cognitive-behavioral intervention for exercise dependence where clients are reinforced for gradually relinquishing exercise time to other activities after being assessed and trained in coping skills.

It has been found that individuals negatively addicted to exercise tend to be well-educated individuals. As a result, they often acknowledge and recognize their symptoms and the negative impact the addiction is having on their lives (Sachs & Pargman, 1984). Still, they do not often seek or accept help readily. This is, in part, due to the belief of exercise addicts that exercise adds something special to their lives. So even though the toll of strenuous training shows in a variety of physical and emotional symptoms noted above, exercise addicts continue to exercise and, in fact, make it a priority in their lives. The central role that exercise can play in the life of an exercise addict is aptly captured in the following quote by Sheehan (1979):

> The world will wait. Job, family, friends will wait: In fact, they must wait on the outcome . . . Can anything have a higher priority than running? It defines me, adds to me, makes me whole. I have a job and family and friends that can attest to that. (p. 49)

Ethical Considerations

Throughout this chapter, we have discussed some of the negative aspects of disordered eating, substance use and abuse, and exercise dependence, but we have neglected to confront some of the touchy ethical issues that surround these areas. Borrowing from the work on personal freedom and the meaning of exercise (see Chapter 14), we should ask the question "Should people be free to choose the type and amount of exercise they desire?" The same question might be posed for the use of drugs as long as they are not illegal or banned by a particular sport. The notion of personal freedom and freedom of choice is paramount with regard to people's exercise choices (Fahlberg & Fahlberg, 1997).

It is not the intent to answer the questions posed above, but we should raise the issue that is not often discussed when referring to exercise. That is, should people be allowed to choose the intensity, frequency, duration, and type of exercise, or whether to exercise at all? On the contrary, should some more autocratic exercise leader, using the guidelines developed by research, prescribe how intensely and for how long a person should exercise, offering exercise prescription, and the need for rigid exercise adherence? These exercise "shoulds" need to be balanced against possible limitations on freedom and empowerment for each individual. For example, should a person be allowed to make the choice to exercise every day and maybe risk becoming negatively addicted to exercise? Should certain eating habits be tolerated even though they might appear to be disordered? Thus, before exercise prescriptions are provided, perhaps the notion of personal freedom should be carefully considered.

Summary

This chapter attempted to focus on various addictive behaviors that have plagued sport and exercise participants (as well as others) in recent years. Starting with disordered eating, anorexia nervosa and bulimia are the two most common eating disorders. Although a variety of characteristics are associated with each of these disorders, anorexia nervosa is characterized by an intense feeling of gaining weight and a distorted body image whereas bulimia is characterized by recurrent episodes of binge eating and regular self-induced vomiting. There are many factors that predispose individuals for

---

Avoiding Negative Addiction to Exercise

We have discussed the problem with negative addiction to exercise along with providing some guidelines for recognizing the symptoms of such an addiction. There are also strategies that an exerciser can follow to help guard against falling into the trap of negative addiction.

- Keep the exercise regimen to around 3–4 times a week, maybe 30 to 60 minutes for each bout. In this way, the person can avoid the everyday exercise typical of exercise addicts.

- Train with hard and easy days. Alternating low-intensity with high-intensity workouts can keep the body from breaking down and also keep things in proper perspective.

- Try to find a partner to work out with who is not obsessed with exercise. This will keep the exerciser from becoming overly obsessed and help him or her stay more realistic.

- Make sure to schedule rest days as part of the exercise regimen. This will allow the body to recuperate and keep the person from exercising when hurt and tired.

- When the exerciser is injured, make sure that he or she has fully recovered before beginning to exercise again.

- Set realistic short- and long-term goals.

developing an eating disorder, ranging from those that are more sociocultural to increased peer pressure and factors associated with sport performance itself, such as weight restrictions and standards and judging criteria. It is difficult to obtain accurate prevalence figures, but it appears that athletes and exercisers are more prone to these disorders. In terms of recognizing eating disorders, the signs are both physical (e.g., weight too low, bloating, swollen salivary glands) and psychological/behavioral (excessive dieting, binge eating, preoccupation with food), and knowledge of these symptoms should assist individuals in getting appropriate specialized assistance. A referral system should be set up to help individuals confidentially and professionally deal with eating-related problems.

Substance abuse is typically related to the continued and recurrent use of psychoactive substances in situations that are either physically hazardous or that are detrimental to an individual's personal or professional life. As in eating disorders, although it is difficult to get exact figures regarding the use of certain drugs, we do know that many athletes and exercisers take both performance-enhancing drugs and recreational drugs, and both have dangerous side effects. Along these lines, athletes and exercisers usually take drugs for physical (e.g., enhance performance), psychological (e.g., relieve stress), or social (e.g., ease social pressure) rea-

sons. Although substance use and abuse can be detected by formal procedures such as drug testing, we are in a better position to employ informal procedures such as observation and listening. Therefore, it is important to be able to recognize the signs and symptoms of substance use and abuse. Several ways have been suggested for preventing substance abuse. These include setting a good example, educating participants about the effects of substance use and abuse, and maybe most important, providing a supportive environment that addresses the reasons individuals take drugs. Finally, new more stringent punishments may be put into place on professional teams due to the steroid abuse scandal that has rocked baseball and other sports

The chapter concluded with a discussion of how positive addiction to physical activity might turn into a negative addiction. Although you might see terms such as dependence, compulsion, and obsession, the exercise psychology literature generally refers to the negative impact exercise can have on one's life as negative addiction. There are both psychological and physiological side effects resulting from this addiction, as exercise overshadows other aspects of people's lives, including personal and work relationships. Several symptoms of exercise addiction were noted as well as suggestions helping to guard against the formation of a negative addiction to exercise.

Can You Define These Terms?

amphetamines

anorexia

bulimia

disordered eating

diuretics

negative exercise addiction

performance-enhancing drugs

positive exercise addiction

recreational drugs

steroids

substance abuse

tolerance

Can You Answer These Questions?

1. Define, compare, and contrast anorexia nervosa and bulimia.

2. How do you recognize individuals with eating disorders? (Describe signs and symptoms.)

3. What is the incidence of eating disorders and eating problems with exercisers/athletes?

4. Discuss three predisposing factors that might increase the frequency of having an eating disorder.

5. If you suspect someone has an eating disorder, how would you approach that person with your concern? What should and should not be done?

6. Define substance abuse. What do the data indicate regarding the use of drugs in sport and exercise?

7. Discuss the physical, psychological, and social reasons exercisers and athletes take drugs.

8. Identify the major categories of performance-enhancing and recreational drugs and their reported effects.

9. What are three strategies professionals in our field can use to prevent and detect substance abuse?

10. What signs and symptoms help identify drug abusers?

11. What is the difference between positive and negative addiction to exercise?

12. Describe the symptoms of someone negatively addicted to exercise.

13. Describe the new drug testing program in the different professional sports.

14. The use of steroids is on the increase for young girls. Describe this increase along with the reasons behind the increase.

15. You are hired as a consultant for a collegiate athletic department. Your main job is to devise a program that will reduce drug and alcohol use by athletes on the campus. Discuss in detail the type of program you would implement showing how it relates to the reasons for substance use.

CHAPTER 17

Gender Issues in Exercise

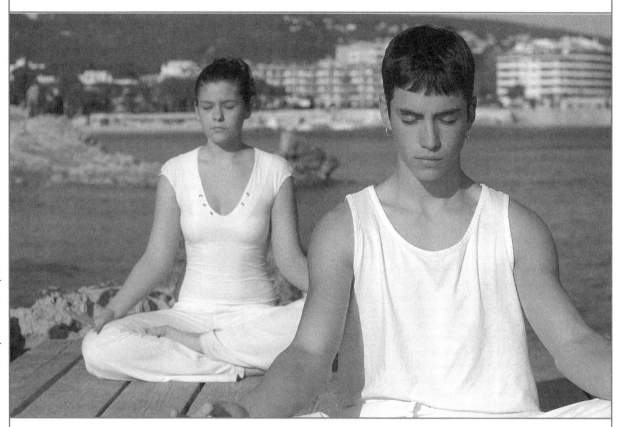

After reading this chapter, you should be able to

- Describe changes in women's opportunities to participate in sport and exercise,

- Identify and discuss gender differences in motivation for exercise,

- Discuss factors that are particularly relevant to participation in exercise by elderly men and women,

- Distinguish between the male and female experiences with body image and weight control,

- Explain the relationship between anorexia nervosa and exercise,

- Define the Adonis syndrome,

- Explain why motherhood can be a barrier to exercise,

- Discuss social physique anxiety as a deterrent to exercise, and

- Explain how exercise influences various feeling states in men and women.

Introduction

The number of women who exercise regularly and compete in organized sports has increased significantly during the past five decades. Dramatic changes in societal values and norms may account for this. Thus, some physical activities that only decades ago were considered inappropriate for females are now acceptable and "par for the course." Until recently, women were not welcome as competitors in 5,000- and 10,000-meter foot races, not to mention the marathon event. Today, they routinely participate in these events at all levels of competition, including the Olympic Games. Women did not play soccer, box, or train with heavy weights until a few years ago. Today, they do and, for the most part, with social approval. Until approximately 30 years ago, women played basketball under rules that were very different from those of today. Even the exercise attire worn now by women is far removed from the long skirts, bloomers, and bathing costumes that inhibited their freedom of movement in previous decades.

Women's Opportunities and Enthusiasm in Exercise

These changes in women's opportunities and enthusiasm for sport and exercise can be considered a result of many factors, including

1. More free time for women and freedom from laborious household chores, to which they were implicitly or explicitly assigned ("women's work"),[1]
2. General relaxation of dress codes,
3. Increased assertiveness of women in their quest for equal opportunity in all areas of life, including sport and exercise,
4. Increased entrepreneurial interest in products, equipment, and facilities used by physically active women, and
5. Improved understanding of the effects of exercise upon females.

To be sure, women have always engaged in recreational and competitive sport at high levels of skill, but only in restricted activities; today, their involvement is in a broader range of activities and is characterized by higher frequencies of participation. Our society has made significant gains in its efforts to provide equal

---

[1] Ironically, women who were able to find freedom from tedious and time consuming household tasks because of technological advancements (such as washing machines), in many cases found it necessary to soon thereafter seek employment outside the home to help make ends meet, thus reducing the amount of available free time.

opportunities for men and women in all aspects of life. Such has not been the case in previous eras of our history. It is unlikely that grandmothers of yesteryear (for example, your grandmother and great-grandmother) participated in aerobic dance, water aerobics, crew, rock climbing, or martial arts. The subservient roles of women, expectations about their achievements, and career options were far different than they are today. Through legislation such as Title IX of the 1972 Education Act and the Civil Rights Restoration Act of 1988, gender parity in educational endeavors has been pursued (Hult, 1999). This, in turn, has had implications for collegiate sport to the extent that many institutions of higher education in the United States now offer organized competitive experiences for women that were simply not available decades ago. And the increase in sport opportunity for women has been reflected in expanded exercise and recreational options. Other recently passed laws are aimed at leveling the playing field in vocational areas.

We have reached a point in our development as a nation where gender inequity is generally considered to be undesirable and unacceptable. However, the notion of equal opportunity does not suggest gender sameness in all dimensions of our being, particularly with regard to anatomical and physiological attributes. As the French say, "*Vive la différence.*" There *are* male-female differences, to be sure; some have little or no bearing upon our interest in exercise, but others are considerably relevant.

Gender Differences and Exercise Behavior

Needless to say, superficial differences exist between men and women. Different structural attributes are apparent. For example, average body weight, skeletal height and framework, amount of stored body fat, cardiac response to rigorous physical activity, and amount of muscle mass are not the same in males and females (Zemra & Rogel, 2001; Clarkson & Hubal, 2001). Males tend to be larger, heavier, and more muscular, and women have approximately 50% to 60% of the average muscle mass of men (Baker, 1987; The & Ploutz-Snyder, 2003). Consequently, men are able to lift a significantly greater amount of weight than women, even when corrections for body mass are incorporated into the comparison (Pincivero, Coelho, & Campy, 2004). Moreover, women expend more energy than men when participating in weight lifting activities despite their overcoming comparable resistances (Pincivero, Coelho, & Campy, 2004). Perhaps less easy to observe with a casual glance are the physiological ways in which males and females differ. Biochemical activity, notably hormonal and metabolic function, vary according to gender (Green, Bishop,

Muir, & Lomax, 2000; Tarnopolsky, Zawada, Richmond, Carter, Shearer, Graham, & Phillips, 2001; Woorons, Mollard, Lamberto, LeTournel, & Richalet, 2005). In addition, sex differences in muscle fatigue have been reported frequently with females generally exhibiting a greater relative fatigue resistance than males (Hicks, Kent-Braun, & Ditor, 2001). Men were observed to run on average 12.4% faster than women in long distances (up to 200 kilometers); the longer the distance, the greater the difference (Coast, Blevisn, & Wilson, 2004). Women reach their peak power more slowly than men, and demonstrate greater fatigability during spring activities, such as cycling (Billant, Giacomoni, & Falgairette, 2003). The latter two functional gender differences may relate to difference in lung volumes, air (oxygen) flow rates, and respiratory control mechanisms (Kilbride, McLoughlin, Gallagher, & Harty, 2003). In these functions, males demonstrate greater capacities than women—both of average fitness levels. However, men exhibit a higher susceptibility to muscle fatigue than females during maximal effort knee extension (Pincivero, Gandaio, and Ito, 2003). This may be due to males having the capacity to execute higher knee extension and torque, and greater amounts of work and expression of power (due most likely to men having greater muscle mass). A host of gender differences have been documented— some impact meaningfully on exercise behavior, and some emphatically do not. One documented gender difference that may have relevance to the domain of exercise and physical activity in general, is the prevalence and severity of self-reported pain (Bingefors & Isacson, 2004). Biological features may partially explain some of the differences, however gender disparities in work, daily living, and expectations between men and women probably account for most.

Many male-female comparisons have questionable bases, and one is tempted to ask why they are pursued in the first place. Therefore, comparative functional achievements and capacities, although of scientific interest, are of modest practical importance (Morgan, Woodruff, & Tiidus, 2003). When contemplating such gender differences, it is helpful to remember that competitively, men and women usually do not oppose one another, although in recreational activities they frequently participate together. In particular is the menstrual cycle (see Case Study 17.1 for scenario). During various phases of the cycle, some females report discomfort associated with bloating, breast tenderness, and distress in the lower back. It appears that cultural stereotypes may influence a woman's expectations about menstruation-related distress, so that women from different parts of the world or from home environments that reflect different cultures may hold different expectations about menstrual discomfort (Anson, 1999; Marvan & Escobedo, 1999; Sveinsdot-

tir, 2000). Presently, we are uncertain as to how a female's perceptions about mood fluctuation possibly affect her motivation to engage in physical activity (Pargman, Urry, & Hutchinson, 2000), but when women report acute menstrual distress, it stands to reason that their perceived readiness for exercise might be compromised. Women in all phases of the menstrual cycle have won medals in the Olympic Games competitions. Thus, while perceptions about discomfort and readiness to perform physically may be negative, actual competitive performance might still occur at a high level.

In law enforcement, firefighting, and the military, it is vital that members of both genders comply with identical standards and confront the same challenges. If a wall is to be scaled, a rope to be climbed, or a heavy weight to be lifted, all participants, whether male or female, may be expected to satisfy the same task demands. At times, gender might exert some influence upon motivation to enter a vocation or profession, but in most cases, its relevance is marginal or largely due to prevailing sociocultural factors rather than physiological or anatomical factors. Gender has

CASE STUDY 17.1

Understanding Menstrual Distress: The Story of Alice

Alice is a member of a women's soccer team that practices three evenings a week and competes on Saturdays in a recreational league. Her premenstrual distress has always been a source of regular discomfort for her. Her symptoms involve a feeling of being bloated and backaches. Some of her teammates are empathetic with her because they also experience similar menstrual distress. They decide to speak with their male coach in order to be certain that he is sensitive to their need for relatively less strenuous activity and enough rest periods. He is a rigorous taskmaster who demands high levels of effort from his athletes during workouts. The women approach the coach after practice one evening and explain their situation. He expresses gratitude for their calling this matter to his attention, saying that he tends not to think about such "women's issues." He assures them that he understands and encourages them to use personal discretion in deciding the level and duration of effort best for them. All's well that ends well.

not been shown to predict success or failure in graduate school or to influence skill in driving a school bus, hanging wallpaper, or operating a computer.

Less ostensible are gender-related psychological differences, some of which appear to be pertinent to sport and exercise participation. Let us now turn to some gender-related attributes that should provide an improved understanding of exercise behavior. In particular, our focus will be upon women. Such comparisons should be meaningful to those who organize, administer, or teach exercise programs insofar as they may bear upon strength of motivation for participation and adherence or avoidance.

Motives for Exercise Participation

In Western culture, concern about body size and shape is more pronounced in women than in men (Markula, 1995). More women are enrolled in the United States in weight-reduction programs and hold memberships in health clubs than men (Arveda, 1991; Bordo, 1989, 1990; Chernin, 1981; Lee & White, 1997; Spitzack, 1990). Most population studies reveal that women, especially middle-aged and elderly women, lead sedentary lives (Stetson, Rahn, Dubbert, Wilner, & Mercury, 1997). Conformity to established models that depict the physically attractive person is emphasized to a greater extent in female exercisers than in males (Spitzack, 1990). Also, women are typically more interested than men in weight regulation (Finkenberg, DiNucci, McCune, & McCune, 1994; Klesges, Mizes, & Klesges, 1987; McDonald & Thompson, 1992). In an attempt to explain this, Markula writes:

> Dieting, thus, is an important part of the disciplinary practices designed to oppress women in this society. The desire to lose weight is maintained through the unobtainable female body ideal: Women are expected to be thin to be considered attractive and accepted in this society. (p. 426)

The very same point is made by Ussher (1989) when she comments about "The perfect body: Achieving the impossible":

> . . . The idea and image of the perfect female body is one which has a pervasive influence on women's consciousness and first creates conflict during puberty. Women in Western cultures are bombarded with images of "ideal" women. An historical analysis will show us that this ideal is wholly socially constructed. . . . As women squeeze, constrict, and pad their bodies in order to comply with some artificial ideal, they are internalizing the message that the natural body is unsightly, not attractive, and needs to be changed. (p. 38)

In this day and age, women are not alone in their quest for the ideal body. Today, men too are availing themselves of cosmetic surgical procedures, hair replacement treatments, and sundry other strategies, in order to conform as closely as possible to idealized standards.

Enhancement of Body Image

Women have lower body-image satisfaction than men, and women are more invested in image attitudes for establishing self-esteem. In other words, as women establish global or overall perspectives of their personal worth, they tend to rely more on perceptions about their bodies (*body image*) than men do. However, women who exercise regularly (e.g., distance running) must deal with lower social approval than men receive (Masters & Lambert, 1989) and, therefore, persevere or overcome greater obstacles than men encounter. More recent data are not yet available, but if the same study were repeated today, it would not be surprising to find that such inequality in social approval has dramatically decreased or no longer exists.

Times are indeed changing. Nonetheless, if exercising women are obliged to meet relatively greater challenges than men, this suggests that women may pursue their exercise program with high levels of intensity—perhaps to the point of exercise dependence. In fact, in one study, women marathon runners reported significantly higher exercise dependence scores than did male runners (Pierce, Rohaly, & Fritchley, 1997). When women do become involved in regular exercise, their commitment tends to be very strong, thereby suggesting a possible link between exercise dependence and gender. However, some published research findings suggest that college males are more likely to experience exercise dependence symptoms than their female counterparts (Hausenblaus & Downs, 2002). On the other hand, in certain kinds of exercise, namely body building, men and women appear to be equally disposed to dependence (Smith & Hale, 2004). It may be that exercise dependence is gender related only in certain activities.

Those who exercise regularly view their bodies more positively and, despite culturally inspired media images of nonmuscular females, women tend to accept muscular shapes (Furnham, Titman, & Sleeman, 1994). In fact, women today increasingly desire not only thinness, but also enough muscularity to appear athletic (Lenart, Goldberg, Bailey, Dallal, & Koff, 1995; Markula, 1995). This is the model (thin/athletic) that today defines the body beautiful and is currently pursued by large numbers of women. It is referred to by Chernin (1981) in the book entitled, *The Obsession: Reflections on the Tyranny of Slenderness*. If and when attained, the body beautiful has, according to Featherstone (1982), *exchange value*. The body beautiful enhances status and enables the perception of youth, health, and happiness. But in the view of Precilla Choi (2003), North American society discourages development of muscularity in women. On the other hand, encouragement is provided to be slender but firm with muscle tone. In a provocative article titled, "Muscle matters: Maintaining visible differences between men and women," Choi argues that even in an activity such as female body building, large muscle development is resisted. As women become more muscular, this resistance becomes greater, since muscularity signifies masculinity and suggests ostensible differences between women and men. According to Choi, this resistance permits the idea of masculinity to be reinforced and time-honored gender stereotyping to be validated. In other words, the woman with large muscular development challenges gender boundaries, which is a clear affront to what Choi refers to as gender order.

Exercise helps us redesign our bodies according to our own image as well as to the societally imposed template. Accordingly, the body carries sociological significance and, as Cole and Stewart (1999) argue, should be an important focus of social scientists as they attempt to understand gender power and politics. According to Maguire and Mansfield (1998), scientists have been remiss in not studying the connection between gender issues—in this case, pursuit of the body beautiful, particularly in females, vis-à-vis factors such as power and their relationship with males. That is, sociologists have ignored the body. Gender relations, according to this perspective, underlie the sociopolitical issues. Thus, to understand the latter, we must get a firm grip on the former. Through exercise, women seek to realign their body shape, empower themselves, and structure their lives. Nonetheless, some evidence exists that women maintain different ideas or *schemas* than men relative to appropriate types of physical activities (Harrison, Lee, & Belcher, 1999).

In a study by Furnham et al. (1994), incentives to exercise varied according to a woman's age, but physical appearance surfaced as an important incentive across all age-groups. As the age of women advances (51–60 years), the most valued exercise incentives were observed to be mental health (e.g., stress management) and affiliation (desire to be with others). In younger women (under 31 years), gaining recognition was reported more frequently than any other reason for exercising. Younger exercisers also reported exercising more as a means to control weight than did the older women in the study (Gill & Overdorf, 1994). Exercise programs for older women should, therefore, emphasize social interaction and stress reduction.

Weight Control

The human form is changeable and can be reshaped, however, exercise will not enable you to increase your skeletal height. The skeletal framework is largely unresponsive to activities such as aerobic dance, swimming, and cycling beyond achievement of maximal maturation. Somewhere between the early and late teen years, we stop growing taller, but fat storage and muscular development (whether our tummies are flat or our waistline is larger than we prefer) are subject to self-regulation. Under most circumstances, through diet and exercise, organically sound individuals can mediate their body's shape and appearance. As Maguire and Mansfield (1998) have so aptly put it, "No-Body's Perfect" (p. 109)—that is, when inspecting and evaluating our physical selves, most of us see room for improvement. Therefore, many of us seek to alter what is perceived as undesirable or unattractive physical characteristics.

The desire for small hips and thighs remains very popular, at least among college women (Lenart et al., 1995), and in North American society the desire to lose weight is considered normative (Cash, Novy, & Grant, 1994) or prevalent among women. In other words, in contrast to men, women exercise more for reasons related to weight concern and appearance

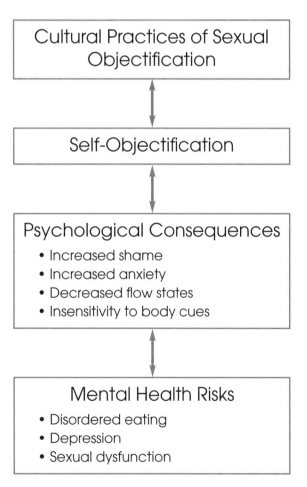

Figure 17.1. Objectification Theory Model (Noll & Frederickson, 1998

(Finkenberg et al., 1994). Although dieting is also prevalent among normal-weight individuals, it is primarily a female phenomenon (Biener & Heaton, 1995), particularly in the American culture. Women especially tend to adopt perspectives about their bodies as held by others. That is, their body image is influenced by others. *Self-objectification* is the term that refers to an experience unique to women and girls and has implications for important psychological consequences. Self-objectification is believed to increase self-monitoring and bear upon:

(1) increased body shame,
(2) increased appearance anxiety,
(3) decreased experiences of flow states, and
(4) decreased sensitivity to internal body states (Greenleaf & McGreer, 2004).

The objectification model is presented in Figure 17.1. Negative perception and body dissatisfaction about the body are enduring and tend to be more common in women than in men (Tiggemann & Ruutel, 2001). Body dissatisfaction has been shown to be stable across age, but consequences of these perceptions such as frequent weighing, high levels of anxiety about the body, and disordered eating tend to decrease with age.

Sexual lifestyle may also interact with weight concern. Lesbians as well as heterosexual women report greater concern with body weight, more body dissatisfaction, and greater frequency of dieting than do gay and heterosexual men. Both lesbian and heterosexual women are influenced by cultural pressures to be thin, but these pressures appear to be greater for heterosexual women (Brand, Rothblum, & Solomon, 1992). Female dieters are also younger than nondieters and are not necessarily overweight. Another observation worth considering is that those involved in programs of restricted food intake for purposes of losing body weight may not be overweight or overfat. This may relate to the tendency of women to distort their own body image to a greater extent than men do (Fallon & Rozin, 1985; Hallinan, Pierce, Evans, DeGrenier, & Anders, 1991). In addition, women are inclined to assess their physical appearance incorrectly (i.e., concluding that they are overly fat or thin when objective measurements reveal otherwise). However, such perceptual misjudgments may be corrected, and certain exercise programs, notably weight training programs, have beneficial influences on body image (Tucker & Mortell, 1993) and self-esteem (Brown & Harrison, 1986).

Anorexia nervosa. In Chapter 16, anorexia was discussed from the perspective of "The Female Triad"—anorexia, amenorrhea, and osteoporosis—three exercise concerns associated with females. Here, we ask you to consider anorexia in terms of gender issues, because it is generally associated with females. We dis-

cuss it briefly as we focus upon differences between male and female exercisers.

Anorexia nervosa entails exaggerated limitation of food intake and often, obsessive participation in rigorous exercise (Klein et al. 2004). This illness is a life-threatening condition that occurs in women more often than in men. However, recently, a form of body dysmorphia referred to as "*Adonis Syndrome*" or "*Adonis Complex*" has received attention (Andersen & Mehler, 1999; Pope, 2000). This condition involves exaggerated dissatisfaction with body size as perceived by males. The "Adonis" is convinced of insufficient muscle mass and strives through unusual devotion to weight training to "get bigger, and bigger, and bigger."

Males also fall prey to disordered eating, apparently in the same way as females (Harvey & Robinson, 2003). In their study of 25 men who met the DSM IV criteria, Olivardia, Pope, Mangweth, and Hudson (1995) observed that "eating disorders, although less common in men than in women appear to display strikingly similar features in affected individuals of the two genders" (p. 1279). Among high school, university, and elite track and field athletes, disordered eating patterns were found to be significantly more prevalent among girls than boys (Hausenblas & McNally, 2004).

As is apparently the case with anorexic women (Hudson, Pope, Jonas, & Yurgelun-Todd, 1983; Gershon et al., 1984), men with disordered eating patterns were found to have had a higher rate of major mood disorder than men who were not anorexic.

Anorexia nervosa has been discussed in medical circles for more than 200 years. It involves abnormal eating behaviors that result in maintenance of body weight at a level beneath 85% of body weight considered desirable for height and age. Also involved is an intense fear of gaining weight or becoming obese. Consequently, anorexic persons are determined not to eat. In women, distorted perceptions of the body are also associated with this eating disorder (Reel & Gill, 1996). It is common for anorexics to complain about being too fat when, in truth, their physical appearance clearly suggests emaciation. *The Diagnostic and Statistical Manual of the Mental Disorders* (DSM IV; American Psychiatric Association, 1994) also lists low self-esteem, depression, perfectionism, and high need for achievement and approval as characteristics of the condition.

Anorexia not only involves unusual eating patterns, but also often a stubborn commitment to grueling exercise that contributes to dangerous loss of body fat, significant loss of muscle mass, and other symptoms such as loss or decrease of libido and abnormal absence or infrequency of menstruation (Romeo, 1993). Adolescent females seem to be at high risk for anorexia because this period involves separation from the nuclear family. As they attempt to cope with feelings of ineffectiveness and powerlessness (C. Johnson & Tobin, 1991), adolescents may exhibit discipline over food intake (Garner & Garfinkel, 1986). In this way, many adolescent girls seek to establish control over their environment (McDonald & Thompson, 1992). There is some evidence that depression is a causal factor among female college students with eating-disordered behaviors. To combat feelings of helplessness associated with negative body image and perceptions of high body-image importance, the eating behaviors of depressed females become disordered (Koenig & Wasserman, 1995). Anorexia may be a consequence. The results of untreated anorexia nervosa (starvation) are often severe, resulting in renal and cardiac complications or even death. By no means is disordered eating restricted to young or college age women. Recent findings indicate that these conditions are occurring with greater frequency in women in middle and late life (Zerbe, 2003).

It may be convenient to describe anorexia as a condition that involves "abnormal" patterns of eating, but a concise definition of "normal" in this context is elusive. Normality, in this case, may best be understood as being person specific. What is appropriate, best, or most healthful for one woman may not be for another. Therefore, deviant patterns of eating are not easy to identify, no less understand. Suffice it to say that many women who are not eating disordered (so-called normal women) may have patterns of behavior and attitudes about eating and their own body weight, as well as views of appropriate frequency and intensity of exercise, that overlap with those of anorexic women (Bunnell, Cooper, Hertz, & Shenker, 1992; Delaney, O' Keefe, & Skene, 1997). It is difficult to draw a clear line between the anorexic and nonanorexic person. In offering their diagnosis, competent clinicians should take into consideration individual as well as cultural, familial, and other contextual factors. Anorexia is a complex and problematic disease. Its diagnosis requires considerable tracing, experience, and insight.

Socioeconomic status and weight control. An interesting link may exist among socioeconomic status (SES), prevalence of dieting, and vigorous exercise for high school girls (but not for boys). Girls coming from more affluent homes seem to be more inclined to diet and participate in exercise. A positive correlation has been observed between each of these two variables and SES of the family (Drenowski, Kurth, & Krahn, 1994). Higher SES was also associated with lower current and desired body weight in both boys and girls. However, girls of higher SES may have greater access to weight-loss programs, health club memberships, and medical care. Thus, they may be identified more often in surveys that investigate such frequencies.

Variation of Exercise Motives With Age

Research into motivation for exercise participation among elderly women has not been extensively conducted. One study by Cousins (1995) concluded that among women aged 70–98 years, social support seems to account for a large share of motivation for exercise. The motives for entering programs of physical activity in elderly sedentary women differ from those of men (Rowland, et al., 2004), however, desire for thinner body shape and physical health and fitness are the most important motives for both (Schuler et al., 2004). Friends and family members were found to be good sources of support (Gill & Overdorf, 1994). Another factor that predicted late-life involvement for female elderly exercisers was childhood encouragement of sport activities (Gill & Overdorf, 1994). Evidently, the nature and intensity of the exercise that elderly women are involved in presently are predictive of the degree to which they will enter and adhere to an exercise regimen in the future. The extent to which they participated in childhood sports is also a good indicator of involvement and compliance. Apparently, childhood sport experiences provide a measure of comfort with physical activity that makes participation in later years attractive, or at least acceptable. Much evidence has been recently forthcoming from gerontologic studies supporting the desirability of elderly men's and women's engagement in regular aerobic as well as resistance exercise (see chapter 19). Suffice it to say that gender differences do not appear to prevail with regard to maintenance of positive self-esteem in older age regular exercisers (65 years and over). In a study by Lampinen and Heikkinen (2002), physically active men and women reported fewer depressive symptoms than their sedentary counterparts at both baseline and follow-up across a variety of physical activities. However, in aged women (65 and older) mental stress responses have been shown to be more pronounced than in young women (Bakke et al., 2004). This suggests a need for caution when leading exercise programs for elderly women, lest their motivation and adherence be compromised.

Deterrents to Exercise

Some factors that tend to inhibit exercise participation in women have also been identified. Let us discuss two of them here: motherhood and social physique anxiety.

Motherhood. Women who have children exercise less than women who do not (Deam, 1982; Verhoef & Love, 1992; Woodward, Green, & Hebron, 1989)—particularly those who are younger than 40 years of age. Moreover, mothers participate with less intensity, frequency, and duration (Verhoef & Love, 1994) when they do engage in exercise. This is most often due to a lack of time, as reported frequently by mothers; a lack of energy may also deter a mother from exercise participation (C. A. Johnson, Corrigan, Dubbert, & Cramling, 1990). In their analysis of more than 13,000 American men and women, Nomaguchi and Bignchi (2004) found that married adults spend less time exercising than unmarried adults, and that having children at home is negatively correlated with exercising. In general, women spend less time exercising than men. Perhaps adequate time for regular exercise is available to women with families if their time management skills could be scrutinized or adjusted. Some women have been shown to harbor misperceptions about time available to them for physical activity (Heesch & Masse, 2004). Despite their reported lower levels of exercise participation, mothers do not differ from women without children with regard to perceived benefits of exercise. This suggests that mothers, although not able to exercise as much as they wish, nonetheless understand the value of participation. Motherhood itself is a barrier to exercising, but the number of children does not further influence this tendency to refrain from exercising; that is, four or five children are no greater obstacles to participation in regular exercise than are two or three (Verhoef & Love, 1994).

Stress. Men and women typically report the same frequency of exposure to stressful events; however, women react to such experiences with greater distress (Solomon & Rothblum, 1986). The very same stressors seem to affect men and women differentially and some evidence suggests that women cope with stressful events less effectively. They tend to use less active, more avoidant strategies than men, whose strategies have greater problem-focus (Solomon & Rothblum, 1986). Hypertension, a major risk factor for heart disease, stroke, and heart failure, increases in prevalence during aging more so in women than in men. Some elderly women have higher blood pressures than men (Hirao-Try, 2003). Prescribed programs of exercise may be helpful to large numbers of elderly women. During times of elevated stress perception (i.e., time pressure, wherein women felt obliged to complete tasks or get things done), exercise adherence decreased. Also, self-efficacy for exercise—that is, the perceived ability to meet upcoming exercise goals—decreased during times of high frequency of stressful events (Stetson et al., 1997). Self-efficacy influences motivation to exercise and will affect mood or emotion associated with it. But

Photo courtesy of © iStockphoto.com

exercise itself may be used to manipulate future assessments of readiness to participate. This was found to be the case in college age women, who when given various kinds of bogus feedback changed their levels of exercise self-efficacies. Their beliefs about their ability to satisfy exercise-related challenges were altered (McAuley & Talbot, 1999).

A note of caution to leaders of exercise programs may be in order. When exercise expectations stemming from inflated self-efficacies in sedentary women are very high and therefore unfulfilled (exercisers reveal an unpreparedness to satisfy task demands), then participants tend to stop exercising or drop out (Sears & Stanton, 2001).

Social physique anxiety. Another inhibiting factor for women is social physique anxiety (SPA). Crawford and Eklund (1994) and Eklund and Crawford (1994) apply this term to feelings of discomfort related to doubt about one's ability to make a desired impression on others. Those who score high on a measure of SPA (i.e., on the Social Physique Anxiety Scale by Hart, Leary, & Rejeski, 1989) tend to be apprehensive about evaluation of their bodies in real or imaginary settings. They, therefore, prefer to exercise in private, rather than public, locations (Spink, 1992). Socioeconomic factors may influence the formation of body image and self-esteem in both men and women. In a study by Snooks and Hall (2002), socioeconomic differences were observed to be more important than ethnic background. Social physique anxiety scores are typically higher in women than in men (Eklund, Kelly, & Wilson, 1997; Frederick & Morrison, 1996; Lantz, Hardy, & Ainsworth, 1997). And sedentary women exercising in front of a mirror reported more negative affect and low exercise efficacy than women in a nonmirrored condition. Those watching themselves perform were significantly less sanguine about their participation (Ginis, Jung, & Gauvin, 2003).

We all desire social approval from others. One source of such recognition is through the presentation of a desirable appearance. Women seek this approval more than men do and experience anxiety when realizing that it may not be forthcoming. This, in turn, may influence them to desist from exercising or refrain from exercising in certain environments. In their sample of 104 women, Crawford and Eklund (1994) observed SPA to be a deterrent to exercising in some settings; that is, if required to exercise when the expectancy for negative response from others about their bodies was high, women in this study experienced anxiety. This suggests that self-presentational concerns, such as SPA, may be a deterrent for exercise participation. It explains why some women are hesitant to enter organized programs of physical activity. Some evidence suggests that women tend to score lower than men on instruments that measure personal satisfaction with the body (*cathexis*). As mentioned previously in this chapter, women focus more on their body weight than men do, and women are also more concerned with lower body parts, such as the thighs, stomach, and hips, than men are (Salusso-Deonier & Schwartzkopf, 1991). Obese women, in particular (both young and old), score higher than nonobese females on SPA (Hart et al., 1989; McAuley, Bane, Rudolf, & Lox, 1995; Spink, 1992; Treasure, Lox, & Lawton, 1998). However, as women age, their scores decrease, thereby suggesting that they expect to become heavier. Perhaps being overweight is more readily acceptable with aging.

On the other hand, a study employing elderly women (ages 70–98 years) revealed that participants who do exercise have more positive views of their own bodies and increased acceptance of muscular body shapes, even though this muscularity diverges from cultural ideals (Furnham et al., 1994). This seems to also be true for younger women as well as for men (Doan & Scherman, 1987; Tucker, 1985). Exercise leaders would do well to attend to their clients' concerns about personal body size and shape because these perceptions may bear heavily upon entry and adherence to the regimen. In addition, they should anticipate a change in their clients' cathexis as a result of participation in an exercise program.

Effects of exercise on women. Is the affective response of women to exercise different from that of men? Results from several studies conducted during the past 10 years suggest that the answer is "yes." However, to adequately understand this issue, familiarity with a number of relevant variables is necessary—namely, exercise dose, baseline feelings of subjects, and feelings of subjects during exercise (Rejeski, Gauvin, Hobson, & Norris, 1995). An inappropriately heavy exercise prescription may generate negative feelings in participants who previously enjoyed physical activity. In other words, too much of a good thing may be bad. Similarly, what the exerciser is thinking while exercising may influence her affective responses to the exercise. If while exercising, one's thoughts center upon frustrating or irreconcilable personal issues, such as financial burdens or relationship problems, the exercise experience may acquire negative overtones and be perceived and reported as a negative experience. Neither age nor menopausal status seems to relate to the beneficial psychological effects of exercise upon women (Pierce

& Pate, 1994; Pronk, Crouse, & Rohack, 1995; Slavin & Lee, 1994). In general, the psychological responses to exercise in women, often assessed by use of the Profile of Mood States (POMS; McNair, Lorr, & Droppleman, 1971), are positive (Slaven & Lee, 1997).

It is possible to extend one's exercise commitment to the extent that dependency upon it develops. Such a condition entails difficulty in disengagement, or not exercising, even when circumstances indicate the appropriateness of doing so. College age men report more exercise dependent behavior than female counterparts (Hausenblas & Downs, 2002). However, it appears that among competitive runners, this is not the case. One fairly recent study was unable to conclude that a difference in running dependence exists between male and female athletes (Kjelsas & Augestad, 2003). Perhaps many (or at least some) of the psychological gender differences observed in sedentary or recreational exercisers are non-existent in highly trained competitive athletes.

Mood alteration associated with exercise is discussed in detail in Chapter 4, where a considerable amount of available evidence linking physical fitness (a consequence of exercise) to mental health is reviewed. Chapter 4 also discusses the mood-enhancement effect of acute bouts of exercise (single, short-term bouts). Because the current chapter addresses women in exercise, a brief comment about the therapeutic effect of exercise upon an unhealthy mental condition, namely clinical depression, is in order. The term *clinical depression* is used to describe persons who worry often and who are preoccupied with things that might go wrong. Clinically depressed individuals are not "down" sporadically or occasionally, but spend long periods of time in this mental framework. Hospitalization is frequently indicated for this serious condition.

It appears that two groups of moderately to severely depressed 18- to 35-year-old women, assigned to either a running or weight-lifting program, experienced a significant reduction in depression without changing their fitness levels (Doyne et al., 1987). Because the fitness levels of the women in this study remained unchanged after 4 weeks (four exercise periods per week), it was concluded that factors other than organic or physiologic improvement were causally related to the significant reduction in depression. Moreover, the reduced depression was sustained throughout a one-year follow-up period. The authors speculate that these striking results may be causally related to a sense of accomplishment and improved self-efficacy that accompanied observable improvements in running or weight-lifting performance. In other words, a feeling of success or accomplishment may explain the observed reduction in depression. No changes were observed in a control group of subjects. Whether these outcomes would also be forthcoming in a sample of males, or older or younger females, remains to be seen. To date, results from a few studies indicate that women may respond more strongly than men in terms of short-term mood benefits (Berger & Owen, 1987; Friedman & Berger, 1991).

Finally, in a study using young adult male and female subjects randomly assigned to a jogging treatment, a bout of jogging was shown to be as effective as the relaxation response for acute reductions of tension, depression, and anger (Berger, Friedmann, & Eaton, 1988).

A second related question: What is the proper exercise prescription for modifying mood? Typically, highly trained individuals respond more positively to more demanding exercise (Farrell, Gustafson, Morgan, & Pert, 1987). That is, the psychological effects of exercise interventions appear to be influenced by level of fitness as well as volume of activity in both males and females. Understandably, the runner who is highly aerobically fit is likely to evaluate a short, slow jog as pleasurable. In contrast, the unfit person would consider the same experience to be taxing and, therefore, very unpleasant.

Exercise is also apt to alter mood to greater extents in participants whose pre-exercise affect was at low to moderate levels. In women, an overly demanding intervention may have a negative impact on psychological states following the activity (Steptoe & Cox, 1988). Moreover, the feelings occurring in women during physical activity as well as their psychological states will bear upon the mental health consequences of exercise. Women with relatively more positive thoughts during exercise reported the highest scores in what Rejeski (1994) referred to as "revitalization" after exercise: "In other words, feelings towards an exercise stimulus are an important aspect in understanding how physical activity influences psychological well-being" (p. 358).

This, therefore, suggests that pre- and mid-exercise affective and cognitive conditions bear not only upon how the exerciser feels about having participated, but also upon the overall feeling states as well. Because women tend to react to emotion-inducing events with greater intensity than men do (Larsen & Diener, 1987), vigorous physical activity that stimulates heightened feelings of pain, discomfort, joy, or pleasure may very well elicit comparatively higher levels of affective response. Exercise leaders as well as participants should understand this in order to establish or sustain optimal exercise regimens.

Summary

Today, women have much more opportunity and social approval to exercise regularly and rigorously than they did a few decades ago. More women than men are enrolled in weight-reduction programs and are members in health clubs. Among numerous reasons for this is that women are more inclined to conform to established models that portray physically attractive people. Women exercise more for reasons related to appearance than men do.

Anorexia nervosa is a disorder that involves deviant eating patterns and sometimes obsessive adherence to exercise regimens. This disorder results in dangerous weight loss, significant loss of muscle tissue, and other negative consequences. Adolescent girls are at high risk for anorexia.

Social support seems to be an important source of motivation for elderly women to exercise. The degree to which they participated in childhood sports is a good predictor of exercise involvement in their elderly years.

Motherhood appears to be associated with lower levels of exercise participation. A lack of time and energy often cause a mother to refrain from exercise. However, women who have children and engage in exercise still appreciate the benefits it produces.

Social physique anxiety may also be a factor in deterring some women from involvement in organized programs of physical activity. Social physique anxiety refers to discomfort associated with insecurity about having the ability to impress others in a positive way.

The way in which women respond emotionally to exercise is contingent upon a number of factors, including level of fitness, volume and intensity of activity, and pre-exercise affect (feelings). Yet another factor—one that requires additional research—is that women rely more than men on body image as they determine personal worth.

Can You Define These Terms?

Adonis syndrome

anorexia nervosa

body cathexis

body image

exchange value

social physique anxiety

Can You Answer These Questions?

1. Identify three factors that have led to improved exercise opportunities for females.
2. Why are more women enrolled in weight-reduction programs than are men?
3. Do motives for women to exercise vary according to age? Explain.
4. What is social physique anxiety?
5. In addition to unusual eating patterns, what other signs are present in anorexia nervosa? Why are adolescent girls, in particular, at risk for this condition?
6. Does participation in exercise always generate positive feelings in women? Explain.

CHAPTER 18

Children and Youth in Exercise

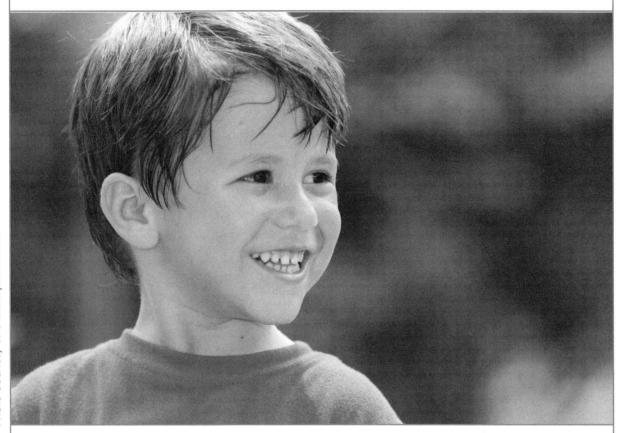

After reading this chapter, you should be able to

- Discuss reasons why it is important for children to exercise with vigor and regularity,

- Identify important motives for children's participation in regular physical activity,

- Discuss adult responsibilities in motivating children to exercise,

- Offer explanations for children's dropping out of exercise programs,

- Identify some age and gender differences in children relative to their participation in physical activity, and

- Discuss approaches for assessing the amount and intensity of exercise participation among children.

Introduction

Words such as "youth," "child," "adolescent," and, of course, the popular term "kid" typically denote a specific age range. They all refer to young individuals. But how young? Are high school seniors still children? At what age does one graduate from childhood? Such questions are not easily answered. Researchers operationally define these terms in order to specifically describe the age of their subject sample. One unfortunate result is that much variation in these operational definitions exists among the many published studies dealing with youth and children. In some studies, high-school-aged boys and girls are referred to as youth; in others, the same is true of college-aged students. Thus, these popular terms may be applied to 14- as well as 18-year-olds. A similar type of confusion may also exist when the word "adult" is used. Drinking age, driving license privileges, eligibility to vote, and joining the armed services are supposedly indicative of adulthood, yet they vary considerably, and the ages associated with them often overlap with ages implied by the terms "children," "youth," and "kids."

Nonetheless, in this chapter, we attempt to clarify issues related to socialization or entry into programs of physical activity, adherence to programs, and dropping out. We elaborate upon why children, youth, kids, or whatever term we happen to use (we use them all) should participate in exercise; why all too many do not; and why they often disengage from it after being involved.

Physical Activity in Children and Adolescents

Physical activity is important throughout the entire life span but is particularly critical during childhood and adolescence for two reasons: (a) it contributes to maintenance of normal growth and development (Bar-Or, 1983) and (b) it establishes lifestyle patterns that will reduce risk factors for health problems in later life (Baranowski et al., 1992). Other benefits are also gained from exercise. Adolescents involved in regular programs of physical activity are less likely to use cigarettes than those who are not involved (Aaron et al., 1995). Also, academic performance (Dwyer, Blizzard, & Dean, 1996; Shephard, 1996b) and creativity (Pargman & Abry, 1997; Tuckman & Hinkle, 1986; Herman-Tofler & Tuckman, 1998) have been observed to be positively related to physical activity in children.

However, the predictive strength of physical activity participation in childhood and adolescence upon similar behaviors in adulthood appears to vary according to age range, gender, and nationality of subjects studied (Anderssen, Wold, & Torshheim, 2005). Exercise participation in children and their level of fitness vary considerably as predictors of adult exercise behavior, although moderate predictive strength has been observed on a year to year basis from early to late childhood. What is disturbing is the conclusion from a number of studies that participation in regular physical activity seems to decline in adolescence (Casperson, Pereira, & Curran, 2000; King & Coles, 1992; Riddoch et al. 2004). In addition, an overview of the literature unfortunately reveals weak or moderate support for the popular contention that generally physically active children become physically active adults (Trudeau, Laurencelle, & Shephard, 2004). However, physical fitness status of children seems to predict physical activity levels in young adulthood (Dennison, Strauss, Mellits, & Charney, 1988).

Children with various physical and psychosocial disabilities benefit from participation in exercise and sport (Dykens, Rosner, & Butterbaugh, 1998). Active arm exercise undertaken by 9- to 12-year-olds with spina bifida—a disease involving the spinal cord—produced significant increases in peripheral vision and various forms of learning (Krebs, Eickelberg, Krobath, & Baruch, 1989). The authors who reported these findings speculated that exercise may increase

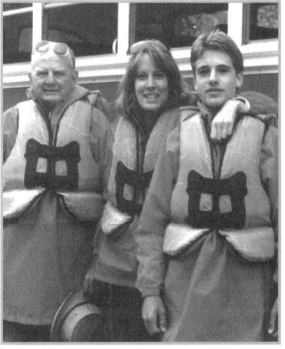

Photo courtesy of Bonnie Berger

blood flow through the lungs, allowing greater oxygen diffusion in the brain, which results in more effective cerebral activity. In another study, educable mentally retarded children were shown to improve their reaction time after participating in a Taekwondo program three times a week for 7 months (Song & Ah, 2004).

Participation in the Special Olympics has resulted in positive changes in perceived self-confidence (Gibbons & Bushakra, 1989) and self-concept (Wright &

Cowden, 1986) among children with mental retardation. As noted in Chapter 4, perceptions about the self are central and critical aspects of our psychology. They relate importantly to well-being and to motivation for a wide variety of activities for interpersonal behavior. In late childhood (years 8–12), comparison with others becomes an important element of the self. (And in early adolescence, these comparisons tend to be most negative [ages 12–14; Linfunen, 1999]). Academic performance has been shown to improve among autistic children who participated in aerobic exercise (Rosenthal-Malek & Mitchell, 1997; Schultheis, Boswell, & Decker, 2000). Some of the stereotyped behaviors (repetitive nonfunctional behaviors such as rhythmic rocking, repetitive jumping, or arm flapping) of autistic children have also been lessened as a consequence of jogging (Levinson & Reid, 1993).

Thus, exercise has proven beneficial for a multitude of youth populations. Yet, there is a marked decline in physical activity with age (Casperson & Merritt, 1995; Telama & Yang, 1999; Van Mechelen, Twisk, Post, Snel, & Kemper, 2000). As we advance chronologically, we tend to be less active.

Play Versus Exercise

Children at play have been studied intensely by scientists for decades. The renowned developmental psychologists Jean Piaget (1932/1965) and Lawrence Kohlberg (1981) understood that play reveals much about the child's moral and cognitive development. However, as discussed in Chapter 1, *play* and *exercise* are not the same. Play does not necessarily incorporate gross motor activity, which is a required component of exercise. Playing house, building sand castles, and making mud pies are playful activities that do not tax the cardiorespiratory mechanisms of the organically healthy child. On the other hand, rigorous physical activity involving large muscle groups is often included in many play activities (Rosenbaum, 1998). Playing "army," "cowboys," or "roughhouse" requires running, fake combat, leaping, and crawling. Many young children find considerable pleasure in such activities. They enjoy running, jumping, spinning, falling, and climbing. Although distinct, play and exercise may overlap in some ways (see Figure 18.1).

Play and exercise often share the element of enjoyment and the requirements of adequate physiological and motor readiness for participation. However, a play experience may not have strategy, rules, or purpose; play is often unscheduled and may happen irregularly or only occasionally. Conversely, exercise, when pursued properly, is done with regularity. An individual bent on deriving the benefits of exercise participates in a specified fashion on a predetermined schedule during prescribed periods of time, with predetermined numbers of repetitions, and against carefully selected levels of

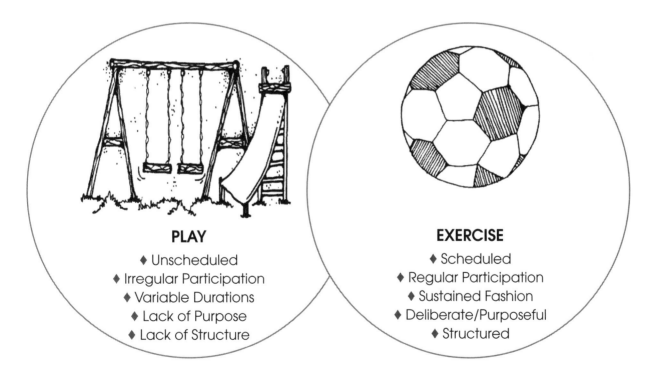

PLAY
- ◆ Unscheduled
- ◆ Irregular Participation
- ◆ Variable Durations
- ◆ Lack of Purpose
- ◆ Lack of Structure

EXERCISE
- ◆ Scheduled
- ◆ Regular Participation
- ◆ Sustained Fashion
- ◆ Deliberate/Purposeful
- ◆ Structured

Figure 18.1. Play versus exercise.
Play and exercise do overlap in some ways, sharing the elements of enjoyment and motor readiness. However, they are distinct and are characterized by different factors.

resistance (as with weight training). To contribute to increased fitness, exercise must be sustained and continuous. Unfortunately, many children who do exercise do not comply with these requirements. The National Children and Youth Fitness Study (Dotson & Ross, 1985; Ross, Dotson, Gilbert, & Katz, 1985; Ross & Gilbert, 1985) concluded that although 82% of 5th through 12th graders in the United States participated in physical activity, only 41% were exerting themselves enough to enhance cardiorespiratory functioning. Parcel et al. (1987) observed that in elementary school physical education classes, students spent only about 6% of class time (less than 2 minutes per 30-minute class) in vigorous, fitness-inducing activity. This is not to suggest that students were entirely inactive 94% of class time—however, a very limited amount of time was devoted to activities of adequate vigor.

Inactivity During Childhood

Children today are not particularly physically active, at least not to the extent that many adults assume they are. And these less than desirable levels of physical activity are not restricted to children in the United States (Elliott, 2004). Canadian, Japanese, Cypriot (Loucaides, Chedzoy, Bennett, & Walshe, 2004), European (Riddoch, Andersen, WedderKopp, Harro, Klasson-Heggeboe, Sardiviah, Cooper, & Ekelund, 2004), and Australian (Barnett, VanBeurden, Zask, Brookes, & Dietrich, 2002) children are also participating in physical activity at less than desirable frequencies, durations, and intensities. Today, school-aged children have more body fat and weight than in previous decades (Corbin & Pangrazi, 1992; Yoshinaga, Shimago, Koriyama, Nomura, Miyata, Hashiguchi, & Arima, 2004). Obesity is also likely to impose a harmful psychological burden on children related to social stigma. Moreover, participation declines dramatically in adolescence (Kann et al., 1996; Myers, Strikmiller, Webber, & Berenson, 1996; Pate, Long, & Heath, 1994; Sallis, 2000a; U.S. Department of Health and Human Services [USDHHS], 1996) so that an improvement in the aforementioned percentages is not forthcoming after the passing of elementary and middle school years. Some studies conclude that this decline is more marked in females than in males; boys are consistently shown to be more active than girls (Casperson, Pereira, & Curran, 2000; Lindquist, Reynolds, & Goren, 1999; Sallis, 1993). Along with smoking and alcohol consumption, physical inactivity has been established as an important mortality risk (Blair et al., 1989). Although exercise is an essential contributor to health throughout the life span, it is especially important to understand why children do or do not participate, for it is during childhood that many patterns of exercise behavior are established (Green-

dorfer, 1983; Pate, Baranowski, Dowda, & Trost, 1996; Telama, Yang, Laasko, & Viikari, 1997). Coronary artery disease, hypertension, diabetes mellitus, and obesity are conditions that are linked to a sedentary lifestyle in adulthood, but believed to originate during childhood (Chandra, 1992). Children are not usually concerned about the future development of disease, but might be encouraged to pursue a lifestyle that could reduce risk factors for chronic diseases. Their level of motor activity also significantly affects children's mental and physical health status and vulnerability to environmental stressors (Bykov, 2001; Vechi, Takenaka, & Oka, 2000). Lower neuroticism scores have been reported in children who are physically active in comparison to those with low activity profiles (Sevcikova, Ruzanska, & Sabalova, 2000).

Motivation for Exercise

Although children believe that frequent activity results in beneficial outcomes, most children are not intrinsically motivated to participate in sustained, rigorous physical activity (Watkins, 1992). In fact, some evidence exists that in North American and some European communities, availability of the home computer may account for decreased participation among children in gross motor activities (Subrahmanyam, Kraut, Greenfield, & Gross, 2000; Caballero, 2004; Licence, 2004). Children do not typically view the aerobic demands and accompanying discomfort associated with aerobic dance, jogging, or distance swimming as "fun." Thus, they participate to very limited degrees in activities that should provide adequate levels of fitness (DiLorenzo et al., 1998; Ross et al., 1985).

Some children may be involved in exercise that is inappropriate for their age or level of development, with injury being an unfortunate consequence (Plumert, 1995). Yet for the aerobic payoff and other positive results to occur, fairly rigorous activities are necessary. The potential health-related benefits of exercise outweigh the risks (Biddle, 1993). Whereas adults may volitionally appreciate the need for aerobic exercise, children may not. This, by no means, suggests that exercise for children must be the aerobic kind. Cardiovascular benefit, muscular strength and endurance gains, and agility and flexibility increases may certainly result from anaerobic activities, but these activities, nonetheless, must be done with regularity and rigor. Also, the activities, although high in the enjoyment component and therefore relatively attractive to children, must challenge their cardiorespiratory and neuromuscular systems. Play, therefore, may also contribute to fitness.

What, then, are reasonably good sources of a child's motivation to exercise regularly and sufficiently? Is fun a strong motive? Will children exercise simply because authority figures such as parents, physicians, or teachers insist, or do they participate because other kids are doing it?

Social support such as parental encouragement and support from friends may be one answer (Weiss, 2000). Children of active parents tend to be more active themselves (Freedson & Evinson, 1991; Moore et al., 1991), and some evidence exists that parental beliefs about their child's competence are related to the child's participation (Kimiecik & Horn, 1998). Parents tend to encourage participation when they sense an affinity for physical activity in their child or when they recognize physical deficiencies or aberrations. Parents, siblings, and friends typically comprise the social support system for youth participation in physical activity. Watching the child participate and providing feedback are two important aspects of the support (Duncan, Duncan, & Strycker, 2005). Another contributing factor may be physical education programs in the schools (Simons-Morton, Simons-Morton, Parcel, & Bunker, 1988). Tragically, the number of physical education offerings (number of times per week, length of period, number of years/semesters for requirement) continues to decrease dramatically.

It appears that enjoyment of physical activity is a consistent predictor of children's participation (Stucky-Ropp, Vanderwal, & Gotham, 1998; Weiss, 2000). Weiss also notes that children wish to demonstrate competence in areas such as appearance, fitness, and acquisition of athletic skills. However, the best answers to questions of motivation are likely to result from a broad interactional approach wherein several influential areas contribute. The studies to date that have examined children's motivation for exercise indicate the influence of three categories of factors: *sociocultural*, *personal*, and *environmental* factors.

From a research perspective, the most helpful and overarching theoretical approach—one that clearly incorporates all three factors—is social cognitive theory (Sallis, Johnson, Calfas, Caparosa, & Nicholls, 1997; Welk, 1999). Social cognitive theory posits that motivational changes for physical activity are influenced by personal factors (such as personality traits), environmental factors (such as peer and parental influences), and aspects of physical activity itself (such as the attractiveness of the exercise). In social cognitive theory, therefore, both internal and external factors

---

CASE STUDY 18.1 The Power of Social Support: Friends Encouraging and Modeling Exercise

Nine-year-old James, much to his parents' disappointment, never displayed an interest in physical activity. He seemed to prefer sedentary afterschool diversions such as computer games and watching television. Although his parents continued to encourage him to become involved in sport or some form of exercise, he resisted their efforts. Both his older brother and younger sister displayed an affinity for physical activity and were enthusiastic participants.

At the commencement of the fourth-grade school year, James befriended two boys in his class. They spent a considerable amount of time together on weekends and after school and soon developed respect, liking, and interest in one another. Their compatibility was uplifting and beneficial for all three boys. However, James soon became aware that his friends were actively involved in a recreational/competitive swim program sponsored by their community's department of recreation. They obviously enjoyed going to swim practice a few times a week and, on occasion, participating in the district age-group competitive meets. The swimmers began a campaign to encourage James to join, insisting that it

was fun, that kids of all ability groups could be accommodated, and that they were becoming skilled swimmers and beginning to notice improvement in their levels of fitness. James's friends began to demonstrate increased commitment to the swimming program, and it soon became obvious to James that decreasing amounts of time were available for the three of them to hang out together. James decided to enter the swim program, and his parents supported and encouraged his decision. His friends eagerly introduced him to an enthusiastic, competent, and understanding coach with whom James immediately developed rapport.

The three boys, now part of a car pool, attended practice together four times a week. Their camaraderie flourished, and James developed swimming skills heretofore not considered attainable by him or his parents. The three friends went on to middle school and high school as excellent swimmers and fine competitors. James wanted to be like his friends, and they thought enough of him to encourage him to participate in an activity that they enjoyed. They talked him into participation, and he let them.

interact. Self-efficacy is the cornerstone of this theory. *Self-efficacy* refers to an individual's belief that he or she has the personal resources to meet the demands of a task (i.e., the physical activity). Bandura (1997) identifies four sources of efficacy formation and modification; that is, four ways by which an individual's beliefs may be altered:

1. *Enactive attainment.* This suggests that the individual's past achievement or history with the task has an impact upon his or her prediction of how well the individual is prepared to meet the same task now.
2. *Modeling or learning by observing others.* This suggests that by observing others engage in the task at hand, the individual develops efficacy for the task; that is, "if he can do it, so can I."
3. *Verbal persuasion.* This source of efficacy influence emphasizes the impact of another person's attempt to convince the performer that she or he indeed can or cannot execute the task. Others may tell those contemplating a certain form or intensity of exercise that it would be easy, difficult, fun, or tiresome.
4. *Physiological and emotional activation.* This influencing factor involves awareness of one's physiological state on behalf of the individual forming predictions about his or her preparedness to participate in exercise. Heightened physiological responses (in contrast to a low level of activation) may be interpreted as nervousness and, thus, unreadiness or inability to participate.

Sociocultural Factors

The influence of friends has also been shown to bear upon exercise involvement in 15- to 16-year-old boys and girls (Vilhjalmsson & Thorlindsson, 1998). Friends not only encourage (or discourage) friends to participate in exercise, but may also serve as models (see Case Study 18.1 for an anecdote portraying the power of encouragement from friends).

In addition, family support exerts influence over a child's motivation for exercise participation (Baranowski & Sallis, 1994). Families serve as important learning environments when children acquire interest in exercise and sport (DiLorenzo et al., 1998; Stucky-Ropp, Renee, & DiLorenzo, 1993). Undoubtedly, perceptions held by children about their home and neighborhood environments are associated with their physical activity behavior (Hume, Salmon, & Ball, 2005; Molner, Gortmeker, Bull, & Buka, 2004).

Single-parent homes may also be an additional sociocultural factor related to activity patterns of children. Researchers have reported higher levels of television viewing, but also higher levels of vigorous exercise, among 6.5- to 13-year-old children from single-parent homes (Lindquist et al., 1999). This sug-

gests that when such children do engage in physical activity, they do so with higher levels of intensity, although with lower frequencies than children from two-parent homes. The reasons for this finding remain unclear, but such results indicate a need for further examination of sociocultural factors as they may relate to exercise among children.

Last, in terms of sociocultural correlates of exercise participation in children, is ethnicity. In one recent study (Neumark-Sztainer, Faulkner, Beuring, & Resnick, 1999), black and Hispanic girls were found to be less likely than white children to diet and exercise. In the same study, all participants (7th-, 9th-, and 11th-grade public school Hispanic, black, and white students) reported that their preferred weight-control method was exercise rather than dieting, but older girls reported less exercise than younger girls reported. This finding is meaningful in that girls who resort to "unhealthy" weight-control behaviors (e.g., disordered eating, starvation, purging) are at greater risk for tobacco, alcohol, and marijuana use, as well as suicide attempts and unprotected sex (Neumark-Sztainer, Dixon, & Murray, 1998).

Similar results were found in a much larger study that employed more than 11,000 12- to 18-year-old high school students (Pate, Heath, Dowda, & Trost, 1996). Those boys and girls reporting low levels of physical activity were associated with cigarette and marijuana use, lower fruit and vegetable consumption, greater TV watching, and failure to wear a seat belt. Socioeconomic factors (race or ethnicity) seemed to affect the relationship between level of physical activity and negative health behaviors.

These social influences on children's (fifth-grade boys and girls) afterschool physical activities may be assessed with a questionnaire developed by Saunders et al. (1997). In their research, the authors found the social influences to be significantly correlated with intention to be physically active as well as with afterschool physical activity participation.

Personal Factors

The perceptions held by children about their motor coordination contribute to their attitude about participation in physical activity as well as to the overall value they place upon themselves as individuals (Craig, Goldberg, & Dietz, 1996; Harter, 1978, 1981; Rainey, McKeow, Sargent, & Valois, 1998). Other psychological variables have also been associated with motivation for exercise in children. Personality, for instance, has been identified as a required match for participation in certain exercise activities. This suggests that the type of exercise a child pursues with high degrees of adherence is associated with his or her personality style. The degree to which fifth and eighth graders believe they

Table 18.1
Habitual Physical Activity Questionnaire

1) What is your main occupation?
2) At work I sit . . . . 1—2—3—4—5
   never/seldom/sometimes/often/always
3) At work I stand . . . . 1—2—3—4—5
   never/seldom/sometimes/often/always
4) At work I walk . . . . 1—2—3—4—5
   never/seldom/sometimes/often/always
5) At work I lift heavy loads . . . . 1—2—3—4—5
   never/seldom/sometimes/often/very often
6) After working I am tired . . . . 5—4—3—2—1
   very often/often/sometimes/seldom/never
7) At work I sweat . . . . 5—4—3—2—1
   very often/often/sometimes/seldom/never
8) In comparison with others of my own age I think my work is
   physically much heavier/heavier/as heavy/lighter/much lighter . . . . . . 5—4—3—2—1
9) Do you play sports?
   yes/no
   If yes:
—which sport do you play most frequently? . . . . Intensity   0.76—1.26—1.76
   —how many hours a week?   <1/1–2/2–3/3–4/>4   Time   0.5—1.5—2.5—3.5—4.5
   —how many months a year?   <1/1–3/4–6/7–9/>9   Proportion 0.04—0.17—0.42—0.67—0.92
   If you play a second sport:
—which sport is it? . . . . Intensity   0.76—1.26—1.76
   —how many hours a week?   <1/1–2/2–3/3–4/>4   Time   0.5—1.5—2.5—3.5—4.5
   —how many months a year?   <1/1–2/2–3/3–4/>4   Proportion 0.04—0.17—0.42—0.67—0.92
10) In comparison with others of my own age I think my
   physical activity during leisure time is . . . . 5—4—3—2—1
   much more/more/the same/less/much less
11) During leisure time I sweat . . . . 5—4—3—2—1
   very often/often/sometimes/seldom/never
12) During leisure time I play sports . . . . 1—2—3—4—5
   never/seldom/sometimes/often/very often
13) During leisure time I watch television . . . . 1—2—3—4—5
   never/seldom/sometimes/often/very often
14) During leisure time I walk . . . . 1—2—3—4—5
   never/seldom/sometimes/often/very often
15) During leisure time I cycle . . . . 1—2—3—4—5
   never/seldom/sometimes/often/very often
16) How many minutes do you walk and/or cycle per day to
   and from work, school, and shopping? . . . . 1—2—3—4—5
   <5/5–15/15–30/30–45/>45

Calculation of the simple sport score (I_q):
(a score of zero is given to people who do not play a sport)

$$I_q = \sum_{i=1}^{2} (\text{intensity} \times \text{time} \times \text{proportion})$$

= 0/0.001 - <4/4-<8/8-<12/≥12

Calculation of scores of the indices of physical activity:
Work index = (I_1 + (6 - I_2) = I_3 + I_4 + I_5 + I_6 + I_7 + I_8)/8
Sport index = (I_q + I_{10} + I_{11} = I_{12})/4
Leisure time index = ((6 - I_{13}) = I_{14} + I_{15} + I_{16})/4

are able to easily regulate their physical activities (perceived behavioral control) has been shown to predict intent to participate (Craig et al., 1996). As is the case with adults, children also become involved in physical activity programs in order to lose weight and increase muscle (McCable & Ricciardel, 2003).

Teachers and parents should assist children in assessing the degree to which they may realistically maximize this control. Some evidence is available that the reasons for adult participation in exercise (ages 18–60) are associated with high levels of extraversion and neuroticism (Davis, Fox, Brewer, & Ratusny, 1995). Additional research conducted with youth subjects is needed to clarify this relationship among children, as very little is presently available. Currently, insufficient evidence is available to speak confidently about a link between personality and exercise choice among children.

A few studies have found perceived physical and athletic competency to be significant predictors of exercise adherence (Douthitt, 1994; Ferer-Caja & Weiss, 2000; Tappe, Duda, & Menges-Ehrnwald, 1990). In the study by Douthitt, the psychological predictors were observed only for females (9th, 10th, and 11th graders) who were queried about adherence in a physical education class setting. Interestingly, the higher the perceived athletic competency, the lower the adherence. This suggests that girls who viewed themselves as physically or athletically competent were not inclined to continue participating in exercise. The implication here is that exercise goals must be continually altered to ensure that they remain challenging. For males in the same study, perceived romantic appeal (looking good so as to be viewed as attractive by females) was found to be a weak but significant predictor of exercise adherence (in the physical education class setting). No psychological variables were predictively significant in the unstructured (out of class setting; on their own) settings for males. For females, however, global self-worth and perceived physical appearance were positively related to adherence. Those girls who viewed themselves as "looking good" were inclined to stay with the exercise program, possibly because they credited it with their perceived attractiveness. Exercise adherence was determined by use of the Habitual Physical Activity Questionnaire (Baecke, Burena, & Frijters, 1982), as presented in Table 18.1.

Douthitt's study suggests that, at least with North American adolescent school children, the psychological determinants of exercise adherence seem to vary between genders. It appears that if gender differences indeed exist, the basis for such differences is likely to be mediated by cultural factors. For instance, in a study by Myers et al. (1996), boys from grades 5 through 8 were more physically active than girls and engaged in more heavy physical activity whereas girls reported a

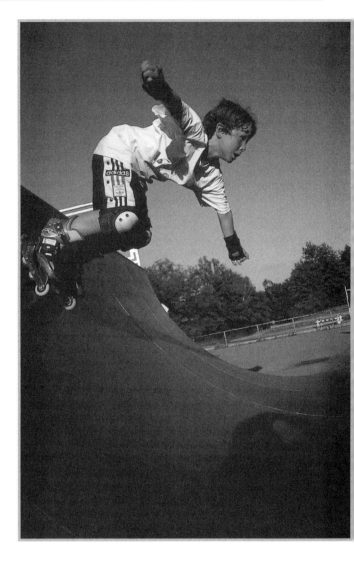

larger percentage of time spent in light and moderate physical activities. In this particular study, black children reported engaging in more sedentary activities than did white children. Cultural factors may also bear upon participatory motivation of children. For example, Chinese-American children report motives for exercising and participating in sport that are different than American children (Yan & McCullagh, 2004).

It is in the preadolescent years (approximately 5–12 years) that attitudes and habits about physical activity are formulated. Regular exercise programs for children in this age-group should therefore occur in the schools as well as in afterschool programs. The former are the responsibility of educators whereas the latter are the responsibility of parents and other adult leaders (i.e., coaches, scout leaders, church leaders, etc.). Children will express preferences and dislikes for some activities; however, their options are typically provided by adults. Organized sport, in particular, is usually within the purview of adults whose leadership styles and skills determine the enthusiasm and regularity with which children participate. Exercise and sport leaders who push children too far, who misinterpret the degree of their capabilities, who compare them unfairly to others, or who fail to reinforce even small gains in achievement undermine children's self-worth. With weakened self-worth, children are not inclined to continue in active participation. On the other hand, children with high perceived confidence are more likely to report that they engage in moderate to vigorous physical activity (Kimiecik, Horn, & Shurin, 1996). Also, some evidence exists that when children perceive that their physical education experiences in the school setting are worthwhile, their motivation for physical activity remains high (Ferer-Caja & Weiss, 2000).

Environmental Influences

Peer and parental support are examples of environmental influences (Martin & Dubbert, 1985), with the former being most powerful in the adolescent stage of development (approximately 13–19 years). Adolescence is a time when high school and college students attempt to resolve personal identity crises. As they at-

tempt to achieve role identity, much of their thinking and behaving are centered upon the question "Who am I?" In trying to answer this question, they seek and honor input from peers—young persons in the same chronological and developmental stage. Adolescents aspire to do what peers do, have identical or similar desires as their peers, and possess the same values. To be unlike one's peers takes courage. Particularly during adolescence, peers are the models most often emulated. Modeling influences dress preferences, hairstyles, use of language, and personal needs and interests. Motivation shifts from the parent or coach to the peer group. Skateboarding, weight lifting, and in-line skating become attractive exercise activities by virtue of the participation of other adolescents. Therefore, adolescents exercise or do not exercise because their friends "do it" or "don't do it" (Vilhjalmsson & Thorlindsson, 1998). Familiar reinforcement of children's participation in worthwhile physical activity programs may reduce sedentary behaviors. Parents, grandparents, and siblings contribute significantly in the initiation and maintenance of motivation to partake of phys-

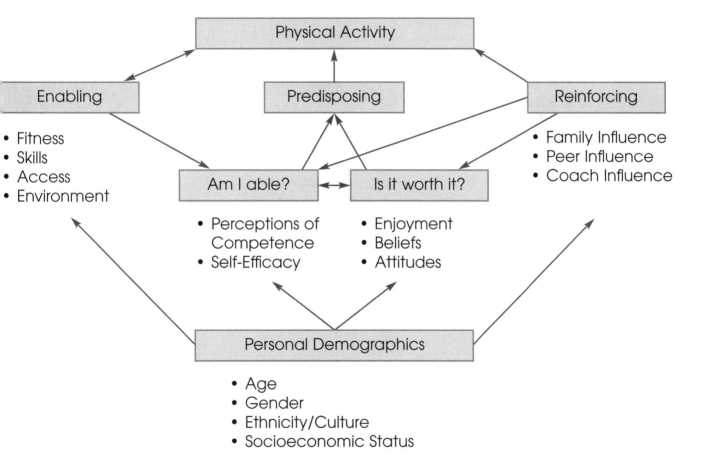

Figure 18.2. Youth Physical Activity Promotion Model.

From "The youth physical activity promotion model: A conceptual bridge between theory and practice", by G. J. Welk, 1999, *Quest, 51*, 5–23. Reprinted with permission.

ical activity of children (Epstein, Paluch, Kilanowkil, & Raynor, 2004; Sallis, Prochaska, Taylor, Hill, & Geraci, 1999).

Children's Attributions and Exercise Adherence

Children look back at their exercise experiences and produce reasons for its enjoyability, difficulty, or unpleasantness. In other words, children who have completed an exercise bout are inclined to conclude that it was fun or not fun "because of the teacher or coach," or that it was unpleasant "because it was too hard." These reasons, called attributions, lead to either a positive or negative emotional reaction and ultimately influence adherence (McAuley, Poag, Gleason, & Wraith, 1990; Vlachopoulos, Biddle, & Fox, 1996). Teachers and exercise leaders should plan, organize, and lead exercise and sport activities for children with an eye toward minimizing negative emotional reactions. Trite as it may seem, it may be concluded that if children enjoy exercise and perceive exercise outcomes positively, they will then tend to adhere to exercise programs.

Youth Physical Activity Promotion Model

A helpful way of understanding why children do or do not enter or adhere to exercise programs is provided by Welk (1999) in his youth physical activity promotion model (see Figure 18.2). The model provides a conceptual framework for the interactions of multiple factors that influence youth participation in exercise. Four broad categories of factors contribute to the model: enabling, predisposing, reinforcing, and personal demographics.

Enabling factors refer to conditions or personal attributes that permit or increase the likelihood of involvement in exercise. Examples include access to equipment, parks, and programs. Other variables relate to the environment such as good weather, physical distance to the exercise facility, and the facility's safety. Enabling factors in the model are in and of themselves not determinants of physical activity, but they are necessary and, according to Welk (1999), are directly related to participation. Biological factors, such as physical skills, fitness, and

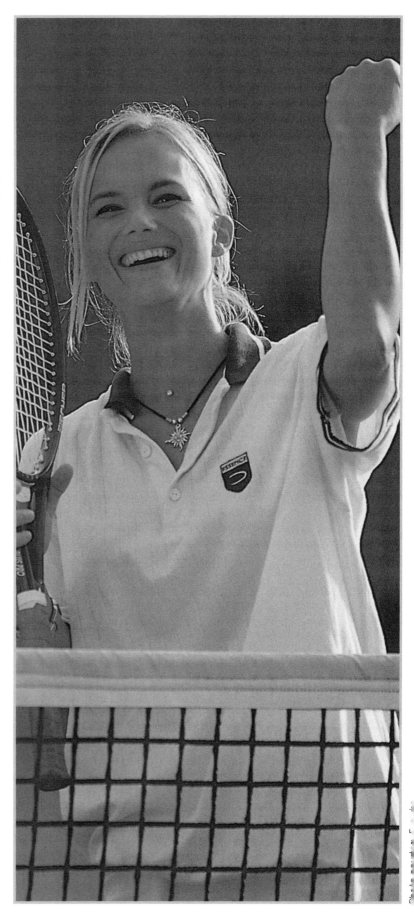

stored body fat, are also considered enabling factors.

Predisposing factors in the model are represented by two basic questions: (a) Is the exercise worth it? and (b) Am I able to do it? The first question relates to issues such as enjoyment or a comparison of costs and benefits. The child, according to the model, is therefore involved cognitively as well as emotionally. The second question involves the youth's perception of self-competence. Accordingly, a child may place high value on exercise, but if he or she feels incapable of performing the activity, the child is not likely to do so. The child who responds affirmatively to both questions (Is it worth it? Am I able?) is likely to be predisposed to an active lifestyle.

Reinforcing factors are sources of support such as parents, peers, and coaches. These are persons in the social and family environment who offer encouragement and reinforcement to the physically active child. Reinforcement may be direct or indirect, blatant or subtle. Either way, the model considers its influences on the involvement of children in physical activity to be strong.

The fourth category is *personal demographics*, which includes age, gender, ethnicity/culture, and socioeconomic status. As previously discussed, children of different ages are more or less attracted to different forms of physical activity. Cultural influences help determine the exercise choices of children—suburban and urban or poor and wealthy children are frequently exposed to different kinds of physical activities (e.g., sailing and golf versus basketball).

Quitting

Martens (1996) suggests three causes of children's disengagement from exercise: incompetent leaders, adult objectives different from those of the children, and vague behavioral programs. Parents play pivotal roles in establishing the motivational level of exercising children. Parental support of urban elementary schoolchildren's physical activity involvement has been shown to be a key factor in their children's liking of sports. Children perceive various forms of social support, and the manner in which they integrate this support is related to their motor competency (Rose, Larkin, & Berger, 1994, 1997). Parents, for instance, can negatively influence their child's self-confidence by expressing anger and excessive concern about clumsiness. Parents who highly value their child's motor ability may be inclined to react to it negatively when their children's performance is less than anticipated (Cratty, 1994). Stress is a likely consequence (Losse et al., 1991), which, in turn, becomes a reason for quitting. Children exposed to strong parental support have higher perceived competence than do those who experienced less parental support (Brustad, 1996).

Some researchers address the issue of exercise dropout or failure to become involved in exercise at all, by studying what they refer to as "barriers to exercise" in youth. Tappe, Duda, and Ehrnwald (1989) reasoned that adolescents (average age approximately 15 years) may be particularly affected by a certain set of barriers that deter or prevent them from participating in regular physical activity. Nine barriers, as perceived by male and female participants in their study, were identified as a result of their research:

1. Desire to do other things with one's time,
2. Lack of interest,
3. Unsuitable weather,
4. No place to exercise and lack of needed equipment,
5. Job responsibilities,
6. School or schoolwork,
7. A boyfriend or girlfriend that kept one from being physically active,
8. Use of alcohol or other drugs, and
9. Feeling sick or having an injury.

When subjects were divided into two groups according to extent of involvement in regular physical activity (high and low active), gender differences were found. Highly active males cited use of alcohol and other drugs and having a girlfriend as the main barriers to exercise. For highly active females, school and school responsibilities were identified. For all subjects (not designated as high or low active), some gender differences were also found. Males reported higher scores for the barriers of "my girlfriend has kept me from being physically active" and "alcohol and drugs." On the other hand, females claimed that they wanted to do other things with time. In addition, females tended to identify the barriers of "unsuitable weather," "lack of desire or interest," and "schoolwork" as reasons for not exercising.

Of importance here is the reporting of at least three barriers to exercise as perceived by adolescents that may be addressed by physical and health educators, parents, and exercise leaders: (a) use of alcohol and other drugs among males, (b) time constraints, and (c) lack of desire or interest among females. Implications for substance abuse and time-management education are evident for the first two, and health education by which young females are introduced to weight-management and psychological benefits of exercise is apparent for the third barrier.

Physical Activity Assessment Among Children

Given the many physical and psychological benefits to children derived from participation in physical activity, assessment and evaluation of their involvement are important. How intensely do children exercise? How often and for how long do children exercise? Very young children may be unable to report the frequencies of their own behavior, and the reliability and credibility of their reports have been taken to task (Bruck, Ceci, & Hembrooke, 1998). Another problem is that parents and teachers may not always be near enough so as to reliably report the degree of the children's participation. To address this issue, Harro (1997) has constructed an instrument for assessing physical activity in preadolescent children. Two questionnaires were validated against data from heart-rate monitors and motion sensors (which assess the quantity and intensity of movements in the vertical plane as reported by the children on a specially constructed questionnaire). The monitors and sensors were attached to 62 kindergarten and first-grade children for 4 consecutive days, from 7:00 am to 8:00 pm. Two other questionnaires were devised—one for parental use and the other for teacher use. Parents and teachers were required to use the instrument to report on (a) physical activities with low to moderate intensity in which heavy breathing was not expected and (b) moderate to vigorous physical activities that caused a child to breathe hard, such as running, jumping, some children's games, aerobic dancing, etc. The intensity of those activities ranged from 5 to 9 metabolic equivalents. The amount of daily moderate to vigorous physical activity was determined in minutes and as a percentage of the child's time awake during the time of monitoring. These two questionnaires (parents and teachers) may be used to provide helpful information about the moderate to vigorous physical activity frequency of 4- to 8-year-old children. However, assessment of physical activity intensity, frequency, and duration requires a good deal of additional methodologically sound research. All too many unanswered questions remain as there is currently no uniform approach to assessing physical activity in children. However, within the past few years, attempts have been made to establish data-collection systems that would eventually yield helpful information about how frequently and intensely (older) children exercise.

Let us now turn our attention to four approaches to surveying physical activity among children and adolescents in the United States, 1990–1997. Exercise leaders working with older clients who are in the upper range of the high school years (seniors) and lower end of college years (freshmen) may find the first three of these instruments particularly helpful.

The first instrument, the National Health Interview Survey, was devised for use with older, youthful subjects 18 years or older in home interviews. Subjects were queried as to whether they had engaged in any of 22 exercises, sports, or physically active hobbies in the previous 2 weeks. Also, respondents were able to report information on two other activities. Frequency, duration, and self-perceived effort associated with par-

ticipation were indicated. Respondents were then grouped according to their patterns:

1. Physically inactive (no leisure-time physical activity);
2. Irregularly active (activity performed less than 3 times per week, less than 20 minutes per occasion, or both);
3. Regularly active, not intense (approximately more than 3 times per week, approximately more than 20 minutes per occasion, and less than 50% of maximal cardiorespiratory capacity); and
4. Regularly active, intense (approximately more than 3 times per week, approximately more than 20 minutes per occasion, approximately more than 50% of maximal cardiorespiratory capacity, and rhythmically contracting large muscle groups).

A second approach, the Behavioral Risk Factor Surveillance System (BRFSS; see Heath & Kendrick, 1989; Simoes, Byers, Coates, & Serdula, 1995; Smith & Remington, 1989), is conducted year-round on a monthly basis through telephone interviews of older adolescents and adults, ages 18 years and older. Subjects are asked about their participation in physical activities or exercise. They are then asked about the frequency and duration of their participation in their two most common physical activities. This information is introduced into a computerized scoring system that yields the participant's estimated maximal cardiorespiratory capacity and calculates an intensity code. Participants are classified in accordance with their level of physical activity. Copies of the surveys are available, and scholars, researchers, and organizers of youth exercise programs, therefore, have at their disposal a potentially helpful source of data.

The National Health Interview Survey—Youth Risk Behavior Survey (NHIS—YRBS; Centers for Disease Control and Prevention, 1992) focused upon youth ages 18–21 years who were not attending school. Answers to the questions asked of respondents were recorded on standardized answer sheets, thus maintaining confidentiality; the questions themselves were administered with portable cassette players, thus eliminating potential difficulties with subjects who were unable to read or write.

A fourth attempt to determine information about youth participation in physical activity is the Youth Risk Behavior Survey (YRBS; Centers for Disease Control and Prevention, 1992). This survey used participants in grades 9–12 at the national, state, and local levels. Although concerned with risk behavior in youth, some of the questions asked on this survey are in reference to exercise, defined as at least 20 minutes of vigorous exercise rather than 30 minutes, as used in the NHIS—YRBS. Also, respondents are asked in two questions about their frequency of attending physical education class every week and the number of minutes spent actually exercising or playing sports in each class.

Many interesting and valuable findings have been obtained from the four survey approaches designed to provide information about physical activity and children in the United States. For instance, males are engaged in regular, vigorous activity to a greater extent (at least up to the year 1992 when the last NHIS—YRBS was conducted) than females. Involvement of male youth was observed to be at 60%, as compared to 47% for females. In addition, declines in participation were less pronounced in males from ages 12 to 21 than for females. Males of differing race and ethnicity status had similar rates for decline, but white, non-Hispanic females reported different decline patterns (less than black and Hispanic females). Also, household income was observed to be related to participation decline in vigorous physical activity. Participation of youth from households with higher incomes decreased less than that of youth from lower income households. Another interesting observation surfacing from surveillance of youth participation in physical activity is that higher participation occurs during May through June than during November and December. Thus, physical activity patterns in American youth relate to sociodemographic and seasonal differences.

Ethnic differences also seem to account for the amount of physical activity performed by 4-year-olds at home (Sallis et al., 1997), as do availability and quality of play spaces and encouragement by friends, parents, and other adults. This finding is compatible with results from research published by Baranowski, Thompson, DuRant, Baranowski, and Puhl (1993).

Summary

Regrettably, children do not participate in physical activity with the adequate intensity and regularity necessary to derive fitness benefits. Although young children often engage in play activity, necessary aerobic demands are often absent. When examining children's motives for participation, researchers report important factors to be enjoyment of the activity, parental encouragement, peer participation, sociocultural factors, and perceptions about their physical selves.

In an effort to understand motives for participation in physical activity by youth, a broad, interactional approach (social cognitive theory) is recommended. This approach incorporates personal, social, and environmental influences and emphasizes modeling and self-efficacy. Another helpful way to examine motivation for exercise among children is use of the youth physical activity promotion model. This model, proposed by Welk (1999), identifies four categories of factors that bear upon physical activity participation in youth: enabling, predisposing, reinforcing, and personal demographic factors.

Lastly, the chapter discusses results from surveys conducted on large samples of children in order to learn about various aspects (frequency, choices, intensity, etc.) of their participation or lack thereof.

Can You Define These Terms?

enactive attainment

exercise

modeling

physiological activation

play

self-efficacy

social cognitive theory

social support

verbal persuasion

Can You Answer These Questions?

1. Why do many children exercise infrequently?

2. As children move from the elementary school years to middle school and high school years, does their participation in physical activity increase or decrease? Why?

3. Why is it important for children to be engaged regularly in vigorous physical activity?

4. How are play and exercise differentiated?

5. Discuss reasons for the disparity in the extent to which boys and girls participate in exercise.

6. Why is social cognitive theory a helpful approach to clarifying motives for exercise participation among children?

7. Describe the youth physical activity promotion model.

8. What are some potential barriers to exercise, according to adolescents?

9. What instruments might be helpful in assessing physical activity among youth?

CHAPTER 19

Exercise for Older Individuals

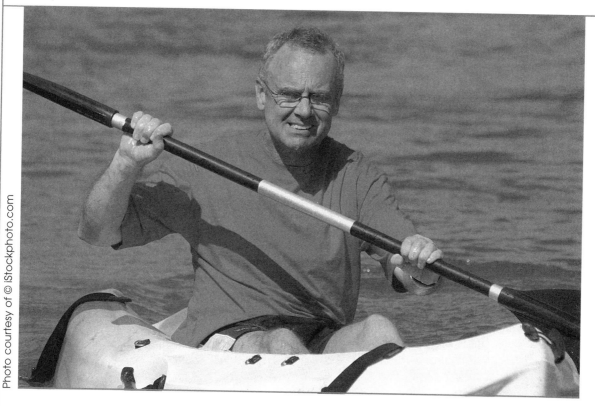

Photo courtesy of © iStockphoto.com

After reading this chapter, you should be able to

- List misconceptions related to exercise held by many elderly persons,

- Discuss deterioration associated with the aging process,

- Provide support for the importance of exercise for the elderly by discussing physiological, psychological, and psychophysiological benefits,

- Differentiate between quantitative and qualitative research designs,

- Offer explanations for problematic research on exercise and the elderly, and

- List distinctions between elderly male and female exercisers.

Introduction

In 1900, those over the age of 65 years comprised only 4% of the population in the United States. Today, roughly 12% of the population exceeds this age, and it is anticipated that by the middle of this century, older adults will constitute approximately 20% of the population (United States Bureau of the Census, July 2002). In a 1996 publication, Caldwell (1996) estimated that there were 30 million Americans over the age of 65. The most rapidly increasing segment of the U.S. population in percentage terms is the 85 and older group (Nickerson, 1998). People are clearly living longer, and aging is in the midst of a dynamic growth spurt.

Paralleling this increase in life expectancy is a surge in related scientific research. There has always been fascination with fountains of youth and other mythical ideas about the prevention of growing old (Gruman, 1966). In recent decades, however, this historic interest has veered in the direction of the psychology of aging, whereas the earlier emphases were more biologically oriented. Today's psychologists are very much focused upon causal factors as well as correlates of the aging process. The precise chronological boundaries for those referred to as "elderly" remain, however, elusive. What are accurate cutoff points for identifying the elderly? When does middle age terminate and yield to old age? Researchers interested in the aging process address these issues by offering operationalized definitions of the term *elderly*—that is, they assign a range of years apropos to only their study and its participants, but such arbitrary designations place serious limitations on their findings. One researcher's "elderly" subjects may be 55 and over; another's may be 60 or 65 years. There is no clear consensus within the psychological research literature for the threshold age at which an individual becomes "elderly" or a "senior citizen." Some studies may use age 65, since this has traditionally been the age at which one becomes eligible for full Social Security benefits. However, according to Dorman:

> There is no biological reason to believe we "become old" at age 65. The reason the age 65 is often used to define "old age" is not because we biologically change at that age, but because the authors of the Social Security Act in 1935 had to pick an age for people to receive Social Security benefits. The authors randomly chose the age of 65 (because few people lived that long in 1935) and this number has been used to define "senior citizens" ever since (1995).

In an attempt to respond to this and related issues, Brown (1992) proposed a three-tiered strategy for describing the elderly. Thus, those between 65 and 74 years of age could be considered "young old"; those 75–84 years, "middle old"; and men and women of 85 or more years would be considered "old-old." The term "Senior Citizen" may also be defined by other criteria, such as whether or not an individual is retired from regular employment; has attained the age of 50 years (American Association of Retired Persons); is receiving Social Security benefits or pension (individuals are eligible for reduced SS benefits at age 62); resides in a nursing home or assisted living facility; uses the services of a Senior Citizen Center; or any number of other factors.

Technological and medical advances continue to improve standards of living, and many recent social reforms and entitlement programs are likely contributors to the greatest presence of elderly citizens in our nation's history. When life is fulfilling, our desire to live as long as possible is strong, and most of us with satisfying, enriched lives strive to extend the number of years available to us. However, to paraphrase the renowned Benjamin Franklin, everyone wants to live long, but no one wants to get old.

In this chapter, we argue that exercise is directly related to life's quality during aging and that it is a necessary experience in the lives of most elderly persons. Unfortunately, as men and women become older, there is a decrease at every age level in reported engagement in strenuous physical activity (Bausell, 1986; Chodzko-Zajko, 1994; Cousins, 1996; Harootyan, 1982; Rudman, 1986; United States Department of Health and Human Services [USDHHS], 1996). Among the elderly, the number of completely sedentary individuals is very large. Only approximately 10% of persons 65 years of age and older exercise regularly (Fiatarone & Garnett, 1997). Dropout rates are high in all age populations; and, as Dishman, Sallis, and Orenstein (1985) suggest, those who are most in need of exercise programs are the ones who typically quit. Physical inactivity is especially prevalent among older age-groups (Owen, Leslie, Salmon, & Fatheringham, 2000). And attitudes about the benefits of regular exercise change with advancing age (Wilcox & Storandt, 1996).

Why the Elderly Do Not Exercise

Although much evidence points to the health benefits of exercise for elderly persons (Brach, Simonsick, Kritchevsky, Yaffe, & Newman, 2004; Cyarto, Moorhead, & Brawn, 2004; Deeg, Kardaun, & Fozard, 1996; Evans & Campbell, 1993; Kamiyama, Kawaguchi, Kanda, Kuno, & Nishijima, 2004; Puggard, 2003; Sinaki, Nwaogwugwu, Phillips, & Mokri, 2001), misconceptions linger that discourage their participation (Cousins, 1996; McPherson, 1984; Ostrow, 1983; Wilcox & Storandt, 1996). Some likely factors involved in declining involvement in exercise are as follows:

1. *Underrating of their physical abilities.* Many elderly persons are convinced that their physical capabilities are compromised to the extent that vigorous activity is not within their reach.

2. *Overestimation of the value of the little exercise they do.* Many elderly individuals exaggerate the degree to which they participate in exercise and believe that they are more active than they actually are.

3. *Exaggeration of the dangers of physical exercise.* Some trepidation about injury, falling, and fatigue are rational because various components of physical fitness are indeed reduced in the elderly. In many cases, however, appropriately selected and properly executed activities can be safe.

4. *Age-role stereotypes that portray the elderly as persons who should simply refrain from rigorous physical activity* (Brown, 1992; Cousins, 1996). Sad to say, 45% of respondents in a study by Biddle (1995) indicated that nothing at all would sustain their motivation to exercise.

When asked why they did not exercise, a sample of 60+ year-old subjects reported that the following incentives would keep them active (Biddle, 1995):

1. 25%—fitness/weight loss
2. 25%—maintain health
3. 45%—nothing would keep them motivated to stay active
4. 5%—other reasons

In their research, Mummery, Schofield, and Caperchione (2002), have found older Australian adults to be motivated to exercise more by health factors than any others and that physical activity is cited by their Australian cohort as a form of stress management. Needless to say, intrinsic motivational factors such as enjoyment contributed significantly to level of involvement in exercise (high, low; Dacey, 2004). Physical health and physical fitness are probably the most important motivations for partaking of regular exercise (Schuler et al., 2004). Older persons have weaker beliefs in their ability to engage in exercise and have lower expectations for exercise's alleged benefits. Such low exercise efficacy appears to be related to age and education; the older one gets, the lower the efficacy, and the more education, the stronger the belief in the benefits of exercise (Netz & Raviv, 2004). Life-events and interpersonal loss will influence participation in exercise class in older adults, particularly for women (Wilcox & King, 2004). In other words, when an elderly person experiences a disturbing event or in some way loses a social relationship, adherence to exercise suffers.

The most highly reported motives for participation in exercise and sport, among elderly Australian women, were found to be fourfold: keeping health, liking the activity, improving fitness, and maintaining joint mobility (Kolt, Driver, & Giles, 2004). It is likely that motives for women in other western world cultures are very similar, if not the same.

In a recent study that incorporated responses from more than 2,000 North American men and women over the age of 55, women reported less leisure-time activity than men did and claimed that lack of an exercise companion was the most important reason for their limited physical activity (Satariano, Haight, & Tager, 2000). Some research findings suggest that for many older women, clothing worn by members of an exercise group can influence the perception held by individuals about themselves as well as the group as a whole. This is particularly relevant for women with high levels of physique anxiety who take note of other women in the group who are wearing "revealing attire" (Sinden, Ginis, & Angove, 2003). See Table 19.1 for a summary of reasons the elderly choose not to exercise.

Exercise is not only appropriate for the elderly, but

Table 19.1
Why the Elderly Do Not Exercise

1. Lack of an exercise companion
2. Too convenient to watch television
3. Fear of being injured
4. Experienced soreness and discomfort when exercised previously
5. Exercise is boring
6. No time available for exercise
7. "I never lose weight by exercising, so why bother?"
8. Exercise is too much like work
9. "I don't feel the need to exercise"

---

also important for their well-being (as it is for persons of all ages). But elderly men and women respond differently to efforts and strategies to recruit them for participation in exercise programs. Results from a study by Rowland et al., (2004) suggest that gender specific recruitment methods should be applied and that those that are effective for elderly men, may not be effective for elderly women.

Older exercisers are also sensitive to the visible attributes of exercise leaders. Leadership is an important factor in adherence and dropping-out. In the view of a group of elderly men and women exercisers interviewed with regard to necessary characteristics of effective physical activity group leaders, three salient features emerged. Allegedly, effective leaders:

(1) Are those whom participants feel are properly qualified.

(3) Are able to develop a personal bond with participants.

(4) Can use their knowledge and the group to demonstrate collective accomplishments (Estabrooks et al., 2004).

The Aging Process

Across the life span, identifiable deterioration occurs in behavioral and biological functioning. These changes typically begin in one's 40s and continue throughout a lifetime. Aging is accompanied by inevitable and somewhat predictable decreases in various capacities, particularly those dependent upon muscular strength (Lemmer et al., 2000). However, these decrements in functioning are highly variable among elderly persons; the time of onset and magnitude of deterioration are specific to each individual (Birren & Schroots, 1996; Chodzko-Zajko, 1996).

Aging is a multifaceted process occurring at molecular, cellular, and organic levels. It involves structural and functional changes in virtually all bodily systems, but not all of these changes are linked to a general decline in physical and mental functions. However, many of these changes occurring in the elderly account for slowness in motor activities as well as in information processing and transmission (Cyarto, Moorhead, & Brown, 2004; Dustman, Emmerson, & Shearer, 1994; Sinaki & Nwaogwugwa, 2001; Smith, 1996; Stones & Kozma, 1996; Weuve, Kang, Manson, Breteler, Ware, & Grodstein, 2004). Age-related decreases in cognitive function are also prevalent (MacKay & Abrams, 1996; Spirduso, 1995; Willis, 1996). These declines happen gradually over many years and do not occur in patterned or systematic ways. Elderly persons who deny such age-related changes, or who do not seek to accommodate them, may hold false expectations for their actions that can result in harmful consequences. It is especially important to recognize this when constructing and administering exercise programs for older persons. Recent research findings suggest that conditions heretofore associated with young women, such as disordered eating, are now occurring with increasing frequency in women in middle and late life as well (Zerbe, 2003).

To understand aging, it is important to distinguish between primary and secondary processes. *Primary aging processes* are highly related to age, but are independent of disease or environmental influence. Primary aging is illustrated by such milestones as puberty and menopause, which have nothing to do with disease or environmental influences. Indications of primary aging include changes in vision, hearing loss, changes in body composition, bone demineralization, and decreases in strength, flexibility, agility, cardiovascular function, and pulmonary function. *Secondary aging processes* include environmental factors (i.e., elevated levels of daily stress, exposure to sunlight, and inhalation of cigarette smoke) as well as the influences of diseases such as diabetes, arthritis, and cancer. Primary and secondary aging processes interact. Aging increases one's vulnerability to environmental stressors and disease. The reverse is also true; disease and environmental stressors can accelerate the primary aging process. In general, aging leads to a general loss of adaptability, functional impairment, and death (Spirduso, 1995). Aging is an inevitable extension of the physiological and psychological processes of growth and development, which begin at birth and end with death.

The extent of psychological and physiological (mental and physical) slowing due to aging is person specific and does not correlate well with age itself. As Scheibel (1996) has said in his introduction to a chapter entitled, "Structural and Functional Changes in the Aging Brain," "However, aging is a coat of many colors. Some individuals, without obvious pathology, are cognitively and emotionally 'showing their age' at 60, whereas others appear vigorous and intellectually vital at 85 or 90" (pp. 105–106). None the less, as task difficulty increases, general slowing in cognitive and motor activities increases concomitantly (Cerella, Poon, & Williams, 1980; Spirduso & MacRae (1990). Specifically, functions of the central nervous system (CNS) are retarded. Less efficient transmission of neural impulses occurs at the synapse with aging (Landfield, McGaugh, & Lynch, 1978) especially when stimuli are presented rapidly. In addition, sensory and motor nerves conduct impulses more slowly in the elderly (Dorfman & Bosley, 1979; Drechsler, 1975; Scheibel, 1996). Lastly, intelligence (fluid as well as crystallized) also decreases with age (Emery & Blumenthal, 1991).

Anxieties expressed by older persons, particularly the fear of falling (Tinetti & Powell, 1993), often relate to their movement abilities. Their steady declining motor capabilities alter their perceptions about their physical selves (Bosscher, 1994). This may be a significant concern for some elderly because movements, particularly activities that move the entire body in space (locomotor), are among the more important ways in which we interact with the physical environment. All of us come to know the physical environment as our bodies move within it. Because advancing age is accompanied by a decline in fat-free body mass (e.g. skeletal muscle), the resting metabolic rate decreases. This suggests that stored body fat increases

(Poehlman, Arciero, & Goran, 1994). During aging, significant decreases in muscular strength, endurance, power, flexibility, and response time occur (Cartee, 1994). By no means completely obliterated, these capacities are, nonetheless, reduced. This realization of deterioration may not only prompt change in self-concept, but may also result in reduced expectations about physical activity as well as the emergence of various negative emotions, and health behaviors in general (Levy, 2004). In North American society, the desire to be thin, enjoy good health, and be fit is not exclusive to youth. The elderly also hold such aspirations (Schuler, Broxon-Hutcherson, Philipp, Isosaari, & Robinson, 2004).

Not all older persons respond in this fashion, but all too many do. For most elderly individuals, the desire for independence in functioning is more important than competitive athletic prowess. Therefore, limited motor capacity may be frustrating in that it inhibits independence and serves as a reminder of advancing age.

Although peak levels of efficiency are short-lived, many individuals function motorically and intellectually at very high levels beyond their 40th year. These decreases need not imply deterioration in overall well-being or lifestyle, despite misconceptions regarding the aging process. In fact, increasing numbers of published studies encourage the conclusion that regular participation in endurance exercise may postpone many of the ravages of time, including diminished central nervous system function (Brach, Simonsick, Kritchevsky, Yaffe, & Newman, 2004; Chodzko-Zajko & Moore, 1994; Cyarto, Moorhead, & Brown, 2004; Puggaard, 2003; Sinaki, Nwaogwugwu, Phillips, & Mokri, 2001; Taylor, 1992). Even a single dose of very low-intensity exercise may have a positive effect on cognitive performance (verbal memory) in the elderly (Fontane, 1996; Molloy, Beerschoten, Borrie, Crilly, & Cape, 1988; Stones & Dawe, 1993). Considerably more research is required before precise doses of exercise may be prescribed for specific neuropsychological function. Additional research is also needed to clarify these beneficial effects on cognitive and psychomotor function.

Beneficial Effects of Exercise on the Elderly

Exercise enhances the longevity and well-being of the elderly in a variety of ways (Brach, 2004; Fox & Stahl, 2002; Washburn, 2000). Most fundamental of all is its capacity to improve the quality of life by preventing undue decline in functional capacity. Thus, when done with vigor and regularity, exercise fosters *functional independence*, or improves one's ability to do things for oneself. The mechanism underlying improved independence may be the enhancement of cardiorespi-

ratory fitness that accrues from increased physical activity (Paterson, Govindasamy, Vidmar, Cunningham, & Koval, 2004). Furthermore, exercise offers the potential for additional physiological and psychological benefits to those involved. One additional observation of note with regard to the link between quality of life / functional independence in the elderly and exercise is that medical expenditures are significantly lower in those who exercise regularly than in those who do not (Kamiyama, Kawaquchi, Kanda, Kuno, &

Table 19.2
Some Psychological and Physiological Changes Due to Aging

1. Slowing in cognitive and motoric activities
2. Decline in central nervous system function
3. Less efficient transmission of neural impulses at the synapse, particularly when stimuli are presented rapidly
4. Slower conduction of sensory and motor nerve impulses
5. Decline in intelligence

Nishijima, 2004; Lee & Anderson, 2004; Martinson, Crain, Pronk, O'Connor, & Maciosek, 2003). Elderly exercisers also report fewer chronic diseases than non-exercisers (Cyarto, Moorhead, & Brown, 2004). In general, in the elderly, exercisers exhibit higher levels of well-being than sedentary persons. This conclusion is drawn by Andrew Wister (2003) in an editorial titled "It's never too late: Healthy lifestyles and aging" in the *Canadian Journal on Aging*.

Sleep Benefits

Exercise has been shown to decrease the time necessary to fall asleep; it has been associated with longer nights of sleep and with the perception of feeling more rested upon awakening (Morgan, 2003; King, Oman, Brassington, Bliwise, & Haskell, 1997). These reported benefits of exercise are considerably noteworthy in that complaints about sleep disturbance are very prevalent among the elderly. More than 50% of adults complain about sleep disturbance (Buchner, 1997).

Of interest is the observation by McAuley and Rudolph (1995) that although involvement in physical activity is associated with improved cardiorespiratory fitness and psychological well-being of older adults, these improvements were not necessarily correlated. In other words, their physical fitness may not have to actually change in order for elderly participants to claim improved well-being. As seductive as the relationship between exercise and mental well-being may appear, it has to date not been shown to be causally connected.

Physiological Benefits

Among the most frequently reported findings from exercise studies is that both elderly male and female subjects experience significant physiological improvements in fitness components as a result of physical training (Buchner, Beresford, Larson, LaCroix, & Wagner, 1992; Emery, Hauck, & Blumenthal, 1992; Mahler, Cunningham, & Curfinan, 1986; Seals & Hagberg, 1984; Shepherd, 1996; Stones & Kozma, 1996; USDHHS, 1996). The parameters that are often improved are cardiovascular function, maximum consumption of oxygen, increased stroke volume, decreased blood pressure, lower resting and submaximal heart rates, decreased body weight, desirable shifts in lean body mass (Buchner et al., 1992), and bone density (Layne & Nelson, 1999). Also, endurance exercise has been shown to have a positive influence on neurotransmitter functioning (Bauer, Rogers, Miller, Bove, & Tyce, 1989). Scientists have concluded that, irrespective of age or gender, exercise is strongly and inversely related to coronary heart disease (Blair, 1994). That is, the more people exercise, the lower their incidence of cardiovascular disease.

One researcher, in particular (Evans, 1999), has concluded that the elderly may benefit more than other age-groups from regular exercise because of their low functional status and high incidence of chronic disease. In the very old, muscle mass, which is responsive to exercise (it increases), is an important determining factor of functional status. Exercise may, therefore, reverse physical frailty so prevalent among the elderly.

The quality of balance regulation decreases as ageing progresses, which results in increased risk of falling. Physical activity and sport program participation has been shown to improve regulation of posture and balance (Godard, Whitman, & Richmond, 2004). Regular physical activity develops or maintains the efficiency of the reflexes involved in the control of posture (Gauchard, Gangloff, Jeandel, & Perrin, 2003).

At a Sports Science Exchange Roundtable discussion entitled," Exercise and Nutrition in the Elderly," scientists who maintain ongoing research interests in this area met to address a series of relevant questions (Blumberg, Kenney, Seals, & Spina, 1992). Although the answers of panel members were qualified and elaborated upon more fully, they were unanimous. Following are four pertinent questions posed to the panel and its consensus responses:

Question 1. Is an individual ever too old to embark on an exercise program?

Answer: No. Exercise can be beneficial at any age. There are no reasons why older individuals should not embark on an exercise program once medical clearance has been obtained.

Question 2. Can elderly persons expect to see the same physiological adaptations as younger persons when they begin an exercise program?

Answer: Some differences are to be expected in cardiovascular adaptations between older women and younger women, and between older women and men. Overall, the adaptations for older persons are quite similar as in young persons. The responses to aerobic and strength training are similar in young and elderly people. Resistance training increases strength in elderly subjects and stimulates muscle hypertrophy, just as in younger subjects.

Question 3: Can an elderly person who begins an exercise program arrest or reverse the progress of any disease?

Answer: There is evidence that exercise can decrease the risk of developing some diseases and be an important component of a program designed to arrest or reverse certain disease conditions.

Question 4: What do current trends indicate about the exercise habits of the elderly?

Answer: A combination of exercise and appropriate diet is effective for optimal strength, health, and physical fitness in the elderly. The onset of certain chronic diseases can be delayed through proper diet and exercise.

Mental Health Benefits

In the general population, physical activity has been shown to be associated with reduced symptoms of clinical depression and anxiety (Camacho, Roberts, Lazarus, Kaplan, & Cohen, 1991; Garcia & Gomez, 2003; Lampinen & Heikkinen, 2002; Ross & Hayes, 1988; Stephens & Craig, 1990). And among the elderly who have been diagnosed with major depressive disorder, and enrolled in programs of exercise therapy, baseline levels of self-reported anxiety and life-satisfaction have been shown to be good predictors of drop-out. Those with high levels of pre-program anxiety and low levels of life-satisfaction are prone to program discontinuation (Herman et al. 2002). Persons with histories of inactivity are twice as likely to show symptoms of depression in comparison to more active persons (USDHHS, 1996). A regular regimen of walking has been associated with a reduced risk of dementia in elderly men (Abbott, White, Ross, Masaki,

Kamal, Curb, & Petrovich, 2004). Berger (1996) has compiled a helpful summary of the mental health benefits of an active lifestyle. In doing so, she indicates the findings that appear consistently in addition to the relationships that remain unclear or unstudied.

Findings are inconsistent with regard to persons who enjoy good mental health. Moreover, many more studies are necessary in terms of the effects of exercise upon the mental health of elderly persons who have no mental disorders. Presently, research in this area has been meager, and the reported findings are mixed (Fontane, 1996). In addition, the precise amounts and intensities of exercise required to produce mental health changes in the elderly have yet to be determined. Age may be a moderating variable in the psychological response to exercise because it may have varying degrees of personal meaning across the adult life span (Cousins, 1996). Gender may also moderate mental health benefits associated with exercise (Brown, 1992). However, psychological factors such as self-esteem, well-being, self-concept, body image, locus of control, anxiety, and depression have been shown to improve among the elderly involved in physical activity (Netz & Jacob, 1994). In addition, a number of researchers have observed that the mental health of older adults is improved as a result of participation in exercise even though their cardiorespiratory fitness remains unchanged (Brown & Wang, 1992; Landers & Petruzzello, 1994; McAuley & Rudolph, 1995).

For instance, Pierce and Pate (1994) administered the Profile of Mood States (POMS) to 16 women (mean age = 64.5 years) before and after a 75-minute aerobic dance session. All of the women had been participating in aerobic dance classes for over 6 months and were therefore considered well trained in the activity. Comparison of pre- and posttest scores showed significant improvements in global mood. Specifically, significant reductions in the POMS subscales of tension, depression, fatigue, and anger occurred following acute exercise; significant increases were reported on the vigor subscale; and no changes occurred on the confusion subscale. Cross cultural effects of exercise upon mood in the elderly or associations between these two variables are also evident. Depressive symptoms have been shown to be lower in elderly Japanese adults (65–79 years) who exercise, in comparison to non-exercisers (Fukukawa, Nakashima, Tsuboi, Kozukai, Doyo, Niino, Ando, & Shimokata, 2004), as well as in elderly Spanish men and women (50–82 years; Garcia-Martin & Gomez, 2004).

In their review of studies examining the effects of exercise on the elderly, Netz and Jacob (1994) report that physical activity has been associated with improvements in happiness, emotional health, self-esteem, well-being, self-concept, body image, locus of

control, anxiety, and depression for healthy, community-dwelling elderly individuals. However, mood benefits associated with physical activity are not likely to occur automatically and may be related to the type of exercise and training (Berger, 1996; Thayer, 1996). This is probably particularly true in the elderly. If, indeed, exercise can result in mood changes in the elderly, what then are the causative factors? We are not sure; however, two plausible explanations are available (Pierce & Pate, 1994):

1. Improvements in mood may be due to distractions from stressful stimuli in the exercising environment, and
2. Decreased levels of b-endorphins produced by the body may account for mood elevations.

Again, reported findings with regard to mood changes in the elderly following exercise are not in agreement, and the underlying mechanisms that may account for observed improvements are not well clarified.

Psychological Benefits

Cognitive function has also been shown to be positively correlated with exercise among the elderly (Emery & Blumenthal, 1991). Long-term regular physical activity, including walking, is associated with significantly better cognitive function and less cognitive decline in older women (Colcombe & Kramer, 2003; Weuve, Kang, Manson, Breteler, Wave, & Grodstein, 2004). Measures of cardiorespiratory fitness appear to be associated with cognitive function and attention; the more fit an elderly person is, the more capable he or she is cognitively and attentionally (Barnes, Yaffee, Satariano, & Tager, 2003). Apparently, such changes do not necessarily occur in institutionalized geriatric or mentally ill elderly populations who, for various reasons, are unable to participate in rigorous exercise.

Regular physical activity in early life seems to be linked with level in information processing speed at older age in men (Dik, Deeg, Visser, & Jonker, 2003). Another way of saying this is that early life physical activity may delay late-life cognitive deficits. Interestingly, the study that generated this positive link did not identify the same association in women.

Exercise environments may offer social opportunities for the elderly that may strengthen their readiness to cope with stressors that diminish their defense systems; this, in turn, may help ward off physical illness (Cassel, 1974). Exercise has also been shown to be positively related to the ability to cope with negative thoughts in the elderly. This finding has implications for developing and applying problem solving and coping strategies (Gyuresik & Estabrooks, 2004). Because a common tendency for older people is to withdraw from society (Shepherd, 1987), exercise may also be beneficial in that it can encourage remaining in the social mainstream.

As mentioned previously, another benefit of participation in an exercise program is a significant increase in self-concept and perceived locus of control (Netz & Jacob, 1994; Perri & Templer, 1984–85). The term *perceived locus of control* refers to the externality or internality of the alleged causes of a behavioral outcome as interpreted by the individual. That is, does a person tend to explain things that have happened to him in terms of factors that are within, or outside of, his control? The degree to which we take responsibility for our health is related to our perceived levels of control. Many elderly often express that, as they age, personal control over their health decreases. Those who believe that their ability to regulate life's many vicissitudes has been compromised tend to relinquish control. However, regular exercise may reverse these perceptions and, consequently, enhance self-concept.

Studies that have investigated mood changes and perceptions about the self in relation to exercise in elderly subjects have also revealed causal relationships. Perceptions about competency in locomotor activity and degree of independence with regard to physical tasks influence the lifestyle and accompanying anxieties in the elderly. Exercise seems to have a positive

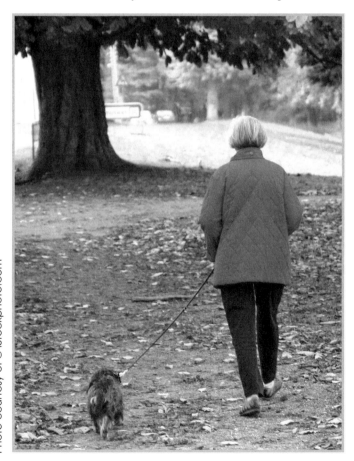

effect on such variables. Moreover, the exercise regimen need not take place in elaborate facilities or be highly rigorous. Neighborhood walking-based programs of low to moderate intensity have been shown to be feasible and beneficial in promoting quality of life among elderly participants (Fisher & Fuzhong, 2004).

Psychophysiological Benefits

It appears that exercise may exert a positive influence on cognitive activity, as well (Molloy et al., 1988; Netz & Jacob, 1994). For instance, cerebral function, including color recognition, has been shown to improve as a consequence of participation in aerobic conditioning classes (Spirduso & MacRae, 1991; Tomporowski & Ellis, 1986). In addition, significant improvements in indicators of fluid intelligence were observed by Dustman et al. (1994), whose subjects participated in 4 months of aerobic exercise at 70 to 80% of heart rate reserve. Although sufficient support of a positive correlation between CNS function and exercise is presently unavailable, it is plausible that such a relationship indeed exists (Brown, 1992). Elsayed, Ismail, and Young (1980) refer to the following mechanisms as reasons that exercise and resultant physical fitness may enhance cognitive functioning: (a) increased oxygen transport to the brain, (b) increased glucose transport to the brain, and (c) increased self-esteem and decreased psychological stress that results in improved performance on complex psychological tasks.

Performance on complex tasks in which qualitative aspects of performance are emphasized does not appear to correlate reliably with fitness levels. Examples of such complex tasks are problem solving, sustained attention, and dual-task performance. It also appears that tasks that demand novel and complex processing are more associated with exercise (Stones & Kozma, 1988). Although available research findings encourage the hypothesis that exercise has positive effects on various psychological functions, it is only fair to conclude that this assertion still remains without affirmation (Chodzko-Zajko, 1991).

Perhaps the lack of conclusive findings is due to other factors, such as education level and socioeconomic status (Dishman, 1989; Stephens, Craig, & Ferris, 1986). In addition, with regard to human subjects, the duration of the training periods in most studies has been abbreviated and is usually no more than a few months in duration. As Chodzko-Zajko and Moore (1994) suggest, this may not allow the impact of exercise upon CNS function to be manifested. It is also important to note that the positive relationship between exercise-related fitness and cognitive function in the elderly derives in large measure from studies that have used speed of response (timing tasks) as the dependent variable, rather than tasks that are highly complex or place emphasis upon attentional demands. Because automatic processes such as free-recall memory, reaction time, and movement time are performed without conscious attention, they are generally not affected by declines in attentional capacity (Hasher & Zacks, 1979).

Research on Exercise and the Elderly

Much more work is needed in the area of psychological benefits of exercise in elderly people. Some of the available findings have not permitted strong and useful conclusions. This may be due, in part, to methodological difficulties facing researchers. Dustman et al. (1994) describe the difficulty as follows:

> Does frequent endurance activity result in positive neurobiological changes in men and women, and with concomitant changes in electrophysiology and behavior?
>
> Obviously invasive procedures cannot be used with healthy humans to investigate possible changes in brain structure, vasculature, and chemistry. One might infer that these kinds of changes had occurred, however, if non-invasive measures of brain functioning consistently revealed that endurance training was positively associated with better performance. (p. 153)

Exercise research in elderly populations encompasses a very broad array of independent and dependent variables. Hypotheses dealing with cognition, psychomotoric response, affect, self-concept, and attributions (among several others) continue to be tested vis-à-vis exercise. Therefore, alternative research strategies are indicated. In recent years, researchers are increasingly turning to qualitative approaches in their efforts to determine relationships between exercise and different psychological variables.

Qualitative and Quantitative Research Designs

As is the case with any body of knowledge that deals with human behavior, what we know about exercise and the elderly derives from scientific studies. These studies are typically conducted by sport or exercise scientists who, more often than not, have employed empirical research (quantitative) approaches. In these studies, selected variables are carefully manipulated or controlled whereas others are permitted to operate freely on subjects or on the environment. The resulting data are then analyzed with appropriate statistical procedures that, in turn, lead to findings that are then interpreted by the researcher. Ultimately, conclusions are drawn that may be applied to the construction,

implementation, or evaluation of exercise programs for the elderly.

In recent years, an alternative research approach has increased in popularity among gerontological researchers. Qualitative research, which uses different strategies than those employed in quantitative research, proceeds through frequent, prolonged, or intense interaction with individuals, groups, or organizations. During this time, the researcher attempts to gain an understanding of "what's going on." The researcher is attentive and empathetic in his or her attempt to identify and find support for themes or perceptions that pervade or underlie the participant's behavior. A fine example of qualitative research design applied to an area within the framework of exercise for older individuals is the work of Duncan, Travis, and McAuley (1995). They explored the meaning and motivations for mall walking among participants over the age of 60. Mall walking has become the activity of choice for many older adults because it is safe, inexpensive, and generally accessible. Findings from this study resulted from personal conversations, guided interviews with the walkers, and observations made by the researchers. It was concluded that older adult mall walkers view this activity as a kind of "work" that replaces that which was lost through retirement. A model was developed by the researchers that will be helpful for leaders who wish to organize such programs for populations of elderly exercise enthusiasts.

Whether the approach is quantitative or qualitative, it is often imperfect in some way. Researchers may move in an inappropriate direction or use an incorrect statistical analysis. Any number of errors or incorrect decisions may be involved. This is particularly true of research related to exercise in the elderly. These weaknesses in formulating hypotheses and collecting, analyzing, or interpreting data make drawing conclusions difficult and inhibit construction of improved programs as well as incorporation of appropriate activities or frequencies and intensities for exercise. Future studies should be planned to examine differences in exercise effects between females and males across various age-groups (LaFontaine et al., 1992).

Methodological Concerns in Research on Exercise and the Elderly

A good portion of the available body of literature derives from methodologically correct research. Unfortunately, a large amount does not. Dishman (1988a) concludes that very few published findings and the lack of standardized research methods make specific functional details of the benefits of exercise for the elderly difficult to determine.

What follows is a brief discussion of shortcomings

of some of the studies with methodological inadequacies that have generated unusable or confusing findings. Another way to consider the following critique is as a partial checklist when conducting future research into exercise in the elderly.

Self-reporting. Numerous published papers dealing with exercise in the elderly employ self-report instruments. Self-report instruments rely upon the respondent's perceptions, recollections, or personal values. Questions included in such tests inquire about what the subject believes he or she has experienced, felt, or accomplished. Sometimes responses are at variance with what objective observers or objectively conducted quantitative assessment procedures would produce. In other words, what the respondent professes may indeed represent an honest viewpoint, but may not be accurate. If a subject's interpretation of a personal experience is the goal of the inquiry, then results are appropriate. On the other hand, if response accuracy is of essence, then clarification of the research question may be inhibited. Response distortion may be due to any number of biases or inclinations held by the respondent.

Sample size. Many of the studies that have tested hypotheses related to exercise in the elderly have employed insufficient numbers of subjects. Although adequate in that these studies may satisfy assumptions for parametric statistical use, the sample sizes may be insufficient to permit helpful generalization of findings. Because so many variables deserve consideration when selecting groups of elderly subjects (gender, race, occupation, level of education, etc.) many subgroups are often necessary, each of which must be adequate in size.

Ages of subjects. Persons 65 years of age are considered to be elderly—but so are those who are 85 years old. As observed earlier in this chapter, researchers accordingly define the term elderly in terms of their study's context. These variations in operational definitions may play havoc with attempts to draw helpful conclusions about the elderly in exercise. Distinctions are frequently made among young old, middle old, and very old subjects. Perhaps a more helpful approach would be to distinguish among subjects according to their physical limitations rather than according to chronological determinants.

Seasonal variations. Level of participation for exercise, energy level, and time available for exercise are variables that may affect exercise duration, frequency, and intensity. These, in turn, are often related to time of year. By and large, such seasonal variations have not been incorporated into research designs used to study elderly subjects in the context of exercise. For instance, inclement weather may influence ease of travel to exercise locations or the availability of exercise facilities or equipment. Climatic conditions can also inhibit participation (e.g., too hot or too cold to jog out of doors). Seasonal allergic reactions to pollen and similar allergens may, in addition, interact with any of the above participation variables. These variables should be considered in research designs.

Subjects' motivation for participation in exercise. In another chapter of this book, we refer to motivation as the fuel or energy within a person underlying his or her behavior. Alternatively, motivation may be viewed as the intensity or direction of behavior. Needless to say, these elements vary within and among exercisers. At times, one's motivation to participate in rigorous physical activity may be at high, moderate, or low levels. These within-person fluctuations may be due to any number of considerations, among them being social, physical, and emotional factors. For instance, enjoyment seems to be an important part of exercise participation (Berger, 1996; Wankel, 1993). Plans for research should appropriately acknowledge the potential interaction of these factors with exercise-related variables. When subjects are observed, evaluated, interviewed, or tested in any manner, their motivation for exercise may be related to their behaviors, achievement, or fashion in which they interpret the ongoing exercise experience.

An interesting line of research has focused upon the prevalence of disability in the elderly (in this case, 65 years or older) during the years preceding death. Those who were regularly physically active were almost twice as likely to die without disability in comparison to sedentary counterparts (Ferrucci et al., 1999; Leveille, Guralnik, Ferrucci, & Langlois, 1999). In other words, a higher level of physical activity is associated with higher quality of life in the years prior to death.

Gender Differences Between Elderly Male and Female Exercisers

In North American society, females begin to outnumber males at the age of 35 and continue this trend into old age. In 1982, there were 1.5 females per each male among persons 65 years of age and older, and in the year 2000, it is estimated that there are 2.34 females for every male between the ages of 85 and 89 years (Dishman, 1988a). In addition, females tend to live longer than males.

It appears that, at all ages, males and females are involved with exercise in different ways (McAuley, Shaffer, & Rudolph, 1995; Spirduso, 1995). For example, Ostrow and Dzewaltowski (1986) observed that elderly subjects of both genders perceive physical activity as more appropriate for males than females. Explanations for this perception remain unclear. Perhaps elderly individuals responding to questionnaires designed to assess perceptions about exercise participants retain gender-related role expectations. Indeed, Stephens and Craig (1990) and Mobily (1987) reported that males participated in exercise more frequently than females did. However, as individuals age, a decline in total physical activity occurs in both sexes (Talbot, Metter, & Fleg, 2000).

At least one reported study attempted to compare the degree to which elderly males and females comply with physician-prescribed exercise regimens. In their sample of 323 men and women (mean age for males = 70.1; for females, 70.8) with documented nonterminal cardiovascular problems, Sharp, Clark, and Janz (1991) observed significantly greater compliance in men than in women. Once again, perhaps the strict gender-based rules governing appropriate physical activity in the early decade of the twentieth century may have inhibited female participation.

In their study of 125 elderly subjects, Mobily and colleagues (1993) found a significant positive correlation between exercise behavior, including frequency and perceptions about competency for physical activity. That is, subjects who expressed confidence in their ability to engage in physical exercise were more inclined to actually do more. Therefore, within segments of a population that has been socialized away from exercise for leisure or health purposes, lower perceptions of competence would be expected. Hence, frequency of participation would be low. Males develop a greater repertoire for leisure physical activity than females do, and males participate more.

Also, older women have reported more dissatisfaction with their bodies than older men have as indicated by the Draw-A-Person test, which measures nonverbal intelligence and screens for emotional or behavioral disorders by analyzing aspects of drawings of body parts, clothing, and so on (Janelli, 1993). Such differences could result in variations in the ways males and females experience mood changes during or after exercise. As mentioned previously in this chapter, some elderly women with elevated levels of physique anxiety may undergo modification of their body image due to other women exercisers who wear "revealing attire" (Sinden, Ginis, & Angove, 2003). Lastly, older women have much more to gain from regular aerobic exercise because they have greater longevity than men do and often experience functional disability in late life (O'Brien & Vertinsky, 1991).

Summary

As the elderly have become the fastest growing age-group in the United States, attention has been afforded to them as a special population in the area of exercise. Unfortunately, fewer than 10% of Americans ages 65 years and older participate in regular, vigorous exercise. They often view the deteriorations that accompany the aging process as barriers to exercise. However, despite the inevitable changes that occur with time, the elderly may greatly benefit from exercise participation.

Fundamentally, exercise improves the quality of life by preventing or slowing further declines in functioning. The elderly may also derive several physiological, psychological, and psychophysiological benefits from exercise. Among these numerous benefits are decreased blood pressure, increased stroke volume, increased self-concept, and increased self-esteem.

Conducting research in exercise with the elderly presents several challenges. Methodological problems often arise through self-reporting, defining the age of elderly persons, and obtaining an adequate sample size. Careful considerations must be made in planning and developing a research design, including devoting attention to seasonal variations and differences in motivation for exercise.

Lastly, gender differences have been observed between male and female elderly exercisers. Elderly men participate in exercise more frequently than elderly females do and also comply with an exercise program more often than elderly females do. However, older females have much more to gain from regular aerobic exercise than males.

Can You Define These Terms?

functional independence

middle old age

old-old age

perceived locus of control

primary aging processes

secondary aging processes

young old age

Can You Answer These Questions?

1. Why do the elderly fail to participate in exercise programs?
2. What changes occur as a result of the aging process?
3. Are adaptations to exercise similar in elderly to those of younger persons?
4. What benefits can the elderly achieve through exercise participation?
5. What are the disadvantages of self-report measures?
6. How do elderly males and females differ with regard to exercise?

CHAPTER 20

Exercise Enjoyment and Mode Considerations: Guidelines for Optimizing Psychological Benefits

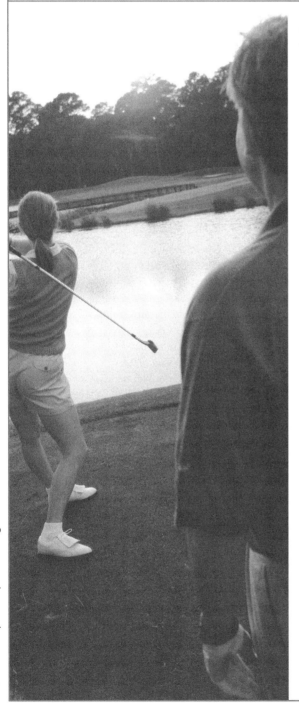

After reading this chapter, you should be able to

- Identify common exercise goals,

- Describe the three broad components of a taxonomy that "maximizes" the psychological benefits associated with exercise,

- Provide contrasting definitions or interpretations of "enjoyment,"

- Explain why enjoyment of an activity is important for the psychological benefits,

- Discuss the possibility that the guideline for aerobic exercise actually may be for abdominal, rhythmical breathing,

- Describe the advantages of de-emphasizing interpersonal competition in physical activity,

- Explain the concept of positive addiction and whether it is desirable,

- Provide the rationale for the benefits of closed, or temporally and spatially certain, activities, and

- Review the possible role of rhythmical and repetitive movements in the psychological benefits of exercise.

Each sport has a rhythm

    of its own

each a lyric quality

    that flows with

        its unique motion

        its unique truth

        its unique emotion

known only within the soul of woman

      as it breaks silence

        with its answer [emphasis added]

(Price, 1983, p. 23)

Introduction

Selecting a specific type of exercise often occurs by accident or chance, rather than by conscious decision making. For example, when you were young, your friends might have played basketball, and you joined them. Today, you may be on an intramural basketball team for similar social reasons. When you were a child, your parents might have enrolled you in ballet classes, swimming lessons at the local YWCA, or lacrosse at a summer sports camp. These choices depended on whether the activities were available in your local community, whether your parents had the time and resources to take you, and whether your parents thought physical activity was important. As you grew older, either you found these activities appealing and continued them, or you dropped out.

Life circumstances such as parental involvement in physical activity, geographical location, socioeconomic status, friendships, and gender strongly influence our exercise patterns. Choices of whether to exercise and even of exercise type and the training parameters are too important to be circumstantial. As future exercise and sport psychologists, physical educators, personal trainers, and sports medicine specialists, you need concrete, research-based information to guide you in facilitating the psychological, as well as the physical, benefits of exercise when designing exercise programs. This information is the focus of the present chapter.

Exercise Considerations for Enhancing Psychological Benefits: A Tentative Taxonomy

Choosing an *enjoyable activity* and an appropriate *mode* or *type* of exercise is an important consideration if the participant is to be successful in reaching her or his exercise goals—both psychological and physical. People have diverse preferences and multiple exercise goals. In addition, exercise enjoyment, mode prefer-

ences, and goals probably change from one exercise activity to another and throughout various stages of an individual's life. Common exercise goals include enjoyment, fun, stress management, improved mood, health, weight loss (or gain), increased muscle definition or bulk, social camaraderie, and even longer-than-normal life span.

Emphasizing the need to find an enjoyable, psychologically satisfying type of activity, philosopher George Sheehan (1992a) reports that a major obstacle to a successful exercise program is boredom:

My object is to suggest to the people in the audience how they can be made to feel at home in a fitness program. *That program, if it is to succeed, must be interesting and satisfying. It should be filled with pleasure and excitement and absorption. It must be place where a person is rarely if ever bored* [italics added].

Can all this be accomplished while doing something boring? Possibly. You might, for instance, try thinking of something interesting while you are doing something boring. *If the running movement can be made automatic, the mind can wander through meadows of thought, completely engrossed in its own activities* [italics added]. This is called dissociation, and most runners do it. When you see them trotting down the road, their minds are usually miles and possibly centuries away.

I find swimming boring because I am unable to dissociate while I swim. The instant I let my mind go off on its own, I sink. I have to attend constantly to the movement of my arms and legs or I flounder in the water. When I run, however, I am able to put my body on automatic pilot and let my mind loose to search for interesting ideas.

. . . If this fails you can try another ploy. Make what is boring interesting. Take an interesting companion on the run. Good talk can halve the distance. You will come to the end of the run feeling as if you had just begun. If you are a gossip, you should run with a gossip. If people form a large part of your world, your fitness world must include them as well.

Another way to make something boring interesting is to make it competitive. (p. 140)

In this chapter, you will examine the importance of exercise enjoyment and exercise mode or type that may enhance the *psychological benefits* of exercise and ultimately the physiological health benefits by facilitating exercise adherence. In the next chapter, you will focus on exercise-training parameters or practice guidelines that may further enhance the psychological benefits of exercise. In general, exercisers who reach their goals, enjoy the activities, and "feel better" after exercising are inclined to be physically active for an extended portion of their lives.

Berger (1983/1984) proposed and subsequently tested a taxonomy or classification system that seems likely to enhance the psychological benefits associated with exercise (e.g., Berger, 2004; Berger & Owen, 1988; Berger & Tobar, in press; Motl, Berger, & Leuschen, 2000). Basic components within the taxonomy include

- Enjoyment of the exercise experience,
- Type of activity, or exercise mode, and
- Practice or training requirements.

The major mode components in the taxonomy are emphasized in Figure 20.1 (e.g., Berger, Grove, Prapavessis, & Butki, 1997; Berger & Owen, 1988, 1992a, 1998). Although Berger and her colleagues continue to test the factors, the components seem to be important considerations in selecting mode and practice conditions to facilitate psychological well-being (e.g., Berger, 2004; Berger & Motl, 2001; Berger & Tobar, in press). The taxonomy components and parameters remain flexible in order to incorporate the latest research results.

Supporting the exercise guidelines in this chapter and in Chapter 21, participants in a conference on exercise and mental health concluded that there was a need to investigate "the *optimal mode, intensity, dura-tion, and frequency* [italics added] of exercise required providing more effective responses to mental stress" (Morgan & Goldston, 1987, p. 157). Ten years later, Morgan (1997a) emphasized in the concluding chapter to his edited book on *Physical Activity and Mental Health* that future research would

> . . . need to address the related issues of *exercise mode* (e.g., running, walking); *intensity* (e.g., low, moderate, high); *duration* (e.g., 15, 30, 45 min); *frequency* (e.g., 1, 3, 5 days per week); *preferred versus prescribed* exertion levels; *personalized prescription* (e.g., based on personality structure); *and lifestyle versus traditional exercise prescription*. . . . (p. 231)

The taxonomy guidelines illustrate the complexity of the relationship between exercise and psychological well-being. Although the taxonomy does not include all components necessary for designing an individualized exercise program to enhance psychological well-being, it provides exercise specialists with basic considerations. This chapter emphasizes that exercise enjoyment and modes are related to the use of exercise to enhance well-being. Some of the information is based on replicable research; other portions are more speculative and in need of further investigation.

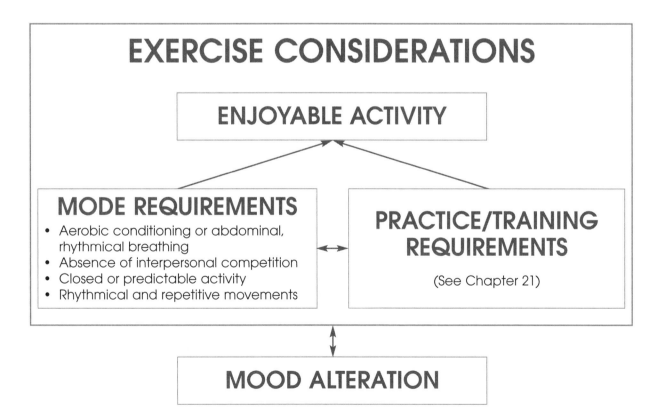

Figure 20.1. Tentative taxonomy for enhancing the psychological benefits of exercise (Berger, 1983/84, 1996; Berger & Motl, 2001; Berger & Owen, 1988, 1992a).

Enjoyment

Enjoyment is the first taxonomy requirement because it can be used to guide the selection of the exercise mode and practice parameters. If exercise is not enjoyable, it is less likely to be associated with desirable psychological changes such as mood enhancement, more positive self-concept, and stress reduction (Berger & Owen, 1988; Motl, Berger & Leuschen, 2000). Miller and colleagues (Miller, Bartholomew, & Springer, 2005) recently tested the influence of exercise enjoyment on the relationship between exercise and mood alteration as hypothesized by Berger and colleagues (e.g., Berger & Motl, 2000; Motl et al., 2000). College students participated in high and low preference exercise modes that were aerobic and rhythmical and reflected common equipment offered to clients in exercise clubs. Exercise modes included using the following equipment: (1) stair stepper, (2) treadmill, (3) rower, (4) stationary cycle ergometer, and (5) cross-country skiing machine (Miller et al., 2005). Results indicated that participants' exercise enjoyment ratings of the exercise mode mediated desirable changes in both positive and negative affect as measured by the Positive Affect Negative Affect Schedule (PANAS; Watson, Clark, & Tellegen, 1988). These findings on the role of enjoyment mediating mood changes replicated the work of Motl and colleagues (2000). In addition to the results for enjoyment, participants exercising in their most preferred exercise mode reported greater improvements in only positive affect than when they participated in their low preference exercise mode. Regardless of mode preferences, exercisers reported similar reductions in negative affect after exercising. It seems that exercise preference was one of many factors that contribute to exercise enjoyment, and additional work is needed to broaden our understanding of how enjoyment contributes to the psychological response to exercise (Miller et al., 2005).

In addition to the direct effects of exercise enjoyment and preference on mood alteration, enjoyment may detract indirectly from the benefits of exercise, because its lack decreases the likelihood of adherence (e.g., Salmon, Owen, Crawford, Bauman, & Sallis, 2003). Most people do not participate in activities on a long-term basis if they do not enjoy them. Thus, lack of enjoyment decreases physiological benefits if the person stops exercising. In his book emphasizing the importance of the joy of exercising, Jay Kimiecik (2002), an exercise psychologist at Miami University of Ohio, emphasizes that

> To become a regular exerciser over a long period of time, you must *learn to love moving your body*. That's it! *And to enjoy moving your body you must develop what I call the* [italics added] *intrinsic*

mindset for changing behavior. Frankly, helping people find the joy or passion in movement is what's missing from most of the programs and books you may have tried. (p. 2)

> Going on sheer willpower or guilt is not enough to make you change. Yet that is the message you typically hear from the health and fitness profession and the media. Instead, *you become an exerciser by finding the joy and fun before, during, and after every exercise experience* [italics added]. (p. 2)

Defining Enjoyment: Not as Easy as It Seems

Before discussing enjoyment, it is important to define what *enjoyment* means. Clarifying the meaning would seem to be an easy undertaking. A dictionary definition of *enjoyment* is "**1 a :** the action or state of enjoying **b :** possession and use <the ~ of civic rights> **2 :** something that gives keen satisfaction <the poorest life has its ~s and pleasures>" (*Merriam-Webster's Collegiate Dictionary*, 2003, p. 414). This dictionary definition refers to *positive affect*, or emotion, and is similar to the following definition by exercise and sport psychologist, Leonard M. Wankel (1993):

> . . . *enjoyment is viewed as a positive emotion, a positive affective state* [italics added]. It may be *homeostatic in nature* [italics added], resulting from the satisfaction of biological needs . . ., or *growth oriented* [italics added], involving a cognitive dimension focused on the perception of successfully applying one's skills to meet environmental challenges. Enjoyment is clearly linked to the concept intrinsic motivation . . . [E]njoyment may be viewed as one dimension of the multi-dimensional construct, intrinsic motivation. (p. 153)

Exercise and sport psychologists have difficulty in agreeing on a definition of enjoyment. Wankel (1993) suggests that enjoyment is one of many factors influencing intrinsic motivation, or the pursuit of an activity for the rewards within the activity itself. However, Scanlan and Simons (1992) present a broader perspective of enjoyment as illustrated in Figure 20.2. Their conception of enjoyment includes *intrinsic and extrinsic factors* as well as *achievement and nonachievement factors* inherent within sport and exercise contexts. Exercise experiences in the four quadrants of Figure 20.2 contribute to the enjoyment of various exercise modes and certainly vary in their importance from one individual to another and from one activity to another. According to the model in Figure 20.2, key influences on exercise enjoyment are:

- The movement experience itself,
- The social and environmental setting,

- Self-reinforced feelings of mastery, competence, and control, and
- Externally reinforced feelings of mastery, competence, and control, such as social recognition.

As Scanlan and Simons noted, their model of enjoyment, which can be applied to exercise, is not predictive of enjoyment, but serves as a base for future studies of the sources of enjoyment in physical activity.

Most definitions of enjoyment suggest that it is a positive affective state that reflects feelings of pleasure, liking, and fun. However, Kimiecik and Harris (1996) suggest, "enjoyment is not an affective product

of experience, but *a psychological process* that *is* the experience" (p. 257; italics added). According to this conceptualization, enjoyment is not the *result* of participating in a physical activity, but enjoyment occurs *during* the physical activity itself. Kimiecik and Harris suggest that enjoyment is similar to the flow experience that, in turn, elicits the affective response of enjoyment. As described over 15 years ago by Csikszentmihalyi (1990), the "father" of flow research,

Enjoyable events [italics added] occur when a person has not only met some prior expectation or satisfied a need or a desire but also gone beyond

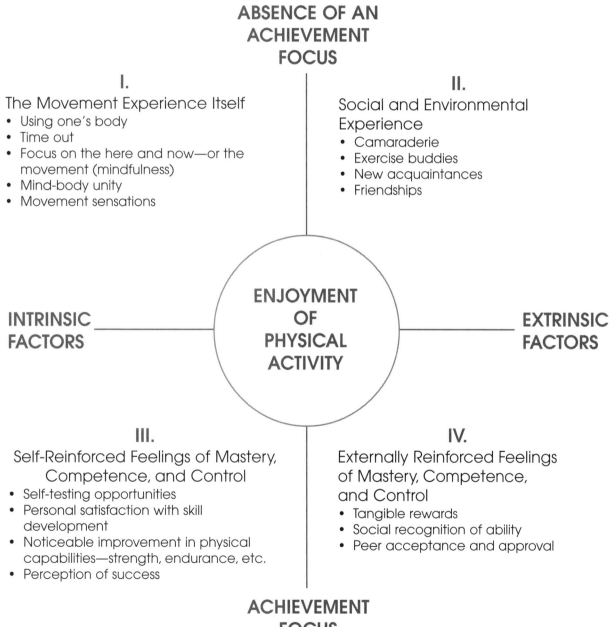

Figure 20.2. Possible sources of enjoyment in physical activity (Scanlan & Simons, 1992).

what she or he has been programmed to do and achieved something unexpected, perhaps something even unimagined before.

Enjoyment is characterized by this forward movement: by a sense of novelty, of accomplishment [italics added]. Playing a close game of tennis that stretches one's ability is enjoyable, as is reading a book that reveals things in a new light.... None of these experiences may have been particularly pleasurable at the time they are taking place, but afterward we think back on them and say, "That really was fun" and wish they would happen again. *After an enjoyable event we know that we have changed, that our self has grown* [italics added]: in some respect, we have become more complex as a result of it. (p. 46)

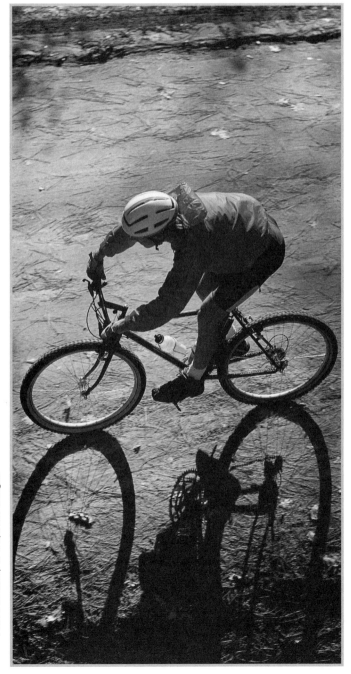

Photo courtesy of © Eyewire Images

In conclusion, the definition of enjoyment used in this chapter is a positive affective response, a process, and part of the larger flow experience. Regardless of how it is defined, enjoyment is a highly sought and valued personal experience (Jackson, 2000). In fact, enjoyment is a major factor in attaining an optimal quality of life, which is characterized by long-term happiness and psychological well-being (Diener, Colvin, Pavot, & Allman, 1991).

The Importance of Enjoyment

Children's enjoyment of physical activity is the most crucial factor in their decisions to remain involved with, or to drop out of, sport and presumably exercise (Fine & Sachs, 1997). In fact, having fun was the primary reason for sport participation in a poll of 2,000 boys and 1,900 girls in grades 7 to 12 when asked what they liked best about sport (American Footwear Association, 1991). Supporting the importance of enjoyment in physical activity, *not having fun*, was the second most important reason provided by adolescents for ceasing their participation in sport according to a poll of 2,700 boys and 3,100 girls. When these same boys and girls were asked what would encourage them to be active again in sport, they responded that they would play if practices were more fun (American Footwear Association). See Table 20.1 for the top 10 reasons for continuing and the top 11 reasons for stopping their participation in school sport. Although these reasons for participating apply to sport, they also appear to be relevant for exercise.

If you enjoy exercise, you are more likely to participate than if you are neutral towards the activity, or even dislike it (e.g., Motl, Dishman, Saunders, Dowda, Felton, & Pate, 2001; Salmon et al., 2003). In a comprehensive study ($N = 1332$ adults) employing behavioral choice theory, the influence of environmental and personal factors on *choice* of participating in either physical activity or sedentary behavior were investigated. Adults randomly selected from the adult Australian population who reported both high exercise enjoyment *and* a preference for physical activity (rather than for sedentary behaviors such as watching TV) were more likely to report high levels of participation in physical activity (Salmon et al., 2003). In addition, adults who reported financial cost, weather conditions, and personal barriers to physical activity were less likely to be physically active than those who did not identify these factors as barriers to physical activity. As Salmon and colleagues (2003) concluded, exercise enjoyment, preference for physical activity, and personal barriers are major factors to consider when designing successful exercise programs for adults.

Habitual participation is important not only to establish fitness, that is, a *product* of exercise, but also

Table 20.1

Reasons That Children Participate and Stop Participating in School Sports (American Footwear Association, 1991)

Reasons for Participating in My Best Sport	Reasons for Ceasing Participation
1. Having fun	1. Losing interest
2. Improving sport skills	2. Not having fun
3. Staying in shape	3. Requiring too much time
4. Doing something I am good at	4. Coach's being a poor teacher
5. Enjoying the excitement	5. Feeling too much pressure
6. Getting some exercise	6. Wanting a nonsport activity
7. Playing as part of a team	7. Being tired of it
8. Meeting the challenge of competition	8. Needing more time to study
9. Learning new skills	9. Coach's playing favorites
10. Winning	10. Finding sport boring
	11. Overemphasizing winning

to facilitate enjoyment of the exercise *process.* Wankel, a noted exercise psychology researcher formerly at the University of Alberta in Canada, has explored the relationship between exercise enjoyment and adherence. Wankel (1993) suggests that enjoyment is influenced by factors such as

- Compatibility of exercise type with specific exercise goals,
- Progress toward reaching one's exercise goals,
- Social interactions within an activity,
- Combination of challenges, feelings of competency, and flow experiences, and
- Individual differences.

Emphasizing the importance of enjoyment in the process of becoming a life-long exerciser, Jay Kimiecik (2002, 2005) suggests that joy and enjoyment are key to becoming an *Intrinsic Exerciser,* a person who exercises for the pure joy/enjoyment of moving his or her body. In fact, as Kimiecik (2002, p. 22) observes, the *Intrinsic Exerciser* celebrates life through exercise. Knowing that research data supports the health benefits of exercise is *insufficient* to help people become regular exercisers. The four steps that facilitate becoming an *Intrinsic Exerciser* include (1) vision, (2) mastery, (3) flow, and (4) inergy (Kimiecik, 2002, pp. 41–47; 2005). Creating *vision,* the first step on the intrinsic path for the exercise experience means that participants use exercise to explore who they are,

and to articulate why they are exercising and what they hope to obtain. Creating a vision of possible selves includes a vision of what exercisers want their bodies to do and how they want to feel when exercising on a path of creating a meaningful exercise program (Kimiecik, 2005). Focusing on *mastery* enables exercisers to draw on their natural desire to improve, to grow, and to accomplish while simultaneously avoiding comparisons with other exercisers. *Flow* and *staying in the moment* is what every exercise session should be about, and "flow or optimal experience is a vital part of being human" (Kimiecik, 2002, p. 44). The final step in becoming an *Intrinsic Exerciser* who enjoys the exercise process is by creating "*inergy,*" an energy that emanates from *in*side the body and results from making connections among one's mind, body, and spirit (Kimiecik, 2002, pp. 44–47).

Inergy, a striving to be whole, balanced, and integrated for optimal functioning and well-being, is very similar to the goals of yoga experts as described by Iyengar (2005). This body-mind-spirit integration for optimal well-being seems to result in enjoyment and is a fascinating concept that continues to emerge in diverse literatures (e.g., Iyengar, 2005; Kimiecik, 2002, 2005). Integration of body-mind-spirit seems to contribute to exercise enjoyment, but at this time remains an ethereal concept. Body-mind-spirit integration is a difficult concept to investigate and is in need of direct investigation.

Measuring Exercise Enjoyment

Enjoyment is in the eye of the beholder; it is difficult to define and measure. Nonetheless, Kendzierski and DeCarlo (1991) have developed the Physical Activity Enjoyment Scale (PACES) to measure this important concept. The PACES includes the 18 bipolar enjoyment-related items as listed in Table 20.2. As reflected in the Table, each item in the inventory is rated on a seven-point scale. You can compute an enjoyment score by summing responses to each of the 18 items.

The PACES is a useful measurement of enjoyment. It has successfully measured enjoyment and subsequent choice of activity in college-aged samples (Kendzierski & DeCarlo, 1991). The college-aged exercisers who had higher enjoyment scores on the PACES when they either were riding an exercise bicycle or jogging on a mini-trampoline on two different occasions selected the more enjoyable activity for participation on a third occasion. Thus, exercise enjoyment scores were related to subsequent choice of activity. This correlation between activity choice and enjoyment scores supports the validity of the PACES as a measure of enjoyment (Kendzierski & DeCarlo, 1991).

A modified version of the PACES was associated with participation in physical activity and sport in a sample of eighth-grade girls (Motl et al., 2001). The minor modifications included deletion of items #5 ("I am very absorbed in the activity") and #11 ("It's very invigorating") and a slight rewording of other items as appropriate for eighth graders. Exercise enjoyment as measured by the slightly modified version of the PACES for eighth-grade children that excluded two of the 18 test items seems to have a unidimensional or a single factor structure that was valid for a large sample ($N = 1797$) of African-American and Caucasian eighth grade girls (Motl et al., 2001).

The PACES also may include several subcomponents such as (1) excitement/sensation aspect of movement, (2) feelings of competence, and (3) a general affect or mood states when measured in youth sport camp participants who ranged between 12 and 16 years of age (e.g., Crocker, Bouffard, & Gessaroli, 1995). Whether the PACES captures a single factor of enjoyment or several sub-components of enjoyment awaits further study before it can be answered. However, it is not surprising that people tend to choose an exercise activity that they enjoy and that those who are physi-

CASE STUDY 20.1 — Examining Your Own Enjoyment of Exercise

Test your own enjoyment of several different physical activities. For comparison purposes, select a *favorite* exercise activity and also one of your *least favorite* exercise activities. Now that you have done this, you are ready to participate in the Case Study.

1) **First, carefully select *one* of your favorite exercise activities.**

   For example, you might choose weight training or jogging. Visualize yourself participating in that activity in one of your favorite places to exercise. Picture how you feel while participating in this exercise activity for a full three to five minutes. Then complete the Physical Enjoyment Activity Scale (PACES) which is contained in Table 20.2 (Kendzierski & DeCarlo, 1991).

2) **Then, pause for a moment after you have rated your favorite exercise activity. Be sure to clear your mind.**

3) **Next, choose another specific type of exercise—this time, one that you do not enjoy.**

   Visualize yourself participating in this activity for another three to five minutes, and get caught up in this exercise mode. Carefully rate this second, disliked type of exercise activity on the PACES.

4) **Score your responses on the PACES for each of the activities.**

   The possible range of scores from 18 to 126 reflects the two extremes of the enjoyment inventory. Your scores for both activities probably are in the middle of the range. The scores for your favorite physical activity should be higher than those for your less enjoyable activity.

5) **Based on your scores, elaborate on the following questions.**

   - How different were your enjoyment scores for the two activities?
   - Do the items in the PACES reflect key aspects of your own enjoyment experiences?
   - What items would you add or delete to accurately reflect your exercise enjoyment?

Table 20.2
Physical Activity Enjoyment Scale (PACES)

Directions: Please rate how you feel *at the moment* about a physical activity (choose a specific activity). Circle your response to each of the following items.

Choice	Response	Opposite Choice
1. I enjoy it.	1 2 3 4 5 6 7	I hate it.
2. I feel bored.	1 2 3 4 5 6 7	I feel interested.
3. I dislike it.	1 2 3 4 5 6 7	I like it.
4. I find it pleasurable.	1 2 3 4 5 6 7	I find it unpleasurable.
5. I am very absorbed in this activity.	1 2 3 4 5 6 7	I am not at all absorbed in this activity.
6. It's no fun at all.	1 2 3 4 5 6 7	It's a lot of fun.
7. I find it energizing.	1 2 3 4 5 6 7	I find it tiring.
8. It makes me depressed.	1 2 3 4 5 6 7	It makes me happy.
9. It's very pleasant.	1 2 3 4 5 6 7	It's unpleasant.
10. I feel good physically while doing it.	1 2 3 4 5 6 7	I feel bad physically while doing it.
11. It's very invigorating.	1 2 3 4 5 6 7	It's not at all invigorating.
12. I am very frustrated.	1 2 3 4 5 6 7	I am not at all frustrated.
13. It's very gratifying.	1 2 3 4 5 6 7	It's not at all gratifying.
14. It's very exhilarating.	1 2 3 4 5 6 7	It's not at all exhilarating.
15. It's not at all stimulating.	1 2 3 4 5 6 7	It's very stimulating.
16. It gives me a strong sense of accomplishment.	1 2 3 4 5 6 7	It does not give me any sense of accomplishment at all.
17. It's very refreshing.	1 2 3 4 5 6 7	It's not at all refreshing.
18. I felt as though I would rather be doing something else.	1 2 3 4 5 6 7	I felt as though there was nothing else I would rather be doing.

Scoring instructions: To determine a score, add the actual numbers you circled for items 2, 3, 6, 8, 12, 15, and 18. The following items are reverse scored: 1, 4, 5, 7, 9, 10, 11, 13, 14, 16, and 17. Thus 1 = 7, 2 = 6, 6 = 2, and 7 = 1. Compute an overall score by summing the total number of points for each of the 18 items.

Note: From "Physical Activity Enjoyment Scale: Two Validation Studies," by D. Kendzierski and K. J. DeCarlo, 1991, *Journal of Sport and Exercise Psychology, 13,* pp. 50–64. Copyright 1991 by Human Kinetics. Adapted with permission.

cally active have higher scores on exercise enjoyment than those who are less active (Dishman et al., 2005).

Take a moment to complete the adult version of the PACES to obtain a firsthand impression of the inventory and its accuracy or validity in capturing exercise enjoyment. See Case Study 20.1 for suggestions for completing the PACES.

You can conduct your own informal analysis of the PACES. As you were measuring enjoyment of your favorite and less favorite exercise activities, did any of the test items seem to be measuring different aspects of enjoyment? If so, how would you describe these subcomponents of enjoyment? Were they the subcomponents of excitement/sensation, accomplishment or competence, and diffuse affective states as identified by Crocker and colleagues (1995)? Did you identify any other subcomponents of enjoyment, or did you think that enjoyment is a single factor as concluded by Motl and colleagues (2001)? Regardless of the measurement issues related to exercise enjoyment, evidence is accumulating that enjoyment is related to mood enhancement (e.g., Miller et al., 2005) and to exercise participation (e.g., Kimiecik, 2002, 2005; Motl et al., 2001; Salmon et al., 2003).

Enjoyment of Diverse Physical Activities: The Research

Racquetball. The enjoyment requirement in the exercise taxonomy adjusts for individual exercise preferences and differences. Illustrating the importance of enjoyment, women and men ranging in age between 18 and 61 years (mean age of 30 years) ranked enjoyment as the most important factor in their attraction to racquetball. Other items included self-satisfaction, challenge, and competition (Battista, 1990). Factors that contribute to enjoyment vary from one type of physical activity to another, and from one person to another. For example, some people might enjoy the social atmosphere and the opportunity to exhibit their attractive bodies when exercising in a busy fitness center. Other individuals might find such an experience to be stress producing. Some people love solitary activities such as running and swimming alone; others find them boring and cannot fathom why anyone would choose to participate in such activities.

Rock climbing and swimming. In an investigation of enjoyment among rock climbers and swimmers, rock climbers enjoyed their activity more than swimmers did (Motl & Berger, 1997). However, the self-selected climbers and swimmers reported greater enjoyment than cyclists and joggers who were randomly assigned to an exercise activity by Kendzierski and DeCarlo (1991). A subsequent study compared enjoyment scores of rock climbers and a comparison group of students in a lecture class that watched a video of climbing (Motl et al., 2000). Rock climbers enjoyed their activity significantly more than did the comparison group. In addition, both enjoyment and type of activity were related to desirable mood changes that included decreases in tension, depression, and total mood disturbance and increases in vigor. Enjoyment appeared to influence the differential mood changes associated with rock climbing and with watching the video of rock climbing.

It still is unclear (a) whether enjoyment causes desirable mood changes or (b) whether experiencing the mood benefits cause enjoyment. However, the study of rock climbers provided some evidence for the first possibility. Regardless of the relationship between enjoyment and mood change, these results support the importance of considering a person's potential enjoyment of an activity when selecting an exercise mode, especially if that particular person wants to "feel better" after exercising.

Highlighting the possible role of enjoyment within the exercise experience, unpleasant weather conditions such as uncomfortable heat or cold may negate the expected mood benefits that often are associated with exercise. This possibility was presented by Berger and Owen (1986) when they tested swimmers on a day that was unbearably hot. Air temperature in the pool area was 106° and the water temperature was unusually warm. These swimmers reported no acute mood changes— either positive or negative. The lack of evidence for mood improvement might be attributed to unpleasant air and water temperature.

Another study of swimmers examining temperature, or "thermogenesis," as a causal factor in the relationship between exercise and mood change has implications for enjoyment (Koltyn, Shake, & Morgan, 1993). Swimmers wearing wet suits that kept them warm reported the mood benefits of decreased state anxiety after swimming in cold water. When swimming in the less enjoyable conditions of cold water without wet suits and in warm water with wet suits, the exercisers reported increases in anxiety. In conclusion, it seems that when exercise experiences are unpleasant, participants do not always "feel better" after exercising. Participants seeking psychological benefits would be well advised to seek alternative forms of exercise if some aspect of that particular activity is unpleasant and cannot be modified (Koltyn et al.).

Enjoyment of Physical Education Classes

Physical education classes in the schools teach movement skills that ideally are used by diverse participants in lifetime personal exercise programs. To establish lifetime exercise patterns, it is important that physical education teachers design activity programs that are enjoyable to establish students' positive perception of diverse exercise modes. As described by Jay Kimiecik (2002) in *The Intrinsic Exerciser*, exercise can be a joyous experience in which participants love moving their bodies. A major question is—how can this joy of movement be imparted to the general population? One avenue of imparting this enjoyment is through physical education classes. Physical education teachers establish multiple goals for their programs, one of which could be the goal of creating intrinsic exercisers by promoting enjoyable physical activity participation.

The goal of creating intrinsic exercisers is particularly important for physical education teachers since enjoyment of physical education classes decreases as students progress through elementary school (Prochaska, Sallis, Slymen, & McKenzie, 2003). In a prospective study that documented changes in physical education enjoyment over time, there was a consistent decline in enjoyment for children (N = 414) as they moved from grade four to six. Enjoyment was measured by a single item, "How do you feel about PE classes," and the response options on a pictorial scale were six "sad/happy" faces. The decline in enjoyment measured in the same students throughout the three-year time period was from 90% to 78%. Since the decline in enjoyment of physical education was strongest for girls, older children, and children not on sports teams, these children could benefit from intervention programs designed to counter dissatisfaction with physical education and possibly with all types of physical activity (Prochaska et al., 2003).

Intervention Program Designed to Increase Exercise Enjoyment

To examine the influence of exercise enjoyment on participation in physical activity, Rod Dishman and colleagues (2005) designed a physical activity intervention program to increase feelings of (1) fun and enjoyment and (2) exercise self-efficacy beliefs in ninth grade girls. Entitled Lifestyle Education for Activity Program (LEAP), the Program emphasized choice of physical activity, gender-separate activities, small group interaction, and inclusivity, and deemphasized competition. LEAP was offered in multiple school settings that included 1049 girls in the experimental group and 1038 girls in a control group. The girls' mean age was 13.6 years and their racial proportions were 46% Caucasian, 50% black, and 4% other.

Results of the intervention program in school-based physical education classes indicated that LEAP influenced the girls' enjoyment of physical education and their physical activity levels. Their enjoyment of physical education influenced their (1) general enjoyment of physical activity as measured by the modified 16-item PACES inventory refined by Motl and colleagues (2001) and (2) exercise-related self-efficacy. Another finding was that by influencing self-efficacy, enjoyment indirectly influenced participation in physical activity. As concluded by Dishman and his colleagues (2005), this is the first randomized, controlled trial that shows that increased enjoyment results in increased physical activity in adolescent girls.

Numerous factors appear to influence exercise enjoyment and those included in the Dishman et al. (2005) study included the following: choice of physical activity, gender-separate activities, small group interaction, inclusiveness, and relative lack of competition. Additional research is needed to identify personal, behavioral, and environmental characteristics that influence specific exercise enjoyment in children as well as adults. The following taxonomy factors of exercise mode and training/practice factors also capture factors that influence exercise enjoyment as reflected by the bi-directional arrows in Figure 20.1.

Exercise Mode Guidelines for Psychological Benefits

In addition to enjoyment, the mode or type of exercise seems likely to influence the relationship between exercise participation and psychological well-being. See Figure 20.1 for the four essential mode characteristics and Table 20.3 for some of the exercise modes, durations, and intensities that have been associated with mood alteration as measured by the Profile of Mood States (POMS; McNair, Lorr, & Droppleman, 1971/1992). Although there may be individual differences, exercise activities that have the following characteristics are good choices for enhancing the psychological benefits of exercise:

- Influence participants' breathing patterns,
- Include relatively little interpersonal competition,
- Are closed, predictable, or temporally and spatially certain, and
- Exhibit rhythmical and repetitive movements.

Aerobic Exercise and Psychological Well-Being: Is It Really Necessary?

Aerobic exercise consists of a continuous, large-muscle activity such as jogging, swimming, and cycling which increases pulmonary and cardiovascular capabilities. Aerobic activities are performed within an individual's aerobic training zone and result in improvements in aerobic fitness. This zone is approximately 60–90% of one's maximal heart rate. Below this intensity, the exercise results in little improvement in aerobic capacity. Exercise above 90% of maximal heart rate is *anaerobic*. Anaerobic exercise is performed without sufficient oxygen, and thus, participants are unable to sustain the activity for the recommended 20 to 30 minutes. In contrast, *nonaerobic* forms of exercise are lower in intensity than the 50 to 90% of maximal heart rate.

There is a general assumption that aerobic exercise is more likely than nonaerobic types of exercise to be associated with psychological well-being—especially with enhanced mood states (e.g., Berger & Tobar, in press; O'Halloran, Murphy, & Webster, 2004). Results

Table 20.3

Acute Mood Changes in a Variety of Exercise Types for Members of Normal Populations

Activities and Authors	Sex[a]	Age (Years)	Duration	Intensity[b]	POMS subscale changes[c,d]
Aerobic Dance					
Dyer & Crouch (1988)	M/F	17 to 26	45 min.	N/A	T, D, V, C
Maroulakis & Zervas (1993)	F	19 to 55; M=28.8	30 min.	60–80% $HR_{reserve}$	T, D, A, V, C
McInman & Berger (1993)	F	15 to 43; M=23.1	45 min.	N/A	T, D, A, V, C
Cycling					
Farrell et al. (1986)	M	M=24.2	30 min.	70% VO_{2max}	T
Steptoe & Cox (1988)	F	18 to 23; M=20.0	8 min.	25 watts	V
				100 watts	T, V, F
Steptoe, Kearsley, & Walters (1993)	M	20 to 35 Active M=26.4 Inactive M=27.3	20 min.	50 & 70% VO_{2max}	T, V
Hatha Yoga					
Berger & Owen (1988)	M/F	Ms=22.8 & 27.2	40 & 80 min.	N/A	T, D, A, F, C
Berger & Owen (1992a)	M/F	M=28.4	60 min.	N/A	T, D, A, F, C
Jogging					
Berger, Friedman, & Eaton (1988)	M/F	M=20.0	20 min	65–80% HR_{max}	T, D, A
Berger & Owen (1998)	M/F	Ms=20.7 to 25.1	20 min.	55, 75, & 79% HR_{max}	T, D, A, V, F, C
Berger et al. (1998)					
Study 1	M/F	18 to 51; M=21.39	15 min.	50, 65, & 80% HR_{max}	T, D, A, V, C (females only)
Study 2	M/F	18 to 45; M=22.22	15 min.	50, 65, & 85% HR_{max}	T, D, A, V, C
Boutcher & Landers (1988)	M	N/A	20 min.	80 to 85% HR_{max}	No changes
Dyer & Crouch (1988)	M/F	17 to 26	30 min.	N/A	T, D, A, V, F, C
Farrell, Gustafson, Morgan, & Pert (1987)	M	M=27.4	80 min. 80 min. 40 min.	40% VO_{2max} 60% VO_{2max} 80% VO_{2max}	No change T T
T Kraemer, Dzewaltowski, Blair, Rinehardt, & Castracane (1990)	M/F	Ms=28.8 to 31.5	30 min.	80% HR_{max}	T, D, A, C, TMD
Rock Climbing					
Motl et al. (2000)	M	18 to 38; M=25.5	10 to 50 min.	N/A	T, D, V, C
Swimming					
Berger et al. (1997)	M/F	12 to 20; M=14.6	3,500–5,000 m 6,000–7,000 m	N/A N/A	T, D, C V, F, TMD
Berger, Owen, & Man (1993)	F	M=22.4 CZ M=20.5 US	60 min. 30 min.	N/A N/A	T, D, A, V, C T, D, A, V, C
Berger & Owen (1988)	M/F	N/A	40 min	N/A	T, C
Berger & Owen (1992a)	M/F	Ms=20.3 & 21.1	25 to 30 min.	N/A	T, D, A, V, C
Tai Chi					
Jin (1992)	M/F	Females: M=37.8 Males: M=34.6	60 min.	N/A	V, TMD
Walking					
Berger & Owen (1998)	M/F	M=22.3	20 min.	55, 75, & 79% HR_{max}	T, D, A, V, F, C
Jin (1992)	M/F	Females: M=34.6 Males: M=37.8	60 min.	6 km/hr.	TMD
Weight Training					
Dyer & Crouch (1988)	M/F	17 to 26	40 min.	N/A	A, V, C

[a] M = Male and F = Female

[b] N/A = Information not available

[c] POMS subscale changes were in both desirable and undesirable directions.

[d] T = Tension, D = Depression, A = Anger, V = Vigor, F = Fatigue, C = Confusion, and TMD = Total Mood Disturbance.

From: "Exercise and Mood: A Selective Review and Synthesis of Research Employing the Profile of Mood States," by B. G. Berger & R. W. Motl, 2000, *Journal of Applied Sport Psychology, 12,* 69–92. Copyright 2000 by the Association for the Advancement of Applied Sport Psychology. Adapted with permission.

of a meta-analysis supports support the superiority of aerobic exercise for reducing anxiety (Petruzzello, Landers, Hatfield, Kubitz, & Salazar, 1991). Others show that both aerobic *and* resistance training have significant effects in reducing depressive symptoms (North, McCullagh, & Tran, 1990) and on well-being in older adults without clinical disorders (Netz, Wu, Becker, & Tenenbaum, 2005). Upon close inspection of the literature, however, there is need for additional investigation before concluding that for psychological benefits, the exercise needs to have aerobic training benefits. Presently the primary evidence for increased benefits of aerobic exercise is demonstrated when it is used for stress management and results in an attenuated stress response as indicated by heart rate (HR) and rate-pressure product (RPP; a product of HR and SBP that indicates workload and myocardial oxygen consumption) (e.g., Spalding, et al., 2004).

The accumulated research appears to be based on a common assumption that the exercise needs to be aerobic. As a result of this assumption, there are relatively few studies of nonaerobic exercise modes. The few studies that have focused on nonaerobic modes of exercise such as weight training, yoga, and qigong support the possibility that diverse exercise modes are associated with diverse psychological benefits (e.g., Berger & Owen, 1988, 1992a; Daubenmier, 2005; Mittelstaedt, Hinton, Rana, Cade, & Xue, 2005; O'Connor, Bryant, Veltri, & Gebhardt, 1993; Tucker, 1987). As concluded by Leith (1994) in *Foundations of Exercise and Mental Health*, "Research has not yet identified one particular type of exercise as being superior in terms of its potential to reduce *depression* [italics added] in the participant. *Both aerobic and anaerobic exercise sessions appear equally effective*" [italics added] (p. 22). Today, there still is a need to examine the psychological benefits of other types of exercise in addition to aerobic activities.

A change in breathing patterns. Rather than the aerobic exercise, it may be a change in breathing patterns that often accompanies aerobic exercise that facilitates feelings of psychological well-being. Studies of hatha yoga and walking lend credence to the possibility that exercising below one's aerobic training zone can promote psychological benefits (e.g., Berger & Owen, 1988, 1992a; Daubenmier, 2005; Thayer, 1987; and Table 20.3). Yoga and walking meet the taxonomy requirements in Table 20.3, except for the aerobic component. They do encourage participants to engage in abdominal, rhythmical breathing. Thus, abdominal (diaphragmatic), rhythmical breathing, a concomitant of aerobic exercise, may be the beneficial factor. Supporting the value of the breathing component, Sheehan (1995), the guru of running, noted, "I know of no better way to find my own genius than running with no companion except the rhythm of my breathing" (p. 18).

Diaphragmatic breathing, or "belly breathing," is receiving considerable attention from psychologists and physicians (e.g., Fried, 1987, 1990, 1993) as well as from yoga experts (Iyengar, 2005; Sovik, 1997a, 1997b). Illustrating a renewed interest and openness in Eastern approaches to health and wellness, the Office of Alternative Medicine at the National Institutes of Health was formed as well as other nongovernmental centers for alternative medicine. Some of these centers include the Columbia Integrative Medicine Program at New York City's Columbia Presbyterian Medical Center (*http://www.columbiasurgery.org/cimp/index.html*; retrieved December 14, 2005) and the University of Michigan Integrative Medicine Clinic (*http://www.med. umich.edu/umim/*; retrieved December 14, 2005). The Columbia Integrative Medicine Program provides *alternative* medicine services that are used to complement standard medical practices in restoring patients' health. These services include the use of yoga and meditation in improving patient psychological and physiological functioning postoperatively. The Columbia Integrative Medicine Program also is sponsoring a pilot study to investigate the effectiveness of a Mindfulness-Based Stress Management Program as "complementary" to standard care for treating a variety of health problems, especially for reducing depression, perceived stress, anxiety, and hostility in patients who are at-risk for developing coronary heart disease. In conclusion, researchers at respected medical centers around the country are investigating holistic approaches to health, psychological well-being, and wellness.

Nearly one-third of the population in the United States was using complementary or integrative health therapies according to a 1993 study published by members of Harvard Medical School in the highly respected *New England Journal of Medicine* (Eisenberg et al., 1993). This is impressive because the patients were spending about $13.7 billion per year, and three-quarters of this amount ($10.3 billion) was paid out of their own pockets for nonreimbursable therapies. The study did not include exercise or prayer for health enhancement. Thus, the statistics would be even higher with their inclusion. Results of a more recent national survey of alternative medicine use indicated that its use increased significantly—from 33.8% of the population in 1990 to 42.1% in 1997 (Eisenberg et al., 1998). This increase in the use of alternative medicine which often includes yoga and other types of Eastern exercise and stress management techniques reflected an increase in the proportion of the population seeking alternative therapies, rather than an increase in the number of visits per patient.

A common focus on breathing: Aerobic exercise, Eastern forms of exercise, and weight training. The growing emphasis on integrating body and mind is leading researchers and health practitioners to explore mind-body benefits of techniques such as the exercise forms of yoga, qigong, and ti chi chan as well as meditation and acupuncture, which have been practiced for centuries in Southeast Asia (e.g., Iyengar with Evans & Abrams; 2005; Patel, 2003; Li, Duncan, Duncan, McAuley, Chaumeton, & Harmer, 2001; Mittelstaedt et al., 2005). Mindfulness (being present in the moment) and an associated awareness of one's breathing patterns, two components of many types of exercise, are integral components of Zen and are under investigation in diverse locations including Columbia Presbyterian Hospital and the Stress Reduction Clinic at the University of Massachusetts Medical Center in Amherst.

Consciously being aware of your breathing patterns and developing skills in changing them are bases in many stress-reduction techniques including yoga, the relaxation response, and biofeedback. However, changes in breathing patterns have generated little objective research until somewhat recently (Fried, 1993). Stressing the importance of breathing for psychological well-being, Jon Kabat-Zinn, director of the Stress Reduction Clinic at the University of Massachusetts Medical Center, employs a technique of mindfully tuning into one's breathing. Mindfulness, practiced by Buddhists for centuries and by many exercisers, is focusing on the present. It consists of being fully aware of the present moment: of your breathing pattern, your posture, the physical sensations in your body, your train of thoughts, your current activity, and your physical surroundings. The practice of mindfulness and being present in the moment while exercising quiets the mind and provides many individuals with an appreciation of living. Awareness of breathing patterns can become an integral part of most exercise sessions as described by Kabat-Zinn (1990):

> The easiest and most effective way to begin practicing mindfulness as a formal meditative practice is to simply focus your attention on your breathing and see what happens as you attempt to keep it here . . . Obviously one is the nostrils . . . [another is] the chest as it expands and contracts, and another is the belly, which moves in and out with each breath if relaxed.

> No matter which location you choose, the idea is to be aware of the sensations that accompany your breathing at that particular place and to hold them in the forefront of your awareness from moment to moment. Doing this, we feel the air as it flows in and out past the nostrils; we feel the movement of the muscles associated with breathing; we feel the belly as it moves in and out.

> . . . Similarly when we focus on our breathing down in the belly, we are tuning to a region of our body that is below the agitation of our thinking mind and is intrinsically calmer. This is a valuable way of establishing inner calmness and balance in the face of emotional upset or when you "have a lot on your mind." (pp. 51–52)

Hatha yoga: An emphasis on breathing. In hatha yoga, participants maintain a series of *asanas* (static stretching poses) and hold the positions for 10 to 20 seconds. The word *hatha* comes from two Sanskrit words: "ha," which means "sun," and "tha," which means "moon." As the term implies, hatha yoga focuses on balancing universal life forces. More concretely, the goal of yoga participants is to balance mind, body, and spirit through physical activity (e.g., Daubenmier, 2005; Iyengar, 2005; Seaward, 1997). As discussed earlier in this chapter, achieving balance of mind, body, and spirit through physical activity is the basis for becoming an *Intrinsic Exerciser* (Kimiecik, 2002). Yoga originated in India approximately 5000 years ago and has certainly passed the test of time. In

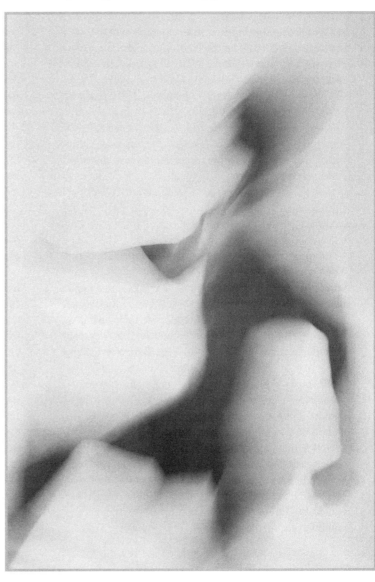

an article on "Yoga's Wider Reach," Biondo (1998) estimated that more than six million Americans participate in yoga. Yoga appeals to nearly all segments of the population for its stress-reduction benefits. It appeals to exercisers who desire its benefits of increased strength, flexibility, and internal awareness, and its enhancement of body-mind unity. Major benefits of hatha yoga are feelings of calmness, mental alertness, increased flexibility, static muscle strength, muscle relaxation, and increased body awareness.

Through the centuries, hatha yoga participants have focused on abdominal breathing and a sequence of poses. Participants direct their attention inward on their bodily sensations while executing the three stages of each asana: moving into, maintaining, and slowly moving out of each pose. A major feature of hatha yoga is coordinating the slow movements with breathing deeply, both with inhalations and exhalations. According to yogic theory, breath is *prana* and is the life force of the person. In each yoga session, there is a constant focus on prana, or controlled breathing, which is performed with conscious effort. Generally, participants inhale when stretching their muscles, hold their breath while maintaining the pose, and exhale when relaxing their muscles. With practice, coordinating the breathing pattern with the asanas becomes almost automatic. Hatha yoga participants have reported a variety of acute mood benefits—primarily decreases in tension, depression, anger, fatigue, and confusion (Berger & Owen, 1988, 1992a). These results support the need for abdominal, rhythmical breathing that occurs in both yoga and swimming rather than the need for an activity to be aerobic or to result in cardiorespiratory fitness.

Absence of Interpersonal Competition—Acceptance of One's Self

You can choose how you exercise, regardless of whether you are aware of the choices and "exercise" them or not. One choice focuses on whether your physical activity is competitive. Exercise can be an arena for competition, or it can provide a measured period of noncompetition, a respite from our typically hectic, often competitive days. An interlude of noncompetitive physical activity enables each of us to focus more thoroughly on the present moment by concentrating on how our bodies are responding to the exercise. The choice about the desirable amount of competition is up to the aware exercise participant.

In noncompetitive activities, the game/match outcome and future are less important to participants than the "here and now." A recent study highlights selected psychological benefits of participating in the noncompetitive, internally-focused, mindful exercise mode

of yoga (Daubenmier, 2005). Daubenmier examined the psychological influences of two types of physical activity that differed in competitiveness: yoga, a noncompetitive exercise mode, and step aerobics which can be somewhat competitive and externally-focused on outward appearances. As hypothesized, the yoga participants ($n = 43$) reported less self-objectification and greater satisfaction with physical appearance than the aerobics participants ($n = 45$) and a group of non-yoga/step aerobics controls ($n = 51$). Yoga participants and members of the control group reported similar levels of disordered eating attitudes, but their levels of disordered eating attitudes were lower than those for the participants in step aerobics.

As reflected by the step-aerobics participants in the study of body awareness and responsiveness to self-objectification (Daubenmier, 2005), no physical activity is totally devoid of competition. Competition certainly can add excitement and zest to our daily lives. Each of us competes with others and with ourselves as we progress throughout the day. Undoubtedly, some of us are more competitive than others.

Competitiveness in youth sport. Recognizing the benefits as well as problems with competition in youth sport, Kimiecik (2002) observes:

> Surveys show that more kids are participating in organized youth sports—such as soccer and basketball—than ever before. . . . Youth sport has a lot of good intentions and can have *many positive effects* [emphasis added].
>
> But I think there's a danger in that it leads to a lot of lazy kids and is partly responsible for this generation of children's low physical activity and fitness levels. *Even worse, youth sport could be detracting from the number of kids who will want to participate in regular exercise as adults* [emphasis added].
>
> In youth sport, almost everything the children do is determined by an outside source. Times for playing are determined by practices and games; the amount of time a child plays is determined by the coach; where a child plays is determined by his or her ability and the coach. Success is based on extrinsic outcomes (won or lost) and trophies and awards are doled out accordingly. *Children can believe that the only time to be physically active is when an adult tells them to or when there is some extrinsic reason for it* [emphasis added].
>
> Once children's physical activity gets tied to extrinsic motivation, what do they do when those external forces are gone? Nothing! . . . This leads to kids who have no ability or desire to initiate their own physical activity. They don't know how. (pp. 37–38)

At the beginning of the previous quotation, Kimiecik (2002) emphasizes that competition has many desirable characteristics. The competitive aspects of physical activity motivate many of us to participate. Competition is enjoyable as we test our skills and challenge ourselves to defeat our opponents. Competition certainly can add fun and excitement to our lives. Taken to an extreme, however, competitiveness detracts from the quality of life by making us feel a need to do "more." Competition does not encourage us to savor the present moment and our current accomplishments. If we wish to maximize the psychological benefits associated with physical activity, a relative absence of competition is desirable.

Noncompetitiveness as a predisposing factor for exercise commitment. William Glasser (1976), a well-known psychologist, has emphasized the importance of noncompetitiveness in his discussion of exercise characteristics leading to positive addictions (PA)—activities in which we participate on a regular basis and which enhance our lives by giving us inner strength. Glasser coined the phrase *positive addiction* to indicate that

- Being unable to exercise can create withdrawal symptoms, but that
- Overall, the addicting activity enhances our quality of life.

It is open to debate, of course, whether any addiction can be positive because addiction takes away individual freedom. Thus use of the word *addiction* in reference to exercise should be avoided. The term *positive addiction* is attention catching, but it might better be named *commitment*, *compulsion*, or *dependence*. Regardless of the terminology employed, the concept of *needing to exercise* is intriguing and captures an experience that many exercisers report. Habitual exercisers miss the benefits of their exercise session when they do not have the opportunity to exercise. Glasser theorized that positive addictions, in contrast to undesirable or negative addictions (drug use, smoking, overeating), lead to highly desirable states such as alertness, confidence, creativity, happiness, health, less anger, self-awareness, and tolerance.

The basic criteria for obtaining exercise commitment are based on Glasser's 22-item questionnaire published in the October 1974 issue of *Runner's World* (Glasser, 1976, p. 101). The questionnaire was completed by nearly 700 runners who considered themselves to be positively addicted. The six criteria in Table 20.4 facilitate positive addiction, but do not guarantee its occurrence. Glasser (1976) theorized that to become committed, the participant has to reach the positive addiction state on a regular basis. "Regular" means several times a week, for several minutes to an hour each time. If this happens, the participant experiences a surge of pleasure that she or he learns to crave.

Three of Glasser's criteria are similar to the exercise mode characteristics in the taxonomy suggested by Berger and colleagues (Berger, 2004; Berger & Owen, 1988, 1992a, 1998; Berger & Motl, 2001; Berger & Tobar, in press). These criteria include the following exercise mode criteria:

- An activity that can be performed alone,
- A noncompetitive activity, and
- An activity performed without self-criticism.

Activities that are performed alone do not involve interaction with others. Thus, they are relatively noncompetitive and generally are "closed" and fairly predictable. In regard to the noncompetitive criterion, Glasser emphasized, "Not only must we not compete with others, we must learn not to compete with ourselves if want to reach the PA state" (1976, p. 57). Glasser's third criterion, performing the activity without self-criticism, also supports a need for a relative absence of competition.

Competition may detract from psychological well-being. A relative absence of interpersonal competition seems to enhance the psychological benefits of physical activity. A poem by Chuang Tzu (Merton, 1965) captures the value of adopting a noncompetitive approach to physical activity. A noncompetitive focus encourages total concentration on the activity itself rather than on the extrinsic rewards often accompanying competition such as brass buckles and gold. Not all competitors focus on winning and external rewards, rather than on the necessary movement skills as described by Chuang Tzu. However, many do and, in the process, experience few if any mood benefits.

The Need to Win

When an archer is shooting for nothing

He has all his skill.

If he shoots for a brass buckle

He is already nervous.

If he shoots for a prize of gold

He goes blind

Or sees two targets—

He is out of his mind!

His skill has not changed. But the prize

Divides him. He cares.

He thinks more of winning

Than of shooting—

And the need to win

Drains him of power.

Chuang Tzu (Merton, 1965, p. 107)

Table 20.4

Criteria for Positive Addiction (Glasser, 1976, p. 93)

Criteria	Description
1. Can be performed alone	Does not depend on others to be able to do it
2. Noncompetitive and freely chosen activity conducted for at least 1 hour a day	Three criteria in one: noncompetitive, freely chosen, and performed 1 hour a day
3. Can be performed without self-criticism	If the participant cannot accept her- or himself while performing the activity, it will not be addicting
4. Can be done easily	Does not require a great deal of mental effort
5. Has some value for the participant	Belief in an activity's physical, spiritual, or mental value
6. Is characterized by the participant's belief that if she or he persists, improvement will occur	The belief is completely subjective

For many reasons, mood benefits may not accompany competitive physical activity. Some of these reasons include the following:

- Losing is not an enjoyable experience,
- Arousal and stress levels are high, and
- Participants tend to push or overuse their bodies in the competitive events themselves and when training for them.

In addition, exercisers who lose tend to criticize their own and their teammates' performance. See Table 20.5 for a summary of typical desirable and undesirable characteristics of interpersonal competition.

Winning and losing. One plausible reason for a lack of desirable mood changes in competitive exercise modes acknowledges that competition results in winning and losing. Losing is not enjoyable and would seem to be related to negative mood states. In any tournament, losing occurs approximately 50% of the time. Research on the interaction between competitive physical activity and psychological well-being supports a need for a relative absence of competition—if mood enhancement is a desired outcome (e.g., Grove & Prapavessis, 1992; Hassmen & Blomstrand, 1995; Kerr & Schaik, 1995).

In a study of male elite rugby players, participants

Table 20.5

Desirable and Undesirable Characteristics of Interpersonal Competition

Desirable Characteristics	Undesirable Characteristics
1. Arousal	1. Criticism of own and/or teammates' performance
2. Enjoyment and fun	2. Focus on outcome, rather than process
3. Excitement	3. Over arousal, stress, and anxiety
4. Winning	4. Losing is not an enjoyable experience
5. Zest	5. Overtraining and staleness
	6. Undesirable changes in mood states

completed measures of mood and stress immediately before and after games (Kerr & Schaik, 1995). After winning, the athlete's stress levels were lower than after losing. Winners also were less serious, more spontaneous, and higher in arousal than losers. In another study of postcompetition mood states, as measured by shortened version of the POMS, women netball players reported similar mood patterns associated with winning and losing (Grove & Prapavessis, 1992). The women's moods as indicated by their total mood disturbance scores on an abbreviated version of the POMS were more negative after losing than after winning. See Figure 20.3 for the netball players' mood scores on the individual subscales that were measured after exercising. All of the subscales except for Fatigue discriminated between winners and losers. This same pattern of results was evident in college-age participants in a single-elimination basketball tournament (Berger et al., 1998). After winning, male and female basketball players reported few, if any, mood benefits.

After losing their game, they reported mood decrements. The relationship between competitive outcome and mood was considerably more negative for the men than for the women who lost. In general, it seems that competitive physical activity is not associated with the mood benefits and that losing may be associated with mood decrements.

A source of stress and anxiety. A second reason for the relative lack of mood benefits after competitive physical activity is that competition increases levels of arousal and is a source of stress and anxiety for many participants. It is important to note, however, that competitive physical activity is appealing to many individuals. Competition is especially appealing to those who are high in *ego orientation* and compare their performances to their competitors', seek heightened stress and thrills, and/or thrive on the exercise intensity necessary for competitive physical activity. Despite a person's choice to participate in competitive activities, a well-established body of research supports the likeli-

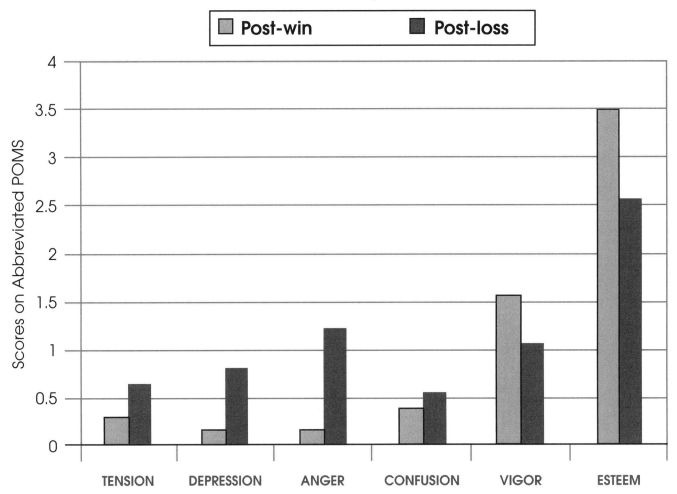

Figure 20.3. Relationship between competitive outcome and mood when measured immediately after exercising (Grove & Prapavessis, 1992).

hood that competition is uncomfortably stressful for many participants. For example, participants in competitive sport "worry" about self-presentational concerns, or how they appear to other people (Wilson & Eklund, 1998). These concerns are both real and imagined and include appearing unskilled, incompetent, and unable to handle stress. Illustrating the stress of competitive environments, exercisers and athletes need familiarity and skill in stress management techniques for both enhanced performance and for enjoyment (e.g., Hackfort & Spielberger, 1989).

Overtraining. A third reason that competitive sport may be counterproductive to enhanced psychological well-being is that many participants tend to *overtrain.* Overtraining is defined as progressively increasing training levels (intensity, duration, and/or frequency) and thus exercising at or near one's physical limits to obtain enhanced performance (Tobar, 2005). Overtraining is an exercise stimulus and is deliberately planned as an integral part of the training process (e.g., Morgan, Brown, Raglin, O'Connor, & Ellickson, 1987; Tobar, 2005). Overtraining for an extended period of time can result in *staleness* as evidenced by long-term performance decrements, mood disturbance, and proneness to illness (Tobar, 2005). As observed by O'Connor (1997), overtraining and staleness often have been ignored in discussions of exercise and mental health. Although overtraining is assumed to be necessary for high-level performance, there is a fine line between overtraining and reaching a point of staleness or burnout, both of which are characterized by decrements in mood. More is not always better. Monitoring exercisers' mood states throughout intense training protocols may be a way to prevent staleness. As suggested in the next chapter on exercise training or practice parameters, the high-intensity and/or long-duration exercise often associated with competition does not appear conducive to desirable changes in mood.

Closed, Predictable, or Temporally and Spatially Certain Activities

Another mode characteristic conducive to desirable mood change focuses on activities that are described as *closed.* This means that they are predictable and *temporally* and *spatially certain.* The timing of the movements is *predictable* and *controllable* as in the exercise modes of figure skating, golf, gymnastics, jogging, swimming, weight training, and yoga. *Spatially,* participants in these activities also encounter few unexpected events. Exercise activities that are not predictable in timing of movements or in space of exertion are defined as *open.* Activities such as tennis and basketball offer open exercise environments. *Open* exercise environments tend to be dual and team

sports activities in which participants must be vigilant and attend to constantly changing environments. In open exercise modes, the movement of the other participants and interactions with them add uncertainty, and require added focus and attention to the rapidly changing environment.

Closed exercise environments tend to occur in individual rather than team activities and allow participants to pre-plan their movement patterns. In *closed* exercise environments, participants do not interact with or respond to their opponents, at least not on a moment-to-moment basis. In *closed* activities, skilled participants encounter few, if any, unexpected events that require careful attention. Thus, participants are free to let their thoughts wander, or even to have a complete absence of thought while exercising. Tuning into inner thoughts during this peace and quiet, or simply having no thoughts at all, may be one reason that joggers frequently report great periods of imagination and creativity while exercising (e.g., Berger & Mackenzie, 1980; Paffenbarger & Olsen, 1996). Of course, some participants in *closed* and predictable exercise modes may find the self-chatter distressing, especially if they recall painful events or focus on endless tasks that need their *immediate* attention. These individuals may need practice in determining and selecting useful or enjoyable topics of self-reflection.

Research evidence supports the psychological value of solitary time for thinking or mental simulation. A primary benefit of mental simulation is having the opportunity to envision new possibilities and solutions to problems, to anticipate and manage associated emotions, and then to develop plans of action to initiate and maintain problem-solving behaviors (Taylor, Pham, Rivkin, & Armor, 1998). Apparently there are "right" and "wrong" ways to use the self-regulatory thinking that tends to occur while exercising. Thinking about the step-by-step *process* such as increasing the amount of exercise, eating less fatty food, and reducing the size of food portions is effective in reaching our goals (Taylor et al.). In contrast, focusing on *desired outcomes* rather than on process does little in helping us reach our goals. Noting the importance of predictability and solitude when exercising and the accompanying creativity, Sheehan (1990) commented, "Where once I found all my good thoughts on the run, I now find them in *other solitary movement* [italics added]. Given the choice I might walk rather than run—or choose to cycle over either one" (p. 210). In summary, "harnessing our imagination" while exercising is an important benefit of participating in closed or predictable forms of physical activity.

Individuals who select closed exercise activities sometimes report that they enjoy the predictability of the activities. Other individuals clearly do not. In fact, some people dislike the solitude of closed activities such as jogging so much that they would rather be inactive than participate. These individuals would be well advised not to force themselves to participate in closed activities and to seek out temporally and spatially uncertain, or open, physical activities based on the primary taxonomy need for the exercise to be enjoyable. To perform well, skilled participants in open environments must temporarily leave behind their daily responsibilities and monitor the immediate sport environment. Their mental focus is on their opponent, anticipating the opponent's strategy, planning the next move, and the temporal and spatial events of the moment. The temporal and spatial uncertainty in open exercise environments adds excitement, but destroys the solitude sought by participants in closed physical activities. The mental health benefits of open sport activities are relatively unexplored and consequently are an inviting area for future research. Since "open" forms of physical activity usually involve competing against others, winning and losing becomes a factor in the participants' moods. Thus, examination of acute mood benefits associated with open exercise modes in both winning situations and losing situations is needed.

In conclusion, it seems that exercise modes that are *closed* and predictable are more likely to be associated with mood benefits than are *open* types of exercise. Some benefits may be related to the opportunities presented by predictable activities to *harness the imagination*, problem solve, and experience related emotions associated with problems, traumatic events, and plans of action. Although the immediate effects of reliving a trauma may decrease emotional regulation, over time, such an activity is beneficial, as evidenced by immune changes and health center visits (Taylor et al., 1998). In contrast to the benefits of *closed* forms of exercise, open activities tend to be competitive, exhilarating, and stress producing. Clearly, different types of physical activity are associated with differing psychological benefits. Participating in physical activity is an individual choice, and participating in *any* type of activity is better than being sedentary due to the broad benefits of exercise.

Rhythmical and Repetitive Movements

Rhythmical and repetitive movements are conducive to mood alteration and closely associated with closed exercise modes. In fact, it is difficult to select an activity that is rhythmical and repetitive that also is not performed alone, and thus is closed. Neither rhythmical and repetitive nor closed types of exercise require close attention from participants. Thus, the exercisers are free to follow their own train of thought and let their minds wander while exercising. The rhythmicity of repetitive movements might encourage introspec-

tive or creative thinking, or both, during participation. Ralph Paffenbarger, a cardiologist and epidemiologist at Stanford University School of Medicine who has run the Boston Marathon 22 times, and Eric Olsen, an award-winning journalist in the area of exercise, fitness, and health, have written a fact-filled book about fitness and health that is tempered by personal insights: *Lifefit: An Effective Exercise Program for Optimal Health and a Longer Life* (1996). Paffenbarger and Olsen report that rhythmical movements can have a hypnotic, relaxing effect and provide opportunities for a wide range of thoughts:

> *Rhythmic large-muscle exercise* [italics added] such as swimming, walking, or jogging can also be *a form of relaxation* [italics added] for many of us. The rhythmic motion of the legs and arms while walking or running can have an almost hypnotic effect, and running long distances at a comfortable pace appears to produce exactly the same changes in brain-wave activity as deep meditation. (p. 200)
>
> *The routine rhythmic motion of running or walking* [italics added], in particular, requires little thought or attention. Anyone who has run or walked regularly for even a few minutes knows *how the mind seems to open to a flood of thoughts and emotions* [italics added]; solutions to nagging problems suddenly appear like flashing 100-watt bulbs. Fantasies arise. You find yourself thinking of all of the smart things you should have said to the cop who gave you that speeding ticket. (p. 225)

Exercisers often allude to the psychological benefits associated with participating in rhythmical, repetitive movements, but such benefits are difficult to investigate. In a phenomenological study of the meaning of jogging to the participant, Berger and MacKenzie (1980) asked a woman jogger, age 35, to keep a personal journal of her thoughts and emotions while completing 32 jogging sessions during a four-month period. As Berger and Mackenzie noted, such research relies on intuitive interview techniques and inferential analysis of interview and journal entries. Thus, the case study needs to be replicated with other joggers and with participants in other types of physical activity.

Interested in answering the broad question "Why is sport meaningful to so many people?" Berger and MacKenzie (1980) asked the jogger what she experienced while jogging. As noted previously in Chapter 6, they suggested the following propositions that were intended as guides for future study. Proposition #2 emphasizes the need for repetitive and rhythmical exercise modes.

- ***Proposition #1.*** The jogger's stream of consciousness reflected a wide spectrum of emotions ranging from agony to ecstasy.

- *Proposition #2.* Repetitive and rhythmical sports such as jogging are conducive to introspection, as well as to thinking in general.
- *Proposition #3.* Engagement in sport satisfies inner psychodynamic needs, and it was related to the jogger's characterological or personality structure and family relationships.
- *Proposition #4.* Exercisers can enhance their self-understanding by the increased awareness of private phenomenological experiences associated with physical activity.

Testing the Exercise Mode Guidelines

Berger and Owen (1988) tested the mode guidelines in their exercise taxonomy and chose swimming, body conditioning, hatha yoga, and fencing to represent various combinations of the characteristics. See the four mode guidelines of the taxonomy and representative activities in Table 20.6. Swimming, jogging, and hatha yoga satisfied all four criteria. The competitive activity of fencing satisfied none of the requirements. Exercisers reported how they felt immediately before and after physical activity on three different days. As anticipated, the competitive fencers who were participating in an open sport reported few changes of the POMS subscales. They reported an increase in Vigor, but no other mood changes. Swimmers reported a decrease in Tension and Confusion after exercising on only the first day. These benefits existed despite the observation that swimmers had the most desirable POMS profiles of all the participants prior to any exercise. Yoga participants in two different classes reported numerous benefits: less Tension, Depression, Fatigue, and, in one class, increased Vigor. Surprisingly, the body-conditioning class, which met most of the taxonomy mode requirements, did not report any changes on mood except for increased Fatigue. Upon examination, it was learned that students in the jogging portion of a body-conditioning class were not jogging. Instead, they used interval training at a very high-intensity level, which was approximately 90% of their age-adjusted maximal heart rate. The relative absence of mood change in this group supported the need for exercise to be pleasing and, as discussed in the next chapter, moderate in intensity.

The same taxonomy mode characteristics were included in a second set of physical activities listed in Table 20.6 (Rudolph & Kim, 1996). Aerobic dance satisfied all four criteria. It is an aerobic activity, noncompetitive, predictable, and repetitive. Bowling was inaccurately described as satisfying none of the criteria. Rudolph and Kim considered bowling to be a "control" activity for a comparison of its benefits to the psychological benefits of other activities that met the taxonomy

Table 20.6
Activities Representing the Exercise Mode Characteristics
(Berger & Owen, 1988; Rudolph & Kim, 1996)

Mode	Abdominal Breathing	Lack of Competition	Closed & Predictable	Rhythmical & Repetitive
Berger & Owen's (1988) categorization of activities (U.S. study)				
Swimming	yes	yes	yes	yes
Body conditioning	yes	yes	yes	yes
Hatha yoga	yes	yes	yes	yes
Fencing	no	no	no	no
Rudolph & Kim's (1996) categorization of activities (Korean study)				
Aerobic dance	yes	yes	yes	yes
Soccer	yes	no	no	no
Tennis	yes	no	no	no
Bowling	yes	no	no (Yes)*	no (Yes)*

* recategorization according to Berger's taxonomy (Berger, 1996, 2004; Berger & Owen, 1988).

requirements. Contrary to the researchers' categorization of bowling, the approach to the foul line and release of the ball are a highly predictable sequence of movements. The steps in the approach remain constant, and they are rhythmical and repetitive. Coordination of the arm swing to the steps remains the same throughout the delivery by skilled bowlers. Bowling participants encounter few unanticipated events, and thus, the activity is highly predictable or closed and repetitive. Soccer and tennis did not meet three of the mode guidelines in the taxonomy. They are competitive, unpredictable or uncertain, and include nonrepetitive movements. See Table 20.6 for a comparison of the categorization of the four activities by Rudolph and Kim and our re-categorization according to Berger's (Berger 1996; Berger & Owen, 1988) taxonomy.

The Korean university students in all four types of physical activities reported few acute mood changes (Rudolph & Kim, 1996). In fact, there were no changes on the Psychological Distress and on the Fatigue subscales of the Subjective Exercise Experience Scale. However, aerobic dance participants and soccer players did report increased Positive Well-Being. These results are difficult to interpret for a variety of reasons. Korean exercisers may respond to exercise and answer mood-related questions in ways that are different from those of their American counterparts. In addition, use of the Subjective Exercise Experiences Scale (SEES) may result in conclusions different from those in studies employing the 65-item POMS with six mood subscales. The SEES has 12 items distributed into the three subscales of Positive Well-Being, Psychological Distress, and Fatigue. These results illustrate the difficulty of comparing results of studies when procedures, measures, and subjects differ. Clearly, there is a need for continued examination of the mode conditions suggested in the taxonomy.

Summary

Because of the large variety of physical activities, it is important to distinguish mode characteristics or types of exercises that are conducive to enhancing psychological well-being. The broad term *psychological well-being* includes such specific benefits as mood alteration, improved self-concept, stress management, and reductions in anxiety and depression, as well as enhanced quality of life. Grouping these psychological benefits is as hazardous as considering all types of physical activity to be the same. Thus, the different chapters in this text have focused on specific psychological benefits.

This chapter, however, highlights the need for the exercise activity to be enjoyable, facilitating the diverse psychological benefits. Enjoyment includes factors that are intrinsic and extrinsic to the exercise experience as well as achievement and nonachievement factors. Basically, enjoyment is highly related to positive emotions based on the movement experience itself; the social setting; feelings of mastery, competence, and control; and social recognition. The guideline for enjoyment accommodates individual preferences for specific types of physical activity.

It seems likely that exercise that is enjoyable and that satisfying the four mode guidelines is conducive to mood enhancement and other psychological benefits. The exercise mode should

- Promote rhythmical, abdominal breathing,
- Be relatively noncompetitive,
- Be closed or predictable, and
- Have rhythmical and repetitive movements.

Rhythmical, abdominal breathing is a key element in many stress-management techniques and may be conducive to feelings of well-being. Noncompetitive types of exercise are recommended for enhancing psychological well-being on a consistent basis, because losing can be related to undesirable changes in mood and is difficult to avoid in competitive activities. Closed, predictable, and temporally and spatially certain activities allow participants to let their thoughts wander. They can tune into their inner dialogue, or even have a moment of silence undistracted by internal chatter. This mental solitude seems to be highly related to psychological well-being. The final mode characteristic of rhythmical and repetitive movements also may encourage introspection and creative thinking, which enhance personal growth and positive moods.

Enjoyment and the four mode guidelines are important for choosing the type of exercise that enhances psychological well-being as well as exercise adherence. However, as suggested in the next chapter, mode characteristics and enjoyment do not function independently, and are closely associated with practice or training guidelines that are identified in the next chapter.

Can You Define These Terms?

abdominal breathing

aerobic exercise

asanas

complementary medicine

closed physical activity

enjoyment

exercise addiction

exercise commitment

exercise dependence

exercise mode

exercise taxonomy

flow

hatha yoga

inergy

integrative medicine

interpersonal competition

intervention programs

intrinsic exerciser

intrinsic and extrinsic motivation

mindfulness

mode guidelines

open physical activity

overtraining

Physical Activity Enjoyment Scale (PACES)

positive addiction

prana

staleness

temporal and spatial certainty

vision

Can You Answer These Questions?

1. How might an exerciser's goals vary across the life span?
2. What are children's major reasons for participating and ceasing participation in school sports? How do these reasons meet with your own experiences?
3. What is the basic structure of the exercise taxonomy designed to enhance the psychological benefits of exercise?
4. What definition of exercise enjoyment is most appealing to you?

5. What exercise modes do you enjoy most? What mode do you enjoy the least? What factors contribute to the differences in your enjoyment levels?

6. Prior to reading this chapter, have you consciously been aware of your breathing patterns during exercise? Describe your general awareness level of your breathing patterns during exercise.

7. Have you participated in an Eastern movement form such as hatha yoga or ti chi chan? Did you enjoy it? Try to capture your experience in a brief description.

8. Why might competition detract from the psychological benefits of exercise? Have you ever experienced this? Describe such a situation.

9. What are some of the benefits of participating in closed and rhythmical/repetitive activities?

10. Do you think that *positive addiction* is a desirable term that can refer to specific exercise? What is the basis for your response?

CHAPTER 21

Practice Guidelines for Optimal Psychological Benefits: Exercise Frequency, Intensity, & Duration

After reading this chapter, you should be able to

- Distinguish between the two sets of fitness training guidelines: physical fitness guidelines and health-related guidelines,

- Explain why exercise frequency is an important consideration for the psychological benefits,

- Discuss the relationship between exercise intensity and the psychological benefits of exercise,

- Explain how "preferred exertion" may influence the relationship between exercise intensity and enhancement of psychological well-being,

- Discuss the relationship between exercise intensity and adherence,

- Explore the possible qualitative differences in psychological benefits when exercising for different durations,

- Review exercise-duration guidelines that may influence the psychological benefits,

- Describe the measurement units and issues for exercise duration, intensity, and frequency,

- Summarize the practice-guideline components and their levels for facilitating optimal psychological benefits.

Introduction[1]

This chapter focuses on exercise practice or training guidelines as key considerations for designing exercise programs to facilitate psychological benefits. In this chapter, you will examine the implications of exercise frequency, intensity, and duration for the psychological benefits of exercise. *Practice guidelines* often are referred to as *training guidelines* and as *exercise prescriptions* by exercise physiologists. This chapter emphasizes *practice guidelines*, instead of training guidelines, to highlight our focus on exercise parameters conducive to the psychological, rather than the physiological, benefits of exercise. Regardless of what the guidelines are called, however, practice guidelines are important considerations. They can facilitate or impede enjoyment of an exercise session, psychological well-being, and ultimately success in reaching specific exercise goals.

For the physiological benefits of exercise, the training considerations of frequency, intensity, and duration are clear, but they continue to evolve as illustrated by a comparison of the guidelines in the two most recent versions of *ACSM's Guidelines for Exercise Testing and Prescription* (American College of Sports Medicine, 2000, 2006). See the chapters on *General Principles of Exercise Prescription.* Physical fitness guidelines abbreviated as FITT (*f*requency, *i*ntensity, and *t*ime—and *t*ype of exercise as identified in Chapter 20) differ according to exercisers' goals. (Please note that the terms *duration* and *time* are synonymous. *Duration* is a component of exercise prescriptions; however, *time* fits the acronym, FITT.) As emphasized throughout this chapter which includes the factors of *f*requency, *i*ntensity and *t*ime, FIT or practice/training guidelines have important implications for the psychological changes associated with physical activity.

Exercisers often set physical activity goals related to health and fitness, appearance, and competitive performance. For these goals, exercisers need to follow the usual physical fitness guidelines and the health-related fitness guidelines. More often, however, exercisers are beginning to set psychological goals. These include mood alteration, stress and tension management, enhanced self-efficacy and self-esteem, experiencing flow-like experiences, and even enhanced self-exploration. To reach these psychological goals, exercisers need to follow another set of practice/training guidelines which are designed to optimize the psychological benefits.

---

[1]The author would like to express appreciation to Lynn A. Darby, PhD, Bowling Green State University, for her helpful comments on an earlier version of this chapter.

—Bonnie Berger

Clarification of Terminology: Exercise Frequency, Intensity, and Duration

Before you analyze exercise practice/training guidelines for optimal psychological benefits, it is important to clarify the meaning and common measures for exercise frequency, intensity, duration, and training. Undoubtedly, you are familiar with these terms. The brief review of exercise frequency, intensity, and duration in this chapter emphasizes a need for an interdisciplinary approach when examining the guidelines. A psychophysiological approach facilitates developing a broad understanding and expertise in exercise psychology, as well as in other exercise science specializations such as exercise physiology, athletic training, coaching, teaching, and personal fitness training. In the following sections, you will review the definitions of some basic terms to facilitate subsequent discussion of the research literature related to the exercise practice guidelines for enhanced psychological well-being.

Exercise Frequency

Frequency is the first consideration in the FIT guidelines. As the word implies, frequency refers to how often an individual exercises. Exercise frequency commonly is expressed as the number of days a week that a person exercises. However, exercise frequency may be several times a day if the participant is separating the recommended 30 minutes of exercise into three 10-minute sessions per day. Frequent training sessions, i.e., exercising most days of the week, are desirable for most exercise participants—if the exercise intensity is moderate to low. At higher exercise intensities, especially those close to maximum, alternate days of rest and exercise may be beneficial.

Recommended exercise frequency varies according to exercise goals such as psychological well-being, weight loss, and cardiovascular endurance as well as sport performance. For individuals who rarely exercise, the most accurate approach to recording exercise frequency is to note the *number of times they exercise each month.* Infrequent exercisers may report only two or three exercise sessions a month. Habitual exercisers, however, usually report the *number of days per week* that they exercise. Thus, in research studies measuring exercise frequency, the participants tested influence selection of a specific measure of duration: days per month, days per week, or even the number of exercise sessions each day.

Exercise Intensity

Exercise intensity refers to how "hard" a person is exercising and varies along a continuum. Anchors of the continuum range from not exercising at all and being sedentary, to the opposite extreme of maximum exertion. Although there are numerous ways to express exercise intensity, five commonly employed techniques are illustrated and compared in Table 21.1. These include percentage of maximal heart rate ($\% HR_{max}$), percentage of heart-rate reserve ($\% HRR$), metabolic equivalent (MET), percentage of maximal oxygen consumed ($\% VO_{2max}$), and rating of perceived exertion (RPE). The various techniques are somewhat independent of one another and can be difficult to equate. However the variables listed in Table 21.1 aid in the quantification of light (low), moderate, and high (hard) intensity exercise (American College of Sports Medicine, 2006, p. 4).

Percentage of maximal heart rate ($\% HR_{max}$). One technique for expressing exercise intensity is as a specific percentage of a participant's maximal heart rate. Exercisers calculate their personal maximal heart rate (HR_{max}) based on a theoretical maximal heart rate for human beings of 220 beats per minute and then subtract their age in years from 220 figure. As noted in Table 21.1, this intensity measure is reflected as a percentage of age-adjusted heart rate max (HR_{max}).

To exercise at a *low/light exercise intensity* that is a percentage of HR_{max}, the participant's heart rate ranges between 50% and 63% of his/her maximal, age-adjusted figure as indicated in Table 21.1. The formula for estimating a needed exercise heart rate when exercising within the range of 50% to 63% of HRmax is as follows:

Training heart rate = (220–age in years) × 50%.
Training heart rate = (220–age in years) × 63%.

For a person who is 20 years old, the formula would be calculated as follows for the lower limit for light intensity exercise: $(220–20 = 200) \times .50$ = a heart rate of 100 beats per minute. A heart rate of 126 beats per minute would be the upper limit for light intensity exercise $[(220–20 = 200) \times .63]$. Low/light intensity exercise range for a target HR is from 100 to 126 beats per minute. Heart rate provides a useful indication of the strenuousness of exercise, but it cannot necessarily be converted directly to oxygen uptake due to influences of psychological characteristics such as anxiety and circulating levels of caffeine and nicotine.

If you are 20 years old and want to estimate your lower and upper HR thresholds for moderate-intensity

Table 21.1

Measures of Exercise Intensity and *Approximate* Equivalency Between Measures[a,b]

Ranges of Intensity	Measures			
Example	% HR$_{max}$	%HRR	METs[c]	RPE

Low/light
   Bowling
   Fishing
   Slow walking
	50–63	~20–39	2.0–5.3	11–12

Moderate
   Brisk walking
   Moderate swimming
	64–76	~40–59	3.1–7.5	13–14

High/hard
   Walking uphill briskly
   Running
	77–93	~60–84	4.1–10.2	15–17+

Maximal	100	100	6–12	20

Note: For more information, see American College of Sports Medicine (2006, pp. 4–5), Corbin and Pangrazi (1996), Wilmore and Costill (2004, 617–624).

[a] Values for ranges are approximate and are based on a 20-year-old exerciser who has a resting heart rate of 75 beats per minute and a VO$_2$ of 46 ml/kg-mg.

[b] These approximations change with the type of exercise, fitness level, gender, and age of the participant.

[c] Ranges reflect METs across all fitness levels (American College of Sports Medicine, 2006, p. 4).

exercise, e.g., at **64% and 76% of HR$_{max}$** as indicated in Table 21.1, you would compute the following calculations.

- **To estimate a target heart rate for exercising at the 64% intensity level,** you calculate your training heart rate as follows: (220–20 years old) × 64%, or (200 × 64%), which equals 128 beats per minute.

- **Similar calculations for the 76% intensity level** are follows: (220–20 years old) × 76%, or (200 × 76%), which equals 152 beats per minute.

A participant exercising within the 64% to 76% heart-rate training zone would be participating in moderate intensity exercise. Based on these calculations, a participant's exercise heart rate at age 20 would be between 128 and 152 beats per minute.

Percentage of heart-rate reserve (%HRR), or the Karvonen method. A more complicated, yet more accurate technique for estimating an appropriate exercise training heart rate involves using a formula developed by Karvonen and colleagues (Karvonen, Kentala, & Mustala, 1957). This method is known as the Karvonen method, or heart-rate reserve method. Maximal heart rate reserve is defined as the difference between age-adjusted maximal heart rate (HR$_{max}$) and resting heart rate (HR$_{rest}$; Wilmore & Costil, 2004, p. 619). The Karvonen method provides a more accurate estimation of exercise heart rate because it adjusts for each exerciser's resting heart rate. This method for calculating training heart rate (THR) includes three primary parts: (1) estimation of the participant's age-adjusted maximal heart rate (220 minus age in years), (2) his/her resting heart rate (HRrest), and (3) a desired training intensity expressed as a percentage.

Take a moment to calculate your own training heart rate according to the Karvonen formula, which is as follows:

Training Heart Rate = [(HR$_{max}$–HR$_{rest}$) × %] + HR$_{rest}$.

If you are 20 years old, have a typical resting heart rate of 75, and want to estimate your exercise training heart rate at **40% and 59% HRR**, the lower and upper thresholds for moderate-intensity exercise as indicated in Table 20.1, you would compute the Karvonen formula in the following manner. (Note that the following calculations include the maximal heart rate of 220 minus age in years e.g., 20, or 200 as the initial figure for heart rate.)

- **For the 40% intensity level**, you calculate your age-adjusted training heart rate as follows: [(200–75) × 40%]+ 75, or (125 × 40%) + 75 which equals 125 beats per minute.

- **Calculations for the 59% intensity level** are follows: [(200–75) × 59%] + 75, or (125 × 59%) + 75, which equals 148.75 which can be rounded to 149 beats per minute.

Based on calculations according to the Karvonen formula, you would be exercising within the moderate heart rate training zone if you maintained a heart rate between 125 and 149 beats per minute while exercising.

When possible, use the Karvonen method, because it includes resting heart rate that can change with fitness level. The heart rate training zones for low, moderate, and high intensity exercise are quite similar when employing the percent HR$_{max}$ and Karvonen methods for determining HR training zones if you employ the percentages listed in Table 21.1. Note that the HR zone for moderate exercise is calculated as ranging between 64% and 76% for percent of HR$_{max}$; it is between 40 and 59% for the Karvonen method. As illustrated for moderate intensity exercise, the exercise training zones would be from 128 to 152 beats per minute for the percent of HR$_{max}$ and 125 to 149 beats per minute for the Karvonen method—when the participant's resting heart rate is a typical 75 beats per minute.

Metabolic equivalent (MET). Another way to indicate exercise intensity is by determining the energy cost of the activity, or its metabolic equivalent (MET). Energy cost is represented by a specific number of milliliters of oxygen consumed per kilogram of body mass per minute, or multiples of resting metabolic rate referred to as METs. A value of one MET represents the approximate rate of oxygen consumption of a seated adult at rest. More specifically, the body uses approximately 3.5 ml of oxygen per kilogram (2.2 lb) of body weight per minute (Wilmore & Costill, 2004, p. 620). Exercising at an intensity of 3 METs requires three times the energy cost of a resting metabolic rate. Although the MET values of specific exercise activities can be reported, they are only approximations since they vary considerably from one person to another and can be affected by changes in environmental conditions and physical conditioning.

Rating of perceived exertion (RPE). Another technique for measuring exercise intensity is by recording exercisers' subjective ratings of how hard they feel they are working, i.e., their rate of perceived exertion (RPE). Perception of effort, as well as physiological change, is an important component of exercise intensity. When estimating RPE, exercisers report their own exertion levels by selecting standardized verbal descriptions from Borg's scale of perceived exertion (American College of Sports Medicine, 2006, pp. 77–78; Borg, 1998). See Table 21.2 for a listing of the standard verbal descriptors. A specific numeral rating listed in Table 21.2 corresponds to the exerciser's perceived intensity of exertion. The additional verbal descriptors in the right column of the table may improve the accuracy of participants' perception when using the scale to regulate exercise intensity (Bayles et al., 1990). The following instructions for using the RPE during exercise testing illustrate the breadth of sensations that RPE reflects.

> During the exercise test we want you to pay close attention to how hard you feel the exercise work rate is. This feeling should reflect your total amount of exertion and fatigue, combining all sensations and feelings of physical stress, effort, and fatigue. *Don't concern yourself with any one factor such as leg pain, shortness of breath or exercise intensity, but try to concentrate on your total inner feeling of exertion* [emphasis added]. Try not to underestimate or overestimate your feelings of exertion; be as accurate as you can. (American College of Sports Medicine, 2006, p. 78)

As illustrated in the RPE table, an exerciser's appraisal of physical activity that is "very light" results in a numerical score of 9; "somewhat hard" results in a numerical score of 13. Borg initially suggested that an exerciser's score of 9 is very roughly equivalent to a

heart rate of 90 beats per minute, and 13 is roughly equivalent to a heart rate of 130 beats per minute (Noble & Robertson, 1996, p. 63). It is important to note, however, that the direct linear relationship between numerical rating and heart rate is inadequate because heart rate is differentially affected by

- Different exercise modes,
- Personal differences in anxiety, fitness levels and age, and
- Environmental conditions (Borg, 1982; Robertson & Noble, 1997).

Exercise characteristics, environmental conditions, and psychological characteristics influence how hard exercisers report their exercise to be (Robertson & Noble, 1997). Some of the psychological characteristics include self-presentational style, association and disassociation, cognitive style, and sex-role typology. The scale numbers that range from 6 to 20 in Table 21.2 remain quite functional in reflecting exercise intensity (Noble & Robertson, p. 67). Exercisers' RPEs are easy to obtain and tend to be similar for women and men.

Borg's scale was developed to help exercise participants determine how intensely they are exercising and

---

Table 21.2
The Borg Scale of Perceived Exertion
(American College of Sports Medicine, 2006, p. 77; Borg, 1998)

Rating[1]	Standard Verbal Descriptors	Additional Verbal Descriptors
6	No exertion at all	Cool
7	Very, very light	No breathing difficulties, no discomfort, and high motivation
8		
9	Very light	
10		
11	Fairly light	
12		Warm
13	Somewhat hard	Minor breathing difficulties, minor discomfort, and moderate motivation
14		
15	Hard	
16		
17	Very hard	
18		Hot
19	Very, very hard	Major breathing difficulties, major discomfort, and low motivation
20	Maximum exertion	

[1] Multiplying the numerical rating by 10 results in an approximate heart rate.

is useful as a rough estimate of exercise intensity. Most exercisers can estimate their RPE accurately and thus can use it to exercise in the broad range of target heart rate zones (Wilmore & Costill, 2004, p., 623). You can find additional information on factors affecting perception of exercise intensity in *Perceived Exertion* (Noble & Robertson, 1996), *Borg's Perceived Exertion and Pain Scales* (Borg, 1998), and *ACSM's Guidelines for Exercise Testing and Prescription* (American College of Sports Medicine, 2006).

General ranges of exercise intensity. For ease of discussion and interpretation of current research studies, it sometimes makes sense to consider broad ranges of exercise intensities rather than specific levels. Three ranges of exercise intensity are low/light, moderate, and high/hard intensity. One purpose of the ranges is to provide a broad rather than narrow target of HR

goals for exercises. Another purpose is to encourage participants to exercise at an intensity that is "good" for them. As they increase their fitness levels, they can change their exercise intensity from the lower to the upper limit of the intensity range.

Low/light-intensity exercise (2 to 5 METs) is below the aerobic training zone for most individuals and reflects exercise that is approximately 50 to 63% of the age-adjusted heart rate maximum (HR_{max}). As noted in Table 21.1, examples include slow walking, stretching, slow cycling on an exercise cycle, fishing (sitting), bowling, and vacuuming a carpet. Although light-intensity exercise may not result in aerobic training and increased cardiorespiratory fitness, the exercise may have health benefits, especially for individuals who have been sedentary. Additional health benefits can be gained by participating in more vigorous exercise of

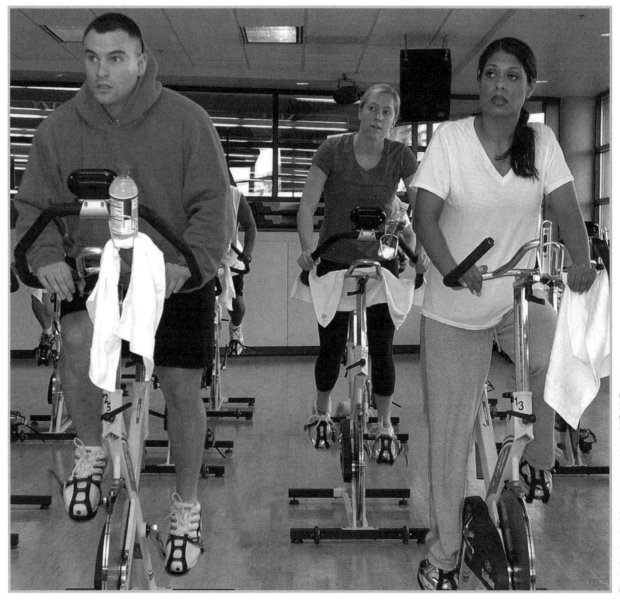

longer duration (American College of Sports Medicine, 2006, p. 6; U.S. Department of Health & Human Services, 1996; Wilmore & Costill, 2004, p. 608). The minimal recommended exercise amount for significant health benefits is for light to moderate exercise "(30 minutes of brisk walking or raking leaves, 15 minutes of running, or 45 minutes of playing volleyball) on most, if not all days of the week" (American College of Sports Medicine, 2006, p. 6; U.S. Department of Health & Human Services, 1996).

Moderate-intensity exercise (3.1 to 7.5 METs) generally begins at the lower end of the aerobic training zone and often is associated with an exercise heart rate of 64 to 76% of HR_{max}. Examples of moderate-intensity activities include walking at a brisk pace, intensely pedaling a bicycle ergometer at speeds that can be maintained for 30 minutes or more, and mowing the lawn by walking behind a power mower.

High/hard-intensity exercise is between 4.1 and 10.2 METs and is 80 to 100% of HR_{max}. High-intensity exercise is characterized by huffing and puffing, perspiring, and perceiving oneself as working hard. Examples of high-intensity activities include walking uphill, jogging, fast cycling, many sport activities, aerobic dance, and mowing the lawn with a hand mower. Exercise above 93% of HR_{max} is very heavy intensity and cannot be sustained for long periods of time (Corbin & Pangrazi, 1996).

Exercise Duration (Time)

Although the word *time* is appropriate for the FIT acronym, *duration* is the word that most aptly captures this exercise component. Duration refers to the length of a single exercise session. Exercise duration is expressed most commonly in minutes. In general, exercise sessions that are 15 minutes in duration or less are considered to be short sessions. Exercise duration of 20 to 30 minutes has been the standard *minimal* recommendation for achieving both the physiological and psychological benefits from exercise (American College of Sports Medicine, 2006, pp. 146–147; Berger, 1984/1997; U.S. Department of Health & Human Services, 1996). Duration between 30 and 60 minutes or as much as 90 minutes per day is recommended for greater health benefits. Longer exercise sessions are recommended for weight control, especially to

- Prevent weight gain,
- Prevent the onset of obesity, and
- Effect weight loss in overweight adults (American College of Sports Medicine, 2006, pp. 6–7, 147, 153).

Exercising for longer than 60 minutes is beyond the duration recommended for *basic* health benefits. However, participants in physical activity who seek weight loss, maintenance of weight loss, enhanced performance, and/or additional psychological benefits often exercise for 60 to 120 minutes or longer per session. Exercise duration beyond 60 minutes, or large exercise volume in general, may be associated with increased risk of injury, especially musculoskeletal and the other accompanying psychological distress (e.g., American College of Sports Medicine, 2006, p. 133). Injury prevention becomes a concern of exercise specialists when advising clients who habitually exercise for a long duration. In addition, exercise that is shorter duration and higher-intensity also is purported to be associated with increased risk of orthopedic injury (American College of Sports Medicine, 2006, p. 141). If lifetime participation in physical activity is a goal, injury prevention is an important consideration. Exercise participants need to listen to their bodies as they exercise and stay within their body's tolerance for exercise in order to continue to exercise throughout their entire lives.

Training Guidelines to Facilitate Physiological Benefits: Two Sets of Guidelines

There are two sets of training guidelines designed to produce different exercise-related physiological goals. The more strenuous training guidelines for physical fitness produce physiological changes that enhance exercise performance and a high level of health. In contrast, the health-related guidelines are less demanding and produce multiple health benefits, but not high-end exercise performance capabilities.

Training Guidelines for Physical Fitness and Exercise Performance

Strenuous training guidelines for physical fitness are designed for recreational exercisers who wish to maximize their exercise performance capabilities. These general guidelines are outlined in Table 21.3. According to these guidelines, exercisers should participate in both aerobic activities and in weight training three to five days a week, at 64% to 93% of maximal heart rate. (See Table 21.1 for the guidelines for light-, moderate-, and high-intensity exercise.) For the cardiorespiratory phase of exercise, the American College of Sports Medicine guidelines (2006, p. 147) suggest including 20 to 60 minutes of continuous activity, or intermittent activity in 10-minute bouts accumulated throughout the day.

Weight training does not have large benefits for cardiorespiratory fitness, the primary focus of the health and exercise performance guidelines. However, weight training should be an integral component of an exercise program as outlined in Table 21.3. These guidelines are provided by the American College of Sports Medicine (2006, pp. 133–173) and reflect desirable exercise requirements for many individuals.

It is important to understand the physiological inter-relationships among exercise frequency, intensity, and duration for obtaining the performance and health benefits. As intensity of exercise increases, duration and frequency can be decreased. As duration increases, exercise intensity and frequency can be decreased. The health benefits of exercise are clear, but the following aspects of the dose-response relationship remain unclear: (1) minimal "dose" of exercise required for the health benefits and (2) what further reductions in disease occur with additional amounts of exercise (American College of Sports Medicine, 2006, p. 7).

Reasons for selecting the strenuous physical fitness-related guidelines rather than the newer and easier health-related guidelines include personal aspirations and exercise performance goals, as well as a desire for high-end health benefits, especially longevity (Blair et al., 1996; Lee, Hsieh, & Paffenbarger, 1995). An underlying premise for each of these goals is that the individual enjoys exercising at this strenuous level in order that the demanding training sessions do not become counterproductive. If participants experience general fatigue, disinterest, burnout, or overuse injuries, they need to reduce their training levels rather than drop out of their exercise programs (Tobar, 2005).

In the past, physically demanding fitness guidelines have been suggested for all individuals regardless of their personal goals. A drawback to these previous guidelines, however, is that they did not allow for individual differences, or for psychological considerations. Physically demanding exercise guidelines seem to be based on the assumption that all individuals seek high levels of physical fitness. This simply is not accurate for many recreational participants who exercise to control their weight, to experience their bodies in movement, to have fun, and/or to interact socially with their friends. Individuals who are not successful in following the physical fitness guidelines and others who do not enjoy following such guidelines often do not look forward to exercising. These people tend to view themselves as never doing "enough," and as exercise failures. People who are neutral towards exercise or even dislike it are less likely to participate in leisure exercise activities, and eventually, become exercise dropouts (e.g., Motl, Dishman, Saunders, Dowda, Felton, & Pate, 2001; Salmon, Owen, Crawford, Bauman & Sallis, 2003). The following more gentle training guidelines for health-related fitness are designed to help sedentary people become physically active, to facilitate exercise enjoyment, and to increase exercise adherence.

Training Guidelines for Health-Related Fitness

Recognizing a need for less stringent exercise guidelines, the U. S. Department of Health and Human Services (USDHHS), Centers for Disease Control,

---

Table 21.3
Training Guidelines for Physical Fitness and Exercise Performance
(ACSM, 2006, pp. 133–173)

Training Factor	Guideline
Mode (or Type):	• **aerobic activities** or "the use of large muscle groups over prolonged periods in activities that are rhythmic and aerobic in nature" (ACSM, 2006, p. 139) • **weight training**: one or more sets of 8 to 12 repetitions of 8 to 10 separate exercises at least two to three nonconsecutive days a week
Frequency:	• **3 to 5 days a week** for exercisers with an ability to participate in moderate-intensity exercise
Intensity:	• **64% to 93% of HR$_{max}$**, or **40% to 84% of HHR** (i.e., moderate- to high-intensity endurance exercise as indicated in Table 21.1)
Duration (or Time):	• **20 to 60 minutes** (in at least 10-minute sessions) of continuous or intermittent aerobic activity accumulated throughout a day for the cardiorespiratory mode

National Center for Chronic Disease Prevention and Health Promotion, and The President's Council on Physical Fitness and Sport have teamed to prepare a report of the Surgeon General entitled *Physical Activity and Health* (USDHHS, 1996). The report contains more flexible, less stringent guidelines to encourage the roughly 40% of American adults who do not participate in any leisure-time physical activity and the 60% of adults who do not exercise sufficiently to adopt more active lifestyles (American College of Sports Medicine, 2006, pp. 5–6; Lee et al., 1995; Schoenborn & Barnes, 2002). The joint recommendation of these organizations is that "every U.S. adult should accumulate 30 minutes or more of moderate-intensity physical activity on most, preferably all, days of the week" (Pate et al., 1995, p. 402). Note that health-related guidelines in general include lower exercise intensity, but higher frequency and longer duration than the physical fitness guidelines. Many adherence experts suggest taking one day a week off from exercising to prevent staleness and to promote exercise enthusiasm.

The newer health-related guidelines are designed to facilitate lifetime physical activity and to enable exercisers to reap substantial health benefits. Some of these benefits include lower rates of all-cause mortality, coronary heart disease and reductions in the risk of type 2 diabetes mellitus, obesity, colon cancer, high blood pressure, osteoporosis, and some forms of can-

cer (American College of Sports Medicine, 2006, pp. 7–10). The more moderate guidelines are health enhancing—primarily for the roughly 40% of the population that is sedentary and participates in no leisure-time physical activity (Schoenborn & Barnes, 2002).

The guidelines for developing health-related fitness reflect the general consensus that some exercise is better than no exercise. The guidelines include daily activities, such as vacuuming and gardening, which can be considered health-related forms of physical activity. See Table 21.4 for a summary of these easier health-related exercise guidelines that include the basic FIT recommendations. Exercisers should participate in both aerobic activities and in weight training for a minimal accumulation of 30 minutes on most, preferably all, days of the week (American College of Sports Medicine, 2006; Pate et al., 1995; U.S. Department of Health and Human Services, 1996). The exercise can be "an accumulation of 30 minutes," but it should be in sessions that are at least 10 minutes each in duration (American College of Sports Medicine, 2006, p. 147).

Conclusion

There are two sets of exercise guidelines: (a) strenuous, physical fitness guidelines for those who enjoy and choose to follow these more demanding parameters that have implications for longevity and (b) a more moderate, health-related set of guidelines designed for

Table 21.4
Training Guidelines for Health-Related Fitness
(U.S. Department of Health and Human Services, 1996)

Training Factor	Guideline
Mode (or Type):	• **aerobic activities** (which include the use of large muscles in the body) • **weight training**: one set of 8–12 repetitions, and 8 to 10 exercises that use major muscle groups
Frequency:	• **most, and preferably all, days of the week**
Intensity:	• **moderate** as represented by 3.1 to 7.5 metabolic equivalents (METs) (One MET is the number of calories expended at rest. Exercise activities measuring 3.1 to 7.5 METs require 3.1 to 7.5 times as much energy as 1 MET and are represented by brisk walking, racquet sports, and mowing the lawn with a power mower that a person walks behind (Corbin & Pangrazi, 1996)
Duration (or Time):	• **30 minutes or more**: These 30 minutes can be distributed throughout a day in sessions that are at least 10 minutes or longer

individuals who have few performance aspirations, but who want to include some exercise in their lives to enhance their overall health. Physiologically, the exercise parameters for various levels of health and fitness are becoming clearer. The more demanding fitness guidelines provide greater physical fitness benefits than do the less-demanding health guidelines, and the fitness guidelines are intended for individuals who are motivated to exercise intensely. However, the strenuous, physical fitness guidelines should not necessarily be espoused as the ultimate exercise goal for all individuals. The less physically demanding health guidelines are beneficial for sedentary individuals and for people who are minimally active. The more moderate exercise guidelines reflect the truism that some exercise is better than none.

Exercise Training/Practice Guidelines to Facilitate Psychological Benefits

Practice guidelines for enhancing the psychological benefits of exercise are becoming clearer—despite the considerable variability in personal preferences. Individual differences in exercise preferences must be acknowledged, because exercise practice/training guidelines are integrally related to exercise enjoyment, personal satisfaction, and the decision to be physically active. See Figure 21.1 for the exercise practice guidelines that compose one of the three major considerations in the taxonomy developed by Berger and her colleagues (Berger, 1996, 2004; Berger & Motl, 2001; Berger & Owen, 1988, 1992b, 1998). As previously suggested in Chapter 20, exercise enjoyment and exercise mode characteristics as well as the practice/training guidelines identified in this chapter seem to influence the relationship between exercise, mood alteration, self-awareness, self-concept, and other psychological benefits.

Familiarity with the psychologically based practice/training guidelines, designed to enhance psychological well-being, will enable you to assist participants in choosing how to exercise on any particular day. Selection of exercise training/practice guidelines as well as type (as identified in Chapter 20) of exercise to facilitate psychological well-being should depend on the participant's exercise goals, physical state that day, and exercise preferences (e.g., Miller, Bartholomew, & Springer, 2005; Salmon et al., 2003).

As an exercise psychologist, exercise physiologist,

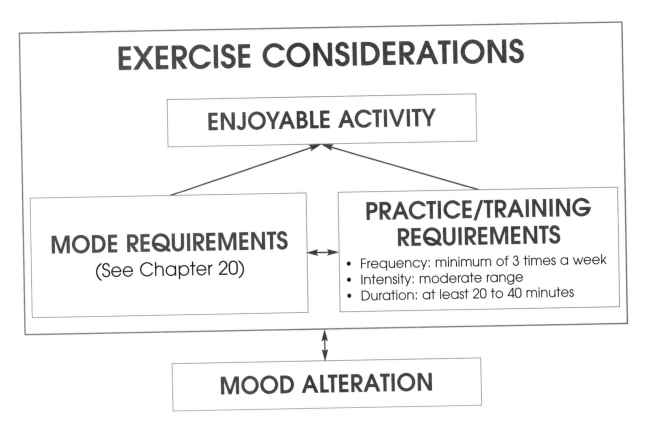

Figure 21.1. Taxonomy for enhancing the psychological benefits of exercise. From "Exercise and Quality of Life," by B. G. Berger and R. W. Motl (2001), *Handbook of sport psychology* (2nd ed.), pp. 636–671. Copyright 2001 by John Wiley & Sons. Adapted with permission.

Table 21.5	
Exercise Practice Guidelines for Optimal Psychological Benefits	
(Berger, 1996; Berger & Motl, 2001)	

Practice Factor	**Guideline**
Frequency	• Minimum of 3 times a week to establish a fitness base for physical comfort
	• Needed to reestablish mood benefits
Intensity	• Moderate-intensity range: approximately 55–75% of HR_{max}
	○ Low-intensity exercise: little available data
	○ High-intensity exercise: can be associated with undesirable mood changes
Duration	• Estimated 20–40 minutes per session
	○ 0–20 minutes: little data available
	○ 40–120 minutes: primarily anecdotal descriptions of benefits
	○ Participants in long-duration competitive swimming report undesirable mood changes

athletic trainer, physical therapist, personal trainer, or movement specialist, you may need to encourage exercisers not to feel guilty if they choose to follow the health-related, rather than the demanding, physical fitness-related guidelines. Subsequent sections in this chapter highlight some of the research concerning the practice guidelines and their implications for psychological well-being (Berger & Motl, 2000; Berger & Tobar, in press). See Table 21.5 for a summary of the practice/training guidelines for optimal psychological benefits.

Frequency of Exercise and the Psychological Benefits

Exercising on a regular basis has implications for the psychological changes associated with exercise. Frequent exercise increases the fitness levels of participants and seems to increase the likelihood that the exercise is enjoyable. Exercising frequently, but not so often as to incur an overuse injury or to become bored, decreases physical discomfort as the conditioning process occurs. Another way frequent exercise serves to decrease physical discomfort is through the self-learning process. Exercisers learn to interpret physical sensations that occur with regular participation. Habitual exercisers become adept at the following:

• Interpreting the meaning of various physical sensations,
• Pacing themselves throughout their exercise session,
• Modifying the exercise session according to the day's needs, and
• Relaxing while exercising.

The need for the exercise frequency guideline tends to be based more on logic or speculation than on research because of the few research studies directly investigating the relationship between exercise frequency and psychological well-being. One of the few investigations of the dose response relationship between exercise and psychological well-being focused on the efficacy of exercise as a treatment for depression (Dunn, Trivedi, Kampert, Clark, & Chambliss, 2005). Initially sedentary participants whose scores on the Hamilton Rating Scale for Depression ($HRSD_{17}$; Hamilton, 1968) indicated that they were mildly or moderately depressed participated in a 12-week exercise program. Participants were randomly assigned to an exercise placebo control group who performed 15 to 20 minutes of flexibility exercises, or to one of four exercise treatment groups. Exercise treatment groups included two exercise frequencies (3 or 5 days/week) and two exercise doses: a low dose (7 kcal/kg/week) or a public health dose (17.5 kcal/kg/week) as established by the American College of Sports Medicine (2000). Participants exercised individually under supervision on a treadmill or stationary bicycle to avoid possible influences of social support. Results indicated that participants in all five groups reported significant decreases in depression. In addition, there was support for a dose effect of caloric expenditure, but not for exercise frequency on lowering exercisers' scores on the $HRSD_{17}$. Regardless of whether they exercised three or five days a week, exercisers in the public health dose reported significantly greater decreases in depression than those in the light dose and the placebo stretching group. Prior to concluding that exercise duration has little influence on the psychological benefits of exercise, studies similar to the one by Dunn and associates (2005) are needed to examine the relationship between various exercise frequencies and psychological well-being for members of the general population.

The Uncertain Role of Physical Fitness

Although there is little research directly examining exercise frequency, there is some related research on psychological well-being and physical fitness, an outcome of habitual exercise as emphasized in the follow-

ing section. Supporting a possible relationship between exercise frequency and the psychological benefits of exercise, exercisers who have high levels of fitness are more likely to report desirable psychological changes after a single exercise session than are those who are less fit. For example, a single, high-intensity (80 to 85% of HR_{max}) session on an exercise treadmill was associated with acute reductions in state anxiety and an increase in alpha power only for those who were fit and had been running 30 miles or more per week for the past two years (Boutcher & Landers, 1988). Novice runners did not report any decreases in anxiety after the same 20 minutes of high-intensity exercise. High-intensity running in the 80 to 85% HR_{max} range probably was not an enjoyable activity for the novice runners. In contrast, other researchers have found that fitness level, which is a reflection of exercise frequency, is not related to the acute mood changes associated with exercise (e.g., Blanchard & Rodgers, 1997). George Sheehan (1992a), the cardiologist who wrote numerous books on the meaning and experiences of his running, captured the difference between being fit and being a recreational athlete or exerciser in the following comment:

Fitness is the ability to do work . . .

Being an athlete is something quite different. Fitness is what you pass through on the way to a superior physical and mental and spiritual state.

Being an athlete is not something I do an hour or so a day. It is something I *am*. Being a runner is something that informs my entire day. My 24 hours is lived as a runner.

Fitness helps you look for the life you should lead. Being an athlete means you have found It [italics added]. (pp. 228–220)

When participating in high-intensity exercise, participants seem to need at least a minimal level of fitness to enjoy the exercise and to "feel better" rather than worse after the physical exertion. This possibility was supported in a meta-analysis of exercise and depression (North, McCullagh, & Tran, 1990). Mental health benefits increased as the length of an exercise program increased. Length of an exercise program was measured by either the number of weeks or the number of sessions. The decreases in depression might be related to accumulative or chronic changes, or they might simultaneously reflect the need for some minimal base of physical conditioning.

Automaticity

Frequent exercise and the resulting increases in physical fitness enable the participant to devote less attention to the actual performance of movement as the movements become more automatically executed. *Automaticity* denotes that the movements in activities such as jogging, swimming, and skiing can be done almost unconsciously, or automatically.

With frequent participation, many types of exercise become almost automatic. With less need to focus on the exercise activity itself, participants can disassociate and follow their own train of thoughts as described in Chapter 20 on selecting type or mode of exercise. Frequent exercise also provides a fitness base and physically the activity becomes easier, less grueling, perhaps more enjoyable, and again more automatic.

Frequency: A Need to Recapture the Psychological Benefits

A totally different reason to exercise frequently is that the mood benefits tend to last for a period between two to four hours after exercising for members of non-clinical populations (Morgan, 1987). The duration of exercise-induced reductions in anxiety (and decreases in systolic blood pressure) after exercising may last up to four hours, and this is considerably longer than the changes associated with simple rest, which were short-lived (Raglin & Morgan, 1987). Other studies also support the conclusion that psychological benefits last beyond the exercise session itself (Bartholomew, 1997; Butki & Rudolph, 1997; Petruzzello & Landers, 1994; Thayer, 1987a). Although the exact time frame for the continuation of the benefits is not clear, the psychological benefits, especially mood changes, do seem to dissipate sometime within four hours of ending an exercise session. Thus, there is a need to exercise on a frequent basis to reestablish the benefits.

Intensity of Exercise and the Psychological Benefits

Exercise intensity, how "hard" one exercises, is a major consideration in designing an exercise program to facilitate psychological benefits. The exercise needs to be of appropriate intensity to be associated with desired changes. Beyond a certain level, however, increasing exercise intensity is counterproductive to "feeling better."

Numerous factors may interact with the relationship between exercise intensity and psychological well-being. Thus, guidelines about the desirability of specific exercise intensities are only general suggestions. Intensity guidelines apply to a broad segment of the population, but they do not apply to all individuals in all situations. For example, the following factors might directly affect the relationship between exercise intensity and psychological well-being:

- **Duration** a person exercises at a particular exercise intensity. Although there is little or no research in the area, exercising at a high intensity level for 5 minutes may have quite different effects on psychological well being than exercising at a high intensity level for 30 minutes.
- **Personal fitness levels.** A person who is highly fit would seem to be have more positive psychological responses to high intensity exercise than a low-fit individual (e.g., Dishman, Farquhar, & Cureton, 1994; Parfitt & Easton, 1995; Steptoe & Bolton, 1988),
- **Personality factors** such as extraversion, optimal stimulation levels, and self-efficacy (e.g., Treasure & Newbery, 1998),
- **Point in time** at which the psychological changes are measured: at various time periods during exercise, immediately after exercising, as well as 30, 60, 180, and 240 minutes or longer after exercising (Bartholomew, Morrison, & Ciccolo, 2005; Dishman, et al., 1994; Roy & Steptoe, 1991; Steptoe & Bolton, 1988; Tate & Petruzzello, 1995), and
- **Preferred levels of exertion.** Some individuals may prefer low intensity exercise; others may consider it a waste of their time. In contrast, some individuals may prefer high intensity exercise, and others may greatly dislike it (e.g., Berger & McInman, 1993; Dishman et al., 1994).

Many of these mediating factors are not included in studies of exercise intensity and mood. Thus, it is difficult to formulate firm conclusions about the relationship between specific exercise intensities and the "feel-better" phenomenon. A preferred or optimal intensity level for one person may not be conducive to psychological well-being for another. Moderate-, high-, and low-intensity exercise levels need to be carefully adjusted and individualized for clients by exercise practitioners based on their own experience. As noted in *ACSM's Guidelines for Exercise Testing and Prescription* (2006), exercise prescription is an art as well as a science. The artistic aspect of exercise prescription lies in individually tailoring an exercise program in accordance with the participant's goals, current fitness level, preferred level of exertion, and personality. As concluded in the following sections, the most advantageous exercise intensity for maximizing the psychological benefits of exercise is unclear. However, moderate-intensity exercise seems to be the "best" choice at the present time. See Table 21.6 for a summary of the intensity guidelines that facilitate the psychological benefits.

Table 21.6

Exercise Intensity and Psychological Benefits

Intensity	Benefits
Low	• Brisk walking associated with mood enhancement • Need further substantiation
Moderate	• Enhances psychological well-being
High	• Associated with no mood changes • Associated with undesirable mood changes • May be mood enhancing for a small subpopulation

Other considerations	• Enjoyment
	• Preferred level of exertion
	• Interactions with exercise frequency and duration
	• Exercise-adherence implications
	• Age adjustments for lifetime participation
	    ○ Young children of various ages
	    ○ Vigorous seniors
	    ○ Frail elderly

Moderate-Intensity Exercise

As Berger (1984/1997) concluded in a chapter on "Running Strategies for Women and Men," moderate-intensity exercise is recommended—if psychological well-being is a major goal. Moderate-intensity exercise in the form of walking rapidly (while swinging one's arms freely and breathing deeply) has been associated with reduced tension and increased energy as measured by the Activation-Deactivation Adjective Checklist in numerous studies (Thayer, 1986, 1987a, 1987b; Thayer, Peters, Takahashi, & Birkhead-Flight, 1993). Results of current research supports the acute psychological benefits of brisk walking as reported by participants with major depressive disorder (e.g., Bartholomew et al., 2005). Walking on a treadmill was performed for 30 minutes at an exercise intensity of 60% to 70% of age-predicted maximal heart rate. Participants in the exercise session reported significantly greater increases in Vigor on the short version of the POMS (McNair, Lorr, & Droppleman, 1972/1992) and increases in Positive Well-Being on the Subjective Exercise Experiences Scale (McAuley & Courneya, 1994) than did the resting-control group. In addition, both exercisers and controls reported reductions in Psychological Distress, Depression, Confusion, Fatigue, Tension, and Anger as measured on the two scales.

When comparing the benefits of walking rapidly and eating a candy bar for energy, the walkers reported higher ratings of energy and lower scores on tension and tiredness than the snackers when measured 30, 60, and 120 minutes after the treatments (Thayer, 1987a). See Figure 21.2 for the advantages of walking in comparison to those of eating a candy bar for reducing tension and in raising energy. As shown in the figure, walkers who exercised in the morning session (open circle) reported more energy than did the morning snack group (open triangle). Likewise, walkers in the evening session (closed circle) had more energy than did evening snackers (closed triangle). After walking, participants reported "calm energy" as reflected in significantly higher energy levels in comparison to their pre-exercise levels. These benefits continued for as long as two hours after the walking sessions. Thayer (1996, p. 184) summarized his research and concluded that "moderate" exercise is one of the best ways to raise energetic arousal and to reduce tension. Although it is difficult to equate walking as suggested by Thayer with a specific heart rate, the brisk and rapid walking probably can be considered to be in the moderate-intensity range.

Additional evidence for the benefits of moderate-intensity exercise is based on a study of sedentary individuals. These nonexercisers were randomly assigned to one of two intensities of cycling or to a control condition (Treasure & Newbery, 1998). One set of exercisers cycled for 15 minutes at moderate intensity (45% to 50% of their age-adjusted heart-rate reserve). Another group cycled for the same amount of time at a high intensity that was 70% to 75% of their age-adjusted heart-rate reserve. The controls sat quietly in the same exercise environment and read while on a stationary cycle. As expected, the exercisers reported greater acute changes in mood than the control group who read. Cyclists exercising at the two intensities also differed from one another. The moderate-intensity exercisers, in contrast to the high-intensity group, reported more positive and fewer negative feeling states both during the exercise as well as for 15 minutes after exercising. During exercise, the moderate-intensity cyclists reported increased revitalization, and the high-intensity cyclists reported decreased revitalization and tranquility as well as increased exhaustion. The moderate-intensity cyclists also reported more benefits when pre- and post-exercise scores were compared. After a 15-

minute rest period, moderate-intensity cyclists were significantly higher in positive engagement, tranquility, and revitalization than the high-intensity cyclists. The only change that high-intensity cyclists reported was an increase in physical exhaustion.

High-Intensity Exercise

Emphasizing the need for moderate-intensity exercise, high-intensity exercise at HRs of 80% of maximum or higher (see Table 21.1) has been associated with inconsistent changes in mood. These include

- **Few changes** (e.g., Berger & Owen, 1988, 1992b),
- **Undesirable changes** (e.g., Berger & Owen, 1992b; Motl, Berger, & Davis, 1997; Motl, Berger, & Wilson, 1996), and
- **Desirable mood changes** (Boutcher & Landers, 1988).

Although high-intensity exercise is required for optimal physical conditioning, consistent overtraining in the form of high-intensity exercise can lead to performance decrements; staleness as characterized by long-term performance decrements; and burnout (O'Connor, 1997; Tobar, 2005). Exercisers and athletes who push the training envelope tend to report decreased Vigor and increased Fatigue. However, undesirable changes in mood, especially on the Tension, Depression, Anger, and Confusion subscales of the POMS, serve as precursors of staleness and as signs that the exerciser needs to reduce the level of training before performance decrements occur (Tobar, 2005). High-intensity exercise is not always desirable—even for highly conditioned, world-class athletes.

Supporting the diminishing returns of high-intensity exercise, Steptoe and colleagues (Roy & Steptoe, 1991; Steptoe & Bolton, 1988; Steptoe & Cox, 1988) compared exercising on a bicycle ergometer at two absolute intensities: 25 watts and 100 watts, which they reported to represent low and high intensity, respectively. Duration varied between 8 and 20 minutes. In all three studies, the cyclists reported benefits of decreased scores on Tension and increased Vigor and Exhilaration in the low-intensity exercise. They also reported mood decrements in high-intensity cycling: increased Tension/Anxiety, and decreased Vigor and Exhilaration. Other studies also support the likelihood of fewer psychological benefits associated with high-intensity exercise. Col-

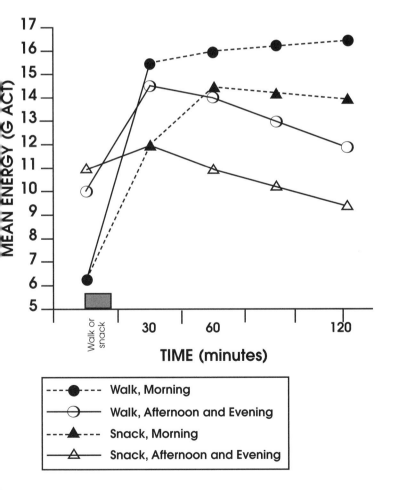

Figure 21.2. Energy states as measured before and after a 10-minute walk or snacking on a candy bar (Thayer, 1987b).

lege students in swimming and in body-conditioning classes exercised at a relatively high intensity of 81% to 90% of HR_{max}. The students also reported no changes in mood—either negative or positive—on any of the POMS subscales, except for an increase in Fatigue (Berger & Owen, 1988, 1992b). It is not exactly clear what qualifies as high-intensity exercise because it changes from one research study to another. Generally, however, high intensity exercise is described as ranging between 80 and 100% of one's age-adjusted maximal heart rate (Corbin & Pangrazi, 1996; McArdle, Katch, & Katch, 1996).

In an investigation of mood changes associated with moderate-, high-, and maximal-intensity exercise, competitive collegiate cyclists reported diverse changes in mood. The trained cyclists reported mood benefits when exercising at a moderate intensity of 69% HR_{max}, a relative absence of mood change at

high-intensity interval training at 90% HR_{max}, and mood decrements at an even higher intensity of 95% HR_{max} (Motl et al., 1996). See Figure 21.3 for a depiction of the mood changes, both desirable and undesirable ones, at the three exercise intensities. Exercising near one's maximal heart rate is not conducive to mood benefits for most people.

Low-Intensity Exercise

In contrast to the developing body of literature on high-intensity exercise and mood, relatively little research has focused on low-intensity exercise and psychological well-being. This lack seems to be based on an assumption that there is an intensity threshold below which exercisers obtain few, if any, psychological benefits (e.g., Dunn et al., 2005). Although there is little experimental evidence of a threshold level of exercise intensity, such an idea is intuitively appealing.

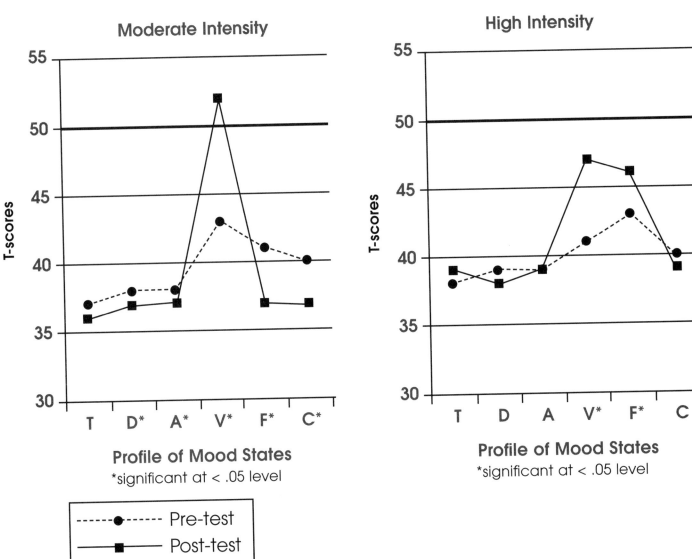

Figure 21.3. Acute changes in mood at three exercise intensities (Motl, Berger, & Wilson, 1996).

As observed by Kirkcaldy and Shephard (1990) in their review of the psychological benefits of exercise,

> Plainly, there is thus no single "exercise hypothesis" that can be tested experimentally. Indeed, there is some evidence that any response to exercise is non-linear; a *threshold dose* [italics added] must be passed in order to yield an effect, while an *excessive dose* [italics added] has adverse physical and psychological consequences. Moreover, both the threshold dose and the safe ceiling of treatment vary widely from one person to another. (pp. 166–167)

In some of the few studies comparing low-intensity exercise to either moderate- or high-intensity exercise, participants in the low-intensity exercise groups have reported more benefits than did members of the other two groups (Berger & Owen, 1998; deVries & Adams,

Maximal Intensity

Profile of Mood States
*significant at < .05 level

------●------ Pre-test
——■—— Post-test

1972; Steptoe & Cox, 1988). When comparing the benefits of low- and high-intensity exercise, Steptoe and Cox reported that eight-minute bouts of low-intensity cycling were associated with desirable increases in Vigor and in Exhilaration. In contrast, the high-intensity exercise on a bicycle ergometer was associated with acute increases in Tension and Fatigue. A classic study of low- and moderate-intensity exercise supported the benefits of low-intensity exercise as indicated by muscle relaxation. Older men and women who walked for 15 minutes at a heart rate of 100 beats per minute significantly reduced the electrical activity in their muscles as recorded using an electromyograph (deVries & Adams). Older participants who exercised at a moderate intensity and maintained a walking heart rate of 120 beats per minute did not evidence the decrease in muscle tension.

In another study of exercise intensity, participants who walked or jogged at a low intensity (55% maximal HR) and a moderate intensity (75% and 79% maximal HR) reported mood benefits (Berger & Owen, 1998). All joggers, regardless of the exercise intensity, reported improved mood states. These included acute reductions in Tension, Depression, Anger, Fatigue, and Confusion, and increased Vigor. Thus, there seems to be some support for reduced muscle tension, and increased feelings of Vigor and Exhilaration while exercising at a low-intensity level. Emphasizing a need for further research concerning the psychological benefits of light-intensity exercise, the results of a recent meta-analysis of the effects of exercise on psychological well-being in advanced age, Netz and her colleagues (2005) concluded that moderate-intensity exercise had the strongest benefit for psychological well-being in older adults, and light-intensity exercise the least.

In contrast to the findings of Netz and colleagues (2005) for older adults, research and writings focusing on the psychological changes associated with Eastern forms of exercise such as hatha yoga, qigong, and ti chi chan as reviewed in the previous chapter on selecting exercise modes support the possibility that low-intensity exercise is associated with increases in diverse aspects of psychological well-being (e.g., Berger & Owen, 1988, 1992a; Daubenmier, 2005; Iyengar with Evans & Abrams, 2005; Li, Duncan, Duncan, McAuley, Chaumeton, & Harmer, 2001; Mittelstaedt, Hinton, Rana, Cade, & Xue, 2005). Clearly, additional research focused directly on the psychological benefits of light-intensity exercise is needed. In conclusion, research focusing on light intensity exercise is greatly needed—especially in view of its appeal to many non-exercisers, and the accumulating research evidence of the health benefits of walking and Eastern forms of exercise (e.g., Daubenmier, 2005; Hakim et al., 1998).

Preferred Level of Exertion

A factor possibly connected with the relationship between exercise intensity and associated psychological benefits is one's preferred level of exercise exertion. Some people like to exercise primarily at a low level of intensity. A low exercise intensity is easy to maintain, involves little pain from exertion, and does not evoke perspiration. Other people prefer a moderate intensity—one that lets the participants know they are doing something "good" for their bodies. Moderate-intensity exercise also is fairly easy to maintain. It is not associated with difficulties in breathing, and does not require careful monitoring of one's physical responses to maintain the fine line between having to stop and being able to continue. Despite the many advantages of moderate-intensity exercise, some individuals prefer a high-intensity level. They seem to feel that if they are not exercising at a high intensity, their exercise session has been a "waste." It is unclear why some people feel that they "must" exercise at high intensity. Perhaps they truly enjoy high-intensity exercise, or they are intent on obtaining the greatest physiological benefits from the exercise sessions. They also may envision themselves as potential elite athletes.

Relatively little is known about factors influencing the fascinating concept of preferred level of exertion or about how preferred exertion might influence the relationship between various exercise intensities and mood alteration (Berger & Motl, 2001). In a recent study that focused directly on preferred exercise intensity, formerly sedentary women participated in a 20-minute exercise session on a treadmill and were allowed to select the speed or exercise intensity they preferred (Lind, Joens-Matre, & Ekkekakis, 2004). Participants also were permitted to adjust the exercise intensity throughout the session. Results indicated that the adult women selected mean exercise intensities within the range of 74% to 83% of maximal HR when measured at various 5-minute intervals throughout the 20-minute session. Their ratings of perceived exertion inceased each 5-minutes of the exercise session and progressed from 10.96 at 5 minutes, to 11.96 at 10 minutes, 13.09 at 15 minutes, and 13.78 at 20 minutes of exercise. Based on the RPE values, the previously sedentary women's preferred exercise intensity was in the low to moderate intensity range as indicated by the parameters in Table 20.1.

Intensity and Enjoyment: Adherence Considerations

Similar to the relationship between exercise intensity and psychological well-being, relationships between exercise intensity, enjoyment, and program adherence await additional experimental exploration for clarification. Illustrating the complex relationship between intensity and adherence, supervised home-based exercise programs that were either moderate intensity (60 to 73% HR $_{peak}$) or high intensity (73 to 88% HR $_{peak}$) did not differ from one another in regard to adherence (King, Haskell, Taylor, Kraemer, & DeBusk, 1991). However, exercisers in both the moderate- and high-intensity home programs had higher adherence than did those in a group-based program who exercised in the same high-intensity range of 73 to 88% HR $_{peak}$. In the second year of the project, the results regarding adherence differed again and indicated the precariousness in forcing any interpretation of the relationship between exercise intensity and adherence to programs (King, Haskell, Young, Oka, & Stefanick, 1995).

Duration of Exercise Sessions and the Psychological Benefits

Exercise duration is another practice factor that appears to be related to the psychological benefits of physical activity. Personal or introspective as well as phenomenological experiences reported when exercising for specific durations indicate that the psychological benefits might change from one duration to another. Exercising for 10, 30, and 120 minutes may be associated with different psychological states (e.g., Mandell, 1979; O'Halloran, Murphy, & Webster, 2004). The mood states associated with various exercise durations also may differ according to the psychological and fitness characteristics of the participant and environmental characteristics. For example, the personality construct of hardiness has been related to the extent of mood decrements associated with an increase in exercise duration (Goss, 1994). Exercising in a rather sterile laboratory environment may be very different from exercising for the same length of time surrounded by the beauty of nature or in an exercise setting with pleasing music engulfing the participant.

The possibility that personal experiences within a single exercise session change as duration increases has been captured in a classic description by Mandell (1979). Arnold Mandell is a psychotherapist and a runner who captured various qualities of his experience in a delightful introspective account:

The *first thirty minutes* [italics added] are tough, old man. Creaks, twinges, pain, and stiffness. A counterpoint of breathless, painful self-depreciation. . . . The first thirty minutes hurt until the body gets the message that you're serious.

Thirty minutes [italics added] out, and something lifts. Legs and arms become light and rhythmic . . . The fatigue goes away and feelings of power begin. I think I'll run twenty-five miles today. I'll double the size of the research grant request. I'll have that talk with the dean . . .

Then, sometime into *the second hour* [italics added] comes the spooky time. Colors are bright and beautiful, water sparkles, clouds breathe, and my body, swimming, detaches from the earth. A loving contentment invades the basement of my mind, and thoughts bubble up without trails. I find the place I need to live if I'm going to live. The running literature says that if you run six miles a day for two months, you are addicted forever. I understand. A cosmic view and peace are located between six and ten miles of running. (p. 57)

Duration of more than 40 minutes

Although there are personal accounts of the psychological experiences associated with exercising for specific durations, few researchers have compared the psychological benefits of exercising for various durations. In a classic study of commitment to running and mental states during a run, Carmack and Martens (1979) surveyed runners who ranged in different ability—from students enrolled in a university conditioning class to those attending an Olympic training clinic. One question pertained to the runners' state of mind during the four quarters of an exercise session. Runners characterized as "under-40-minute runners" and those characterized as "over-40-minute runners" reported opposing patterns during four quarters of their exercise sessions. The under-40-minute runners reported feelings of psychological uneasiness during the first half and last quarter of their run. In contrast, the over-40-minute runners reported feelings of psychological well-being during the same periods. Both fitness groups reported a different set of experiences during the third quarter. The under-40-minute runners had feelings of well-being. The over-40-minute runners had feelings of psychological uneasiness during the third quarter, but they also reported more altered mental states as poetically described by Mandell (1979). These experiences tended to occur more often during the last half of the run. The results of Carmack and Martens (1979) support the possibility that runners and other exercisers experience different mental states during various segments of an exercise session. This possibility awaits further investigation.

Regular-length and abbreviated training distances have been differentially related to mood alteration in young competitive swimmers (Berger, Grove, Prapavessis, & Butki, 1997). Collegiate swimmers also have reported mood decrements after long-duration sessions (Morgan, Costill, Flynn, Raglin, & O'Connor, 1988). Both studies showed significant interactions between the duration of swimming and acute changes in mood. The young swimmers reported mood improvement after shortened or tapered practice sessions (between 3500 and 5000 meters) held prior to competition as indicated by decreases in Total Mood Disturbance Scores (Berger et al., 1997). Total Mood Disturbance (TMD) is a single composite score, which combines the six subscales of the Profile of Mood States. After the tapered sessions, the young swimmers reported less Depression and Confusion, but still not the broader-based benefits that recreational participants usually report.

In contrast to the shorter duration exercise sessions, swimmers' TMD scores increased when measured immediately before and after normal-distance practice sessions of 6000 and 7000 meters that were over 40 minutes in length. They reported increased Fatigue and decreased Vigor. Competitive swimming was associated with mood benefits only when distances or durations were considerably shorter than usual (Berger et al., 1997). These results agree with those of Morgan and colleagues (1988), who also investigated swimmers who swam various durations. Intensity was high, approximately 94% VO_2 max, and swimming distance increased from 4000 to 9000 meters. As expected, the highly fit collegiate swimmers reported significant increases in Depression, Anger, Fatigue, and TMD scores in the longer duration practices. Beyond a certain duration of exercise, the typical mood benefits of exercise do not exist. Either there are no mood changes, or they become negative. As clarified in a recent review of overtraining and staleness, psychological monitoring with the Profile of Mood States (POMS: McNair, Lorr, & Droppleman, 1972/1992) can be employed to prevent staleness from occurring (Tobar, 2005).

Psychological Benefits and an Exercise Duration of less than 40 minutes: 20 to 39 minutes

Exercising for more than 40 minutes is not always desirable. As previously indicated, it can lead to staleness, and some individuals simply do not enjoy the physical/psychological experience of exercising. They may wish to obtain the health benefits but to minimize the length of time they exercise. As a result, the question arises, what is the minimal amount of exercise that is needed to reach specific goals? If health—both physical and psychological—is the primary reason for exercising, then, the Surgeon General's recommendation of 30 minutes most days of the week becomes the guideline for exercise duration. In addition, long-duration exercise sessions in excess of 40 minutes present scheduling problems to busy people. Long-duration exercise sessions also may exacerbate exercise-related injuries. Thus, for practical considerations, it is important to examine the psychological benefits of exercising less than 40 minutes.

In a meta-analysis that focused on the anxiety-reducing effects of acute and chronic exercise,

Petruzzello, Landers, Hatfield, Kubitz, and Salazar (1991) observed that decreases in anxiety were related to duration of exercise. Exercise sessions between 0 and 20 minutes in duration were not as conducive to reductions in anxiety as sessions longer than 20 minutes. However, subsequent analyses of the same data, which included only pre- and post-exercise anxiety scores, prompted Petruzzello and colleagues to conclude that both 1 to 20 minutes and 20 to 30 minutes of exercise were associated with significant reductions in state anxiety. Supporting the benefits of both durations of exercise, the magnitude of the anxiety changes for the two categories of exercise duration was also similar (Petruzzello & Landers, 1994; Petruzzello et al., 1991).

In a recent investigation of mood states during a 60-minute treadmill run, 80 regular runners completed the b-form of the POMS (1) prior to the run (2) during the run at 10-, 25-, 40-, and 55-minutes, and (3) 10-minutes after completing a 60-minute walk/run session on a treadmill (O'Halloran et al., 2004). Exercise intensity was described as low to moderate and reflected 70% of participants' age-predicted maximum heart rate. After 40 minutes of exercise, runners reported less Anxiety (increased composure), less Confusion (increased mental clarity), and increased Energy. However 10-minutes after completing the 60-minute running session, participants' Energy and Confusion returned to baseline levels. These results support the psychological benefits of running durations of 40 minutes for trained runners and fewer psychological benefits at a 55-minute duration.

Duration of less than 40 minutes: 5 to 19 minutes

The Surgeon General's Report (U.S. Department of Health and Human Services, 1996) recommends 30 minutes of exercise most days of the week and indicates that the 30 minutes of exercise can be completed in three 10-minute blocks of time. Thus the psychological benefits, as well as the physiological benefits, of the 10-minute exercise sessions are of particular interest.

A study of affective changes in exercisers who ran on a treadmill in a laboratory setting for 15 or for 30 minutes supports the possibility that exercising for both durations of exercise (when performed at 75% of VO_2max) is associated with significant reductions in state anxiety (Petruzzello & Landers, 1994). Surprisingly, neither the 15 minutes nor the 30 minutes of exercise were associated with changes in either positive or negative affect when measured by the Positive Affect-Negative Affect Scale (PANAS; Watson, Clark, & Tellegen, 1988). A lack of change in affect is difficult to explain. Perhaps there were no changes, or perhaps the PANAS is not sensitive enough to detect changes as measured before and after a single exercise session (Petruzzello & Landers, 1994).

To examine the influence of the current health-related recommendation for 30 minutes of exercise accumulated throughout the day in sessions that are at least 10 minutes in duration on mood state, the mood benefits of 10-, 20-, and 30-minute exercise sessions were compared with one another and with a placebo condition of sitting quietly for 30 minutes (Hansen, Stevens, & Coast, 2001). College students ($N = 21$) rode a bicycle ergometer and exercised alone (to prevent social interaction) for each of the three time periods that were randomly assigned on three different days. The students completed the Profile of Mood States with the "how do you feel right now" instructional set immediately before and after each session that included a 10-minute cool down period after each of the assigned exercise durations. Exercise intensity in each of the three durations was at a moderate exercise intensity of approximately 60% of estimated VO_{2max} as indicated the use of heart rate monitors. Exercisers reported significant decreases in Fatigue and Total Negative Mood, and increases in Vigor after the 10-minute session. After the 20-minute session, they reported the same benefits as previously and also a decrease in Confusion. They reported the same, but no additional benefits after 30 minutes of exercise. These results indicate that in this college student population, there were mood benefits after as little as 10-minutes of moderate intensity exercise with additional benefits after 20 minutes, but no additional benefits after 30 minutes of aerobic exercise.

Conclusions: Current duration guidelines

Various durations of activity may be associated with differing psychological benefits as reflected in phenomenological accounts such as the one by Mandell (1979). However, quantative studies employing standardized anxiety and mood measures have not yet captured these changes. Qualitative studies using phenomenological reports and interviews are needed to understand possible differences between psychological states associated with exercising for various durations. In conclusion, there is a consensus that exercise sessions of 20 minutes to 40 minutes in duration are conducive to acute psychological changes (e.g., Berger, 1984/1997; Dishman, 1986). This conclusion, however, is somewhat premature and warrants continued investigation. Until there is additional information, exercising for at least 20 minutes seems to be an effective and somewhat cautious approach. Exercising for 40 minutes or longer may produce additional qualitative benefits such as those of detachment, contentment, and finding one's special "place" as described by Mandell (1979).

Exercising for as little as 5 or 10 minutes also may be associated with the calm-energy benefits illustrated in the work of Thayer (1987a, 1987b; Thayer et al., 1993). After 10 minutes of exercise, walkers reported feeling calm-energy as reflected by more energy and less tension and tiredness after exercising in comparison to how they felt before. These psychological changes persisted 30, 60, and 120 minutes after the walking sessions. In another study, running on a treadmill for either 10, 15, or 20 minutes was associated with decreases in perceived psychological distress and increases in well-being at 5 and 20 minutes after exercising (Butki & Rudolph, 1997). It seems that as little as 10 minutes of exercise might be associated with desirable changes in affective states. Such results suggest a continued need to clarify the role of exercise duration in enhancing psychological well-being.

Summary

There clearly is a need for additional research on psychological well-being and the practice/training conditions of exercise frequency, intensity, and duration/time as well as possible mediating factors such as fitness level, age, preferred level of exertion, and environmental influences (Berger, 1996; Morgan, 1997a; Spirduso & Cronin, 2001). As concluded in their review of exercise dose-response effects on quality of life and independent living in older adults, Spirduso and Cronin (2001) concluded that older adults who are physically active report higher levels of well-being and physical functioning, but that exercise intervention studies do not *always* support the psychological benefits of aerobic exercise and/or strength training. In addition, there was little evidence that exercise intensity operated in a dose-response relationship to increase the quality of life for adults who were 65 years or older (Spirduso & Cronin, 2001). Although there may not be a direct dose-response relationship with the training factors of intensity, duration, and frequency in older adults—or in individuals of any age group—the training/practice factors are important considerations. Exercise frequency, intensity, and duration influence exercise enjoyment, the quality of the exercise experience, and exercise adherence.

Ideally, the frequency rate should be daily because mood benefits tend to last between two and four hours. Exercise on most days of the week also is in agreement with the Surgeon General's recommendations for exercise frequency (U.S. Department of Health & Human Services, 1996). Other psychological benefits such as enhanced self-concept and quality of life and decreases in clinical anxiety and depression tend to be more lasting than the mood benefits (e.g., Dunn et al., 2005). Still, exercisers who seek psychological benefits should exercise frequently to re-establish and maintain the benefits. Frequent if not daily exercise also would seem to be closely connected to being able

to exercise for various duration and intensities and to finding the exercise an enjoyable experience. Habitual exercise allows the participant to have sufficient fitness to avoid the discomfort of beginning exercisers.

Exercise intensity probably should be in the moderate range since the predominance of research supports this exercise intensity for the psychological benefits (e.g., Netz et al., 2005). Some individuals who greatly prefer high intensity or low intensity exercise sessions may choose to adjust their exercise intensity according to preferred level of exertion. Those who prefer low intensity exercise can exercise at the low end of the moderate exercise intensity range; those who prefer high intensity exercise can exercise at the high end of the moderate intensity range.

Preliminary evidence indicates that low-intensity exercise such as hatha yoga is associated with mood alteration, feelings of relaxation and revitalization as participants balance mind, body, and spirit through physical activity (e.g., Berger & Owen, 1988, 1992a; Daubenmier, 2005; Iyengar with Evans & Abrams, 2005). Although the benefits of low-intensity exercise has been questioned in a recent meta-analysis focusing on older adults (Netz et al., 2005), there remains a need for additional research regarding the potential psychological benefits of this exercise intensity.

High-intensity exercise for most individuals, including highly fit athletes, is related to undesirable mood changes. Highly fit exercisers report either no mood changes or mood decrements after high-intensity exercise (e.g., Motl et al.,1996). In fact, mood decrements are markers for overtraining and staleness (Tobar, 2005). It also is important to note that high-intensity exercise is related to the increased likelihood of injury (ACSM, 2006, p. 141). Overuse injuries preclude the continuation of the psychological benefits. Injury also is associated with undesirable symptoms of exercise withdrawal as discussed in Chapter 10, "Exercise-Related Injury."

For the psychological benefits, exercise duration should be between 10 and 20 minutes (e.g., Hansen et al., 2001) until more support is available for both shorter and longer durations. These exercise durations are somewhat in agreement with the recommendations in the Surgeon General's Report; however, according to these guidelines, the exercise should be for a minimum of 30 minutes (U.S. Department of Health and Human Services, 1996).

Anecdotal reports as well as some research studies support the possibility that exercising for various exercise durations may be associated with different psychological experiences (e.g., Hansen et al., 2001; Mandell, 1979). Some benefits such as calm-energy may occur as soon as 10 minutes into an exercise session. Additional benefits may be associated with the often-cited 20 minutes of exercise. Exercisers may

CASE STUDY 21.1

Creating an Exercise Program for a Golfer Who Dislikes Exercise Programs.

Background

Chris was a highly skilled golfer who loved to play golf, but who did not enjoy other types of exercise. Thus, he had a difficult time including exercise in his daily activities. Chris knew that he "should" exercise on a regular basis, but just could not bring himself to do so. He knew habitual exercise would improve his golf by increasing his stamina and strengthening his back muscles, which are sorely taxed by golf, and that exercise even might help him regulate his mood states, especially during the occasional poor performance in a tournament. Despite this knowledge about the benefits of exercise, Chris just could not bring himself to participate in any types of exercise, other than golf. He did not consider his lack of exercise to be any sort of a problem or concern, and he definitely was in the precontemplation stage of exercise as described in chapter 11 on models of exercise behavior.

The Presenting Problems: Tiredness, Mild Depression, and Back Pain

During one of his regularly scheduled sessions with a sport psychologist, however, Chris mentioned his physical tiredness and mild depression at the end of many tournaments and his concern about recent back pain. His sport psychologist had some background both in exercise physiology and in exercise psychology. Thus, she decided to assist Chris in including exercise as a part of his daily activities. Chris was quite receptive to her suggestions because she already had helped him improve his mental concentration during tournaments. Based on Berger's (1996, 2004) exercise taxonomy, the sport psychologist considered the factors of exercise enjoyment, exercise mode, and practice/training factors.

Selecting Appropriate Exercise Guidelines

Enjoyment and Mode Guidelines

The enjoyment issue was a major hurdle for Chris because he disliked jogging, an activity that would have enhanced his ability to walk the golf course. Jogging reminded him of unpleasant experiences when he was in the Navy. Chris also disliked walking because it was too mundane.

Although it did not readily appear to be related to building up endurance for golf, Chris found weight training somewhat appealing, and he was willing to give it a try. Weight training also satisfied many of the mode considerations in the taxonomy. It emphasized rhythmical breathing patterns in response to the extension and contraction portions of the movements. Weight training was not competitive because Chris was not planning to enter a competitive weight-lifting event. Weight training also was temporally and spatially certain because it involved no team interactions or a moving ball, and it included repetitive and rhythmical movements.

Training/Practice Guidelines

The sport psychologist was a bit perplexed, however, at how to combine the training guidelines for physical fitness, which Chris needed, with the practice guidelines for psychological benefits. She knew that Chris greatly needed a physical fitness base. She also thought that Chris would appreciate the mood benefits of exercise that might offset his occasional state of depression that was exacerbated by his occasional poor golf performance. After considerable time spent reading about the various exercise guidelines in the physiology and exercise psychology literature, the sport psychologist initially decided to suggest to Chris that he follow the practice guidelines for enhanced psychological well-being. The practice guidelines were needed to treat Chris's tiredness and mild depression. They also were less taxing than the sport-related physical fitness guidelines and thus appeared to be an ideal way to get Chris started on the road to fitness.

An Exercise Plan

Together, the exercise psychologist and Chris designed an exercise plan that included a weight-training frequency of three days a week and an intensity of 8 to 12 repetitions at weights sufficient to result in Chris's inability to perform more than 12 repetitions. Initially there were 10 upper- and lower-body exercises on the weight-training equipment at a local exercise studio. A few weeks later, Chris chose to add 20 minutes on a bicycle ergometer on alternating days to his exercise sessions. He chose the exercise stu-

CASE STUDY 21.1 (cont.)

dio specifically because it was not the training location for the serious bodybuilders in town. Initially the duration of his sessions was 25 to 30 minutes, and thus Chris easily could work them into his schedule on his way home from work.

Successful Results

We are pleased to report that Chris has been successful with his weight training and cycling program for approximately seven months. He continues to occasionally fine-tune his program during sessions with his exercise and sport psychologist. A major factor that has encouraged Chris to continue with his exercise program is that he notices a big improvement in his golf game. Chris has more energy, especially at the end of the round, and notices that the pain he occa-sionally had in his back has nearly disappeared.

A bonus to his exercise program is that he feels more enthusiastic about his game and has more energy for his daily activities. Chris has become an exercise enthusiast who actually enjoys his sessions and looks forward to them at the end of his workday. He has passed the difficult six-month period that is characterized by a high exercise-dropout rate (Dishman, 1988b), and it is likely that Chris will continue to exercise. In fact, recently Chris has begun to exercise nearly every day of the week by including the leg and arm portions of his workout on alternate days. As long as his exercise sessions are only 30 minutes in duration for the weight portion of his program, and 50 minutes for the weights and cycling sessions, Chris finds no trouble in scheduling them in his hectic day.

reap other benefits such as altered states of consciousness and flow-like states at durations of 40 minutes and longer. Beyond a certain duration, which may vary according to fitness levels, exercisers may not experience any mood changes, and with even longer duration, may start to report undesirable changes in mood (Berger & Motl, 2001).

Personal factors and characteristics of specific studies may influence the relationship between psychological well-being and exercise at various frequencies, intensity levels, and duration. One of the personal factors is the fitness level of the exerciser. Individuals who are more fit may be more likely to experience desirable psychological changes (e.g., Dishman et al., 1994; Steptoe & Bolton, 1988). However, other investigators have not shown such a relationship (e.g., Steptoe, Kearsley, & Walters, 1993). The time-line of the measurement of mood following cessation of exercise (i.e., immediately after exercise, or 5-minutes, 20-minutes, and 40-minutes after exercise) is another consideration that might affect the findings (e.g., Miller et al., 2005). Mood benefits associated with low- and moderate-intensity exercise seem to last between two and four hours and then dissipate. Mood decrements, sometimes associated with high-intensity exercise, may be evident during and immediately after exercising and may taper off 30 to 60 minutes following cessation. During the exercise recovery period, the negative changes, particularly anxiety, may decrease and become even more positive than they were at the beginning of the exercise session (Tate & Petruzzello, 1995). Such changes would be missed if mood, affect, and other measures of well-being were measured only immediately following the exercise sessions.

At the present time, knowledge about the need for enjoyment and the influence of exercise mode and practice conditions on psychological changes associated with physical activity is developing rapidly. The information presented in Chapter 20 on type of exercise and in this chapter on training/practice guidelines for optimal psychological benefits undoubtedly will be refined as new studies emerge. The exercise taxonomy developed by Berger and colleagues (e.g., Berger, 1996, 2004; Berger & Owen, 1988, 1998; Berger & Motl, 2000) includes some of the components necessary for exercise psychologists and other exercise science practitioners to design individualized exercise programs for their clients. These components include exercise enjoyment, mode or type of activity, and practice guidelines.

As illustrated in Case Study 21.1, creating an exercise program remains an art (American College of Sports Medicine, 2006, p. 136). However program design also needs to be heavily based on the best available research evidence. The FITT considerations identified in Chapters 20 and 21 illuminate the key considerations. As reviewed in the case study, the exercise needs to be enjoyable and satisfy the mode characteristics of encouraging rhythmical breathing, being relatively low in interpersonal competition, closed or predictable and include rhythmical and repetitive movements. The training/practice considerations include a minimum frequency of three times a week, moderate intensity, and at least 20 minutes in duration.

The practice/training guidelines have implications for the psychological changes associated with exercise. They also differ across the exercise mode characteristics explored in Chapter 20 and have implications for exercise enjoyment. As emphasized throughout the text, many areas of investigation need further research. Thus, the design of exercise programs for maximizing psychological well-being remain a combination of an art and science, much like the exercise prescriptions for physiological benefits (American College of Sports Medicine, 2006, p. 136).

We wish you great success as you design your own personal exercise programs and those for students and clients as you in continue in your profession. Our goal of writing this text is to facilitate your leadership in helping individuals of all ages to become *Ultimate Exercisers* who

- Enjoy the exercise process,
- Reach their exercise goals,
- Find pleasure and personal meaning in the exercise experience, and
- Continue to exercise throughout their lives.

Can You Define These Terms?

automaticity
_____

exercise duration
_____

exercise frequency
_____

exercise intensity
_____

heart rate reserve (HRR)
_____

Karvonen method of determining exercise HR
_____

low-, moderate-, and high-intensity exercise
_____

maximum heart rate (HR_{max})
_____

metabolic equivalent (MET)
_____

practice/training guidelines for optimal psychological benefits
_____

preferred level of exertion
_____

rating of perceived exertion (RPE)
_____

training guidelines for health-related fitness
_____

training guidelines for physical fitness and exercise performance
_____

threshold dose of exercise
_____

Can You Answer These Questions?

1. In what ways do the training guidelines for physical fitness and more moderate training guidelines for health-related fitness differ?

2. What proportion of American adults do not exercise sufficiently for health benefits?

3. What does the term MET represent?

4. Can you provide the MET equivalencies of low-, moderate-, and high-intensity exercise?

5. Based on your experiences, what factors might influence the relationship between exercise intensity and psychological well-being?

6. What are the major implications of exercise intensity for psychological well-being?

7. Can you elaborate on the ways in which exercise intensity, duration, and frequency might be related to exercise adherence?

8. How might the first 30 minutes of exercise compare to the second hour of exercise? Would fitness level affect these experiences?

9. How has training duration or distance been related to mood in swimmers?

10. Do you think that exercise frequency is related to the relationship between exercise and psychological well-being? How did you come to this conclusion?

11. Can you identify other training/practice factors that might be related to the exercise-psychological well-being relationship?

12. What do you consider to be the primary factors in helping a student or client plan an exercise program for psychological well-being?

END NOTE

EXERCISE PSYCHOLOGY: WHAT IS IT ALL ABOUT?

Exercise is different from sport and play and yet all three activities can be integrated into a single movement experience. A playful approach supports an individual's

- Enjoyment of the exercise experience,
- Likelihood of becoming an Intrinsic Exerciser who exercisers for pleasure, and
- Continuation of physically activity throughout our lives.

Exercise psychology focuses on enhancing the psychological benefits of exercise, and on further developing the scientific base for applied practice in the scientist-practitioner model. Throughout the world, exercise psychologists are exploring the role of exercise in enhancing participants' quality of life, self-concept and self-esteem, mood states, stress levels, eustress, and peak moments and flow experiences. These highly sought-after benefits and experiences tend to occur both for women and men throughout their lives from childhood to an advanced age.

The benefits of exercise are not automatic and tend to occur when exercise occurs in specific types or modes and under specific practice guidelines. Despite the many desirable psychological benefits, exercise can have a dark side. It can be associated with undesirable changes in psychological well-being, overuse injuries, heart attacks, eating disorders, substance abuse, and exercise dependence. These undesirable effects emphasize the importance of the exercise mode and practice guidelines when designing exercise programs for diverse participants.

Low rates of participation in physical activity are a major public health concern in industrialized countries. Despite the well-documented benefits of exercise, approximately 40% of the adult population is sedentary and engages in no leisure-time physical activity (e.g., Schoenborn & Barnes, 2002). A challenge to us all as exercise and health specialists is to identify exercise approaches and programs that encourage sedentary individuals and others who are insufficiently active to contemplate, initiate, and maintain personally successful exercise programs. Throughout this text, we have identified the often immediate psychological benefits of exercise as a way to encourage exercise specialists to design programs that might encourage more people to be physically active. By focusing on the more immediate psychological benefits in addition to the more long-term physical health benefits, people may discover that the exercise experience itself is rewarding and even enjoyable.

The benefits of exercise are closely aligned with the personal meaning of exercise to participants. Some of these include extreme dislike as well as fun and enjoyment, personal freedom, improved health and appearance, time alone, continuity and predictability of life, self-exploration, communing with nature, spirituality, postponement of death with immortality projects, and moving for the sheer pleasure of moving.

You now have a firm grasp of the psychological changes associated with exercise. As illustrated throughout the chapters, the benefits of exercise outweigh possible undesirable changes. It is important, however, to maintain a balanced perspective of both desirable and undesirable effects of exercise.

We hope that you have enjoyed exploring the psychological changes associated with exercise and will use this information in your own personal and professional exercise lives. As future movement professionals, we hope that you will use this information with your students and clients. Keep a watchful eye on new research as it develops, and modify the information in this text accordingly. We invite you to use the gymnasium, practice field, pool, rehabilitation settings, and other movement spaces as real-life laboratories to test these concepts and alter them according to your own professional needs.

We have enjoyed visiting with you throughout this book and hope you have enjoyed reading. If you have thoughts and ideas that you would like to share, we would be pleased to hear from you at the e-mail addresses listed below.

Happy Trails,

Bonnie Berger, bberger@bgnet.bgsu.edu

David Pargman, dpargman@lsi.fsu.edu

Bob Weinberg, weinber@muohio.edu

REFERENCES

American College of Sports Medicine. (2006). *ACSM's guidelines for exercise testing and prescription* (7th ed.). Philadelphia, PA: Lippincott, Williams & Wilkins.

Aaron, D. J., Dearwater, S. R., Anderson, R. D., Olsen, T., Kriska, A. M., & Laporte, R. E. (1995). Physical activity and the initiation of high-risk health behaviors in adolescents. *Medicine and Science in Sports and Exercise, 27,* 1639–1645.

Abbott, R. D., White, L. R., Ross, G. W., Masaki, K. H., Kamal, H., Curb, J. D., & Petrovich, H. (2004). Walking and dementia in physically capable elderly men. *Journal of the American Medical Association, 292*(12), 1447–1453.

Achterberg, J. (1991, May). *Enhancing the immune function through imagery.* Paper presented to the Fourth World Conference on Imagery, Minneapolis, MN.

Achterberg, J., Kenner, C., & Lawlis, G. F. (1988). Severe burn injury: A comparison of relaxation, imagery and biofeedback for pain management. *Journal of Mental Imagery, 12,* 71–87.

Adams, J., & Kirkby, R. J. (1998). Exercise dependence: A review of its manifestation, theory and measurement. *Sports Medicine, Training and Rehabilitation, 8,* 265–376.

Aidman, E., & Wollard, S. (2003). The influence of self-reported exercise addiction on acute emotional and physiological responses to brief exercise deprivation. *Psychology of Sport and Exercise, 4,* 225–236.

Airhihenbuwa, C. O., Kumanyika, S., Agurs, T. D., & Lowe, A. (1995). Perception and beliefs about exercise, rest, and health among African-Americans. *American Journal of Health Promotion, 9,* 426–429.

Ajzen, I. (1985). From intentions to action: A theory of focus on these important subgroups. In J. Kuhl & J. Beckman (Eds.), *Action-control: From cognition to behavior* (pp. 11–39). Heidelberg: Springer.

Ajzen, I., & Fishbein, M. (1980). *Understanding attitudes and predicting social behavior.* Englewood Cliffs, NJ: Prentice Hall.

Ajzen, I., & Madden, T. J. (1986). Prediction of goal-directed behavior: Attitudes, intentions and perceived behavioral control. *Journal of Experimental Social Psychology, 22,* 453–474.

Albright, C. L., King, A. C., Taylor, C. B., & Haskell, W. L. (1992). Effect of a six-month aerobic exercise training program on cardiovascular responsivity in healthy middle-aged adults. *Journal of Psychosomatic Research, 36,* 25–36.

Alfermann, D., & Stoll, O. (2000). Effects of physical exercise on self-concept and well-being. *International Journal of Sport Psychology, 31,* 47–65.

Allen, R. M., Haupt, T. D., & Jones, W. (1964). An analysis of peak experiences reported by college students. *Journal of Clinical Psychology, 20,* 207–212.

Alzado, L. (1991, July). I'm sick and I'm scared. *Sports Illustrated, 75,* 21–25.

American College of Sports Medicine. (1991). *Guidelines for graded exercise testing and prescription* (pp. 93–119). Philadelphia: Author.

American College of Sports Medicine. (2000). *ACSM's guidelines for exercise testing and prescription* (6th ed.). Baltimore, MD: Lippincott, Williams & Wilkins.

American College of Sports Medicine. (2006). *ACSM's guidelines for exercise testing and prescription* (7th ed.). Philadelphia, PA: Lippincott, Williams & Wilkins.

American Diabetes Association. Retrieved December 5, 2005, from http://www.diabetes.org.

American Footwear Association. (1991). *American youth and sports participation: A study of 10,000 students and their feelings about sports.* North Palm Beach, FL: American Footwear Association.

American Psychiatric Association. (1994/2000). *Diagnostic and statistical manual of mental disorders (DSM-IV)* (4th ed., text revision). Washington, DC: Author.

American Psychological Association, Division 47. (2003, Fall). APA—approved: A proficiency in sport psychology: Division 47 Education Committee report. *ESPNews, 17(3),* 13.

American Psychological Association, Division 47. (2005, Spring). Congratulations to Amy Latimer. *ESPNews, 19*(1), 11.

Andersen, A. E., & Mehler, P. S. (1999). *Eating disorders: A guide to medical care and complications.* Baltimore, MD: Johns Hopkins University Press.

Anderson, D. F., & Cychosz, C. M. (1994). Development of an exercise identity scale. *Perceptual and Motor Skills, 78,* 747–751.

Anderssen, N., Wold, B., & Torsheim, T. (2005). Tracking of physical activity in adolescence. *Research Quarterly for Exercise and Sport, 76,* 119–129.

Andrews, F. M., & Whithey, S. B. (1976). *Social indicators of well-being: America's perception of life quality.* New York: Plenum.

Anshel, M. (2001). Drug use in sport: Causes and cures. In J. Williams (Ed.), *Applied sport psychology: Personal growth to peak performance.* (4th ed., pp. 436–444). Mountain View, CA: Mayfield.

Anshel, M. (2003). *Sport psychology: From theory to practice.* San Francisco: Benjamin Cummings.

Anshel, M. (2005). Substance use: Chemical roulette in sport. In S. Murphy (Ed.), *The sport psych handbook* (pp. 255–276). Champaign, IL: Human Kinetics.

Anton, S., Perri, M., Riley, J., Kanasky, W., Rodrigue, J., Sears, S., & Martin, D. (2005). Differential predictors of adherence in exercise programs' levels of intensity and frequency. *Journal of Sport and Exercise Psychology, 27,* 171–187.

Arai, Y., & Hisamichi, S. (1998). Self-reported exercise frequency and personality: A population-based study in Japan. *Perceptual and Motor Skills, 87,* 1371–1375.

Ardell, D. B. (1996). *The book of wellness: A secular approach to spirit, meaning, and purpose.* Amherst, NY: Prometheus Books.

Armstrong, L., & Jenkins, S. (2000). *It's not about the bike: My journey back to life.* New York: G. P. Putnam's Sons.

Arveda, K. E. (1991). One size does not fit all, or how I learned to stop dieting and love the body. *Quest, 43,* 135–147.

Asci, F. H. (2003). The effects of physical fitness training on trait anxiety and physical self-concept on female university students. *Psychology of Sport and Exercise, 4*(3), 255–264.

Association for the Advancement of Applied Sport Psychology. (1989). *Journal of Applied Sport Psychology, 1,* 1–51.

Association for the Advancement of Applied Sport Psychology. (2005, Summer). *Congratulations! Newsletter, 20*(2), 16.

Atlantis, E., Chow, C.-M., Kirby, A., & Singh, M. F. (2004). An effective exercise-based intervention for improving mental health and quality of life measures: A randomized controlled trial. *Preventive Medicine, 39,* 424–434.

AuBuchon, B. (1991, May). *The effects of positive mental imagery on hope, coping, anxiety, dypsnea, and pulmonary function in persons with chronic obstructive pulmonary disease: Tests of a nursing intervention and a theoretical model.* Paper presented to the Fourth World Conference on Imagery, Minneapolis, MN.

Babkes, M. L., & Weiss, M. R. (1999). Parental influence on children's cognitive and affective responses to competitive soccer participation. *Pediatric Exercise Science, 11,* 44–62.

Bacon, V., Lerner, B., Trembley, D., & Seestedt, M. (2005). Substance abuse. In J. Taylor & G. Wilson (Eds.), *Applying sport psychology: Four approaches* (pp. 229–248). Champaign, IL: Human Kinetics.

Baecke, J. A. H., Burema, J., & Frijters, J. E. R. (1982). A short questionnaire for the measurement of habitual physical activity in epidemiological studies. *American Journal of Clinical Nutrition, 36*, 936–942.

Bahrke, M. S., & Morgan, W. P. (1978). Anxiety reduction following exercise and meditation. *Cognitive Therapy and Research, 2*, 323–333.

Bakeland, F. (1970). Exercise deprivation: Sleep and psychological reactions. *Archives of General Psychiatry, 22*, 365–369.

Baker, M. A. (Ed.). (1987). *Sex differences in human performance.* New York: John Wiley & Sons.

Balogun, J. A. (1987). The interrelationships between measures of physical fitness and self-concept. *Journal of Human Movement Studies, 13*, 255–265.

Bandura, A. (1977). Self-efficacy: Toward a unifying theory of behavioral change. *Psychological Review, 84*, 191–215.

Bandura, A. (1986). *Social foundations of thought and action: A social cognitive theory.* Englewood Cliffs, NJ: Prentice Hall.

Bandura, A. (1995) On rectifying conceptual ecumenism. In J. Maddux (Ed.), *Self-efficacy, adaptation, and adjustment: Theory, research, and application* (pp. 347–375). New York: Plenum Press.

Bandura, A. (1997). *Self-efficacy: The exercise of control.* New York: W. H. Freeman and Company.

Baranowski, T., & Sallis, J. F. (1994). Family determinants of childhood physical activity: A social-cognitive model. In R. K. Dishman (Ed.), *Advances in exercise adherence* (pp. 319–342). Champaign, IL: Human Kinetics.

Baranowski, T., Bouchard, C., Bar-Or, O., Bricker, T., Heath, G., Kimm, S. Y. S., Malina, R., Obarzanek, E., Pate, R., Strong, W. B., Truman, B., & Washington, R. (1992). Assessment, prevalence, and cardiovascular benefits of physical activity and fitness in youth. *Medicine and Science in Sports and Exercise, 24*, S237–247.

Baranowski, T., Thompson, W. O., DuRant, R. H., Baranowski, J., & Puhl, J. (1993). Observations on physical activity in physical locations: Age, gender, ethnicity, and month effects. *Research Quarterly for Exercise and Sport, 64*, 127–133.

Barber, T. X. (1978). Hypnosis, suggestions and psychosomatic phenomena: A new look from the standpoint of recent experimental studies. *The American Journal of Clinical Hypnosis, 21*, 13–27.

Barber, T. X., Chauncey, H. M., & Winer, R. A. (1964). The effect of hypnotic and nonhypnotic suggestions on parotid gland response to gustatory stimuli. *Psychosomatic Medicine, 26*, 374–380.

Barnes, D. E., Yaffee, K., Satariano, W. A., & Tager, I. B. (2003). A longitudinal study of cardiorespiratory fitness and cognitive function in healthy older adults. *Journal of the American Geriatrics Society, 51* (4), 459–465.

Barnett, L. M., VanBeurden, E., Zask, A., Brooks, L.O., & Dietrich, U.C. (2002). How active are rural children in Australian physical education? *Journal of Science and Medicine in Sport, 5*, 253–265.

Baron, R., & Byrne, D. (1991). *Social psychology: Understanding human interaction* (6th ed.). Boston: Allyn & Bacon.

Bar-Or, O. (1983). *Pediatric sports medicine for the practitioner: From physiologic principles to clinical application.* New York: Springer Verlag.

Barr, K., & Hall, C. (1992). The use of imagery by rowers. *International Journal of Sport Psychology, 23*, 243–261.

Barrett, K. C., & Campos, J. J. (1991). A diacritical function approach to emotions and coping. In E. M. Cummings, A. L. Greene, & K. H. Karraker (Eds.), *Life-span developmental psychology: Perspectives on stress and coping* (pp. 21–41). Hillsdale, NJ: Lawrence Erlbaum.

Bartholomew, J. B. (1997). Post exercise mood: The effect of a manipulated pre-exercise mood state [Abstract]. *Journal of Sport & Exercise Psychology, 9* (Suppl.), S29.

Bartholomew, J. B., Morrison, D., & Ciccolo, J. T. (2005). Effects of acute exercise on mood and well-being in patients with major depressive disorder. *Medicine and Science in Sports and Exercise, 37*, 2032–2037.

Battista, R. R. (1990). Personal meaning: Attraction to sports participation. *Perceptual and Motor Skills, 70*, 1003–1009.

Bauer, B. A., Rogers, P. J., Miller, T. O., Bove, A. A., & Tyce, G. M. (1989). Exercise training produces changes in free and conjugated catecholamines. *Medicine and Science in Sports and Exercise, 21*, 558–562.

Bausell, R. B. (1986). Health-seeking behavior among the elderly. *The Gerontologist, 26*, 556–559.

Bayles, C. M., Metz, K. F., Robertson, J. R., Goss, F. L., Cosgrove, J., & McBurney, D. (1990). Perceptual regulation of prescribed exercise. *Journal of Cardiopulmonary Rehabilitation, 10*, 25–31.

Becker, M. H., & Maiman, L. A. (1975). Socio-behavioral determinants of compliance with health care and medical care recommendations. *Medical Care, 13*, 10–24.

Becker, M. H., Nathanson, C. A., Drachman, M. D., & Kirscht, J. P. (1977). Mothers' health beliefs and children's clinic visits: A prospective study. *Journal of Community Health, 3*, 125–135.

Bednarowicz, E. (2004). The amen of running. In G. Battista (Ed.), *The runner's high: Illumination and ecstasy in motion* (pp. 17–21). Halcottsville, NY: Breakaway Books.

Benson, H. (1984). The relaxation response and stress. In J. D. Matarazzo, S. M. Weiss, J. A. Herd, N. E. Miller, & S. M. Weiss (Eds.), *Behavioral health: A handbook of health enhancement and disease prevention* (pp. 326–337). New York: John Wiley & Sons.

Benyo, R. (1990). *The exercise fix.* Champaign, IL: Human Kinetics.

Berg, F. M. (2000). *Women afraid to eat: Breaking free in today's weight-obsessed world.* Hettinger, ND: Healthy Weight Network.

Berger B. G., & Motl, R. W. (2000). Exercise and mood: A selective review and synthesis of research employing the Profile of Mood States. *Journal of Applied Sport Psychology, 12*, 69–92.

Berger, B. G. (1983/1984). Stress reduction through exercise: The mind-body connection. *Motor skills: Theory into practice, 7*, 31–46.

Berger, B. G. (1984/1997). Running strategies for women and men. In M. L. Sachs & G. W. Buffone (Eds.), *Running as therapy* (pp. 23–62). Northvale, NJ: Jason Aronson.

Berger, B. G. (1994). Coping with stress: The effectiveness of exercise and other techniques. *Quest, 46*, 100–119.

Berger, B. G. (1996). Psychological benefits of an active life style: What we know and what we need to know. *Quest, 48*, 330–353.

Berger, B. G. (2004). Subjective well-being in obese individuals: The multiple roles of exercise. *Quest, 56*, 50–76.

Berger, B. G., & Mackenzie, M. (1981). A case study of a woman jogger: A psychodynamic profile. In M. H. Sacks & M. L. Sachs (Eds.), *Psychology of running* (pp. 99–112). Champaign, IL: Human Kinetics Publishers.

Berger, B. G., & Mackenzie, M. M. (1980). A case study of a woman jogger: A psychodynamic analysis. *Journal of Sport Behavior 3*, 3–16.

Berger, B. G., & McInman, A. (1993). Exercise and the quality of life. In R. N. Singer, M. Murphey, & L. K. Tennant (Eds.), *Handbook of research on sport psychology* (pp. 729–760). New York: Macmillan.

Berger, B. G., & Motl, R. W. (2000). Exercise and mood: A subjective review and synthesis of research employing the Profile of Mood States. *Journal of Applied Sport Psychology, 12*, 69–92.

Berger, B. G., & Motl, R. W. (2001). Exercise and the quality of life. In R. N. Singer, H. A. Hausenblas, & C. M. Janelle (Eds.), *Handbook of sport psychology* (2nd ed.) (pp. 636–671). New York: John Wiley & Sons.

Berger, B. G., & Owen, D. R. (1983). Mood alteration with swimming—swimmers really do "feel better." *Psychosomatic Medicine, 45*, 425–433.

Berger, B. G., & Owen, D. R. (1986). Mood alteration with swimming: A re-evaluation. In L. Vander Veldon & J. H. Humphrey (Eds.), *Current selected research in the psychology and sociology of sport* (Vol. 1, pp. 97–114). New York: AMS Press.

Berger, B. G., & Owen, D. R. (1987). Anxiety reduction with swimming: Relationship between exercise and state, trait, and somatic anxiety. *International Journal of Sport Psychology, 18*, 286–302.

Berger, B. G., & Owen, D. R. (1988). Stress reduction and mood enhancement in four exercise modes: Swimming, body conditioning, hatha yoga, and fencing. *Research Quarterly for Exercise and Sport, 59*, 148–159.

Berger, B. G., & Owen, D. R. (1992a). Mood alteration with yoga and swimming: Aerobic exercise may not be necessary. *Perceptual and Motor Skills, 75*, 1331–1343.

Berger, B. G., & Owen, D. R. (1992b). Preliminary analysis of a causal relationship between swimming and stress reduction: Intense exercise may negate the effects. *International Journal of Sport Psychology, 23*, 70–85.

Berger, B. G., & Owen, D. R. (1998). Relation of low and moderate intensity exercise with acute mood change in college joggers. *Perceptual and Motor Skills, 87*, 611–621.

Berger, B. G., & Tobar, D. (2006). Physical activity and quality of life. In G. Tenenbaum & R. C. Eklund (Eds.), *Handbook of Sport Psychology* (3rd ed.). New York: John Wiley & Sons.

Berger, B. G., Butki, B. D., & Berwind, J. S. (1995). Acute mood changes associated with competitive and non-competitive physical activities. *Journal of Applied Sport Psychology, 7*, S41.

Berger, B. G., Friedman, E., & Eaton, M. (1988). Comparison of jogging, the relaxation response, and group interaction for stress reduction. *Journal of Sport and Exercise Psychology, 10*, 431–447.

Berger, B. G., Grove, J. R., Prapavessis, H., & Butki, B. D. (1997). Relationship of swimming distance, expectancy, and performance to mood states of competitive athletes. *Perceptual and Motor Skills, 84*, 1119–1210.

Berger, B. G., Owen, D. R., & Man, F. (1993). A brief review of literature and examination of acute mood benefits of exercise in Czechoslovakian and United States swimmers. *International Journal of Sports Psychology, 24*, 130–150.

Berger, B. G., Owen, D. R., Motl, R. W., & Parks, L. (1998). Relationship between expectancy of psychological benefits and mood alteration in joggers. *International Journal of Sport Psychology, 29*, 1–16.

Berger, B., & Motl, R. (2001). Physical activity and quality of life. In R. N. Singer, H. A. Hausenblas, & C. M. Janelle (Eds.), *Handbook of sport psychology* (2nd ed., pp. 636–671). New York: John Wiley.

Berk, L. S., Nieman, D. C., Youngberg, W. S., Arabatzis, K., Simpson-Westerberg, M., Lee, J. W., Tan, S. A., & Eby, W. C. (1990). The effect of long endurance running on natural killer cells in marathoners. *Medicine and Science in Sports and Exercise, 22*, 207–212.

Biddle, S. J. (1993). Children, exercise and mental health. *International Journal of Sport Psychology, 24*, 200–216.

Biddle, S. J. H. (1995). *European perspectives on exercise and sport psychology*. Exeter, England: Human Kinetics.

Biddle, S., & Mutrie, N. (2001). *Psychology of physical activity*: Determinants, well-being and interventions. London: Routledge.

Biddle, S., Goudas, M., & Page, A. (1994). Social-psychological predictors of self-reported actual and intended physical activity in a university workforce sample. *British Journal of Sports Medicine, 28*, 160–163.

Biener, L., & Heaton, A. (1995). Women dieters of normal weight: Their motives, goals, and risks. *American Journal of Public Health, 85*, 714–717.

Billaut, F., Giacomoni, M., & Falgairette, G. (2003). Maximal intermittent cycling exercise: Effects of recovery duration and gender. *Journal of Applied Physiology, 95*(4), 1632–1637.

Biondo, B. (1998, March 27–29). Yoga's wider reach. *USA Weekend's*, p. 12.

Birch, I. L., & Fisher, J. O. (1998). Development of eating behaviors among children and adolescents. *Pediatrics, 101*, 325–244.

Birren, J. E., & Schroots, J. J. F. (1996). History, concepts, and theory in the psychology of aging. In J. E. Birren, K. W. Schaie, R. P. Abeles, M. Gatz, & T. A. Salthouse (Eds.), *Handbook of the psychology of aging* (4th ed., pp. 3–23). San Diego: Academic Press.

Blair, S. H., Kohl, H. W., Paffenbarger, R. S., Clark, D. G., Cooper, K. H., & Gibbons, L. W. (1989). Physical fitness and all-cause mortality: A prospective study of healthy men and women. *Journal of the American Medical Association, 262*, 2395–2401.

Blair, S. N. (1994). Physical activity, fitness, and coronary heart disease. In C. Bouchard, R. J. Shepherd, & T. Stephens (Eds.), *Physical activity, fitness, and health: International proceedings and consensus statement* (pp. 579–590). Champaign, IL: Human Kinetics.

Blair, S. N., Clark, D. G., Cureton, K. J., & Powell, K. E. (1989). Exercise and fitness in childhood: Implications for a lifetime of health. In C. V. Gisolfi & D. R. Lamb (Eds.), *Perspectives in exercise and sports medicine:* Vol. 2: *Youth, exercise and sport* (pp. 401–430). Indianapolis: Benchmark Press.

Blair, S. N., Kampert, J. B., Hohl, H. W. III, Barlow, C. E., Macera, C. A., Paffenbarger, R. S. Jr., & Gibbons, L. W. (1996). Influences of cardiorespiratory fitness and other precursors on cardiovascular disease and all-cause mortality in men and women. *Journal of the American Medical Association, 276*, 205–210.

Blair, S. N., LaMonte, M. J., & Nichaman, M. Z. (2004). The evolution of physical activity recommendations: How much is enough? *American Journal of Clinical Nutrition, 79* (Suppl.), 913S–920S.

Blamey, A., Mutrie, N., & Aitchison, T. (1995). Health promotion by encouraged use of stairs. *British Medical Journal, 311*, 289–290.

Blanchard, C., & Rodgers, W. (1997). The effects of exercise intensity and fitness level on mood states [Abstract]. *Journal of Sport & Exercise Psychology, 9* (Suppl.), S32.

Blascovich, J., & Katkin, E. S. (Eds.). (1993). *Cardiovascular reactivity to psychological stress and disease*. Washington, DC: American Psychological Association.

Blumberg, J., Kenney, W., Seals, D., & Spina, R. (1992). Exercise and nutrition in the elderly. *Gatorade Sports Science Institute: Sports Science Exchange Roundtable, 3*(4), RT #10.

Blumenthal, J. A., Emery, C. F., Madden, D. J., George, L. K., Coleman, R. E., Riddle, M. W., McKee, D. C., Reasoner, J., & Williams, R. S. (1989). Cardiovascular and behavioral effects of aerobic exercise training in healthy older men and women. *Journal of Gerontology: Medical Sciences, 44*, M147–M157.

Blumenthal, J. A., Emery, C. F., Walsh, M. A., Cox, D. K., Kuh, C. M., Williams, R. B., & Williams, R. S. (1988). Exercise training in healthy Type A middle-aged men: Effects on behavioral and cardiovascular responses. *Psychosomatic Medicine, 50*, 418–433.

Bock, B. C., Albrecht, A. E., Traficante, R. M., Clark, M. M., Pint, B. M., Tilkemeier, P., & Marcus, B. H. (1997). Predictors of exercise adherence following participation in a cardiac rehabilitation program. *International Journal of Behavioral Medicine, 4*, 60–75.

Bond, G., Aiken, L., & Somerville, S. (1992). The health belief model and adolescents with insulin-dependent diabetes mellitus. *Health Psychology, 11*, 190–198.

Bonheim, J. (1992). *The serpent and the wave: A guide to movement meditation*. Berkley, CA: Celestial Arts.

Booth, M., Owen, N., Bauman, A., Cavisi, O., & Leslie, E. (2000). Social-cognitive and perceived environment influences associated with physical activity in older Australians. *Preventive Medicine, 31*, 15–22.

Bordo, S. (1989). The body and the reproduction of femininity: A feminist appropriation of Foucault. In A. M. Jagger & S. R. Bordo (Eds.), *Gender/body/knowledge: Feminist reconstructions of being and knowing* (pp. 13–33). New Brunswick, NJ: Rutgers University Press.

Bordo, S. (1990). Reading the slender body. In M. Jacobus, E. Fox Keller, & S. Shuttleworth (Eds.), *Body/politics: Women and the discourse of science* (pp. 83–112). New York: Routledge.

Bordo, S. (1993). *Unbearable weight: Feminism, western culture and the body*. Los Angeles: University of California Press.

Borg, G. A. V. (1982). Psychological bases of physical exertion. *Medicine and Science in Sports and Exercise, 14*, 377–381.

Borg, G. A. V. (1998). *Borg's perceived exertion and pain scales*. Champaign, IL: Human Kinetics.

Bortz, W. M., II (1996). *Dare to be 100*. New York: Fireside.

Bosscher, R. J. (1994). Self-efficacy expectations. In D. J. H. Deeg & M. Westendorp-de Seriere (Eds.), *Autonomy and well-being in the aging population: Report from the Longitudinal Aging Study 1992–1993* (pp. 45–51). Amsterdam: VU University Press.

Bouchard, C. (1997). Biological aspects of the active living concept. In J. E. Curtis & S. J. Russell (Eds.), *Physical activity in human experience: Interdisciplinary perspectives* (pp. 11–58). Champaign, IL: Human Kinetics.

Bouchard, T. J., & Loehlin, J. C. (2001). Genes, evolution, and personality. *Behavioral Genetics, 31*, 243–273.

Boutcher, S. H., & Landers, D. M. (1988). The effects of vigorous exercise on anxiety, heart rate, and alpha activity of runners and nonrunners. *Psychophysiology, 25*, 696–702.

Boyd, M. P., & Yin, Z. (1996). Cognitive-affective sources of sport enjoyment in adolescent sport participants. *Adolescence, 31*, 383–395.

Brach, J. S., Simonsick, E. M., Kritchevsky, S., Yaffe, K., & Newman, A. B. (2004). The association between physical function and lifestyle activity and exercise in the health, aging, and body composition study. *Journal of the American Geriatrics Society, 52*(4), 502–509.

Bracken, B. A. (1992). *Multidimensional Self Concept Scale*. Austin, TX: Pro-Ed.

Bradburn, N. M. (1969). *The structure of psychological well-being*. Chicago: Aldine.

Brahmi, Z., Thomas, J. E., Park, M., & Dowdeswell, I. A. G. (1985). The effect of acute exercise on natural killer-cell activity of trained and sedentary human subjects. *Journal of Clinical Immunology, 5*, 321–328.

Brand, P. A., Rothblum, E. D., & Solomon, L. J. (1992). A comparison of lesbians, gay men, and heterosexuals on weight and restrained eating. *International Journal of Eating Disorders 11*, 253–259.

Bray, S., Millen, A., Eidsness, J., & Leuzinger, C. (2005). The effects of leadership style and exercise program choreography on enjoyment and intentions to exercise. *Psychology of Sport and Exercise, 6*, 415–425.

Breathnach, S. B. (1998). *Something more: Excavating your authentic self*. New York: Warner Books.

Brettschneider, W. D., & Heim, R. (1997). Identity, sport and youth development. In Fox, K. R. (Ed.), *The physical self: From motivation to well-being* (pp. 205–227). Champaign, IL: Human Kinetics.

Breus, M. J., & O'Connor, P. J. (1998). Exercise-induced anxiolysis: A test of the "time out" hypothesis in high anxious females. *Medicine & Science in Sports & Exercise, 30*, 1107–1112.

Brewer, B. W., & Petrie, T. A. (2002). Psychopathology in sport and exercise. In B. W. Brewer & J. Van Raalte (Eds.), *Advances in sport and exercise psychology* (2nd ed.). Washington, DC: American Psychological Association.

Brice, C. F. & Smith, A. P. (2002). Effects of caffeine on mood and performance: A study of realistic consumption. *Psychopharmacology, 164*, 188–192.

Briggs, J. D. (1994). An investigation of participant enjoyment in the physical activity setting. *Journal of Physical Education, Recreation, and Dance, 65*, 213–221.

Brink, N. E. (1989). The power struggle of Workers Compensation: Strategies for intervention. *Journal of Applied Rehabilitation Counseling, 20*, 25–28.

Brone, R., & Reznikoff, M. (1989). Strength gains, locus of control, and self-description of college football players. *Perceptual and Motor Skills, 69*, 483–493.

Brosschot, J. F., & Thayer, J. F. (1998). Anger inhibition, cardiovascular recovery, and vagal function: A model of the line between hostility and cardiovascular disease. *Annals of Behavioral Medicine, 20*, 326–332.

Brosschot, J. F., & Thayer, J. F. (2003). Heart rate response is longer after negative emotions than after positive emotions. *International Journal of Psychophysiology, 50*, 181–187.

Brosschot, J. F., & Thayer, J. F. (2004). Worry, perseverative thinking and health. In Nyklicek, I., Temoshok, L. R., Vingerhoets, A. J. J. M. (Eds.), *Emotional expression and health: Advances in theory, assessment and clinical applications* (pp. 99–115). London, UK: Taylor and Francis.

Brosschot, J. F., Pieper, S., & Thayer, J. F. (2005). Expanding stress theory: Prolonged activation and perseverative cognition. *Psychoneuroendocrinology, 30*, 1043–1049.

Brown, D. R. (1992). Physical activity, aging, and psychological well-being: An overview of the research. *Canadian Journal of Sport Sciences, 17*, 185–193.

Brown, D. R., & Blanton, C. J. (2002). Physical activity, sports participation, and suicidal behavior among college students. *Medicine and Science in Sports and Exercise, 34*, 1087–1096.

Brown, D. R., & Wang, Y. (1992). The relationship among exercise training, aerobic capacity, and psychological well-being in the general population. *Medicine, Exercise, Nutrition and Health, 3*, 125–142.

Brown, D. R., Wang, Y., Ward, A., Ebbeling, C. B., Fortalage, L., Puleo, E., Benson, H., & Rippe, J. M. (1995). Chronic psychological effects of exercise and exercise plus cognitive strategies. *Medicine and Science in Sports and Exercise, 27*, 765–775.

Brown, J. D. (1991). Staying fit and staying well: Physical fitness as a moderator of life stress. *Journal of Personality and Social Psychology, 60*, 555–561.

Brown, J. D., & McGill, K. L. (1989). The cost of good fortune: When positive life events produce negative health consequences. *Journal of Personality and Social Psychology, 57*, 1103–1110.

Brown, J. D., & Siegel, J. M. (1988). Exercise as a buffer of life stress: A prospective study of adolescent health. *Health Psychology, 7*, 341–353.

Brown, J. D., Wang, Y., Ward, A., Ebbeling, C. B., Fortalage, L., Puleo, E., Benson, H., & Rippe, J. M. (1995). Chronic psychological effects of exercise and exercise plus cognitive strategies. *Medicine and Science in Sports and Exercise, 27*, 765–775.

Brown, R., & Harrison, J. (1986). The effects of a strength training program on the strength and self-concept of two female age groups. *Research Quarterly for Exercise and Sports, 57*, 315–320.

Browne, M. A., & Mahoney, M. J. (1984). Sport psychology. *Annual Review of Psychology, 35*, 606–607.

Brownell, K., Stunkard, A., & Albaum, J. (1980). Evaluation and modification of exercise patterns in the natural environment. *American Journal of Psychiatry, 137*, 1540–1545.

Bruck, M., Ceci, S. J., & Hembrooke, H. (1998). Reliability and credibility of young children's reports. *American Psychologist, 53*, 136–151.

Brustad, R. (1997). A critical-postmodern perspective on knowledge development in human movement. In J. Fernandez-Balboa (Ed.),

Critical postmodernism in human movement, physical education, and sport (pp. 87–98). Albany, NY: State University of New York Press.

Brustad, R. J. (1996). Attraction to physical activity in urban school children: Parental socialization and gender influences. *Research Quarterly for Exercise and Sport, 67,* 316–323.

Buchner, D. M. (1997). Physical activity and quality of life in older adults. *Journal of the American Medical Association, 277,* 64–66.

Buchner, D. M., Beresford, S. A., Larson, E. B., LaCroix, A. Z., & Wagner, E. H. (1992). Effects of physical activity on health status in older adults 2: Intervention studies. *Annual Review of Public Health, 13,* 469–488.

Buckworth, J., & Dishman, R. (2002). *Exercise psychology.* Champaign, IL: Human Kinetics.

Buckworth, J., & Dishman, R. K. (1999). Determinants of physical activity: Research to application. In J. Rippe (Ed.), *Lifestyle medicine* (pp. 1016–1027). Malden, MA: Blackwell Science Inc.

Buckworth, J., & Dishman, R. K. (2002). *Exercise psychology.* Champaign, IL: Human Kinetics.

Bunnell, D. W., Cooper, P. J., Hertz, S., & Shenker, I. R. (1992). Body shape concerns among adolescents. *International Journal of Eating Disorders, 11,* 79–83.

Burckes-Miller, M. E., & Black, D. R. (1988). Male and female college athletes: Prevalence of anorexia nervosa and bulimia nervosa. *Athletic Training, 23,* 137–140.

Burke, K. L., Sachs, M. L., & Smisson, C. P. (2004). *Directory of graduate programs in applied sport psychology* (7th ed.). Morgantown, WV: Fitness Information Technology.

Butki, B. D. (1998). The relationship between physical activity and multidimensional self-concept among adolescents. *Dissertation Abstracts International Section A: Humanities and Social Sciences, 59*(5-A), 1506.

Butki, B. D., & Rudolph, D. L. (1997). Self efficacy and affective responses to short bouts of exercise [Abstract]. *Journal of Sport & Exercise Psychology, 9* (Suppl.), S38.

Bykov, E.V. (2001). Individual health status indices in schoolchildren of big cities depending on the way of life. *Human Physiology, 27,* 129–131.

Byrne, B. M. (1984). The general/academic self-concept nomological network: A review of construct validation research. *Review of Educational Research, 54,* 427–456.

Caballero, B. (2004). Obesity prevention in children: Opportunities and challenges. *International Journal of Obesity, 28,* 590–595.

Cacioppo, J. T., Berntson, G. G., Klein, D. J., & Poehlmann, K. M. (1998). Psychophysiology of emotion across the life span. In K. W. Schaie & M. P. Lawton (Eds.), *Annual review of gerontology and geriatrics: Focus on emotion and adult development.* (Vol. 17, pp. 27–74). New York: Springer.

Cairney, J., Faught, B. E., Hay, J., Wade, T. J., & Corna, L. M. (2005). Physical activity and depressive symptoms in older adults. *Journal of Physical Activity and Health, 2,* 98–114.

Caldwell, J. R. (1996). Exercise in the elderly: An overview. *Activities, Adaptation, and Aging, 20,* 3–8.

Calfas, K. J., & Taylor, W. C. (1994). Effects of physical activity on psychological variables in adolescents. *Pediatric Exercise Science, 6,* 406–423.

Camacho, T. C., Roberts, R. E., Lazarus, N. B., Kaplan, G. A., & Cohen, R. D. (1991). Physical activity and depression: Evidence from the Alameda County Study. *American Journal of Epidemiology, 134,* 220–231.

Cameron, J. (1992). *The artist's way: A spiritual path to higher creativity.* New York: Jeremy P. Tarcher/Putnam.

Campbell, D. (1997). The Mozart effect: Tapping the power of music to heal the body, strengthen the mind, and unlock the creative spirit. New York: Avon.

Campbell, R. N. (1984). *The new science: Self-esteem psychology.* Lanham, MD: University Press of America.

Canadian Fitness and Lifestyle Research Institute. (1996). *Progress in prevention.* Bulletin no. 2.

Cardinal, B. (1999). Extended stage model for physical activity behavior. *Journal of Human Movement Sciences, 37,* 37–54.

Cardinal, B. J. (1997). Construct validity of stages of change for exercise behavior. *American Journal of Health Promotion, 12,* 68–74.

Carels, R. A., Berger, B. G., & Darby, L. A. (in press). The association between mood states and physical activity in postmenopausal, obese, sedentary women: A preliminary investigation. *Journal of Aging and Physical Activity.*

Carliss, R. (2001, April 23). The power of yoga. *Time, 157,* 54–62.

Carmack, M. A., & Martens, R. (1979). Measuring commitment to running: A survey of runners' attitudes and mental states. *Journal of Sport Psychology, 1,* 25–42.

Carpenter, P. J., & Coleman, R. (1998). A longitudinal study of elite cricketers' commitment. *International Journal of Sport Psychology, 29,* 195–210.

Carr, C., Kennedy, S., & Dimick, K. (1990). Alcohol use among high school athletes: A comparison of alcohol use and intoxication in male and female high school athletes and non-athletes. *Journal of Alcohol and Drug Education, 27,* 13–25.

Carron, A., Hausenbas, H., & Estabrooks, P. (2003). *The psychology of physical activity.* New York: McGraw Hill.

Carron, A., Hausenblas, H., & Mack, D. (1996). Social influence and exercise: A meta-analysis. *Journal of Sport and Exercise Psychology, 18,* 1–16.

Cartee, G. D. (1994). Aging skeletal muscle: Response to exercise. In J. O. Holloszy (Ed.), *Exercise and sport sciences reviews* (Vol. 22, pp. 91–120). Baltimore: Williams & Wilkins.

Cash, T. F., Novy, P. L., & Grant, J. L. (1994). Why do women exercise? Factor analysis and further validation of the reasons for exercise inventory. *Perceptual and Motor Skills, 78,* 539–544.

Caspersen, C. J., & Merritt, R. K. (1995). Physical activity trends among 26 states, 1986–1990. *Medicine and Science in Sport and Exercise, 27,* 713–720.

Casperson, C. J., Pereira, M. A., & Curran, K. M. (2000). Changes in physical activity patterns in the United States, by sex and cross-sectional age. *Medicine and Science in Sports and Exercise, 32,* 1601–1609.

Cassel, J. (1974). An epidemiological perspective of psychological factors in disease etiology. *American Journal of Public Health, 64,* 1040–1043.

Cattell, R. B. (1973). *Personality and mood by questionnaire.* New York: Jossey Bass.

Cattell, R. B., & Eber, H. W. (1961). *The Sixteen Personality Factor Questionnaire.* Champaign, IL: Institute for Personality and Ability Testing.

Cattell, R. B., Eber, H. W., & Tatsuoka, M. M. (1980). *Handbook for the Sixteen Personality Factor Questionnaire.* Champaign, IL: Institute for Personality and Ability Testing.

Centers for Disease Control. (1997). Guidelines for school and community programs to promote lifelong physical activity among young people. *Morbidity and Mortality Weekly Report, 46* (no. RR-6), 1–37.

Centers for Disease Control and Prevention. (1992). *National Health Interview Survey—Youth Risk Behavior Survey.* (Machine readable data file and documentation). Atlanta, GA: U.S. Department of Health and Human Services, Public Health Service, Centers for Disease Control and Prevention, National Center for Health Statistics.

Cerella, J., Poon, L. W., & Williams, D. M. (1980). Age and the complexity hypothesis. In L.W. Poon (Ed.), *Aging in the 1980's: Psychological issues* (pp. 332–340). Washington, DC: American Psychological Association.

Chaiken, T., & Telander, R. (1988, October). The nightmare of steroids. *Sports Illustrated, 72,* 84–93, 97–98, 100–102.

Chan, C. (1986). Addicted to exercise. In *Encyclopedia Britannica Medical and Health Annual* (pp. 429–432).

Chandra, R. K. (1992). Primary prevention of cardiovascular disease in childhood: Recent knowledge and unanswered questions. *Journal of the American College of Nutrition, 11,* 3S–7S.

Chappel, J. N. (1987). Drug use and abuse in the athlete. In J. R. May & M. J. Asken (Eds.), *Sport psychology: The psychological health of the athlete* (pp.187–211). New York: PMA.

Chernin, K. (1981). *The obsession: Reflections on the tyranny of slenderness.* New York: Harper & Row.

Chiodo, J., & Latimer, P. R. (1983). Vomiting as a learned weight-control technique in bulimia. *Journal of Behavior Therapy and Experimental Psychiatry, 14,* 131–135.

Chodzko-Zajko, W. J. (1991). Physical fitness, cognitive performance, and aging. *Medicine and Science in Sports and Exercise, 23,* 868–872.

Chodzko-Zajko, W. J. (1994). Assessing physical performance in older adult populations. *Journal of Aging and Physical Activity, 2,* 103–104.

Chodzko-Zajko, W. J. (1996). The physiology of aging: Structural changes and functional consequences. Implications for research and clinical practice in the exercise and activity sciences. *Quest, 48,* 311–329.

Chodzko-Zajko, W. J., & Moore, K. A. (1994). Physical fitness and cognitive functioning in aging. In J. O. Holloszy (Ed.), *Exercise and sport sciences reviews* (Vol. 22, pp. 195–220). Baltimore: Williams & Wilkins.

Chung, C. (1996). Sport and exercise psychology in Korea. *Journal of Applied Sport Psychology* [Abstract], *8* (Suppl.), S4.

Ciarrochi, J., Deane, F. P., & Anderson, S. (2002). Emotional intelligence moderates the relationship between stress and mental health. *Personality and Individual Differences, 32,* 197–209.

Clark, D. M., & Teasdale, J. D. (1985). Constraints on the effects of mood on memory. *Journal of Personality & Social Psychology, 48,* 1595–1608.

Clarkson, R. M., & Hubal, M. J. (2001). Are women less susceptible to exercise-induced muscle damage? *Current Opinion in Clinical Nutrition and Metabolic Care, 4*(6), 527–531.

Claytor, R. P. (1991). Stress reactivity: Hemodynamic adjustments in trained and untrained humans. *Medicine and Science in Sports and Exercise, 23,* 873–881.

Clingman, J. M., & Hilliard, V. D. (1990). Race walkers quicken their step by tuning in, not stepping out. *The Sport Psychologist, 4,* 25–32.

Coast, J. R., Blevins, J. S., & Wilson, B. A. (2004). Do gender differences in running performance disappear with distance? *Canadian Journal of Applied Physiology Review, 24*(2), 139–145.

Cogan, K. (2005). Eating disorders: When rations become irrational. In S. Murphy (Ed.). *The sport psych handbook* (pp. 237–253). Champaign, IL: Human Kinetics.

Cohen, J., & Hansel, M. (1956). *Risk and gambling.* London: Longmans, Green and Company.

Cohen, S., & Rodriguez, M. S. (1995). Pathways linking affective disturbances and physical disorders. *Health Psychology, 14,* 374–380.

Cohen, S., & Williamson, G. M. (1991). Stress and infectious disease in humans. *Psychological Bulletin, 109,* 5–24.

Cohen, S., Kessler, R. C., & Gordon, L. U. (Eds.). (1995). *Measuring stress: A guide for health and social scientists.* New York: Oxford University Press.

Colcombe, S., & Kramer, A. F. (2003). Fitness effects on the cognitive function of older adults: A meta-analytic study. *Psychological Science, 14*(2), 125–130.

Cole, E. R., & Stewart, A. J. (1999). Meanings of political participation among black and white women: Political identity and social responsibility. In L. A. Peplau, S. C. DeBro, et al. (Eds.), *Gender, culture, and ethnicity: Current research about women and men* (pp. 153–172). Mountain View, CA: Mayfield Publishing.

College of Human Medicine, Michigan State University (1985, June*). The substance use and abuse habits of college student-athletes.* Paper presented at the NCAA Drug Education Committee, Michigan State University.

Columbia Integrative Medicine Program. Retrieved December 14, 2005, from http://www.columbiasurgery.org/cimp/index.html.

Cooke, D. (1993). State of the Sport Psychology Academy message. *Sport Psychology Academy Newsletter, 14,* 1–2.

Cooper, J., & Croyle, R. T. (1984). Attitudes and attitude change. *Annual Review of Psychology, 35,* 395–426.

Corbin, C. B., & Pangrazi, R. D. (1992). Are American children and youth fit? *Research Quarterly for Exercise and Sport, 63,* 96–106.

Corbin, C. B., & Pangrazi, R. P. (1996). How much physical activity is enough? *Journal of Physical Education, Recreation, and Dance, 67 (4),* 33–37.

Costill, D. (1986). *Inside running: Basics of sport physiology.* Indianapolis: Benchmark.

Courneya, K. S., & Hellsten, L. (1998). Personality correlates of exercise behavior, motives, barriers, and preferences: An application of the five-factor model. *Personality and Individual Differences, 24,* 625–633.

Courneya, K., & McAuley, E. (1993). Can short-range intentions predict physical activity participation? *Perceptual and Motor Skills, 77,* 115–122.

Courneya, K., Friedenreich, C., Arthur, K., & Bobick, T. (1999). Understanding exercise motivation in colorectal cancer patients: A prospective design using the theory of planned behavior. *Rehabilitation Psychology, 44,* 68–84.

Courneya, K., Vallance, J., Jones, L., & Reiman, T. (2005). Correlates of exercise intentions in non-Hodgkins lymphoma survivors: An application of the Theory of Planned Behavior. *Journal of Sport and Exercise Psychology, 27,* 335–349.

Cousins, S. O. (1995). Social support for exercise among elderly women in Canada. *Health Promotion International, 10,* 273–282.

Cousins, S. O. (1996). Exercise cognition among elderly women. *Journal of Applied Sport Psychology, 8,* 131–145.

Crabbe, J. B., & Dishman, R. K. (2004). Brain electrocortical activity during and after exercise: A quantitative synthesis. *Psychophysiology, 41,* 563–574.

Craft, L. L., & Landers, D. M. (1998). The effect of exercise on clinical depression and depression resulting from mental illness: A meta-analysis. *Journal of Sport & Exercise Psychology, 20,* 339–357.

Craig, S., Goldberg, J., & Dietz, W. H. (1996). Psychosocial correlates of physical activity among fifth and eighth graders. *Preventive Medicine, 25,* 506–513.

Cratty, B. J. (1994). *Clumsy child syndromes: Descriptions, evaluation, and remediation.* Chur: Harwood Academic.

Cratty, B. J., & Vanek, M. (1970). *Psychology and the superior athlete.* New York: Macmillan.

Crawford, J. R., & Henry, J. D. (2004). The Positive and Negative Affect Schedule (PANAS): Construct validity, measurement properties and normative data in a large non-clinical sample. *British Journal of Clinical Psychology, 43,* 245–265.

Crawford, S., & Eklund, R. C. (1994). Social physique anxiety, reasons for exercise, and attitudes toward exercise settings. *Journal of Sport & Exercise Psychology, 16,* 70–82.

Crews, D. J., & Landers, D. M. (1987). A meta-analytic review of aerobic fitness and reactivity to psychosocial stressors. *Medicine and Science in Sports and Exercise, 19,* 114–120.

Crocker, P. R. E., Bouffard, M., & Gessaroli, M. E. (1995). Measuring enjoyment in youth sport settings: A confirmatory factor analysis of the Physical Activity Enjoyment Scale. *Journal of Sport and Exercise Psychology, 17,* 200–205.

Crone-Grant, D. U., & Smith, R. A. (1999). Broadening horizons: A qualitative inquiry into the experiences of patients on an exercise prescription scheme. *Journal of Sports Sciences, 17,* 12.

Csikszentmihalyi, M. (1975). *Beyond boredom and anxiety.* San Francisco, CA: Josey-Bass Publishers.

Csikszentmihalyi, M. (1975). Play and intrinsic rewards. *Journal of Humanistic Psychology, 15,* 41–63.

Csikszentmihalyi, M. (1990/1991). *Flow: The psychology of optimal experience.* New York: Harper & Row.

Csikszentmihalyi, M. (1993). *The evolving self.* New York: Harper & Row.

Csikszentmihalyi, M. (1997). Activity, experience, and personal growth. In J. E. Curtis & S. J. Russell (Eds.), *Physical activity in human experience: Interdisciplinary perspectives* (pp. 61–88). Champaign, IL: Human Kinetics.

Csikszentmihalyi, M. (1997). *Finding flow: The psychology of engagement with everyday life.* New York: Basic Books.

Csikszentmihalyi, M. (1999). If we are so rich, why aren't we happy? *American Psychologist, 54,* 821–827.

Culos-Reed, S., Gyurcsik, N., & Brawley, L. (2001). Using theories of motivated behavior to understand physical activity: Perspectives on their influence. In R. N. Singer, H. A. Hausenblas, & C. M. Janelle (Eds.), *Handbook of research on sport psychology* (2nd ed., pp. 695–717). New York: Wiley.

Cunningham, L. S. (1997). (Ed.). *A search for solitude: Pursuing the monk's true life.* San Francisco: Harper Collins.

Cureton, T. K. (1963). Improvement of psychological states by means of exercise-fitness programs. *Journal of the Association for Physical and Mental Rehabilitation, 17,* 14–17.

Cyarto, E. V., Moorhead, G. E., & Brown, W. J. (2004). Updating the evidence relating to physical activity intervention studies in older people. *Journal of Science and Medicine in Sport, 7*(1), 30–38.

Dacey, M. L. (2004). Physical activity motivation across stages of change in older adults. *Dissertation Abstracts International, Section A: Humanities and Social Sciences, 64* (8-A), 2821.

Daley, A. J., & Buchanan, J. (1999). Aerobic dance and physical perceptions in female adolescents: Some implications for physical education. *Research Quarterly for Exercise and Sport, 70,* 196–200.

Daniel, M., Martin, A. D., & Carter, J. (1992). Opiate receptor blockade by Naltrexone and mood state after acute physical activity. *British Journal of Sports Medicine, 26,* 111–115.

Daubenmier, J. J. (2005). The relationship of yoga, body awareness, and body responsiveness to self-objectification and disordered eating. *Psychology of Women Quarterly, 29,* 207–219.

Davidson, R. J. (1994). On emotion, mood, and related affective constructs. In P. Ekman & R. J. Davidson (Eds.), *The nature of emotion: Fundamental questions* (pp. 51–55). New York: Oxford University Press.

Davidson, R. J., & Schwartz, G. E. (1976). The psychobiology of relaxation and related states: A multi-process theory. In D. I. Mostofsky (Ed.). *Behavior control and the modification of physiological activity* (pp. 399–442). Englewood Cliffs, NJ: Prentice Hall.

Davis, C. (1997). Eating disorders and hyperactivity: A psychobiological perspective. *Canadian Journal of Psychiatry, 42,* 168–175.

Davis, C. (2000). Exercise abuse. *International Journal of Sport Psychology, 31,* 278–287.

Davis, C., Claridge, G., & Brewer, H. (1996). The two faces of narcissism: Personality dynamics of body esteem. *Journal of Social and Clinical Psychology, 15,* 153–166.

Davis, C., Fox, J., Brewer, H., & Ratusny, D. (1995). Motivations to exercise as a function of personality characteristics, age, and gender. *Personality and Individual Differences, 19,* 165–174.

de la Torre, J. (1995). Mens sana in corpore sano, or exercise abuse? Clinical considerations. *Bulletin of the Menninger Clinic, 59,* 15–31.

Deam, R. (1982). Women, leisure and inequality. *Leisure Studies, 1,* 29–46.

Deci, E. L., & Ryan, R. M. (1985). *Intrinsic motivation and self-determinism in human behavior.* New York: Plenum Press.

Deci, E. L., & Ryan, R. M. (1991). A motivational approach to self: Integration in personality. In R. A. Dienstbier (Ed.), *Nebraska symposium on motivation 1991: Vol. 38. Perspectives on motivation: Current theory and research in motivation* (pp. 237–238). Lincoln, NE: University of Nebraska Press.

Deeg, D. J., Kardaun, J. W. P. F., & Fozard, J. L. (1996). Health, behavior, and aging. In J. E. Birren, K. W. Schaie, R. P. Abeles, M. Gatz, & T. A. Salthouse (Eds.), *Handbook of the psychology of aging* (4th ed., pp. 129–149). San Diego: Academic Press.

Delaney, M. E., O' Keefe, L. D., & Skene, K. M. L. (1997). Development of a sociocultural measure of young women's experiences with body weight and shape. *Journal of Personality Assessment, 69,* 63–80.

DeLongis, A., Coyne, J., Dakof, G., Fortman, S., & Lazarus, R. S. (1982). Relationship of daily hassles, uplifts, and major life events to health status. *Health Psychology, 1,* 119–136.

Demo, D. H. (1985). The measurement of self-esteem: Refining our methods. *Journal of Personality and Social Psychology, 48,* 1490–1502.

Dennison, B. A., Straus, J. H., Mellits, E. D., & Charney, E. (1988). Childhood physical fitness test: Predictor of adult physical activity levels? *Pediatrics, 82,* 324–330.

Denollet, J. (1993a). Emotional distress and fatigue in coronary heart disease: The Global Mood Scale (GMS). *Psychological Medicine, 23,* 111–121.

Denollet, J. (1993b). Sensitivity of outcome assessment in cardiac rehabilitation. *Journal of Consulting and Clinical Psychology, 61,* 686–695.

DeSensi, J. T. (1996). Virtue, knowledge, and wisdom: Proclaiming the personal meanings of movement. *Quest, 48,* 518–530.

deVries, H. A., & Adams, G. M. (1972). Electromyographic comparisons of single doses of exercise and meprobamate as to the effect on muscle relaxation. *American Journal of Physical Medicine, 51,* 130–141.

Diener, E. (1994). Assessing subjective well-being: Progress and opportunities. *Social Indicators Research, 31,* 103–157.

Diener, E., & Lucas, R. E. (1999). Personality and subjective well-being. In D. Kahneman, E. Diener, & N. Schwarz (Eds.), *Well-being: The foundations of hedonic psychology* (pp. 213–229). New York: Russell Sage Foundation.

Diener, E., & Suh, M. E. (1998). Subjective well-being and age: An international analysis. In K. W. Schaie & M. P. Lawton (Eds.), *Annual review of gerontology and geriatrics: Focus on emotion and adult development.* (Vol. 17, pp. 304–324). New York: Springer.

Diener, E., Colvin, C. R., Pavot, W. G., & Allman, A (1991). The psychic costs of intense positive affect. *Journal of Personality and Social Psychology, 61,* 492–503.

Diener, E., Emmons, R. A., Larson, R. J., & Griffin, S. (1985). The satisfaction with life scale. *Journal of Personality Assessment, 49,* 71–75.

Dienstbier, R. A. (1989). Arousal and physiological toughness: Implications for mental and physical health. *Psychological Review, 96,* 84–100.

Dienstbier, R. A. (1991). Behavioral correlates of sympathoadrenal reactivity: The toughness model. *Medicine and Science in Sports and Exercise, 23,* 846–852.

Dienstbier, R. A. (1997). The effect of exercise on personality. In M. L. Sachs & G. W. Buffone (Eds.), *Running as therapy: An integrated approach* (pp. 253–272). Lincoln, NE: University of Nebraska Press.

Digman, J. M. (1990). Personality structure: Emergence of the five-factor model. *Annual Review of Psychology, 41,* 417–440.

DiLorenzo, T. M., Bargman, E. P., Stucky-Ropp, R., Brassington, G. S., Frensch, P. A., & LaFontaine, T. (1999).

Long-term effects of aerobic exercise on psychological outcomes. *Preventive Medicine: An International Devoted to Practice & Theory, 28 (1)*, 75–85.

DiLorenzo, T. M., Stucky-Ropp, R. C., Vander Wal, J. S., & Gothan, H. J. (1998). Determinants of exercise among children. II. A longitudinal analysis. *Preventive Medicine, 27*, 470–477.

Dishman, R. K. (1981). Biologic influences on exercise adherence. *Research Quarterly for Exercise and Sport, 52*, 143–159.

Dishman, R. K. (1982). Compliance/adherence in health-related exercise. *Health Psychology, 1*, 237–267.

Dishman, R. K. (1986). Mental health. In V. Seefeldt (Ed.), *Physical activity and well-being* (pp. 303–341). Reston, VA: American Alliance for Health, Physical Education, Recreation, and Dance.

Dishman, R. K. (1988). Behavioral barriers to health-related physical fitness. In L. K. Hall & G. C. Meyer (Eds.), *Epidemiology, behavior change and intervention in chronic disease: Lacrosse, exercise and health series* (pp. 49–83). Champaign, IL: Life Enhancement Publications.

Dishman, R. K. (1988b). Overview. In R. K. Dishman (Ed.), *Exercise adherence: Its impact on public health* (pp. 1–9). Champaign, IL: Human Kinetics.

Dishman, R. K. (1989). Determinants of physical activity and exercise for persons 65 years of age or older. In W. W. Spirduso & H. M. Eckert (Eds.), *Physical activity and aging* (pp. 140–162). Champaign, IL: Human Kinetics.

Dishman, R. K. (1993). Exercise adherence In R. N. Singer, M. Murphey, & L. K. Tennant (Eds.), *Handbook of research in sport psychology* (pp.779–798). New York: Macmillan.

Dishman, R. K. (1994). *Advances in exercise adherence.* Champaign, IL: Human Kinetics.

Dishman, R. K. (1997). Adherence to physical activity. In W. P. Morgan (Ed.), *Physical activity and mental health* (pp. 63–80). Philadelphia, PA: Taylor & Francis.

Dishman, R. K., & Buckworth, J. (1996). Increasing physical activity: A quantitative synthesis. *Medicine and Science in Sports and Exercise, 28*, 706–719.

Dishman, R. K., & Buckworth, J. (1997). Adherence to physical activity. In W. P. Morgan (Ed.), *Physical activity and mental health* (pp. 63–80). Englewood, NJ: Taylor & Francis.

Dishman, R. K., & Sallis, J. F. (1994). Determinants and interventions for physical activity and exercise. In C. Bouchard, R. Sheppard, & T. Stephens (Eds.), *Physical activity, fitness, and health: International proceedings and consensus statement* (pp. 214–238). Champaign, IL: Human Kinetics.

Dishman, R. K., & Steinhardt, M. (1988). Reliability and concurrent validity for a seven-day recall of physical activity in college students. *Medicine and Science in Sports and Exercise, 20*, 14–25.

Dishman, R. K., & Steinhardt, M. (1990). Internal health locus of control predicts free-living, but not supervised, physical activity: A test of exercise-specific control and outcome expectancy hypothesis. *Research Quarterly for Exercise and Sport, 61*, 383–394.

Dishman, R. K., Farquhar, R. P., & Cureton, K. J. (1994). Responses to preferred intensities of exertion in men differing in activity levels. *Medicine and Science in Sports and Exercise, 26*, 783–790.

Dishman, R. K., Motl, R. W., Saunders, R., Felton, G., Ward, D. S., Dowda, M., & Pate, R. R. (2005). Enjoyment mediates effects of a school-based physical-activity intervention. *Medicine and Science in Sports and Exercise, 37*, 478–487.

Dishman, R. K., Sallis, J. F., & Orenstein, D. O. (1985). The determinants of physical activity and exercise. *Public Health Reports, 100*, 158–171.

Dishman, R., Oldenburg, B., O'Neal, H., & Sheppard, R. (1998). Worksite physical activity interventions. *American Journal of Preventive Medicine, 15*, 344–361.

Doan, R., & Scherman, A. (1987). The therapeutic effect of physical fitness on measures of personality: A literature review. *Journal of Counseling and Development, 66*, 28–36.

Dorfman, L. J., & Bosley, T. M. (1979). Age-related changes in peripheral and central nerve conduction in man. *Neurology, 29*, 38–44.

Dorman, D., Price, C., Alley, H. (1995). *Senior Sense: Vol. 3, No. 2.* Athens, GA: University of Georgia, Cooperative Extension Service.

Dortch, S. (1997, June). America weighs in. *American Demographics*, 1–6.

Dotson, C. O., & Ross, J. G. (1985). The National Children and Youth Fitness Study: Relationships between activity patterns and fitness. *Journal of Physical Education, Recreation and Dance, 56*, 86–90.

Douillard, J. (1994). *Body, mind, and sport: The mind-body guide to lifelong fitness and your personal best.* New York: Crown.

Douthitt, V. L. (1994). Psychological determinants of adolescent exercise adherence. *Adolescence, 29*, 711–722.

Doyne, E. J., Chambless, D. L., & Beutler, L. E. (1983). Aerobic exercise as a treatment for depression in women. *Behavioral Therapy, 14*, 434–440.

Doyne, E. J., Ossip-Klein, D. G., Bowman, E. D., Osborn, K. M., McDougall-Wilson, I. B., & Neimayer, R. A. (1987). Running versus weightlifting in the treatment of depression. *Journal of Consulting and Clinical Psychology, 5*, 748–754.

Drechsler, F. (1975). Sensory action potentials of the median and ulnar nerves in aged persons. In K. Kunze & J. E. Desmedt (Eds.), *Studies on neuromuscular diseases* (pp. 232–235). Basel: Karger.

Drenowski, A., Kurth, C. L., & Krahn, D. D. (1994). Body weight and dieting in adolescence: Impact of socioeconomic status. *International Journal of Eating Disorders, 16*, 61–65.

Drewe, S. B. (2003). *Why sport? An introduction to the philosophy of sport.* Toronto: Thompson Educational Publishing.

Ducharme, K. A., & Brawley, L. R. (1995). Predicting the intentions and behavior of exercise initiates using two forms of self-efficacy. *Journal of Behavioral Medicine, 18*, 479–497.

Duda, J. L., Smart, A. E., & Tappe, M. K. (1989). Predictors of adherence in the rehabilitation of athletic injuries: An application of personal investment theory. *Journal of Sport and Exercise Psychology, 11*, 367–381.

Duncan, H. H., Travis, S. S., & McAuley, W. J. (1995). An emergent theoretical model for interventions encouraging physical activity (mall walking) among older adults. *Journal of Applied Gerontology, 14*, 64–77.

Duncan, M. C., & Robinson, T. T. (2004). Obesity and body ideals in the media: Health and fitness practices of young African-American women. *Quest, 56*, 77–104.

Duncan, S.C., Duncan, T.E., & Strycker, L.A. (2005). Sources and types of social support in youth physical activity. *Health Psychology, 24*, 3–10.

Duncan, T. E., McAuley, E., Stoolmiller, M., & Duncan, S. C. (1993). Serial fluctuations in exercise behavior as a function of social support and efficacy cognitions. *Journal of Applied Social Psychology, 23*(18), 1498–1523.

Dunn, A. L., Reigle, T. G., Youngstedt, S. D., Armstrong, R. B., & Dishman, R. (1996). Brain norepinephrine and metabolites after treadmill training and wheel running in rats. *Medicine & Science in Sports & Exercise, 28*, 204–209.

Dunn, A. L., Trivedi, M. H., Kampert, J. B., Clark, C. G., & Chambliss, H. O. (2005). Exercise treatment for depression: Efficacy and dose response. *American Journal of Preventative Medicine, 28*, 1–8.

Dunning, E., & Rojek, C. (1992). Introduction: Sociological approaches to the study of sport and leisure. In E. Dunning & C. Rojek (Eds.), *Sport and leisure in the civilizing process: Critique and counter-critique* (pp. xi–xix). Toronto, Canada: University of Toronto Press.

Durden, A. E. (1994). *Risk appraisal and sensation-seeking traits of female recreational athletes*. Unpublished master's thesis, Florida State University, Tallahassee, FL.

Dustman, R. E., Emmerson, R., & Shearer, D. C. (1994). Physical activity, age, and cognitive-neuropsychological function of older individuals. *Neurobiology of Aging, 5*, 35–42.

Dwyer, T., Blizzard, L., & Dean, K. (1996). Physical activity and performance in children. *Nutritional Reviews, 54*, S27–31.

Dyer, J. B., III, & Crouch, J. G. (1988). Effects of running and other activities on moods. *Perceptual and Motor Skills, 67*, 43–50.

Dykens, E. M., Rosner, B. A., & Butterbaugh, G. (1998). Exercise and sports in children and adolescents with developmental disabilities: Positive physical and psychosocial effects. *Child and Adolescent Psychiatric Clinics of North America, 7*, 757–771.

Dzewaltowski, D. A., Noble, J. M., & Shaw, J. M. (1990). Physical activity participation: Social cognitive theory versus the theories of reasoned action and planned behavior. *Journal of Sport and Exercise Psychology, 12*, 388–405.

Eid, M., & Diener, E. (2004). Global judgments of subjective well-being: Situational variability and long-term stability. *Social Indicators Research, 65*, 245–277.

Eisenberg, D. M., Davis, R. B., Ettner, S. L., Appel, S., Wilkey, S., Van Rompay, M., & Kessler, R. C. (1998). Trends in alternative medicine use in the United States, 1990–1997. *Journal of the American Medical Association, 280*, 1569–1575.

Eisenberg, D. M., Kessler, R. C., Foster, C., Norlock, F. E., Calkins, D. R., & Delbanco, T. L. (1993). Unconventional medicine in the United States: Prevalence, costs, and patterns of use. *The New England Journal of Medicine, 328*, 246–252.

Ekkekakis, P., & Lind, E. (in press). Exercise does not feel the same when you are overweight: The impact of self-selected and imposed intensity on affect and exertion. *International Journal of Obesity*.

Ekkekakis, P., Hall, E. E., VanLanduyt, L. M., & Petruzzello, S. J. (2000). Walking in (affective) circles: Can short walks enhance affect? *Journal of Behavioral Medicine, 23*, 245–275.

Eklund, R. C., & Crawford, S. (1994). Active women, social physique anxiety and exercise. *Journal of Sport and Exercise Psychology, 16*, 431–448.

Eklund, R. C., Kelley, B., & Wilson, P. (1997). The social physique anxiety scale: Men, women, and the effects of modifying item 2. *Journal of Sport and Exercise Psychology, 19*, 188–196.

Eklund, R. C., Mack, D., & Hart, E. (1996). Factorial validity of the Social Physique Anxiety Scale for Females. *Journal of Sport and Exercise Psychology, 18*, 281–295.

Ekman, P. (1994). All emotions are basic. In P. Ekman & R. J. Davidson (Eds.), *The nature of emotion: Fundamental questions* (pp. 15–19). New York: Oxford University Press.

Elliott, E. (2004). Advocating for increased physical activity for children: The role of the physical education teacher. *Teaching Elementary Physical Education, 15*, 46–48.

Elsayed, M., Ismail, A. H., & Young, R. J. (1980). Intellectual differences of adult men related to age and physical fitness before and after an exercise program. *Journal of Gerontology, 35*, 383–387.

Elster, J. (2004). Emotions and rationality. In A. S. R. Manstead, N. Frijda, & A. Fischer (Eds.), *Feelings and emotions: The Amsterdam symposium* (pp. 30–49). Cambridge: Cambridge University Press.

Emery, C. F., & Blumenthal, J. A. (1991). Effects of physical exercise on psychological and cognitive functioning of older adults. *Annals of Behavioral Medicine, 13*, 99–107.

Emery, C. F., Hauck, E. R., & Blumenthal, J. A. (1992). Exercise adherence or maintenance among older adults: 1-year follow-up study. *Psychology and Aging, 7*, 466–470.

Emery, C. F., Schein, R. L., Hauck, E. R., & MacIntyre, N. R. (1998). Psychological and cognitive outcomes of a randomized trial of exercise among patients with chronic obstructive pulmonary disease. *Health Psychology, 17*, 232–240.

Endler, N. S., & Magnusson, D. (1976). *Interactional psychology and personality*. New York: Wiley.

Engebretson, T. O., Clark, M. M., Niaura, R. S., Phillips, T., Albrecht, A., & Tilkemeier, P. (1999). Quality of life and anxiety in a phase II cardiac rehabilitation program. *Medicine and Science in Sports and Exercise, 31*, 216–223.

Epstein, L. H., Wing, R. R., Thompson, J. K., & Griffiths, M. (1980). Attendance and fitness in aerobics exercise: The effects of contract and lottery procedures. *Behavior Modification, 4*, 465–479.

Epstein, L. H., Paluch, R. A., Kilanowski, C. K., & Raynor, H. A. (2004). The effect of reinforcement or stimulus control to reduce sedentary behavior in the treatment of pediatric obesity. *Health Psychology, 23*, 371-380

Erling, J., & Oldridge, N. B. (1985). Effect of a spousal support program on compliance with cardiac rehabilitation. *Medicine and Science in Sport and Exercise, 17*, 284.

European Federation of Sport Psychology. (1996). Position statement of the European Federation of Sport Psychology (FEPSAC): I. Definition of sport psychology. *The Sport Psychologist, 10*, 221–223.

Evans, L., & Hardy, L. (1995). Sport injury and grief responses: A review. *Journal of Sport and Exercise Psychology, 17*, 227–245.

Evans, L., Hardy, L., & Fleming, S. (2000). Intervention strategies with injured athletes: An action research study. *Sport Psychologist, 14*, 188–206.

Evans, M., Weinberg, R., & Jackson, A. (1992). Psychological factors related to drug use in college athletes. *The Sport Psychologist, 6*, 24–41.

Evans, W. J. (1999). Exercise training guidelines for the elderly. *Medicine and Science in Sports and Exercise, 31*, 12–17.

Evans, W. J., & Campbell, W. W. (1993). Sarcopenia and age-related changes in body composition and functional capacity. *Journal of Nutrition, 123*, 465–468.

Eyler, A. A., Baker, E., Cromer, L., King, A. C., Brownson, R. C., & Donatelle, R. J. (1998). Physical activity and minority women: A qualitative study. *Health Education and Behavior, 25*, 640–652.

Eysenck, H. J., & Eysenck, S. B. G. (1991). *Manual of the Eysenck Personality Scales*. London: Hodder and Stoughton.

Eysenck, S. B. G. (1983). One approach to cross-cultural studies of personality. *Australian Journal of Psychology, 35*, 381–391.

Fahlberg, L. L., & Fahlberg, L. A. (1990). From treatment to health enhancement: Psychosocial considerations in the exercise components of health promotion programs. *The Sport Psychologist, 4*, 168–179.

Fahlberg, L. L., & Fahlberg, L. A. (1994). A human science for the study of movement: An integration of multiple ways of knowing. *Research Quarterly for Exercise and Sport, 65*, 100–109.

Fahlberg, L. L., & Fahlberg, L. A. (1997). Health, freedom, and human movement in the postmodern era. In J. Fernandez-Balboa (Ed.), *Critical postmodernism in human movement, physical education, and sport* (pp. 65–86). Albany, NY: State University of New York Press.

Fairburn, C. G., Welch, S. L., & Doll, H. A. (1997). Risk factors for bulimia nervosa: A community-based case-control study. *Archives of General Psychiatry, 54*, 509–517.

Fairburn, G., & Wilson, G. T. (1993). *Binge eating*. New York: Guilford.

Fallon, A. E., & Rozin, P. (1985). Sex differences in perception of desirable body shape. *Journal of Abnormal Psychology, 94*, 102–105.

Farrell, P. A. (1985). Excercise and endorphins—male responses. *Medicine and Science in Sports and Exercise, 17*(1), 89–93.

Farrell, P. A., Gustafson, A. B., Garthwaite, T. L., Kalkhoff, R. K., Cowley, A. W., & Morgan, W. P. (1986). Influence of endogenous opioids on the response of selected hormones to exercise in humans. *Journal of Applied Physiology, 61*, 1051–1057.

Farrell, P. A., Gustafson, A. B., Morgan, W. P., & Pert, C. B. (1987).

Enkephalins, catecholamines, and psychological mood alterations: Effects of prolonged exercise. *Medicine and Science in Sports and Exercise, 19,* 347–353.

Featherstone, M. (1982). The body in consumer culture. *Theory, Culture and Society, 1,* 18–33.

Feldman, L. A. (1995). Variations in the circumplex structure of mood. *Personality and Social Psychology Bulletin, 21,* 806–817.

Feltz, D. L., & Landers, D. M. (1983). The effects of mental practice on motor skill learning and performance: A meta-analysis. *Journal of Sport Psychology, 5,* 25–27.

Ferer-Caja, E., & Weiss, M. R. (2000). Predictors of intrinsic motivation among adolescent students in physical education. *Research Quarterly for Exercise and Sport, 71,* 267–279.

Fernandez-Balboa, J. (1997). Physical education teacher preparation in the postmodern era: Toward a critical pedagogy. In J. Fernandez-Balboa (Ed.), *Critical postmodernism in human movement, physical education, and sport* (pp. 121–138). Albany, NY: State University of New York Press.

Ferrari, M., & Sternberg, R. J. (Eds.). (1998). *Self-awareness: Its nature and development.* New York: Guilford.

Ferrucci, L., Izmerlian, G., Leveille, S. G., Phillips, C. L., Corti, M. C., Brock, D. B., & Guralnik, J. M. (1999). Smoking, physical activity and active life expectancy. *American Journal of Epidemiology, 149(7),* 645–653.

Fiatarone, M. A., & Garnett, L. R. (1997). Keep on keeping on. *Harvard Health Letter, 22,* 4.

Field, L., & Steinhart, M. (1992). The relationship of internally directed behavior to self-reinforcement, self-esteem, and expectancy values for exercise. *American Journal of Health Promotion, 7,* 21–27.

Figler, S. K., & Whitaker, G. (1991). *Sport and play in American life: A textbook in the sociology of sport* (2nd ed.). Dubuque, IA: Brown Publishers.

Fine, A. H., & Sachs, M. L. (1997). *The total sports experience—for kids: A parent's guide to success in youth sports.* South Bend, IN: Diamond Communications.

Finger, A., & Guber, L. G. (1984). *Yoga moves with Alan Finger.* New York: Simon & Schuster.

Fink, E. (1979). The ontology of play. In E. W. Gerber & W. J. Morgan (Eds.), *Sport and the body: A philosophical symposium* (2nd ed., pp. 73–83). Philadelphia: Lea & Febiger.

Finkenberg, M. E., DiNucci, J. M., McCune, S. L., & McCune, E. D. (1994). Analysis of course type, gender, and personal incentives to exercise. *Perceptual and Motor Skills, 78,* 155–159.

Fischer, A. C., & Zwart, E. F. (1982). Psychological analysis of athletes' anxiety responses. *Journal of Sport Psychology, 4,* 139–158.

Fishbein, M., & Ajzen, I. (1975). *Belief, attitude, intention, and behavior: An introduction to theory and research.* Reading, MA: Addison-Wesley.

Fisher, A. C., Domm, M. A., & Wuest, D. A. (1988). Adherence to sports injury rehabilitation programs. *The Physician and Sportsmedicine, 16,* 47–52.

Fisher, J. K., & Fuzhong, L. (2004). A community-based walking trial to improve neighborhood quality of life in older adults: A multilevel analysis. *Annals of Behavioral Medicine, 28(3),* 186–194.

Fixx, J. (1977). *The complete book of running.* New York: Random House.

Flint, F. A. (1991). *The psychological effects of modeling in athletic injury rehabilitation.* (Doctoral dissertation, University of Oregon, 1991). (Microform Publications No. BF 357)

Focht, B. C., & Hausenblas, H. A. (2003). State anxiety responses to acute exercise in women with high social physique anxiety: Influence of perceived evaluative threat and self-selected vs. prescribed intensity. *Journal of Sport and Exercise Psychology, 25,* 123–144.

Focht, B. C., & Hausenblas, H. A. (2004). Perceived evaluative threat and state anxiety during exercise in women with social physique anxiety. *Journal of Applied Sport Psychology, 16,* 361–368.

Folkman, S. (1991). Coping across the life span: Theoretical issues. In E. M. Cummings, A. L. Greene, & K. H. Karraker (Eds.), *Life-span developmental psychology: Perspectives on stress and coping* (pp. 3–19). Hillsdale, NJ: Lawrence Erlbaum.

Folkman, S., & Moskowitz, J. T. (2000). Positive affect and the other side of coping. *American Psychologist, 55,* 647–654.

Fontane, P. E. (1996). Exercise, fitness, and feeling well. *American Behavioral Scientist, 39,* 288–305.

Ford, H. T., Jr., Puckett, J. R., Blessing, D. L., & Tricker, L. A. (1989). Effects of selected physical activities on health-related fitness and psychological well-being. *Psychological Reports, 64,* 203–208.

Fox, K. R. (2000). Self-esteem, self-perceptions and exercise. *International Journal of Sport Psychology, 31,* 228–240.

Fox, K. R. (Ed.). (1997). *The physical self: From motivation to well-being.* Champaign, IL: Human Kinetics.

Fox, K. R., & Corbin, C. B. (1989). The Physical Self-Perception Profile: Development and preliminary validation. *Journal of Sport and Exercise Psychology, 11,* 408–430.

Fox, K. R., & Stahi, A. (2002). Physical activity and mental health in older adults: Current evidence and future perspectives. *Psychology: The Journal of Hellenic Psychological Society. Special Issues of Psychology of Exercise and Sport, 9(4),* 563–580.

Fox, K., Rejeski, J., & Gauvin, L. (2000). Effects of leadership style and group dynamics on enjoyment of physical activity. *American Journal of Health Promotion, 14,* 277–283.

Frank, M. G., Ekman, P., & Friesen, W. V. (1997). Behavioral markers and recognizability of the smile of enjoyment. In P. Ekman & E. L. Rosenberg (Eds.), *What the face reveals: Basic and applied studies of spontaneous expression using the Facial Action Coding System (FACS)* (pp. 217–242). New York: Oxford University Press.

Franklin, B. A. (1984) Exercise program compliance. In J. Storlie & H. A. Jordan (Eds.), *Behavioral management of obesity* (pp. 105–135). New York: Spectrum Press.

Frederick, C. M., & Morrison, C. S. (1996). Social physique anxiety: Personality constructs, motivations, exercise attitudes, and behaviors. *Perceptual and Motor Skills, 82,* 963–972.

Fredrickson, B. L., Roberts, T. A., Noll, S. M., Quinn, D. M., & Twenge, J. M. (1998). That swimsuit becomes you: Sex differences in self-objectification, restrained eating, and math performance. *Journal of Perspectives in Social Psychology, 75(1),* 269–284.

Freedson, P. S., & Evinson, S. K. (1991). Familial aggregation and physical activity. *Research Quarterly for Exercise and Sport, 62,* 384–389.

Fried, R. (1987). *The hyperventilation—Research and clinical treatment.* Baltimore: Johns Hopkins University Press.

Fried, R. (1990). *The breath connection.* New York: Insight/Plenum.

Fried, R. (with Grimaldi, J.) (1993). *The psychology and physiology of breathing in behavioral medicine, clinical psychology, and psychiatry.* New York: Plenum Press.

Fried, R., & Berkowitz, L. (1979). Music hath charms and can influence helpfulness. *Journal of Applied Social Psychology, 9,* 199–208.

Friedman, E., & Berger, B. G. (1991). Influence of sex, masculinity and femininity on the effectiveness of three stress reduction techniques: Jogging, relaxation response and group interaction. *Journal of Applied Sport Psychology, 3,* 61–86.

Fries, J. F. (1980). Aging, natural death, and the compression of morbidity. *New England Journal of Medicine, 303(3),* 130–135.

From FSU Star to Olympic Gold Hero. (2000, October 2). *Tallahassee Democrat,* p.1.

Fromm, E. (1969). *Escape from freedom.* New York: Avon Books.

Fukukawa, Y., Nakashima, C., Tsuboi, S., Kozukai, R., Doyo, W., Niino, N., Ando, F., & Shimokata, H. (2004). Age differences in the effect of physical activity on depressive symptoms. *Psychology of Aging, 19(2),* 346–351.

Furlong, W. B. (1976, June). The fun in fun. *Psychology Today, 10,* 35–38, 80.

Furnham, A., Titman, P., & Sleeman, E. (1994). Perception of female body shapes as a function of exercise. *Journal of Social Behavior and Personality, 9*(2), 335–352.

Gallup, G., Jr., & Castelli, J. (1989). *The people's religion.* New York: Macmillan.

Gallwey, W. T. (1982). *The inner game of tennis.* Toronto: Bantam Books.

Garcia-Martin, M. A., Gomez-Jacinto, L., & Martimportugues-Goyenecha, L. (2004). A structural model of the effects of organized leisure activities on the well-being of elder adults in Spain. *Activities, Adaptation, and Aging, 28*(3), 19–34.

Garner, D. M. (1991). *Eating Disorders Inventory-2.* Odessa, FL: Psychological Assessment Resources Inc.

Garner, D. M., & Garfinkel, P. E. (1979). The eating attitudes test: An index of the symptoms of anorexia nervosa. *Psychological Medicine, 9,* 273–279.

Garner, D. M., & Garfinkel, P. G. (Eds.) (1986). *Handbook of psychotherapy for anorexia nervosa and bulimia.* New York: Guilford Press.

Garner, D. M., & Rosen, L. W. (1991). Eating disorders among athletes: Research and recommendations. *Journal of Applied Sport Science Research, 5,* 100–107.

Gaston, L., Crombez, J., & Dupuis, G. (1989). An imagery and meditation technique in the treatment of psoriasis: A case study using an A-B-A design. *Journal of Mental Imagery, 13*(1), 31–38.

Gatch, C. L., & Kendzierski, D. (1990). Predicting exercise intentions: The theory of planned behavior. *Research Quarterly for Exercise and Sport, 61,* 100–102.

Gauron, E. F., & Bowers, W. A. (1984). Pain control techniques in college-age athletes. *Psychological Reports, 59,* 1163–1169.

Gauvin, L., & Rejeski, W. J. (1993). The Exercise-induced Feeling Inventory: Development and initial validation. *Journal of Sport & Exercise Psychology, 15,* 403–423.

Gauvin, L., Levesque, L., & Richard, L. (2001). Helping people initiate and maintain a more active lifestyle: A public health framework for physical activity promotion research. In R. Singer, H. Hausenblas, & C. Janelle (Eds.), *Handbook of sport psychology* (2nd ed., pp. 695–717). New York: John Wiley.

Gauvin, L., Rejeski, W. J., & Reboussin, B. A. (2000). Contributions of acute bouts of vigorous physical activity to explaining diurnal variations in feeling states in active, middle-aged women. *Health Psychology, 19,* 365–375.

Gavin, J. (1987). *The Psychosocial Activity Dimensions Profile. Some observations on the relationship between activity preferences, participation, and personal profiles* [technical manuscript.] Montreal: Concordia University.

Ghoncheh, S., & Smith, J. C. (2004). Progressive muscle relaxation, yoga stretching, and ABC relaxation theory. *Journal of Clinical Psychology, 60,* 131–136.

Giacobbi, P. R., Hausenblas, H. A., & Frye, N. (2005). A naturalistic assessment of the relationship between personality, daily life events, leisure-time exercise, and mood. *Psychology of Sport & Exercise, 6,* 67–81.

Gibbons, S. L., & Bushakra, F. B. (1989). Effects of Special Olympics participation on the perceived competence and social acceptance of mentally retarded children. *Adapted Physical Activity Quarterly, 6,* 40–51.

Gill, K. S., & Overdorf, V. (1994). Incentives for exercise in younger and older women. *Journal of Sport Behavior, 17,* 87–97.

Girdano, D. A, Everley, G. S., Jr., & Dusek, D. E. (1997). *Controlling stress and tension* (5th ed.). Boston: Allyn & Bacon.

Glasser, W. (1976). *Positive addiction.* New York: Harper & Row.

Godin, G. (1994). Social cognitive models. In R. K. Dishman (Ed.), *Advances in exercise adherence* (pp. 113–136). Champaign, IL: Human Kinetics.

Godin, G., & Kok, G. (1996). The theory of planned behavior: A review of its applications to health-related behaviors. *American Journal of Health Promotion, 11,* 87–98.

Godin, G., & Shephard, R. J. (1990). Use of attitude-behavior models in exercise promotion. *Sports Medicine, 10,* 103–121.

Godin, G., Valois, P., & Lepage, L. (1993). The pattern of influence of perceived behavioral control upon exercising behavior: An application of Ajzen's theory of planned behavior. *Journal of Behavioral Medicine, 16,* 81–102.

Gohm, C. L., & Clore, G. L. (2000). Individual differences in emotional experience: Mapping available scales to processes. *Personality and Social Psychology Bulletin, 26,* 679–697.

Golden, R. N., Gaynes, B. N., Ekstrom, R. D., Hamer, R. M., Jacobsen, F. M., Suppes, T., et al. (2005). The efficacy of light therapy in the treatment of mood disorders: A review and meta-analysis of the evidence. *American Journal of Psychiatry, 162,* 656–662.

Goldsmith, D. J. (1994). The role of facework in supportive communication. In B. R. Burleson, T. L. Albrecht, & I. G. Sarason (Eds.), *Communication of social support: Messages, interactions, relationships, and community* (pp. 29–49). Thousand Oaks, CA: Sage.

Goodman, E. (1999, May 28). Eating disorders: The Columbine for girls. *Boston Globe.*

Gorley, T., & Gordon, S. (1995). An examination of the transtheoretical model and exercise behavior in older adults. *Journal of Sport & Exercise Psychology, 17,* 312–324.

Gorsch, R. L., Baumeister, R. F., Cameron, N. M. S., Collins, R. L., Connors, G. J., DeGruy, F., Elinwood, Jr., E., Glaser, F. B., Hill, P. C., Holder, H. D., Hood, R. W., Idler, E., Josephson, A. M., Longabaugh, R., MacNutt, F. S., Martin, J. E., Pargament, K. I., VanLeeuwen, M. S., Weaver, A. J., Williams, D. R., & Whitehorse, P. J. (1998). Definitions of religion and spirituality. In D. B. Larson, J. P. Swyers, and M. E. McCullough (Eds.), *Scientific research on spirituality and health: A consensus report* (pp. 14–30). Rockville, MD: National Institute for Healthcare Research.

Goss, J. D. (1994). Hardiness and mood disturbances in swimmers while overtraining. *Journal of Sport & Exercise Psychology, 16,* 135–149.

Goss, J., Cooper, S., Stevens, D., Croxon, S., & Dryden, N. (2005). Eating disorders. In J. Taylor & G. Wilson (Eds.), *Applying sport psychology: Four perspectives* (pp. 207–228). Champaign, IL: Human Kinetics.

Gottlieb, B. H. (1988). Support interventions: A typology and agenda for research. In S. W. Duck (Ed.), *Handbook of personal relationships: Theory, research and interventions* (pp. 519–541). New York: John Wiley & Sons.

Gould, D., Jackson, S., & Finch, L. (1993). Life at the top: The experience of U.S. national champion figure skaters. *The Sport Psychologist, 7,* 354–374.

Goyeche, J. R. (1979). Yoga as therapy in psychosomatic medicine. *Psychotherapy and Psychosomatics, 31,* 373–381.

Grassi, K., Gonzales, M.G., Tello, P., & He, G. (1999). La Vida Caminando: A community-based physical activity program designed by and for rural Latino families. *Journal of Health Education, 30* (Suppl.), S13–17.

Green, E. K., Burke, K. I., Nix, C. L., Lambrecht, K. W., & Mason, D. C. (1996). Psychological factors associated with alcohol use by high school athletes. *Journal of Sport Behavior, 18,* 195–208

Green, J. M., Bishop, P. A., Muir, I. H., & Lornax, R. G. (2000). Gender differences in sweat lactate. *European Journal of Applied Physiology, 82*(3), 230–235.

Greenberg, J. S. (1985). Health and wellness: A conceptual differentiation. *Journal of School Health, 55,* 403–406.

Greendorfer, S. L. (1983). Shaping the female athlete: The impact of the family. In M. Boutslier & L. San Giovani (Eds.), *The sporting woman* (pp. 135–155). Champaign, IL: Human Kinetics.

Greenleaf, C., & McGreer, R. (2004). Examining objectification theory among female college exercisers and non-exercisers. Presented at the annual meeting of the Association for the Advancement of Applied Sport Psychology, Minneapolis, MN.

Greensberg, J. S. (1998). *Health education: Learner-centered instructional strategies.* Boston: WCB McGraw-Hill.

Greenwald, A. G., & Pratkanis, A. R. (1984). The self. In R. S. Wyer & T. K. Srull (Eds.), *Handbook of social cognition* (Vol. 3, pp. 129–178). Hillsdale, NJ: Erlbaum.

Griest, J. H., Klein, M. H., Eischens, R. R., Faris, J., Gurman, A. S., & Morgan, W. P. (1979). Running as treatment for depression. *Comprehensive Psychiatry, 20,* 41–54.

Griffin, J., & Harris, M. B. (1996). Coaches' attitudes, knowledge, experiences, and recommendations regarding weight control. *The Sport Psychologist, 10,* 180–194.

Griffith, C. R. (1926). *Psychology of coaching.* New York: Charles Scribner.

Griffith, C. R. (1928). *Psychology of athletics.* New York: Charles Scribner.

Gronwall, D. M. A., & Sampson, H. (1974). *The psychological effects of concussion.* Auckland, NZ: Auckland University Press.

Grossman, A., & Sutton, J. R. (1985). Endorphins: What are they? How are they measured? What is their role in exercise? *Medicine and Science in Sports and Exercise, 17*(1), 74–81.

Grove, J. R., & Prapavessis, H. (1992). Preliminary evidence for the reliability and validity of an Abbreviated Profile of Mood States. *International Journal of Sport Psychology, 23,* 93–109.

Grove, J. R., Bahnsen, A., & Eklund, R. (1997). Neuroticism, injury severity, and coping with rehabilitation. In R. Lidor & Bar-Eli (Eds.), *Innovations in sport psychology: Linking theory and practice.* Proceedings, International Society of Sport Psychology, IX World Congress of Sport Psychology, Israel, July 5–9, 1997.

Gruman, G. J. (1966). *A history of the ideas about the prolongation of life: The evolution of prolongevity hypotheses to 1800.* Philadelphia: American Philosophical Society.

Guest, R. S., Klose, K. J., Needhamshropshire, B. M., & Jacobs, P. L. (1997). Evaluation of a training program for persons with SCI paraplegia using the Parastep (R) 1 ambulation system, 4. Effect on physical self-concept and depression. *Archives of Physical Medicine and Rehabilitation, 78,* 804–807.

Guttmann, A. (1988). *A whole new ballgame: An interpretation of American sports.* Chapel Hill, NC: The University of North Carolina Press.

Gyurcsik, N., Culos, S., Bray, S., & DuCharme, K. (1998). Instructor efficacy: Third-party influence of exercise adherence. *Journal of Sport and Exercise Psychology, 20* (Suppl.), S9.

Gyursik, N. C., & Estabrooks, P. A. (2004). Acute exercise thoughts, coping, and exercise intention in older adults. *Journal of Applied Social Psychology, 34*(6), 1131–1146.

Hackfort, D., & Spielberger, C. D. (Eds.). (1989). *Anxiety in sports: An international perspective.* New York: Hemisphere.

Hahn, S. E. (2000). The effects of locus of control on daily exposure, coping and reactivity to work interpersonal stressors: A diary study. *Personality and Individual Differences, 29,* 729–748.

Hakim, A. A., Petrovitch, H., Burchfiel, C. M., Ross, G. W., Rodriguez, B. L., White, L. R., Yano, K., Curb, J. D., & Abbott, R. D. (1998). Effects of walking on mortality among nonsmoking retired men. *The New England Journal of Medicine, 338,* 94–99.

Hall, C., Pongrac, J., & Buckholz, E. (1985). The measurement of imagery ability. *Human Movement Science, 4,* 107–118.

Halliburton, S., & Sanford, S. (1989a, July). Making weight becomes torture for UT swimmers. *Austin American-Statesman,* pp. D1, D7.

Halliburton, S., & Sanford, S. (1989b, July). Being thin turns grim at Texas. *Austin American-Statesman,* pp. D1, D8

Hallinan, C. J., Pierce, E. F., Evans, J. E., DeGrenier, J. D., &

Anders, F. F. (1991). Perceptions of current and ideal body shape of athletes and non-athletes. *Perceptual and Motor Skills, 72,* 123–130.

Hamilton, M. (1968). Development of a rating scale for depressive illness. *British Journal of Social Clinical Psychology, 6,* 278–296.

Hanley, G. L., & Chinn, D. (1989). Stress management: An integration of multidimensional arousal and imagery theories with case study. *Journal of Mental Imagery, 13*(2), 107–118.

Hansel, T. (1979). *When I relax, I feel guilty.* Elgin, IL: David C. Cook.

Hansen, C. J., Stevens, L. C., & Coast, J. R. (2001). Exercise duration and mood state: How much is enough to feel better? *Health Psychology, 20,* 267–275.

Hardy, C. J., & Crace, R. K. (1991). Social support within sport. *Sport Psychology Training Bulletin, 3*(1), 1–8.

Hardy, C. J., Burke, K. L., & Crace, R. K. (1999). Social support and injury: A framework for social support-based interventions with injured athletes. In D. Pargman (Ed.), *Psychological bases of sport injuries* (2nd ed., pp. 175–198). Morgantown, WV: Fitness Information Technology.

Hardy, C. J., Rejeski, W. J. (1989). Not what, but how one feels: The measurement of affect during exercise. *Journal of Sport and Exercise Psychology, 11,* 304–317.

Harootyan, R. A. (1982). The participation of older people in sports. In R. M. Panking (Ed.), *Social approaches to sport* (pp. 122–197). East Brunswick, NJ: Associated University Press.

Harris, D. (1973). *Involvement in sport: A somatopsychic rationale for physical activity.* Philadelphia: Lea & Feiberger.

Harris, M. B., & Greco, D. (1990). Weight control and weight concern in competitive female gymnasts. *Journal of Sport and Exercise Psychology, 12,* 427–433.

Harrison, L., Lee, A. M., & Belcher, D. (1999). Race and gender differences in sport participation as a function of self-schema. *Journal of Sport and Social Issues, 23*(3), 287–307.

Harro, M. (1997). Validation of a questionnaire to assess physical activity of children ages 4–8 years. *Research Quarterly for Exercise and Sport, 68,* 259–268.

Hart, E. A., Leary, M. R., & Rejeski, W. J. (1989). The measurement of social physique anxiety. *Journal of Sport and Exercise Psychology, 11,* 94–104.

Hart, S. G., & Staveland, L. E. (1988). Development of NASA TLX (Task Load Index): Results of empirical and theoretical research. In P. A. Hancock & N. Meshkati (Eds.), *Human mental workload* (pp. 139–183). Amsterdam: Elsevier.

Harter, S. (1978). Effectance motivation reconsidered: Toward a developmental model. *Human Development, 1,* 34–64.

Harter, S. (1981). A model of intrinsic mastery motivation in children: Individual differences and developmental change. In W. A. Collins (Ed.), *Minnesota symposium on child psychology* (Vol. 14, pp. 215–255). Hillsdale, NJ: Erlbaum.

Harter, S. (1990). Causes, correlates, and the functional role of global self-worth: A life-span perspective. In R. J. Sternberg & J. Kolligan, Jr., *Competence considered* (pp. 67–97). New Haven, CT: Yale University Press.

Harter, S. (1990). Self and identity development. In S. S. Feldman & G. R. Elliot (Eds.), *At the threshold: The developing adolescent* (pp. 352–387). Cambridge, MA: Harvard University Press.

Hasher, L., & Zacks, R. T. (1979). Automatic and effortful processes in memory. *Journal of Experimental Psychology, 108,* 356–388.

Hassmen, P., & Blomstrand, E. (1995). Mood state relationships and soccer team performance. *The Sport Psychologist, 9,* 297–308.

Hausenblas, H. A., Brewer, B. W., & Van Raalte, J. L. (2004). Self-presentation and exercise. *Journal of Applied Sport Psychology, 16,* 3–18.

Hausenblas, H., & Carron, A. (1999). Eating disorder indices with athletes: An integration. *Journal of Sport and Exercise Psychology), 21,* 230–258.

Hausenblas, H., & Symons Downs, D. (2002a). Exercise dependence: A systematic review. *Psychology of Sport and Exercise, 3*, 89–123.

Hausenblas, H., & Symons Downs, D. (2002b). How much is too much? The development and validation of the Exercise Dependence Scale. *Psychology and Health: An International Journal, 16*, 387–404.

Hausenblas, H., Nigg, C., Dannecker, E., Symons, D., Ellis, S., Fallon, E., Focht, B., & Loving, M. (2001). A missing piece of the transtheoretcal model applied to exercise: Development and validation of the Exercise Temptation Scale. *Psychology and Health: An International Journal, 16*, 381–390.

Hausenblau, H. A., & Symons Downs, D. (2002). Relationship among sex, imagery, and exercise dependence symptoms. *Psychology of Addictive Behaviors, 16*(2), 169–172.

Hawkes, C. H. (1992). Endorphins: The bases of pleasure. *Journal of Neurology, Neurosurgery, and Psychiatry (Editorial), 55*, 247–250.

Hayden, R. M., Allen, C. J., & Camaione, D. N. (1986). Some psychological benefits resulting from involvement in an aerobic fitness class from the perspectives of participants and knowledgeable informants. *Journal of Sports Medicine and Physical Fitness, 26*, 67–76.

Hays, K. F. (1998). (Ed.). *Integrating exercise, sports, movement and mind: Therapeutic unity.* New York: The Haworth Press.

Hays, K. F. (1999). *Working it out: Using exercise in psychotherapy.* Washington, DC: American Psychological Association.

Hays, K. F., & Brown, Jr., C. H. (2004). *You're on! Consulting for peak performance.* Washington, DC: American Psychological Association.

Hayslip, B., Weigand, D., Weinberg, R., Richardson, P., & Jackson, A. (1996). The development of new scales for assessing health belief model constructs in adulthood. *Journal of Aging and Physical Activity, 4*, 307–324.

Heaney, C., & Goetzel, R. (1997). A review of health-related outcomes of multi-component worksite health promotion programs. *American Journal of Health Promotion, 11*, 290–307.

Heath, G. W., & Kendrick, J. S. (1989). Outrunning the risks: A behavioral risk profile of runners. *American Journal of Preventive Medicine, 5*, 347–352.

Heck, T. A., & Kimiecik, J. C. (1993). What is exercise enjoyment: A qualitative investigation of adult exercise maintainers. *Wellness Perspectives, 10*, 3–21.

Heil, J. (1993). *The psychology of sport injury.* Champaign, IL: Human Kinetics.

Heil, J., & Fine, P. G. (1999). Pain in sport: A biopsychological perspective. In D. Pargman (Ed.), *Psychological bases of sport injuries* (2nd ed., pp. 13–28). Morgantown, WV: Fitness Information Technology.

Helson, R., Kwan, V. S. Y., John, O. P., & Jones, C. (2002). The growing evidence for personality change in adulthood: Findings from research with personality inventories. *Journal of Research in Personality, 36*, 287–306.

Henning, A. D. (1987). Exercise at work? I don't have time. *Fitness in Business, 2*, 68–69.

Herberman, R. B., & Ortaldo, J. R. (1981). Natural killer cells: Their role in defenses against disease. *Science, 214*, 24–30.

Herman-Tofler, L. R., & Tuckman, B. W. (1998). The effects of aerobic training on children's creativity, self-perception, and aerobic power. *Child and Adolescent Psychiatry Clinics of North America, 7*, 773–790.

Hittleman, R. (1969). *Richard Hittleman's yoga: 28 day exercise plan.* New York: Workman.

Hobfoll, S. E. (1989). Conservation of resources: A new attempt at conceptualizing stress. *American Psychologist, 44*, 513–524.

Hobfoll, S. E. (1998). *Stress, culture, and community: The psychology and philosophy of stress.* New York: Plenum Press.

Hobfoll, S. E., & Stephens, M. A. P. (1990). Social support during extreme stress: Consequences and intervention. In B. R. Sarason & G. R. Pierce (Eds.), *Social support: An interactional view* (pp. 454–481). New York: John Wiley & Sons.

Hobson, C. J., Hoffman, J. J., Corso, L. M., & Freismuth, P. K. (1987). Corporate fitness: Understanding and motivating employee participation. *Fitness in Business, 2*, 80–85.

Hofstetter, C., Howell, M., Macera, C., Sallis, J., Spry, V., Barrington, E., & Callender, C. (1991). Illness, injury, and correlates of aerobic exercise and walking: A community study. *Research Quarterly for Exercise and Sport, 62*, 1–9.

Hollander, B. J., & Seraganian, P. (1984). Aerobic fitness and psychophysiological reactivity. *Canadian Journal of Behavioral Science, 16*, 257–261.

Hollander, D. B., & Acevedo, E. O. (2000). Successful English Channel swimming: The peak experience. *The Sport Psychologist, 14*, 1–16.

Holmes, D. S., & Roth, D. L. (1985). Association of aerobic fitness with pulse rate and subjective responses to psychological stress. *Psychophysiology, 22*, 525–529.

Holmes, T. H., & Rahe, R. H. (1967). The Social Readjustment Rating Scale. *Journal of Psychosomatic Research, 11*, 213–218.

Holowchak, M. A. (2002). Philosophy of sport: Critical readings, crucial issues. Upper Saddle River, NJ: Prentice Hall.

Hong, S., Farag, N. H., Nelesen, R. A., Ziegler, M. G., & Mills, P. J. (2004). Effects of regular exercise on lymphocyte subsets and CD621L after psychological vs. physical stress. *Journal of Psychosomatic Research, 56*, 363–370.

Hooper, S. L., Mackinnon, L. T., & Hanrahan, S. (1997). Mood states as an indication of staleness and recovery. *International Journal of Sport Psychology, 28*, 1–12.

Hoyt, M. F., & Janis, I. L. (1975). Increasing adherence to a stressful decision via a motivational balance-sheet procedure: A field experiment. *Journal of Personality and Social Psychology, 35*, 833–839.

Hughes, J., Smith, T. W., Kosterlitz, H. W., Fothergill, L. A., Morgan, B. A., & Morris, H. R. (1975). Identification of two related pentapeptides from the brain with potent opiate agonist activity. *Nature, 258*, 577–579.

Huizinga, J. (1955). *Homo ludens: A study of the play element in culture.* Boston: Beacon.

Hult, J. S. (1999). NAGWS and AIAW: The strange and wondrous journey to the athletic summit, 1950–1990. *Journal of Physical Education, Recreation and Dance, 70*, 24–31.

Hume, C., Salmon, J., Ball, K. (2005). Children's perceptions of their home and neighborhood in a national sample of girls and boys in grades 4 through 12. *Health Psychology, 18*, 410–415.

International Society of Sport Psychology (1992). Physical activity and psychological benefits: A position statement from the International Society of Sport Psychology. *Journal of Applied Sport Psychology, 4*, 94–98.

Isen, A. M. (2004) Some perspectives on positive feelings and emotions: Positive affect facilitates thinking and problem solving. In A. S. R. Manstead, N. Frijda, & A. Fischer (Eds.), *Feelings and emotions: The Amsterdam symposium* (pp. 263–282). Cambridge: Cambridge University Press.

Ismail, A. H., & Trachtman, L. E. (1973, March). Jogging the imagination. *Psychology Today, 6*, 1973.

Iyengar, B. K. S. (with Evans, J. J., & Abrams, D.) (2005). Light on life: The yoga journey to wholeness, inner peace, and ultimate freedom. Emmaus, PA: Rodale.

Izard, C. E., & Ackerman, B. P. (1998). Emotions and self-concepts across the life span. In K. W. Schaie & M. P. Lawton (Eds.), *Annual review of gerontology and geriatrics: Focus on emotion and adult development* (Vol. 17, pp. 1–26). New York: Springer.

Jackson, S. A. (2000). Joy, fun, and flow state in sport. In Y. L. Hanin (Ed.), *Emotions in Sport* (pp.135–155). Champaign, IL: Human Kinetics.

Jackson, S. A., & Eklund, R. C. (2004). *The flow scales manual.* Morganton, WV: Fitness Information Technology.

Jackson, S. A., & Marsh, H. W. (1996). Development and validation of a scale to measure optimal experience: The Flow State Scale. *Journal of Sport & Exercise Psychology, 18,* 17–35.

Jackson, S. A., Thomas, P. R., Marsh, H. W., & Smethurst, C. J. (2001). Relationships between flow, self-concept, psychological skills, and performance. *Journal of Applied Sport Psychology, 13,* 129–153.

Jackson, S., & Csikszentmihalyi, M. (1999). *Flow in sports: The keys to optimal experiences and performances.* Champaign, IL: Human Kinetics.

Jackson, S., & Marsh, H. W. (1986). Athletic or antisocial: The female sport experience. *Journal of Sport Psychology, 8,* 198–211.

Jacobson, E. (1976). You must relax: Practical methods for reducing the tensions of modern living (5th ed.). New York: McGraw-Hill Paperback.

Jakicic, J., Wing, R., Butler, B., & Robertson, R. (1995). Prescribing exercise in multiple short bouts versus one continuous bout: Effects on adherence, cardiorespiratory fitness and weight loss in overweight women. *International Journal of Obesity, 19,* 893–901.

Janelli, L. M. (1993). Are there body image differences between older men and women? *Western Journal of Nursing Research, 15,* 327–329.

Janz, K., Dawson, J., & Mahoney, L. (2000). Tracking physical fitness and physical activity from childhood to adolescence: The Muscatine study. *Medicine and Science in Sports and Exercise, 32,* 1250–1257.

Janz, N. K., & Becker, M. H. (1984). The health belief model: A decade later. *Health Education Quarterly, 11,* 319–333.

Jemmott, J. B. III, & Magloire, K. (1988). Academic stress, social support and secretory immunoglobulin A. *Journal of Personality and Social Psychology, 55,* 803–810.

Jin, P. (1992). Efficacy of tai chi, brisk walking, meditation, and reading in reducing mental and emotional stress. *Journal of Psychosomatic Research, 36,* 361–370.

Johnsgard, K. W. (1989). *The exercise prescription for depression and anxiety.* New York: Plenum Press.

Johnsgard, K. W. (2004). *Conquering depression and anxiety through exercise.* Amherst, NY: Prometheus Books.

Johnson, C. A., Corrigan, S. A., Dubbert, P. M., & Cramling, S. E. (1990). Perceived barriers to exercise and weight control practices in community women. *Women and Health, 16,* 177–192.

Johnson, C., & Pure, D. L. (1986). Assessment of bulimia: A multidimensional model. In K. D. Brownell & J. P. Foreyt (Eds.), *Handbook of eating disorders: Physiology, psychology and treatment* (pp. 405–449). New York: Basic Books.

Johnson, C., & Tobin, D. L. (1991). The diagnosis and treatment of anorexia nervosa and bulimia among athletes. *Athletic Trainer, 26,* 119–128.

Johnson, W., McGue, M. & Kreuger, R. F. (2005). Personality stability in late adulthood: A behavioral genetic analysis. *Journal of Personality, 73*(2), 523–551.

Johnson-Kozlow, M. F., Sallis, J. F., & Calfas, K. J. (2004). Does life stress moderate the effects of a physical activity intervention? *Psychology and Health, 19,* 479–489.

Jonah, B. A., & Dawson, N. E. (1987). Youth and risk: Age differences in risky driving, risk perception, and risk utility. *Alcohol, Drugs and Driving, 3*(3–4), 13–29.

Jones, D. J., Bromberger, J. T., Sutton-Tyrrell, K., & Matthews, K. A. (2003). Lifetime history of depression and carotid atherosclerosis in middle-aged women. *Archives of General Psychiatry, 60,* 153–160.

Jorm, A. F. (1989). Modifiability of trait anxiety and neuroticism: A meta-analysis of the literature. *Australian and New Zealand Journal of Psychiatry, 23,* 21–29.

Kabat-Zinn, J. (1982). An outpatient program in behavioral medicine for chronic pain patients based on the practice of mindfulness meditation: Theoretical considerations and preliminary results. *General Hospital Psychiatry, 4,* 33–47.

Kabat-Zinn, J. (1990). *Full catastrophe living: Using the wisdom of your body and mind to face stress, pain, and illness.* New York: Delacorte.

Kabat-Zinn, J., Lipworth, L., & Burney, R. (1985). The clinical use of mindfulness meditation for the self-regulation of chronic pain. *Journal of Behavioral Medicine, 8,* 163–190.

Kahneman, D., Diener, E., & Schwarz, N. (Eds.). (1999). *Well-being: The foundations of hedonic psychology.* New York: Russell Sage Foundation.

Kamiyama, Y., Kawaguchi, T., Kanda, A., Kuno, S., & Nishijima, T. (2004). Effect of muscle exercise on reduction in medical expenditures among elderly. *Japanese Journal of Physical Fitness and Sports Medicine, 53*(2), 205–210.

Kanfer, F. H., & Gaelick, L. (1986). Self-management methods. In F. H. Kanfer & A. P. Goldstein (Eds.), *Helping people change: A textbook of methods* (pp. 283–345). New York: Pergamon Press.

Kann, L., Warren, C. W., Harris, W. A., Collins, J. L., Williams, B. I., Ross, J. G., & Kolbe, L. J. (1996). Youth risk behavior surveillance—United States, 1995. *Morbidity and Mortality Weekly Report, 45,* 1–84.

Kanner, A. D., Coyne, J. C., Schaefer, C., & Lazarus, R. S. (1981). Comparisons of two modes of stress measurement: Daily hassles and uplifts versus major life events. *Journal of Behavioral Medicine, 4,* 1–39.

Kaplan, R. M. (1994). The Ziggy Theorem: Toward an outcomes-focused health psychology. *Health Psychology, 13,* 451–460.

Kaplan, R. M., Ries, A. L., Prewitt, L. M., & Eakin, E. (1994). Self-efficacy expectations predict survival for patients with chronic obstructive pulmonary disease. *Health Psychology, 13,* 366–368.

Karvonen, M., Kentala, K., & Mustala, O. (1957). The effects of training on heart rate: A longitudinal study. *Annales Medicinae Experimentalis et Biologiae Fenniae, 35,* 307–315.

Kawachi, I., Sparrow, D., Vokonas, P. S., & Weiss, S. T. (1994). Symptoms of anxiety and risk of coronary heart disease: The normative aging study. *Circulation, 90,* 2225–2229.

Keller, S., & Seraganian, P. (1984). Physical fitness level and autonomic reactivity to psychosocial stress. *Journal of Psychosomatic Research, 28,* 279–287.

Kelly, C. H. (1971). Stress, trait-anxiety, and type of coping process. *Dissertation Abstracts International, 31*(9-B), 5627–5628.

Kendzierski, D. (1988). Self-schemata and exercise. *Basic and Applied Social Psychology, 9,* 45–59.

Kendzierski, D. (1990). Exercise self-schemata: Cognitive and behavioral correlates. *Health Psychology, 9,* 69–82.

Kendzierski, D. (1994). Schema theory: An information processing focus. In R. K. Dishman (Ed.), *Advances in exercise adherence* (pp. 137–159). Champaign, IL: Human Kinetics.

Kendzierski, D., & DeCarlo, K. J. (1991). Physical Activity Enjoyment Scale: Two validation studies. *Journal of Sport & Exercise Psychology, 13,* 50–64.

Kenyon, G. S., & Grogg, T. M. (Eds.). (1970). *Contemporary psychology of sport: Proceedings of the Second International Congress of Sport Psychology.* Chicago: The Athletic Institute.

Kernis, M. H., & Goldman, B. M. (2003). In M. R. Leary & J. P. Tangney (Eds.), *Handbook of self and identity* (pp. 106–127). New York: Guilford Press.

Kerr, J. H., & Schaik, P. (1995). Effects of game venue and outcome on psychological mood states in rugby. *Personality and Individual Differences, 19,* 407–410.

Ketterer, M. W. (1993). Secondary prevention of ischemic heart disease: The case for aggressive behavioral monitoring and intervention. *Psychosomatics 34,* 478–484.

Keutzer, C. S. (1978). Whatever turns you on: Triggers to transcendent experiences. *Journal of Humanistic Psychology, 18,* 77–80.

Keyes, C. L. M. (2005). Mental illness and/or mental health? Investigating axioms of the complete state model of health. *Journal of Consulting and Clinical Psychology, 73,* 530–548.

Keyes, C. L. M., & Haidt, J. (Eds.). (2003). *Flourishing: Positive psychology and the life well-lived.* Washington, DC: American Psychological Association.

Kilbride, E., McLoughlin, P., Gallagher, C. G., & Harty, H. R. (2003). Do gender differences exist in ventilatory response to progressive exercise in males and females of average fitness? *European Journal of Applied Physiology, 89* (6), 595–602.

Kimiecek, J. C. (1993). Commentary on Dzewaltowski's commentary. *Journal of Sport and Exercise Psychology, 15,* 101–105.

Kimiecik, J. C. (1998, March). The path of the intrinsic exerciser. *IDEA Health and Fitness Source,* 34–42.

Kimiecik, J. C. (2002). *The intrinsic exerciser: Discovering the joy of exercise.* Boston: Houghton Mifflin.

Kimiecik, J. C. (2005). Phat exercise: How young adults enjoy and sustain physical activity. *Journal of Physical Education, Recreation, and Dance, 76 (8),* 19–21, 30.

Kimiecik, J. C., & Harris, A. T. (1996). What is enjoyment? A conceptual/definitional analysis with implications for sport and exercise psychology. *Journal of Sport and Exercise Psychology, 18,* 247–263.

Kimiecik, J. C., & Horn, T. S. (1998). Parental beliefs and children's moderate-to-vigorous physical activity. *Research Quarterly for Exercise and Sport, 69,* 163–175.

Kimiecik, J. C., & Stein, G. L. (1992). Examining flow experiences in sport contexts: Conceptual issues and methodological concerns. *Journal of Applied Sport Psychology, 4,* 144–160.

Kimiecik, J. C., Horn, T. S., & Shurin, C. S. (1996). Relationships among children's beliefs, perceptions of their parents' beliefs, and their moderate-to-vigorous physical activity. *Research Quarterly for Exercise and Sport, 67,* 324–336.

King, A. C. (1994). Clinical and community interventions to promote and support physical activity participation. In R. K. Dishman (Ed.), *Advances in exercise adherence.* Champaign, IL: Human Kinetics.

King, A. C., & Frederiksen, L. W. (1984). Low-cost strategies for increasing exercise behavior: Relapse preparation training and social support. *Behavior Modification, 8,* 3–21.

King, A. C., Blair, S. N., & Bild, D. (1992). Determinants of physical activity and interventions in adults. *Medicine and Science in Sport and Exercise, 24* (Suppl.), S221–S236.

King, A. C., Carl, F., Birkel, L., & Haskell, W. L. (1988). Increasing exercise among blue-collar employees: The tailoring of work-site programs to meet specific needs. *Preventive Medicine, 17,* 357–365.

King, A. C., Castro, C., Wilcox, S., Eyler, A. A., Sallis, J. F., & Brownson, R. C. (1999). Personal and environmental factors associated with physical inactivity among different racial-ethnic groups of U.S. middle-aged and older-aged women. *Health Psychology, 19,* 354–364.

King, A. C., Haskell, W. L., Taylor, C. B., Kraemer, H. C., & DeBusk, R. F. (1991). Group- vs home-based exercise training in healthy older men and women. *Journal of the American Medical Association, 266,* 1535–1542.

King, A. C., Haskell, W. L., Young, D. R., Oka, R. K., & Stefanick, M. L. (1995). Long-term effects of varying intensities and formats of physical activity on participation rates, fitness, and lipoproteins in men and women aged 50 to 65 years. *Circulation, 91,* 2596–2604.

King, A. C., Kiernan, M., Oman, R. F., Kraemer. H. C., Hull, M., & Ahn, D. (1997). Can we identify who will adhere to long-term physical activity? Signal detection methodology as a potential aid to clinical decision making. *Health Psychology, 16,* 380–389.

King, A. C., Oman, R. F., Brassington, G. S., Bliwise, D. L., & Haskell, W. L. (1997). Moderate-intensity exercise and self-rated quality of sleep in older adults. *Journal of the American Medical Association, 277,* 32–37.

King, A. C., Taylor, C. B., & Haskell, W. L. (1993). Effects of differing intensities and formats of 12 months of exercise training on psychological outcomes in older adults. *Health Psychology, 12,* 292–300.

King, A. C., & Coles, B. (1992). *The health of Canadians. Views and behaviors of 11, 13, and 15 year olds from 11 countries.* Ottawa, Ontario, Canada: Minister of Supply and Services Canada.

Kirkcaldy, B. D., & Shephard, R. J. (1990). Therapeutic implications of exercise. *International Journal of Sport Psychology, 21,* 165–184.

Kleiber, D. A., & Kirshnit, C. E. (1991). Sport involvement and identity formation. In L. Diamant (Ed.), *Mind-body maturity: Psychological approaches to sports, exercise, and fitness* (pp. 193–211). New York: Hemisphere.

Klesges, R. C., Mizes, J. S., & Klesges, L. M. (1987). Self-help dieting strategies in college males and females. *International Journal of Eating Disorders, 6,* 409–417.

Knapen, J., Vande Viliet, P., Van coppenolle, H., David, A., Peuskens, J., Knapen, K., & Pieters, G. (2003). The effectiveness of two psychomotor therapy programs on physical fitness and physical self-concept in non psychotic psychiatric patients in a randomized controlled trial. *Clinical Rehabilitation, 17*(6), 637–647.

Knapp, D. (1988). Behavioral management techniques and exercise promotion. In R. K. Dishman (Ed.), *Exercise adherence: Its impact on public health* (pp. 203–235). Champaign, IL: Human Kinetics.

Knapp, D., Gutmann, M., Squires, R. A., & Pollack, M. (1983). Exercise adherence among coronary artery bypass surgery (CABS) patients. *Medicine and Science in Sports and Exercise, 15,* S120.

Koenig, L., & Wasserman, E. L. (1995). Body image and dieting failure in college men and women: Examining links between depression and eating problems. *Sex Roles, 32,* 225–249.

Kohlberg, L. (1981). *Essays on moral development, Volume 1: The philosophy of moral development.* San Francisco: Harper & Row.

Kolyton, K. F., Shake, C. L., & Morgan, W. P. (1993). Interaction of exercise, water temperature and protective body apparel on body awareness and anxiety. *International Journal of Sport Psychology, 24,* 297–305.

Korn, E. R. (1983). The use of altered states of consciousness and imagery in physical and pain rehabilitation. *Journal of Mental Imagery, 7*(1), 25–34.

Kouvonen, A., Kivimaki, M., Elovainio, M., Virtanen, M., Linna, A., & Vahtera, J. (2005). Job strain and leisure-time physical activity in female and male public sector employees. *Preventative Medicine, 41,* 532–539.

Kraemer, R. R., Dzewaltowski, D. A., Blair, M. S., Rinehardt, K. F., & Castracane, V. D. (1990). Mood alteration from tread mill running and its relationship to beta-endorphin, corticotrophin, and growth hormone. *Journal of Sports Medicine and Physical Fitness, 30,* 241–246.

Kramer, A. F., Colcombe, S. J., McAuley, E., Eriksen, K. I., Scalf, P., Jerome, G. J., Marquez, D. X., Elavsky, S., & Webb, A. G. (2003). Enhancing brain and cognitive function of older adults through fitness training. *Journal of Molecular Neuroscience, 20*(3), 213–221.

Krebs, P., Eickelberg, W., Krobath, H., & Baruch, I. (1989). Effects of physical exercise on peripheral vision and learning in children with spina bifida manifesta. *Perceptual and Motor Skills, 68,* 167–174.

Kyllo, L. B., & Landers, D. M. (1995). Goal setting in sport and exercise: A research synthesis to resolve the controversy. *Journal of Sport and Exercise Psychology, 17,* 117–137.

Labbate, L. A., & Miller, R. W. (1990). A case of malingering. *American Journal of Psychiatry, 47,* 257–258.

LaFontaine, T. P., DiLorenzo, T. M., Frensch, P. A., Stucky-Ropp, R. C., Bargman, E. P., & McDonald, D. G. (1992). Aerobic exercise and mood: A brief review, 1985–1990. *Sports Medicine, 13,* 160–170.

Lampinen, P., & Heikkinen, R. L. (2002). Gender differences in depressive symptoms and self-esteem in different physical activity categories among older adults. *Women in Sport and Physical Activity Journal, 11*(2), 171–197.

Landers, D. M., & Petruzzello, S. J. (1994). Physical activity, fitness and anxiety. In C. Bouchard, R. J. Shepherd, & T. Stephens (Eds.), *Physical activity, fitness and health: International proceedings and consensus statement* (pp. 868–882). Champaign, IL: Human Kinetics.

Landers, D., & Arent, S. M. (2001). Physical activity and mental health. In R. N. Singer, H. A. Hausenblas, & C. M. Janelle (Eds.), *Handbook of sport psychology* (2nd ed., pp.740–765). New York: John Wiley.

Landfield, P. W., McGaugh, J. L., & Lynch, G. (1978). Impaired synaptic potentiation processes in the hippocampus of aged, memory-deficient rats. *Brain Research, 150*, 85–101.

Langens, T. A., & Stucke, T. S., (2005). Stress and mood: The moderating role of activity inhibition. *Journal of Personality, 73*, 47–78.

Lantz, C. D., Hardy, C. J., & Ainsworth, B. E. (1997). Social physique anxiety and perceived exercise behavior. *Journal of Sport Behavior, 20*, 83–93.

Larsen, R. J., & Diener, E. (1987). Affect intensity as an individual difference characteristic: A review. *Journal of Research in Personality, 21*, 1–39.

Lasco, R. A., Curry, C. R. H., Dickson, V. J., Powers, J., Menes, S., & Merritt, R. K. (1989). Participation rates, weight loss, and blood pressure changes among obese women in a nutrition-exercise program. *Public Health Reports, 104*, 640–646.

Laski, M. (1962). *Ecstasy: A study of some secular and religious experiences*. Bloomington, IN: Indiana University Press.

Lawther, J. D. (1951). *The psychology of coaching*. Englewood Cliffs, NJ: Prentice Hall.

Layne, J. E., & Nelson, M. E. (1999). The effects of progressive resistance training on bone density: A review. *Medicine and Science in Sports and Exercise, 31*, 25–30.

Lazarus, R. S. (1999). *Stress emotion: A new synthesis*. New York: Springer Publishing.

Lazarus, R. S., & Folkman, S. (1986). Cognitive theories of stress and the issue of circularity. In M. H. Appley & R. Trumbull (Eds.), *Dynamics of stress: Physiological, psychological, and social perspectives* (pp. 63–80). New York: Plenum Press.

Lazarus, R. S., DeLongis, A., Folkman, S., & Gruen, R. (1985). Stress and adaptational outcome: The problem of confounded measures. *American Psychologist, 40*, 770–779.

Leach, D. (1963). Meaning and correlates of peak experience. *Dissertation Abstracts, 24*, 180.

Leary, M. R. (1992). Self-presentational processes in exercise and sport. *Journal of Sport & Exercise Psychology, 14*, 339–351.

Leary, M. R., Tchividjian, L. R., & Kraxberger, B. E. (1999). Self-presentation can be hazardous to your health: Impression management and health risk. In R. F. Baumeister (Ed.), *The self in social psychology* (pp. 69–77). Philadelphia, PA: Psychology Press.

LeDoux, J., & Armony, J. (1999). Can neurobiology tell us anything about human emotion? In D. Kahneman, E. Diener, & N. Schwarz (Eds.), *Well-being: The foundations of hedonic psychology* (pp. 489–499). New York: Russell Sage Foundation.

Lee, C., & White, S. W. (1997). Controlled trial of a minimal-intervention exercise program for middle-aged working women. *Psychology and Health, 12*, 361–374.

Lee, I., & Paffenbarger, R. S., Jr. (1996). Do physical activity and physical fitness avert premature mortality? *Exercise and Sport Sciences Reviews, 24*, 135–171.

Lee, I., Hsieh, C., & Paffenbarger, R. S. (1995). Exercise intensity and longevity in men: The Harvard alumni health study. *Journal of the American Medical Association, 273*, 1179–1184.

Lee, S. M., & Anderson, D. R. (2004). Assessing the association of walking with health services use and costs among socioeconomically disadvantaged older adults. *American Journal of Health Promotion, 18*, 400.

Lees-Haley, P. R. (1986). Psychological malingerers. *Trial, 21*, 68–69.

Legwold, C. (1987). Incentives for fitness programs. *Fitness in Business, 2*, 131–133.

Lehrer, P. M., & Woolfolk, R. L. (1984). Are stress reduction techniques interchangeable, or do they have specific effects?: A review of the comparative empirical literature. In R. L. Woolfolk & P. M. Lehrer (Eds.), *Principles and practice of stress management* (pp. 404–477). New York: The Guilford Press.

Leith, L. M. (1994). *Foundations of exercise and mental health*. Morgantown, WV: Fitness Information Technology.

Lemmer, J. F., Hurlbut, D. E., Martel, G. F., Tracy, B. L., Ivey, F. M., Metter, E. J., Fozard, J. L., Fleg, J. L., & Hurley, B. F. (2000). Age and gender responses to strength training and detraining. *Medicine and Science in Sports and Exercise, 32*, 1505–1512.

Lenart, E. B., Goldberg, J. P., Bailey, S. M., Dallal, G. E., & Koff, E. (1995). Current and ideal physique choices in exercising and nonexercising college women from a pilot athletic image scale. *Perceptual and Motor Skills, 81*, 831–848.

Leonard, G. (1975/1977). *The ultimate athlete: Re-visioning sports, physical education, and the body*. New York: Avon.

Leonard, G. (1988). *Walking on the edge of the world*. Boston: Houghton Mifflin.

Leonard, G., & Murphy, M. (1995). *The life we are given: A long-term program for realizing the potential of body, mind, heart, and soul*. New York: G. P. Putnam's Sons.

Leslie, E., Fotheringham, M., Owen, N., & Bauman, A. (2001). Age-related differences in physical activity levels of young adults, *Medicine and Science in Sports and Exercise, 33*, 255–258.

Leslie, E., Owen, N., Salmon, J., Bauman, A., Sallis, J., & Lo, S. (1999). Insufficiently active Australian college students: Perceived personal, social, and environmental influences. *Preventive Medicine, 28*, 20–27.

Leveille, S. G., Guralnik, J. M., Ferrucci, L., & Langlois, X. X. (1999). Aging successfully until death. *American Journal of Epidemiology, 149*(7), 654–664.

Leventhal, H., Patrick-Miller, L., Leventhal, E. A., & Burns, E. A. (1998). Does stress-emotion cause illness in elderly people? In K. W. Schaie & M. P. Lawton (Eds.), *Annual review of gerontology and geriatrics: Focus on emotion and adult development* (Vol. 17, pp. 138–184). New York: Springer.

Levinson, L. J., & Reid, G. (1993). The effects of exercise intensity on the stereotypic behaviors of individuals with autism. *Adapted Physical Activity Quarterly, 10*, 255–268.

Levy, B. R., & Myers, L. M. (2004). Preventative health behaviors influenced by self-perceptions of aging. *Preventative Medicine: An International Journal Devoted to Practice and Theory, 39*(3), 625–629.

Li, F., Duncan, T. E., Duncan, S., McAuley, E., Chaumeton, N. R., & Harmer, P. (2001). Enhancing psychological well-being of elderly individuals through tai-chi exercise. *Structural Equation Modeling, 8*, 53–83.

Licence, K. (2004). Promoting and protecting the health of children and young people. *Child Care, Health, & Development, 30*, 623–635.

Lind, E., Joens-Matre, R. R., & Ekkekakis, P. (2004). What intensity of physical activity do previously sedentary middle-aged women select? Evidence of a coherent pattern from physiological, perceptual, and affective markers. *Preventative Medicine, 40*, 407–419.

Linden, W., Earle, T. L., Gerin, W., & Christenfeld, N. (1997). Physiological stress reactivity and recovery: Conceptual siblings separated at birth? *Journal of Psychosomatic Research, 42*, 117–135.

Lindquist, C. H., Reynolds, K. D., & Goren, M. I. (1999). Sociocultural determinants of physical activity among children. *Preventive Medicine, 29*, 305–312.

Linengar, J., Chesson, C., & Niuce, D. (1991). Physical fitness gains following simple environmental change. *American Journal of Preventive Medicine, 7*, 298–310.

Lintunen, T. (1999). Development of self-perceptions during the school years. In Y. Vauden Auweele (Ed.), *Psychology for Physical Educators*, pp. 115–134. Champaign, IL: Human Kinetics.

Linville, P. W. (1987). Self-complexity as a cognitive buffer against stress-related illness and depression. *Journal of Personality and Social Psychology, 52*, 663–676.

Lippe, S., Zioegelmann, J., & Schwarzer, R. (2005). Stage-specific adoption and maintenance of psychical activity: Testing a three-stage model. *Psychology of Sport and Exercise, 6*, 585–603.

Locke, E. A., & Latham, G. P. (1990). A *theory of goal setting and task performance.* Englewood Cliffs, NJ: Prentice Hall.

Loeser, J. (1982). A multifaceted model of the components of pain. In M. Stanton-Hicks & R. A. Boas, *Chronic low back pain* (p. 146). New York: Raven Press.

Loftus, E. F., & Loftus, G. R. (1980). On the permanence of stored information in the human brain. *American Psychologist, 35*, 409–420.

Lohman, T., & Wright, J. (2004). Maintenance of long-term weight loss: Future directions. *Quest, 56*, 105–119.

Lombard, D. N., Lombard, T. N., & Winett, R. A. (1995). Walking to meet health guidelines: The effect of prompting frequency and prompt structure. *Health Psychology, 14*, 164–179.

Long, B. C. (1991). Physiological and psychological stress recovery of physically fit and unfit women. *Canadian Journal of Behavioral Science, 23*, 53–65.

Long, B. C. (1993). Aerobic conditioning (jogging) and stress inoculation interventions: An exploratory study of coping. *International Journal of Sport Psychology, 24*, 94–109.

Long, B. C., & van Stavel, R. (1995). Effects of exercise training on anxiety: A meta-analysis. *Journal of Applied Sport Psychology, 7*, 167–189.

Lorr, M., McNair, D. M., & Heuchert, J. W. P. (1980/2003). *Profile of Mood States Bi-polar manual supplement.* North Tonawanda, NY: Multi-Health Systems (MHS).

Losse, A., Henderson, S. E., Elliman, D., Hall, D., Knight, E., & Jongmans, M. (1991). Clumsiness in children—Do they grow out of it? A 10-year follow-up study. *Developmental Medicine and Child Neurology, 33*, 55–68.

Loucaides, C. A., Chedzoy, S. M., Bennett, N., & Walshe, K. (2004). Correlates of physical activity in a Cypriot sample of sixth grade children. *Pediatric Exercise Science, 16*, 25–36.

Lovallo, W. R. (2005). *Stress and health: Biological and psychological interactions* (2nd ed.). Thousand Oaks, CA: Sage.

Lox, C.L., McAuley, E., & Tucker, R. (1995). Exercise as an intervention for enhancing subjective well-being on an HIV-1 population. *Journal of Sport and Exercise Psychology, 17*, 345–362.

Lubin, B., & Zuckerman, M. (1999). *Manual for The Multiple Affect Adjective Check List—Revised.* San Diego, CA: Educational and Industrial Testing Service.

Lubin, B., & Van Whitlock, R. V. (1998). A grade four reading level key for the MAACL-R. *Perceptual and Motor Skills, 86*, 119–125.

Lubin, B., Van Whitlock, R. V., & Rea, M. R. (1995). A grade six reading level key for the MAACL-R. *Perceptual and Motor Skills, 81*, 883–889.

Lubin, B., Van Whitlock, R.V., Reddy, D., & Petren, S. (2001). A comparison of the short and long forms of the MAACL-R. *Journal of Clinical Psychology, 57*, 411–416.

Luepker, R., Perry, C., & Mackinlay, S. (1996). Outcomes of a field trial to improve children's dietary patterns and physical activity: The child and adolescent trial for cardiovascular health (CATCH). *Journal of the American Medical Association, 275*, 768–776.

MacKay, D. G., & Abrams, L. (1996). Language, memory and aging: Distributed deficits and the structure of new-versus-old connections. In J. E. Birren, K. W. Schaie, R. P. Abeles, M. Gatz, & T. A. Salthouse (Eds.), *Handbook of the psychology of aging* (4th ed., pp. 251–265). San Diego: Academic Press.

Mackinnon, L. T. (1992). *Exercise and immunology: Current issues in exercise science* (Monograph No. 2). Champaign: Human Kinetics.

Maddux, J. (1997) Health, habit, and happiness. *Journal of Sport and Exercise Psychology, 19*, 331–346.

Maguire, J., & Mansfield, L. (1998). "No-Body's Perfect": Women, aerobics, and the body beautiful. *Sociology of Sport Journal, 15*, 109–137.

Mahler, D. A., Cunningham, L. N., & Curfinan, G. D. (1986). Aging and exercise performance. *Clinical Geriatric Medicine, 2*, 433–452.

Maier, S. F., Watkins, L. R., & Fleshner, M. (1994). Psychoneuroimmunology: The interface between behavior, brain, and immunity. *American Psychologist, 49*, 1004–1017.

Malina, R. (2001). Adherence to physical activity from childhood to adulthood: A perspective from tracking studies. *Quest, 53*, 346–355.

Mandell, A. (1979). The second second wind. *Psychiatric Annals, 9*, 57–68.

Manstead, A. S. R., Frijda, N., & Fischer, A. (Eds.). (2004). *Feelings and emotions: The Amsterdam symposium.* Cambridge: Cambridge University Press.

Marcus, B. H., Banspach, S. W., Lefebvre, R. C., Rossi, J. S., Carelton, R. A. & Abrams, D. B. (1992). Using the stages of change model to increase the adoption of physical activity among community participants. *American Journal of Applied Social Psychology, 24*, 489–508.

Marcus, B. H., Dubbert, P. M., Forsyth, L. H., McKenzie, T. L., Stone, E. J., Dunn, A. L., & Blair, S. N. (2000). Physical activity behavior change: Issues in adoption and maintenance. *Health Psychology, 19*, 42–56.

Marcus, B. H., Emmons, K. M., Simkin-Silverman, L. R., Linnan, L. A., Taylor, E. R., Bock, B. C., Roberts, M. B., Rossi, J. S., & Abrams, D. B. (1998). Evaluation of motivationally tailored vs. standard self-help physical activity interventions at the workplace. *American Journal of Health Promotion, 12*, 246–253.

Marcus, B. H., Pinto, B. M. Simkin, L. R., Audrain, J. E., & Taylor, E. R. (1994). Application of theoretical models to exercise behavior among employed women. *American Journal of Health Promotion, 9*, 49–55.

Marcus, B. H., Rossi, J. S., Selby, V. C., Niaura, R. S., & Abrams, D. B. (1992). The stages and processes of exercise adoption and maintenance in a worksite sample. *Health Psychology, 11*, 386–395.

Marcus, B., Dubbert, P., Forsyth, L., McKenzie, T., Stone, E., Dunn, A., & Blair, S. (2000). Physical activity behavior change: Issues in adoption and maintenance. *Health Psychology, 19*, 32–41.

Marcus, B., Owen, N., Forsyth, L., Cavill, N., & Fridinger, E. (1998). Physical activity interventions using mass media, print media, and information technology. *American Journal of Preventive Medicine, 15*, 362–378.

Markland, D., Emberton, M., & Tallon, R. (1997). Confirmatory factor analysis of the Subjective Exercise Experiences Scale among children. *Journal of Sport & Exercise Psychology, 19*, 418–433.

Markula, P. (1995). Firm but shapely, fit but sexy, strong but thin: The postmodern aerobicizing female bodies. *Sociology of Sport Journal, 12*, 424–453.

Markus, H., & Wurf, E. (1987). The dynamic self-concept: A social psychological perspective. *Annual Review of Psychology, 38*, 299–337.

Maroulakis, E., & Zervas, Y. (1993). Effects of aerobic exercise on mood of adult women. *Perceptual and Motor Skills, 76*, 795–801.

Marsh, H. W. (1990). A multidimensional, hierarchical self-concept:

Theoretical and empirical justification. *Educational Psychology Review, 2,* 77–172.

Marsh, H. W. (1994). The importance of being important: Theoretical models of relations between specific and global components of physical self-concept. *Journal of Sport and Exercise Psychology, 16,* 306–325.

Marsh, H. W. (1997). The measurement of physical self-concept: A construct validation approach. In K. R. Fox (Ed.), *The physical self: From motivation to well-being* (pp. 27–58). Champaign, IL: Human Kinetics.

Marsh, H. W., & Jackson, S. A. (1999). Flow experience in sport: Construct validation of multidimensional, hierarchical state and trait responses. *Structural Equation Modeling, 6,* 343–371.

Marsh, H. W., & Peart, N. (1988). Competitive and cooperative physical fitness programs for girls: Effects on physical fitness and on multidimensional self-concepts. *Journal of Sport and Exercise Psychology, 10,* 390–407.

Marsh, H. W., & Redmayne, R. S. (1994). A multidimensional physical self-concept and its relations to multiple components of physical fitness. *Journal of Sport and Exercise Psychology, 16,* 43–55.

Marsh, H. W., & Shavelson, R. J. (1985). Self-concept: Its multifaceted, hierarchical structure. *Educational Psychologist, 20,* 107–125.

Marsh, H. W., Richards, G., & Barnes, J. (1986a). Multidimensional self-concepts: A long-term follow-up of the effect of participation in an Outward Bound program. *Personality and Social Psychology Bulletin, 12,* 475–492.

Marsh, H. W., Richards, G., & Barnes, J. (1986b). Multidimensional self-concepts: The effect of participation in an Outward Bound program. *Journal of Personality and Social Psychology, 45,* 173–187.

Martin, J. E., & Dubbert, P. M. (1985). Adherence to exercise. *Exercise and Sport Science Reviews, 13,* 137–167.

Martin, J., Dubbert, P. M., Katell, A. D., Thompson, J. K., Raczynski, J. R., Lake, M., Smith, P. O., Webster, J. S., Sikora, T., & Cohen, R. E. (1984). The behavioral control of exercise in sedentary adults: Studies 1 through 6. *Journal of Consulting and Clinical Psychology, 52,* 795–811.

Martin, K. A., Rejeski, W. J., Leary, M. R., McAuley, E., & Bane, S. M. (1997). Is the Social Physique Anxiety Scale really multidimensional? Conceptual and statistical arguments for a unidimensional model. *Journal of Sport and Exercise Psychology, 19,* 359–367.

Martin, M., & Anshel, M. (1991). Attitudes of elite junior athletes on drug-taking behaviors: Implications for drug prevention programs. *Drug Education Journal of Australia, 5,* 223–238.

Martin-Ginnis, K. A., Jung, M., & Gauvin, L. (2003). To see or not to see: The effects of exercising in mirrored environments on sedentary women's feeling states and self-efficacy. *Health Psychology, 22,* 354–361.

Martinsen, E. W. (1993). Therapeutic implications of exercise for clinically anxious and depressed patients. *International Journal of Sport Psychology, 24,* 185–199.

Martinsen, E. W., & Morgan, W. P. (1997). Antidepressant effects of physical activity. In W. P. Morgan (Ed.), *Physical activity and mental health* (pp. 93–106). Washington, DC: Taylor & Francis.

Martinsen, E. W., & Stranghelle, J. K. (1997). Drug therapy and physical activity. In W. P. Morgan (Ed.), *Physical activity and mental health* (pp. 81–90). Washington, DC: Taylor & Francis.

Martinsen, E. W., Hoffart, A., & Solberg, O. (1989). Aerobic and non-aerobic forms of exercise in the treatment of anxiety disorders. *Stress Medicine, 5,* 115–120.

Martinson, B. L., Crain, A. L., Pronk, N. P., O'Connor, P. J., & Maciosek, M. V. (2003). Changes in physical activity and short-term changes in health care changes: A prospective cohort study of older adults. *Preventative Medicine: An International Journal Devoted to Practice and Theory, 37*(4), 319–326.

Maslow, A. H. (1962/1968). *Toward a psychology of being.* Princeton, NJ: D. Van Nostrand.

Maslow, A. H. (1970). *Religions, values, and peak-experiences.* New York: Viking Press.

Maslow, A. H. (1971). *The farther reaches of human nature.* New York: Viking Press.

Masters, K. S. (1992). Hypnotic susceptibility, cognitive dissociation, and runner's high in a sample of marathon runners. *American Journal of Clinical Hypnosis, 34,* 193–201.

Masters, K. S., & Lambert, M. J. (1989). On gender comparison and construct validity: An examination of the commitment to running scale in a sample of marathon runners. *Journal of Sport Behavior, 12,* 196–203.

Matthews, G., Jones, D. M., & Chamberlain, A. G. (1990). Refining the measurement of mood: The UWIST Mood Adjective Checklist. *British Journal of Psychology, 81,* 17–42.

Matthews, K. A. (2005). Psychological perspectives on the development of coronary heart disease. *American Psychologist, 60,* 783–796.

Matthews, K. A., Räikkönen, K., Sutton-Tyrrell, K., & Kuller, L. H. (2004). Optimistic attitudes protect against progression of carotid atherosclerosis in healthy middle-aged women. *Psychosomatic Medicine, 66,* 640–644.

May, J., & Johnson, H. (1973). Psychological activity to internally elicited arousal and inhibitory thoughts. *Journal of Abnormal Psychology, 82,* 239–245.

May, P. (1974). Foreword. In T. Schoop, *Won't you join in the dance?*. Palo Alto, CA: National Press Books.

Mayer, J. D. (2005). Can a new view of personality help integrate personality? *American Psychologist, 60*(4), 294–307.

McArdle, W. D, Katch, F. I., & Katch, V. L. (1996). *Exercise physiology: Energy, nutrition, and human performance* (4th ed.). Baltimore: Williams and Wilkins.

McAuley, E. (1993a). The role of efficacy cognitions in the prediction of exercise behavior in middle-aged adults. *Journal of Behavioral Medicine, 15,* 65–88.

McAuley, E. (1993b). Self-efficacy and the maintenance of exercise participation in older adults. *Journal of Behavioral Medicine, 16,* 103–113.

McAuley, E. (1994). Physical activity and psychosocial outcomes. In C. Bouchard, R.J. Shepherd, & T. Stephens (Eds.), *Physical activity, fitness, and health: International proceedings and consensus statement* (pp. 551–568). Champaign, IL: Human Kinetics.

McAuley, E. K., & Courneya, S. (1994). The subjective exercise experiences scale (SEES): Development and preliminary validation. *Journal of Sport and Exercise Psychology, 16,* 163–177.

McAuley, E., & Blissmer, G. (2002). Self-efficacy and attributional processes in physical activity. In T. Horn (Ed.), *Advances in sport psychology* (2nd ed. pp. 185–206). Champaign, IL: Human Kinetics Press.

McAuley, E., & Blissmer, G. (2003). Self-efficacy and attributional processes in physical activity. In T. Horn (Ed.), *Advances in sport psychology* (2nd ed.). Champaign, IL: Human Kinetics.

McAuley, E., & Courneya, K. (1993) Adherence to exercise and physical activity as health-promoting behaviors: Attitudinal and self-efficacy influence. *Applied and Preventive Psychology, 2,* 65–77.

McAuley, E., & Courneya, K. S. (1992). Self-efficacy relationships with affective and exertion responses to exercise. *Journal of Applied Social Psychology, 22,* 312–326.

McAuley, E., & Courneya, K. S. (1994). The Subjective Exercise Experiences Scale (SEES): Development and preliminary validation. *Journal of Sport & Exercise Psychology, 16,* 67–96, 163–177.

McAuley, E., & Katula, J. (1998). Physical activity interventions in the elderly: Influence on physical health and psychological function. In R. Schulz, M. P. Lawton, & G. Maddux (Eds.), *Annual review of gerontology and geriatrics* (Vol. 18, pp. 115–154). New York: Springer Publishing.

McAuley, E., & Mihalko, S. (1998). Measuring exercise-related self-efficacy. In J. L. Duda (Ed.), *Advances in sport and exercise psychology measurement* (pp. 371–390). Morgantown, WV: Fitness Information Technology.

McAuley, E., & Rudolph, D. (1995). Physical activity, aging, and psychological well-being. *Journal of Aging and Physical Activity, 3,* 67–96.

McAuley, E., Bane, S. M., Rudolf, D. L., & Lox, C. L. (1995). Physique anxiety and exercise in middle-aged adults. *Journal of Gerontology, 5,* 229–235.

McAuley, E., Courneya, K. S., Rudolph, D. L., & Lox, C. L. (1994). Enhancing exercise adherence in middle-aged males and females. *Preventative Medicine, 23,* 498–506.

McAuley, E., Poag, K., Gleason, A., & Wraith, S. (1990). Attrition from exercise programs: Attributional and affective perspectives. *Journal of Social Behavior and Personality, 5,* 591–602.

McAuley, E., Shaffer, S. M., & Rudolph, D. (1995). Affective responses to acute exercise in elderly impaired males: The moderating effects of self-efficacy and age. *International Journal of Aging and Human Development, 41,* 13–27.

McCabe, M.P., Ricciardelli, L.A. (2003). Body image and strategies to lose weight and increase muscle among boys and girls. *Health Psychology, 22,* 39–46.

McCarthy, T. (1981). *The critical theory of Jürgen Habermas.* Cambridge, MA: MIT Press.

McClenney, B. N. (1969). *A comparison of personality characteristics, self-concepts, and academic aptitude of selected college men classified to performance on a test of physical fitness.* Unpublished doctoral dissertation, University of Texas, Austin, TX.

McCrae, R. R., & Costa, P. T., Jr. (1997). Personality trait structure as a human universal. *American Psychologist, 52,* 509–516.

McCullagh, P., Weiss, M. R., & Ross, D. (1989). Modeling considerations in motor skill acquisition and performance: An integrated approach. In K. B. Pandolf (Ed.), *Exercise and sport sciences reviews* (Vol. 17, pp. 475–513). Baltimore: Williams & Wilkins.

McDonald, K., & Thompson, J. K. (1992). Eating disturbance, body image dissatisfaction, and reasons for exercising: Gender differences and correlational findings. *International Journal of Eating Disorders, 11*(3), 289–292.

McElroy, M. (2002). School physical education in crisis. In M. McElroy, *Resistance to exercise: A social analysis of inactivity* (pp. 137–171). Champaign, IL: Human Kinetics.

McEwen, B. S. (1998). Stress, adaptation, and disease—allostasis and allostatic load. *Neuroimmunomodul, 840,* 33–44.

McGuigan, F. J. (1992). *Calm down: A guide to stress and tension control* (2nd ed.). Dubuque, IA: Kendall/Hunt.

McInman, A. D., & Berger, B. G. (1993). Self-concept and mood changes associated with aerobic dance. *Australian Journal of Psychology, 45,* 134–140.

McInman, A. D., & Grove, J. R. (1991). Peak moments in sport: A literature review. *Quest, 43,* 333–351.

McInman, A., & Berger, B. G. (1993). Self-concept and mood changes associated with aerobic dance. *Australian Journal of Psychology, 45,* 134–140.

McKenzie, T. L., & Rushall, B. S. (1974). Effects of self-recording on attendance and performance in a competitive swimming training environment. *Journal of Applied Behavioral Analysis, 7,* 199–206.

McKinney, C. H., Antoni, M. H., Kumar, M., Tims, F. C., & McCabe, P. M. (1997). Effects of guided imagery and music (GIM) therapy on mood and cortisol in healthy adults. *Health Psychology, 16,* 390–400.

McLafferty, C. L., Wetzstein, C. J., & Hunter, G. R. (2004). Resistance training is associated with improved mood in healthy older adults. *Perceptual and Motor Skills, 98*(3), 947–957.

McNair, D. M., & Heuchert, J. W. P. (2003/2005). *Profile of Mood States technical update.* North Tonawanda, NY: Multi-Health Systems (MHS).

McNair, D. M., & Lorr, J. (1980/2003). *POMS bi form.* North Tonawanda, NY: Multi-Health Systems (MHS).

McNair, D. M., Lorr, J., & Droppleman, L. F. (1971/2003). *POMS standard form.* North Tonawanda, NY: Multi-Health Systems (MHS).

McNair, D. M., Lorr, J., & Droppleman, L. F. (1972/1992). *Manual for the Profile of Mood States.* San Diego, CA: EdITS/Educational and Industrial Testing Service.

McNair, D. M., Lorr, J., & Droppleman, L. F. (1989/2003). *POMS brief form.* North Tonawanda, NY: Multi-Health Systems (MHS).

McNair, D. M., Lorr, M., & Droppleman, L. F. (1971). *Manual: Profile of Mood States.* San Diego: Educational and Industrial Testing Service.

McNair, D.M., Lorr, J., & Droppleman, L. F. (1971/1992). *Manual: Profile of Mood States, Revised 1992.* San Diego: Educational and Industrial Testing Service.

McPherson, B. D. (1984). Sport participation across the life cycle: A review of the literature and suggestions for future research. *Sociology of Sport Journal, 1,* 213–230.

Melamed, B. G. (1995). Introduction to the special section: The neglected psychological-physical interface. *Health Psychology, 14,* 371–373.

Melia, P., Pipe, A., & Greenberg, L. (1996). The use of anabolic-androgenic steroids by Canadian students. *Clinical Journal of Sports Medicine, 6,* 9–14.

Melzack, R., & Wall, P. D. (1965). Pain mechanisms: A new theory. *Science, 150,* 971–979.

Merriam-Webster's Collegiate Dictionary (11th ed.). (2003). Springfield, MA: Merriam-Webster.

Merton, T. (1965). *The way of Chuang Tzu.* New York: New Directions.

Middleman, A. B., & DuRant, R. H. (1996). Anabolic steroid use and associated health risk behaviors. *Sports Medicine, 21,* 251–255.

Miller, B. M., Bartholomew, J. B., & Springer, B. A. (2005). Post-exercise affect: The effect of mode preference. *Journal of Applied Sport Psychology, 17,* 263–272.

Miller, J. L., & Levy, G. D. (1996). Gender role conflict, gender-typed characteristics, self-concepts, and sport socialization in female athletes and non-athletes. *Sex Roles: A Journal of Research, 35,* 111–123.

Miller, W. R., & Thoresen, C. E. (1999). Spirituality and health. In W. R. Miller (Ed.), *Integrating spirituality into treatment: Resources for practitioners* (pp. 3–18). Washington, DC: American Psychological Association.

Mischel, W., & Shoda, Y. (1995). A cognitive-affective system theory of personality: Reconceptualizing situations, dispositions, dynamics, and invariance in personality structure. *Psychological Review, 102*(2), 246–268.

Mittelstaedt, R. D., Hinton, J., Rana, S., Cade, D., & Xue, S. (2005). Qigong and the older adult: An exercise to improve health and vitality. *Journal of Physical Education, Recreation, and Dance, 76 (4),* 36–44.

Mobily, K. E. (1987). Leisure, lifestyle, and lifespan. In R. D. MacNeil & M. L. Teague (Eds.), *Aging and leisure: Vitality in later life* (pp. 155–180). Englewood Cliffs, NJ: Prentice-Hall.

Mobily, K. E., Lemke, J. H., Ostiguy, L. J., Woodard, R. J., Griffen, T. I., & Pickens, L. C. (1993). Leisure repertoire in a sample of Midwestern elderly: The case for exercise. *Journal of Leisure Research, 25,* 84–99.

Mokdad, A. H., Serdula, M. K., Dietz, W. H., Bowman, B. A., Marks, J. S., & Koplan, J. P. (1999). The spread of the obesity epidemic in the United States, 1991–1998. *Journal of the American Medical Association, 282,* 1519–1522.

Molloy, D. W., Beerschoten, D. A., Borrie, M. J., Crilly, R. G., & Cape, R. D. T. (1988). Acute effects of exercise on neuropsychological function in elderly subjects. *Journal of the American Geriatrics Society, 36,* 29–33.

Molnar, B. E., Gortmaker, S. L., Bull, F. C., & Buka, S. L. (2004). Unsafe to play? Neighborhood disorder and lack of safety predict reduced physical activity among urban children and adolescents. *American Journal of Health Promotion, 18,* 378–386.

Mom's rule on life jackets saves her young son's life. (2000, June 24). *The Atlanta Journal-Constitution,* p. C7.

Moore, L. L., Lombardi, D. A., White, M. J., Campbell, J. L., Olivera, S. A., & Ellison, R. C. (1991). Influence of parent's physical activity levels on activity levels of young children. *Journal of Pediatrics, 118,* 215–219.

Morgan, B., Woodruff, S. J., & Tiidus, P. M. (2003). Gender differences in aerobic energy expenditure during resistance exercise. *Canadian Journal of Applied Physiology Revue, 20,* 584.

Morgan, K. (2003). Daytime activity and risk factors for late-life insomnia. *Journal of Sleep Research, 12*(3), 231–238.

Morgan, W. P. (1978, November). The mind of the marathoner. *Psychology Today, 11,* 38–40, 43, 45–46, 49.

Morgan, W. P. (1979). Negative addiction in runners. *Physician and Sportsmedicine, 7,* 56–63, 67–70.

Morgan, W. P. (1980). The trait psychology controversy. *Research Quarterly for Exercise and Sport, 51,* 50–76.

Morgan, W. P. (1987). Reduction of state anxiety following acute physical activity. In W. P. Morgan & S. E. Goldston (Eds.), *Exercise and mental health* (pp. 105–109). Washington, DC: Hemisphere.

Morgan, W. P. (Ed.). (1997a). Conclusion: State of the field and future research. In W. P. Morgan (Ed.), *Physical activity and mental health* (pp. 227–232). Washington, DC: Taylor & Francis.

Morgan, W. P. (Ed.). (1997b). *Physical activity and mental health.* Washington, DC: Taylor & Francis.

Morgan, W. P., & Goldston, S. E. (Eds.). (1987). *Exercise and mental health.* New York: Hemisphere.

Morgan, W. P., & Pollack, M. L. (1977). Psychologic characterization of the elite distance runner. *Annals of the New York Academy of Sciences, 301,* 382–403.

Morgan, W. P., Brown, D. R., Raglin, J. S., O'Connor, P. J., & Ellickson, K. A. (1987). Psychological monitoring of overtraining and staleness. *British Journal of Sports Medicine, 21,* 107–114.

Morgan, W. P., Costill, D. L., Flynn, M. G., Raglin, J. S., & O'Connor, P. J. (1988). Mood disturbance following increased training in swimmers. *Medicine and Science in Sports and Exercise, 20,* 408–414.

Morgan, W. P., Horstman, D., Cymerman, A., & Stokes, J. (1983). Facilitation of physical performance by means of a cognitive strategy. *Cognitive Therapy and Research, 7*(3), 251–264.

Morris, W. N. (1989). *Mood: The frame of mind.* New York: Springer-Verlag.

Morris, W. N. (1999). The mood system. In D. Kahneman, E. Diener, & N. Schwarz (Eds.), *Well-being: The foundations of hedonic psychology* (pp. 169–189). New York: Russell Sage Foundation.

Morrow, J. (1988, October). *A cognitive-behavioral interaction for reducing exercise addiction.* Paper presented at the annual meeting of the Association for the Advancement of Applied Sport Psychology, Nashua, NH.

Motl, R. W., & Berger, B. G. (1997). Enjoyment of rock-climbing and recreational swimming: Possible personality influences [Abstract]. *Journal of Applied Sport Psychology, 9* (Suppl.), S134.

Motl, R. W., Berger, B. G., & Davis, S. L. (1997). High-intensity exercise and the acute mood states of trained cyclists. *Journal of Sport & Exercise Psychology, 19* (Suppl.), S91.

Motl, R. W., Berger, B. G., & Leuschen, P. S. (2000). The role of enjoyment in the exercise-mood relationship. *International Journal of Sport Psychology, 31,* 347–363.

Motl, R. W., Berger, B. G., & Wilson, T. E. (1996). Exercise intensity and the acute mood states of cyclists. *Journal of Sport & Exercise Psychology, 18* (Suppl.), S59.

Motl, R. W., Dishman, R. K., Saunders, R., Dowda, M., Felton, G.,

& Pate, R. R. (2001). Measuring enjoyment of physical activity in adolescent girls. *American Journal of Preventative Medicine, 21,* 110–117.

Mroczek, D. K., & Kolarz, C. M. (1998). The effect of age on positive and negative affect: A developmental perspective on happiness. *Journal of Personality and Social Psychology, 75,* 1333–1349.

Mummery, K., Schofield, G., & Caperchione, C. (2002). Physical activity and mental health status in a population of older adults. *Journal of Science and Medicine in Sport, 5* (4), 114.

Mummery, W. K., & Wankel, L. M. (1999). Training adherence in adolescent competitive swimmers: An application of the theory of planned behavior. *Journal of Sport and Exercise Psychology, 21,* 313–328.

Murphy, M. (1972). *Golf in the kingdom.* New York: Viking.

Murphy, M. (1977). Sport as yoga. *Journal of Humanistic Psychology, 17,* 21–23.

Murphy, M. (1992). *The future of the body: Explorations into future evolution of human nature.* New York: G. P. Putnam's Sons.

Murphy, M., & White, R. (1995). *In the zone: Transcendent experience in sports.* New York: Penguin/Arkana.

Mutrie, N. (2005). The somatopsychic rationale revisited. In B. Berger (Chair), *Increasing physical activity in sedentary individuals: In search of the golden fleece.* Symposium conducted at the 11th World Congress of Sport Psychology, Sydney, Australia.

Myers, L., Strikmiller, P. K., Webber, L. S., & Berenson, G. S. (1996). Physical and sedentary activity in school children grades 5–8: The Bogalusa Heart Study. *Medicine and Science in Sports and Exercise, 28,* 852–859.

Nagel, J. J. (1998). Injury and pain in performing musicians: A psychodynamic diagnosis. *Bulletin of the Menninger Clinic, 62,* 83–95.

Nagy, S., & Frazier, S. (1988). The impact of exercise on locus of control, self-esteem and mood states. *Journal of Social Behavior and Personality, 3,* 263–268.

National Center for Health Statistics (Centers for Disease Control and Prevention). Prevalence of Overweight and Obesity among Adults in the United States. Retrieved December 5, 2005, from *http://www.cdc.gov/nchs/products/pubs/pubd/hestats/3and4/over weight.htm.*

National Heart, Lung, and Blood Institute. (1998). *Clinical guidelines on the identification, evaluation, and treatment of overweight and obesity in adults: The evidence report.* Bethesda, MD: National Institutes of Health.

National Institute on Drug Abuse (2000). *Anabolic steroid abuse.* Bethesda, MD: National Institutes of Health.

Nelson, D. L., & Burke, R. J. (Eds.) (2002). *Gender, work stress, and health.* Washington, DC: American Psychological Association.

Nelson, S. (2004). Mind wide open. In G. Battista (Ed.), *The runner's high: Illumination and ecstasy in motion* (pp. 53–58). Halcottsville, NY: Breakaway Books.

Nelson, T. F., & Morgan, W. P. (1994). Acute effects of exercise on mood in depressed female students. *Medicine and Science in Sports and Exercise, 26* (Suppl.), 156.

Netz, Y., & Jacob, T. (1994). Exercise and the psychological state of institutionalized elderly: A review. *Perceptual and Motor Skills, 79,* 1101–1118.

Netz, Y., Wu, M.-J., Becker, B. J., & Tenenbaum, G. (2005). Physical activity and psychological well-being in advanced age: A meta-analysis of intervention studies. *Psychology and Aging, 20,* 272–284.

Neumark-Sztainer, D. S. M., Dixon, L. B., & Murray, D. M. (1998). Adolescents engaging in unhealthy weight control behaviors: Are they at risk for other health-compromising behaviors? *American Journal of Public Health, 88,* 952–955.

Neumark-Sztainer, D. S. M., Faulkner, N. H., Beuring, T., & Resnick, M. (1999). Sociodemographic and personal characteristics of adolescents engaged in weight loss and weight/muscle gain behaviors: Who is doing what? *Preventive Medicine, 28,* 40–50.

Nicholson, N. (1989). The role of drug education. In S. Haynes & M. Anshel (Eds.), *Proceedings of the 1989 National Drugs in Sport Conference: Treating the causes and symptoms* (pp. 48–57). Wollongong, NSW, Australia: University of Wollongong.

Nickerson, R. S. (1998). Applied experimental psychology. *Applied Psychology: An International Review, 47,* 155–173.

Nicol, M. (1993). Hypnosis in the treatment of repetitive strain injury. *Australian Journal of Clinical and Experimental Hypnosis, 21* (special issue), 121–126.

Niemand, D. (1978). *Attitudes about risk and preferences for physical risk and vertigo risk among participants in selected sports.* Unpublished doctoral dissertation, University of Northern Colorado, Greeley, CO.

NIH Consensus Conference. (1996). Physical activity and cardiovascular health. *Journal of the American Medical Association, 276,* 241–246.

Noble, B. J., & Robertson, R. J. (1996). *Perceived exertion.* Champaign, IL: Human Kinetics.

Nolen-Hoeksema, S., & Rusting, C. L. (1999). Gender differences in well-being. In D. Kahneman, E. Diener, & N. Schwarz (Eds.), *Well-being: The foundations of hedonic psychology* (pp. 330–350). New York: Russell Sage Foundation.

Noll, S. M., & Fredrickson, B. L. (1998). A mediational model linking self-objectification, body shame, and disordered eating. *Psychology of Women Quarterly, 22,* 623–636.

North American Society for the Psychology of Sport and Physical Activity. (2004). *NASPSPA Newsletter, 29*(3), 25.

North, T. C., McCullagh, P., & Tran, Z. V. (1990). Effect of exercise on depression. In K. B. Pandolf & J. O. Holloszy (Eds.), *Exercise and sport sciences reviews* (Vol. 18, pp. 379–415). Baltimore: Williams & Wilkins.

North, T. C., McCullaugh, P., & Tran, Z. V. (1990). Effect of exercise on depression. *Exercise & Sport Science Reviews, 18,* 379–415.

Norwegian Confederation of Sports. (1984). *Physical activity in Norway, 1983.* Oslo.

O'Brien, S. J., & Vertinsky, P. A. (1991). Unfit survivors: Exercise as a resource for aging women. *The Gerontologist, 31,* 347–357.

O'Conner, P. J. (1997). Overtraining and staleness. In W. P. Morgan (Ed.), *Physical activity and mental health* (pp.145–160). Washington, DC: Taylor & Francis.

O'Connor, P. J., & Puetz, T. W. (2005). Chronic physical activity and feelings of energy and fatigue. *Medicine and Science in Sports and Exercise, 37,* 299–305.

O'Connor, P. J., & Smith, J. C. (1999). Physical activity and eating disorders. In J. M. Rippe (Ed.), *Lifestyle management* (pp. 1005–1013). Cambridge, MA: Blackwell Science.

O'Connor, P. J., Lewis, R. D., & Kirchner, E. M. (1995). Eating disorders in female college gymnasts. *Medicine and Science in Sports and Exercise, 27,* 550–555.

O'Connor, P. J., Lewis, R. D., Kirchner, E. M., & Cook D. B. (1996). Eating disorders in former college gymnasts: Relations with body composition. *American Journal of Clinical Nutrition, 64,* 840–843.

O'Connor, P. J., Raglin, J. S., & Martinsen, E. W. (2000). Physical activity, anxiety, and anxiety disorders. *International Journal of Sport Psychology, 31,* 136–155.

O'Halloran, P. D., Murphy, G. C., & Webster, K. E. (2004). Mood during a 60-minute treadmill run: Timing and type of mood change. *International Journal of Sport Psychology, 35,* 309–327.

O'Neal, H. A., Dunn, A. L., & Martinsen, E. W. (2000). Depression and exercise. *International Journal of Sport Psychology, 31,* 110–135.

O'Connor, P. J., Bryant, C. X., Veltri, J. P., & Gebhardt, S. M. (1993). State anxiety and ambulatory blood pressure following resistance exercise in females. *Medicine and Science in Sports and Exercise, 25,* 516–521.

Ogilvie, B., & Tutko, T. (1966). *Problem athletes and how to handle them.* London: Pelham Books.

Oishi, S., Diener, E. F., Lucas, R. E., & Suh, E. M. (1999). Cross-cultural variations in predictors of life satisfaction: Perspectives from needs and values. *Personality and Social Psychology Bulletin, 25,* 980–990.

Okwumabua, T. M., Meyers, A. W., Schleser, R., & Cooke, C. J. (1983). Cognitive strategies and running performance: An exploratory study. *Cognitive Therapy and Research, 7*(4), 363–370.

Oldridge, N. B., & Jones, N. L. (1983). Improving patient compliance in cardiac rehabilitation: Effects of written agreement and self-monitoring. *Journal of Cardiac Rehabilitation, 3,* 257–262.

Oldridge, N. B., & Streiner, D. L. (1990). The health belief model: Predicting compliance and dropout in cardiac rehabilitation. *Medicine and Science in Sports and Exercise, 22,* 678–683.

Oldridge, N. B., Donner, A. P., Buck, C. W., Jones, N. L., Andrew, G. M., Parker, J. O., Cunningham, D. A., Kavanagh, T., Rechnitzer, P. A., & Sutton, J. R. (1983). Predictors of dropouts from cardiac exercise rehabilitation: Ontario exercise-heart collaborative study. *American Journal of Cardiology, 51,* 70–74.

Oldridge, N. B., Guyatt, G. H., Fischer, M. E., & Rimm, A. A. (1988). Cardiac rehabilitation after myocardial infarction: Combined experience of randomized clinical trials. *Journal of the American Medical Association, 260,* 945–950.

Olson, J. M., & Zanna, M. P. (1982). *Predicting adherence to a program of physical exercise: An empirical study.* Report to the Government of Ontario, Canada, Ontario Ministry of Tourism and Recreation.

Oman, R. F., & King, A. C. (2000). The effect of life events and exercise program format on the adoption and maintenance of exercise behavior. *Health Psychology, 19,* 605–612.

Oman, R. F., & McAuley, E. (1993). Intrinsic motivation and exercise behavior. *Journal of Health Education, 24,* 232–238.

Ornish, D. (1990). *Dr. Dean Ornish's program for reversing heart disease.* New York: Ballantine.

Osei-Tutu, K. B. & Campagna, P. D. (2005). The effects of short- vs. long-bout exercise on mood, VO_2max, and percent body fat. *Preventive Medicine, 40,* 92–98.

Ostrow, A. C. (1983). Age-role stereotyping—Implications for physical activity participation. In G. D. Rowles & R. J. Ohta (Eds.), *Aging and milieu: Environmental perspectives on growing old* (pp. 153–170). New York: Academic Press.

Ostrow, A. C. (Ed.). (1996). *Directory of psychological tests in the sport and exercise sciences.* Morgantown, WV: Fitness Information Technology, Inc.

Ostrow, A. C., & Dzewaltowski, D. A. (1986). Older adults' perceptions of physical activity participation based on age role and sex role appropriateness. *Research Quarterly for Exercise and Sport, 57,* 167–169.

Owen, N., Leslie, E., Salmon, J., & Fatheringham, M. (2000). Environmental determinants of physical activity and sedentary behavior. *Exercise and Sport Science Reviews, 28,* 153–158.

Paffenbarger, R. S. Jr., & Olsen, E. (1996). *Lifefit: An effective exercise program for optimal health and a longer life.* Champaign, IL: Human Kinetics.

Panzarella, R. (1980). The phenomenology of aesthetic peak experiences. *Journal of Humanistic Psychology, 20,* 69–85.

Parcel, G. S., Simons-Morton, B. G., O'Hara, N. M., Baranowski, T., Kolbe, L. J., & Bee, D. E. (1987). School promotion of healthful diet and exercise behavior: An integration of organizational change and social learning theory interventions. *Journal of School Health, 57,* 150–156.

Parfitt, G., & Easton, R. (1995). Changes in ratings of perceived exertion and psychological affect in the early stages of exercise. *Perceptual and Motor Skills, 80,* 259–266.

Pargman, D. (1999). *Psychological bases of sport injuries* (2nd ed.). Morgantown, WV: Fitness Information Technology.

Pargman, D., & Abry, D. (1997). Scores on emotional self-control of elementary school children after a five-week running program. *Perceptual and Motor Skills, 5,* 694.

Pargman, D., & Baker, M. (1980). Running high: Enkephalin indicted. *Journal of Drug Issues, 10*(3), 341–349.

Pargman, D., Urry, S., & Hutchinson, J. (2000). A model for clarifying psychological mediators of menstrual distress in female athletes. *Science in the Olympic Sports, Special Issue,* 40–45.

Parsons, R. D., Hinson, S. L., & Sardo-Brown, D. (2001). *Educational psychology: A practitioner-researcher model of teaching.* Belmont, CA: Wadsworth/Thomson Learning.

Pate, R. R., Baranowski, T., Dowda, M., & Trost, S. G. (1996). Tracking of physical activity in young children. *Medicine and Science in Sports and Exercise, 28,* 92–96.

Pate, R. R., Heath, G. W., Dowda, M., & Trost, S. G. (1996). Associations between physical activity and other health behaviors in a representative sample of US adolescents. *American Journal of Public Health, 86,* 1577–1581.

Pate, R. R., Long, B. J., & Heath, G. (1994). Descriptive epidemiology of physical activity in adolescents. *Pediatric Exercise Science, 6,* 434–447.

Pate, R. R., Pratt, M., Blair, S. N., Haskell, W. L., Macera, C. A., Bouchard, C., Buchner, D., Ettinger, W., Heath, G. W., King, A. C., Kriska, A., Leon, A. S., Marcus, B. H., Morris, J., Paffenbarger, R. S. Jr., Patrick, K., Pollock, M. L., Rippe, J. M., Sallis, J., & Wilmore, J. H. (1995). Physical activity and public health: A recommendation from the Centers for Disease Control and Prevention and the American College of Sports Medicine. *The Journal of the American Medical Association, 273,* 402–407.

Patel, C. (1973). Yoga and biofeedback in the management of hypertension. *Lancet, ii,* 1053–1055.

Patel, C. (1975a). Yoga and biofeedback in the management of hypertension. *Journal of Psychosomatic Research, 19,* 355–360.

Patel, C. (1975b). Twelve-month follow-up of yoga and biofeedback in the management of hypertension. *Lancet, i,* 62–64.

Patel, D. R., & Roth, A. E. Pediatric athletes with physical disabilities. *Athletic Therapy Today, 9,* 11–15.

Patel, N. (2003). *Total yoga.* San Diego: Thunder Bay.

Pavot, W., & Diener, E. F. (1993). Review of the Satisfaction With Life Scale. *Psychological Assessment, 5,* 164–172.

Pavot, W., Diener, E., Colvin, C. R., & Sandvik, E. (1991). Further validation of the Satisfaction With Life Scale: Evidence for the cross-method convergence of well-being measures. *Journal of Personality Assessment, 57,* 149–161.

Paxton, S. J., Browning, C. J., & O'Connell, G. (1997). Predictors of exercise program participation in older women. *Psychology and Health, 12,* 543–552.

Pedic, F. (1989). Effect on social esteem of nationalistic appeals in corporate image advertisements. *Australian Journal of Psychology, 41,* 37–47.

Pelletier, K. (1977). *Mind as healer, mind as slayer.* New York: Dell.

Peper, E., & Holt, C. F. (1993). *Creating wholeness: A self-healing workbook using dynamic relaxation, images, and thoughts.* New York: Plenum Press.

Perkins, K. A., Dubbert, P. M., Martin, J. E., Faulstich, M. E., & Harris, J. K. (1986). Cardiovascular reactivity to psychological stress in aerobically trained versus untrained mild hypertensives and normotensives. *Health Psychology, 5,* 407–421.

Perri, S., & Templer, D .I. (1984–85). The effects of an aerobic exercise program on psychological variables in older adults. *International Journal of Aging and Human Development, 20,* 167–172.

Peterson, C., & Seligman, M. E. P. (2004). *Character strengths and virtues: A handbook and classification.* Washington, DC: American Psychological Association.

Peterson, S. (1993, December). Qualities to look for in an exercise leader. *Fitness Management, 52,* 32–33.

Petrie, T. A., Diehl, N., Rogers, R. L., & Johnson, C. L. (1996). The Social Physique Anxiety Scale: Reliability and construct validity. *Journal of Sport and Exercise Psychology, 18,* 420–425.

Petruzzello, S. J., & Landers, D. M. (1994). Varying the duration of acute exercise: Implications for changes in affect. *Anxiety, Stress, and Coping, 6,* 301–310.

Petruzzello, S. J., Landers, D. M., Hatfield, B. D., Kubitz, K. A., & Salazar, W. (1991). A meta-analysis on the anxiety reducing effects of acute and chronic exercise: Outcomes and mechanisms. *Sports Medicine, 11,* 142–182.

Petruzzello, S. J., Landers, D. M., Hatfield, B., D., Kubitz, K. A., & Salazar, W. (1991). A meta-analysis on the anxiety-reducing effects of acute and chronic exercise. *Sports Medicine, 11,* 143–182.

Piaget, J. (1954). *The construction of reality in the child* (M. Cook, Trans.). New York: Basic Books.

Piaget, J. (1965). *The moral judgment of the child.* (M. Gabin, Trans.). New York: Free Press. (Original work published 1932).

Pierce, E. F., & Morris, J. T. (1998). Exercise dependence among competitive power lifters. *Perceptual and Motor Skills, 86,* 1097–1098.

Pierce, E. F., & Pate, D. (1994). Mood alterations in older adults following acute exercise. *Perceptual and Motor Skills, 79,* 191–194.

Pierce, E. F., Rohaly, K. A., & Fritchley, B. (1997). Sex differences on exercise dependence for men and women in a marathon road race. *Perceptual and Motor Skills, 84,* 991–994.

Pincivero, D. M., Coelho, A. J., & Campy, R. M. (2004). Gender differences in perceived exertion during fatiguing knee extensions. *Medicine & Science in Sports and Exercise, 36*(2), 109–117.

Pincivero, D. M., Gandaio, C. B., & Ito, Y. (2003). Gender-specific knee extensor torque, flexor torque, and muscle fatigue responses during maximal effort contractions. *European Journal of Applied Physiology and Occupational Physiology, 89,* 134–141.

Plante, T., G., Coscarelli, L., & Ford, M. (2001). Does exercising with another enhance the stress-reducing benefits of exercise? *International Journal of Stress Management, 8,* 201–213.

Plotnikoff, R. C., Brez, S., & Hotz, S. B. (2000). Exercise behavior in a community sample with diabetes: Understanding the determinants of exercise behavioral change. *Diabetes Educator, 26,* 450–459.

Plumert, J. M. (1995). Relations between children's overestimation of their physical abilities and accident proneness. *Developmental Psychology, 31,* 866–876.

Plummer, D. K., & Koh, Y. D. (1987). Effect of "aerobics" on self-concepts of college women. *Perceptual and Motor Skills, 65,* 271–275.

Poag-DuCharme, K. A., & Brawley, L. R. (1994). Perceptions of the behavioral influence of goals: A mediational relationship to exercise. *Journal of Applied Sport Psychology, 6,* 32–50.

Poehlman, E. T., Arciero, P. J., & Goran, M. I. (1994). Endurance exercise in aging humans: Effects on energy metabolism. In J. O. Holloszy (Ed.), *Exercise and sport sciences reviews* (Vol. 22, pp. 251–284). Baltimore: Williams and Wilkins.

Pollock, M. L., Foster, C., Salisbury, R., & Smith, R. (1982). Effects of a YMCA starter fitness program. *Physician and Sportsmedicine, 10,* 89–100.

Pope, H. (2000). *The Adonis Complex: The secret crisis of male body obsession.* New York: Free Press.

Pope, H. G., Katz, D. L., & Hudson, J. I. (1993). Anorexia nervosa and "Reverse Anorexia" among 108 male bodybuilders. *Comprehensive Psychiatry, 34,* 406–409.

Post-White, J. (1991, May). *The effects of mental imagery on emotions, immune function and cancer outcome.* Paper presented to the Fourth World Conference on Imagery, Minneapolis, MN.

Potgieter, J. R., & Venter, R. E. (1995). Relationship between adherence to exercise and scores on extraversion and neuroticism. *Perceptual and Motor Skills, 81,* 520–522.

Power, T. G. (2000). *Play and exploration in children and animals.* Mahwah, NJ: Lawrence Erlbaum Associates.

Powers, P. S., Schocken, D. D., & Boyd, F. F. (1998). Comparison of habitual runners and anorexia nervosa patients. *International Journal of Eating Disorders, 23,* 133–143.

Price, L. E. (1983). *The wonder of motion: A sense of life for woman* (3rd printing). Reston, VA: The American Alliance for Health, Physical Education, Recreation and Dance.

Privette, G. (1964). Factors associated with functioning which transcends model behavior. *Dissertation Abstracts, 25,* 3406.

Privette, G. (1965). Transcendent functioning. *Teachers College Record, 66,* 733–737.

Privette, G. (1968). Transcendent functioning: Full use of potentialities. In H. Otto & J. Mann (Eds.), *Ways of growth: Approaches to expanding awareness* (pp. 213–223). New York: Grossman Press.

Privette, G. (1981). The phenomenology of peak performance in sports. *International Journal of Sport Psychology, 12,* 51–60.

Privette, G. (1982). Peak performance in sports: A factorial topology. *International Journal of Sport Psychology, 13,* 242–249.

Privette, G. (1983). Peak experience, peak performance and flow: A comparative analysis of positive human experiences. *Journal of Personality and Social Psychology, 45,* 1361–1368.

Privette, G. (1984). *Questionnaire: Peak performance and peak experience.* Pensacola, FL: University of West Florida.

Privette, G., & Bundrick, C. M. (1987). Measurement of experience: Construct and content validity of the Experience Questionnaire. *Perceptual and Motor Skills, 65,* 315–332.

Privette, G., & Bundrick, C. M. (1989). Effects of triggering activity on construct events: Peak performance, peak experience, flow, average events, misery, and failure. *Journal of Social Behavior and Personality, 4,* 299–306.

Privette, G., & Bundrick, C. M. (1991). Peak experience, peak performance, and flow: Correspondence of personal descriptions and theoretical constructs. *Journal of Social Behavior and Personality, 6,* 169–188.

Privette, G., & Bundrick, C. M. (1997). Psychological processes of peak, average, and failing performance in sport. *International Journal of Sport Psychology, 28,* 323–334.

Privette, G., & Landsman, T. (1983). Factor analysis of peak performance: The full use of potential. *Journal of Personality and Social Psychology, 44,* 195–200.

Prochaska, J. J., Sallis, J. F., Slymen, D. J., & McKenzie, T. L. (2003). A longitudinal study of children's enjoyment of physical education. *Pediatric Exercise Science, 15,* 170–178.

Prochaska, J. O., & DiClemente, C. C. (1983). Stages and processes of self-change of smoking: Toward an integrative model of change. *Journal of Consulting & Clinical Psychology, 51,* 390–395.

Prochaska, J. O., & DiClemente, C. C. (1986). Toward a comprehensive model of change. In W. R. Miller & N. Heather (Eds.), *Testing addictive behaviors*: *Processes of change* (pp. 3–27). New York: Plenum.

Prochaska, J. O., & Velicer, W. F. (1997). Misinterpretations and misapplications of the transtheoretical model. *American Journal of Health Promotion, 12,* 11–12.

Prochaska, J. O., DiClemente, C. C., & Norcross, J. C. (1992). In search of how people change. *America Psychologist, 47,* 1102–1114.

Prochaska, J. O., Norcross, J. C., & DiClemente, C. C. (1994). *Changing for good.* New York: William Morrow.

Prochaska, J. O., Velicer, W. F., DiClemente, C. C., & Fava, J. (1988). Measuring processes of change: Application to the cessation of smoking. *Journal of Consulting and Clinical Psychology, 56,* 520–528.

Prochaska, J., & Velicer, W. (1997). The transtheoretical model of health behavior change. *American Journal of Health Promotion, 12,* 38–48.

Pronk, N. P., Crouse, S. F., & Rohack, J. J. (1995). Maximal exercise and acute mood response in women. *Physiology and Behavior, 57,* 1–4.

Pucher, J., & Lefevre, C. (1996). *The urban transportation crisis in Europe and North America.* London: Macmillan.

Puggaard, L. (2003). Effects of training on functional performance in 65, 75, 85 year old women: Experience deriving from community based studies in Odense, Denmark. *Scandinavian Journal of Medicine and Science in Sports, 13*(1), 70–76.

Raglin, J. S. (1997). Anxiolytic effects of physical activity. In W. P. Morgan (Ed.), *Physical activity and mental health* (pp. 107–126). Washington, DC: Taylor & Francis.

Raglin, J. S., & Morgan, W. P. (1987). Influence of exercise and quiet rest on state anxiety and blood pressure. *Medicine and Science in Sports and Exercise, 19,* 456–463.

Rahe, R. H. (1990). Life change, stress responsivity, and captivity research. *Psychosomatic Medicine, 52,* 373–396.

Rainey, C. J., McKeow, R. E., Sargent, R. G., & Valois, R. F. (1998). Adolescent athleticism, exercise, body image, and dietary practices. *American Journal of Health Behavior, 22,* 193–205.

Rapid increase in the prevalence of obesity in elementary school children. *International Journal of Obesity, 28,* 494–499.

Rappaport, J. (1981). In praise of paradox: A social policy of empowerment over prevention. *American Journal of Community Psychology, 9,* 1–25.

Redding, C., & Rossi, J. (1999). Testing a model of situational self-efficacy for safer sex among college students: Stages of change and gender-based differences. *Psychology and Health, 14,* 467–486.

Reel, J. J., & Gill, D. L. (1996). Psychological factors related to eating disorders among high school and college female cheerleaders. *The Sport Psychologist, 10,* 195–206.

Rejeski, W .J., Gauvin, L., Hobson, M. L., & Norris, J. L. (1995). Effects of baseline responses, in-task feelings, and duration of activity on exercise-induced feeling states in women. *Health Psychology, 14,* 350–359.

Rejeski, W. J. (1994). Dose-response issues from a psychological perspective. In C. Bouchard, R. J. Shephard, & T. Stephens (Eds.), *Physical activity, fitness, and health: International proceedings and consensus statement* (pp. 1040–1053). Champaign, IL: Human Kinetics.

Rejeski, W. J., Gregg, E., Thompson, A., & Berry, M. (1991). The effects of varying doses of acute aerobic exercise on psychophysiological stress responses in highly trained cyclists. *Journal of Sport and Exercise Psychology, 13,* 188–199.

Rejeski, W. J., Thompson, A., Brubaker, P. H., & Miller, H. S. (1992). Acute exercise: Buffering psychosocial stress responses in women. *Health Psychology, 11,* 355–362.

Remington, N. A., Fabrigar, L. R., & Visser, P. S. (2000). Reexamining the circumplex model of affect. *Journal of Personality & Social Psychology, 79,* 286–300.

Rhodewalt, F., & Zone, J. B. (1989). Appraisal of life change, depression, and illness in hardy and nonhardy women. *Journal of Personality and Social Psychology, 56,* 81–88.

Ricciardelli, L. A., & McCabe, M. P. (2001). Children's eating concerns and eating disturbances: A review of the literature. *Clinical Psychology Review, 21,* 325–244.

Richman, J. M., Rosenfeld, L. B., & Hardy, C. J. (1993). The Social Support Survey: An initial evaluation of a clinical measure and practice model of the social support process. *Research on Social Work Practice, 3,* 288–311.

Riddoch, C. J., Andersen, L. B., Wedderkopp, N., Harrow, M., Klasson-Heggeboe, L., Sardinah, L. B., Cooper, A. R., & Ekelund, U. (2004). Physical activity levels and patterns of 9 and 15 year old European children. *Medicine and Science in Sports and Exercise, 36,* 86–92.

Riggs, C. E. (1981). Endorphins, neurotransmitters, and/or neuromodulators and exercise. In M. H. Sacks & M. L. Sachs (Eds.), *Psychology of running* (pp. 224–230). Champaign, IL: Human Kinetics.

Rippere, V. (1977). "What's the thing to do when you're feeling depressed?"—A pilot study. *Behaviour Research and Therapy, 15,* 185–191.

Robbins, R. W., Noffle, E. E., Trzesniewski, K. H., & Roberts, B. W. (2005). Do people know how their personality has changed? Correlates of perceived and actual personality change in young adulthood. *Journal of Personality, 73*(2), 489–521.

Roberts, B. W. (1997). Plaster or plasticity: Are work experiences associated with personality change in women? *Journal of Personality, 65*, 205–232.

Roberts, B. W., Robbins, R. W., Caspi, A., & Trzeniewski, K. (2003). Personality trait development in adulthood. In J. Mortimer & M. Shanahan (Eds.), *Handbook of the Life Course* (pp. 579–598). New York: Klewer Academic.

Roberts, B. W., Wood, D, & Smith, J. L. (2005). Evaluating five factor theory and social investment perspectives on personality trait development. *Journal of Research in Personality, 39*(10), 166–184.

Robertson, R. J., & Noble, B. J. (1997). Perception of physical exertion: Methods, mediators, and applications. *Exercise and Sport Science Review, 25*, 407–452.

Rodgers, W. M., & Brawley, L. R. (1996). The influence of outcome expectancy and self-efficacy on the behavioral intentions of novice exercisers. *Journal of Applied Social Psychology, 26*, 618–634.

Rogers, R. (1990). Development of a new classification model of malingering. *Bulletin of the American Academy of Psychiatry and the Law, 18*, 323–333.

Romeo, F. F. (1993). Anorexia nervosa on college campuses. *College Student Journal, 27*, 437–440.

Rook, K. S. (1992). Detrimental aspects of social relationships: Taking stock of an emerging literature. In H. O. F. Veiel & U. Baumann (Eds.), *The meaning and measurement of social support* (pp. 157–169). New York: Hemisphere Publishing.

Rosch, P. J. (1986). Forword. In J. H. Humphrey (Ed.), *Human stress: Current selected research* (Vol. 1, pp. ix–xi). New York: AMS Press.

Rose, B., Larkin, D., & Berger, B. G. (1994). Perceptions of social support in children of low, moderate, and high levels of coordination. *ACHPER Healthy Lifestyles Journal, 41*, 18–21.

Rose, B., Larkin, D., & Berger, B. G. (1997). Coordination and gender influences on the perceived competence of children. *Adapted Physical Activity Quarterly, 14*, 210–221.

Rosenbaum, P. (1998). Physical activity play in children with disabilities: A neglected opportunity for research? *Child Development, 69*, 607–608.

Rosenstock, I. M. (1974). Historical origins of the health belief model. *Health Education Monographs, 2*, 328–335.

Rosenthal-Malek, A., & Mitchell, S. (1997). Brief report: The effects of exercise on the self-stimulatory behaviors and positive responding of adolescents with autism. *Journal of Autism and Developmental Disorders, 27*, 193–202.

Roskies, E., Seraganian, P., Oseasohn, R., Hanley, J. A., Collu, R., Martin, N., & Smilga, C. (1986). The Montreal Type A intervention project: Major findings. *Health Psychology, 5*, 45–69.

Ross, C. (2000). Walking, exercising, and smoking: Does neighborhood matter? *Social Science and Medicine, 51*, 265–274.

Ross, C. E., & Hayes, D. (1988). Exercise and psychologic well-being in the community. *American Journal of Epidemiology, 127*, 762–771.

Ross, J. G., & Gilbert, G. G. (1985). The National Children and Youth Fitness Study: A summary of findings. *Journal of Physical Education, Recreation and Dance, 56*, 45–50.

Ross, J. G., Dotson, C. O., Gilbert, G. G., & Katz, S. J. (1985). The National Children and Youth Fitness Study: Physical activity outside of physical education programs. *Journal of Physical Education, Recreation and Dance, 56*, 35–39.

Rostad, F. G., & Long, B. C. (1996). Exercise as a coping strategy for stress: A review. *International Journal of Sport Psychology, 27*, 197–222.

Rotella, R. J., Ogilvie, B. C., & Perrin, D. H. (1999). The malingering athlete: Psychological considerations. In D. Pargman (Ed.), *Psychological bases of sport injury* (2nd ed., pp. 111–122). Morgantown, WV: Fitness Information Technology.

Roth, D. L. (1989). Acute emotional and psychophysiological effects of aerobic exercise. *Psychophysiology, 26*, 593–602.

Roth, D. L., Wiebe, D. J., Fillingim, R. B., & Shay, K. A. (1989). Life events, fitness, hardiness, and health: A simultaneous analysis of proposed stress-resistance effects. *Journal of Personality and Social Psychology, 57*, 136–142.

Rothermund, K., & Meninger, C. (2004). Stress-buffering effects of self-complexity: Reduced affective spillover or self-regulatory processes? *Self and Identity, 3*(3), 263–281.

Rowlinson, R. T., & Felner, R. D. (1988). Major life events, hassles, and adaptation in adolescence: Confounding in the conceptualization and measurement of life stress and adjustment revisited. *Journal of Personality and Social Psychology, 55*, 432–444.

Roy, M., & Steptoe, A. (1991). The inhibition of cardiovascular responses to mental stress following aerobic exercise. *Psychophysiology, 28*, 689–700.

Rudman, R. J. (1986). Life course socioeconomic transitions and sport involvement: A theory of restricted opportunity. In B. D. McPherson (Ed.), *Sport and aging* (pp. 25–35). Champaign, IL: Human Kinetics.

Rudolph, D. L., & Kim, J. G. (1996). Mood responses to recreational sport and exercise in a Korean sample. *Journal of Social Behavior and Personality, 11*, 841–849.

Russell, J. A., & Carroll, J. M. (1999). On the bipolarity of positive and negative affect. *Psychological Bulletin, 125*, 3–30.

Ruuskanen, J., & Puoppila, I. (1995). Physical activity and psychological well-being among people aged 64–85 years. *Age and Aging, 24*, 292–296.

Ryska, T. A. (1998). Cognitive-behavioral strategies and precompetitive anxiety among recreational athletes. *Psychological Record, 48*, 697–708.

Sachs, M. L. (1980). *On the tail of the runner's high: A descriptive and experimental investigation of characteristics of an elusive phenomenon.* Unpublished doctoral dissertation, Florida State University.

Sachs, M. L. (1984). The mind of the runner: Cognitive strategies used during running. In M. L. Sachs & G. W. Buffone (Eds.), *Running as therapy: An integrated approach* (pp. 288–303). Lincoln, NE: University of Nebraska Press.

Sachs, M. L. (1984). The runner's high. In M. L. Sachs & G. W. Buffone (Eds.), *Running as therapy* (pp. 273–287). Lincoln, NE: Nebraska University Press.

Sachs, M. L. (1997). The runner's high. In M. L. Sachs & G. W. Buffone (Eds.), *Running as therapy: An integrated approach* (pp. 273–287). Lincoln, NE: University of Nebraska Press.

Sachs, M. L., & Buffone, G. W. (Eds.) (1984). *Running as therapy: An integrated approach.* Lincoln, NE: University of Nebraska Press.

Sachs, M. L., & Buffone, G. W. (Eds.). (1997). *Running as therapy: An integrated approach.* Northvale, NJ: Jason Aronson.

Sachs, M. L., & Pargman, D. (1984). Running addiction, In M. L. Sachs & G. W. Buffone (Eds.), *Running as therapy: An integrated approach* (pp. 231–253). Lincoln, NE: University of Nebraska Press.

Sacks, M. H., & Sachs, M. L. (Eds.). (1981). *Psychology of running.* Champaign, IL: Human Kinetics.

Sallis, J. F. (1993). Epidemiology of physical activity and fitness in children and adolescents. *Critical Reviews in Food, Science and Nutrition, 33*, 405–408.

Sallis, J. F. (2000). Age-related decline in physical activity: A synthesis of human and animal studies. *Medicine and Science in Sports and Exercise, 32*, 1598–1600.

Sallis, J. F. (2000). Environmental influences on physical activity: Applying ecological models. *Journal of Sport and Exercise Psychology, 22*, S1.

Sallis, J. F., & Hovell, M. F. (1990). Determinants of exercise behavior. *Exercise and Sport Science Review, 18*, 307–330.

Sallis, J. F., & Owen, N. (1999). *Physical activity and behavioral medicine.* Thousands Oaks, CA: Sage.

Sallis, J. F., Calfas, K. J., Alcaraz, J. E., Gehrman, C., & Johnson, M. F. (1999). Potential mediators of change in a physical activity promotion course for university students: Project GRAD. *Annals of Behavioral Medicine, 21*, 149–158.

Sallis, J. F., Haskell, W. F., Fortmann, S. P., Vranzan, K. M., Taylor, C. B., & Solomon, D. S. (1986). Predictors of adoption and maintenance of physical activity in a community sample. *Preventive Medicine, 15*, 331–341.

Sallis, J. F., Hovell, M. F., Hofstetter, C. R., & Barrington, E. (1992). Explanation of vigorous physical activity during two years using social learning variables. *Social Science & Medicine, 34*, 25–32.

Sallis, J. F., Hovell, M. F., Hofstetter, C. R., Faucher, P., Elder, J. P., Blanchard, J., Caspersen, C. J., Powell, K. E., & Christenson, G. M. (1989). A multivariate study of determinants of vigorous exercise in a community sample. *Preventive Medicine, 18*, 20–34.

Sallis, J. F., Howell, M. F., Hofstetter, C. R., Elder, J. P., Hackley, M., Caspersen, C. J., & Powell, K. E. (1990). Distance between homes and exercise facilities related to frequency of exercise among San Diego residents. *Public Health Reports, 105*, 179–180.

Sallis, J. F., Johnson, M. F., Calfas, K. J., Caparosa, S., & Nicholls, J. F. (1997). Assessing perceived physical environmental variables that may influence physical activity. *Research Quarterly for Exercise and Sport, 68*, 345–351.

Sallis, J. F., Prochaska, J. J., Taylor, W. C., Hill, J. O., & Geraci, J. C. (1999). Correlates of physical activity in a national sample of girls and boys in grades 4 through 12. *Health Psychology, 18*, 410–415.

Sallis, J., Prochaska, J., Taylor, W., Hill, J., & Geraci, J.C. (1999). Correlates of physical activity in a national sample of girls and boys in grades 4 through 12. *Health Psychology, 18*, 410–415.

Salmon, J., Owen, N., Crawford, D., Bauman, A., & Sallis, J. F. (2003). Physical activity and sedentary behavior: A population-based study of barriers, enjoyment, and preference. *Health Psychology, 22*, 178–188.

Salusso-Deonier, C. J., & Schwartzkopf, R. J. (1991). Sex differences in body-cathexis associated with exercise involvement. *Perceptual and Motor Skills, 73*, 139–145.

Sanborn, C., Horea, M., Siemers, B., & Dieringer, K. (2000). Disordered eating and the female athlete triad. *Clinics in Sports Medicine, 19*, 199–213.

Sanford-Martens, T., Davidson, M., Yakushko, O., Martens, M., Hinton, P., & Beck, N. (2005). Clinical and subclinical eating disorders: An examination of collegiate athletes. *Journal of Applied Sport Psychology, 17*, 79–86.

Sarason, I. G. (1980). Life stress, self-occupation, and social supports. In I. G. Sarason & C. D. Spielberger (Eds.), *Stress and anxiety* (Vol. 7, pp. 73–92). Washington, DC: Hemisphere.

Sarason, I. G., Johnson, J. H., & Siegel, J. M. (1978). Assessing the impact of life changes: Development of the Life Experiences Survey. *Journal of Consulting and Clinical Psychology, 46*, 932–946.

Sarason, I. G., Sarason, B. R., & Pierce, G. R. (1990). Social support, personality and performance. *Journal of Applied Sport Psychology, 2*, 117–127.

Satariano, W. A., Haight, F. J., & Tager, I. B. (2000). Reasons given by older people for limitation or avoidance of leisure time physical activity. *Journal of American Geriatrics Society, 48*, 505–512.

Saunders, R. P., Pate, R. R., Felton, G., Dowda, M., Weinrich, M. C., Ward, D. S., Parsons, M. A., & Baranowski, T. (1997). Development of questionnaires to measure psychosocial influences on children's physical activity. *Preventive Medicine, 26*, 241–247.

Scanlan, T. K., & Simons, J. P. (1992). The construction of sport enjoyment. In G. C. Roberts (Ed.), *Motivation in sport and exercise* (pp. 199–215). Champaign, IL: Human Kinetics.

Scanlan, T. K., Stein, G. L., & Ravizza, K. (1989). An in-depth study of former elite figure skaters: II. Sources of enjoyment. *Journal of Sport & Exercise Psychology, 11*, 65–83.

Schaie, K. W., & Lawton, M. P. (1998). Preface. In K. W. Schaie & M. P. Lawton (Eds.), *Annual review of gerontology and geriatrics: Focus on emotion and adult development.* (Vol. 17, pp. xi–xvi). New York: Springer.

Scheibel, A. B. (1996). Structural and functional changes in the aging brain. In J. E. Birren, K. W. Schaie, R. P. Abeles, M. Gatz, & T. A. Salthouse (Eds.), *Handbook of the psychology of aging* (4th ed., pp. 105–128). San Diego: Academic Press.

Scherf, J., & Franklin, B. (1987). Exercise compliance: A data documentation system. *Journal of Physical Education, Recreation, and Dance, 58*, 26–28.

Schimmack, U., Oishi, S., Diener, E., & Suh, E. (2000). Facets of affective experiences: A framework for investigations of trait affect. *Personality and Social Psychology Bulletin, 26*, 655–668.

Schmitz, K. L. (1979). Sport and play: Suspension of the ordinary. In E. W. Gerber & W. J. Morgan (Eds.), *Sport and the body: A philosophical symposium* (2nd ed., pp. 22–29). Philadelphia: Lea & Febiger.

Schnirring, L. (1998). ACSM makes exercise advice more flexible: Fitness recommendations updated. *The Physician and Sportsmedicine, 26*, 16–17.

Schoenborn, C. A., & Barnes, P. M. (2002). Leisure-time physical activity among adults: Advanced Statistics from Vital and Health Statistics No. 325, April 7, 2002. United States, 1997–1998.

Schomer, H. H. (1986). Mental strategies and perceptions of effort of marathon runners. *International Journal of Sport Psychology, 17*, 41–59.

Schomer, H. H. (1987). Mental strategies programme for marathon runners. *International Journal of Sport Psychology, 18*, 133–151.

Schuler, P. B., Broxon-Hutcherson, A., Philipp, S. F., Isosaari, R. M., & Robinson, D. (2004). Body-shape perceptions in older-adults and motivations for exercise. *Perceptual and Motor Skills, 98*(3), 1251–1260.

Schultheis, S.F., Boswell, B.B., & Decker, J. (2000). Succesful physical activity programming

Schwartzer, R., & Leppin, A. (1989). Social support and health: A meta-analysis. *Psychology and Health: An International Journal, 3*, 1–15.

Scott, J. (1971). *The athletic revolution.* New York: The Free Press.

Seals, D. R., & Hagberg, J. M. (1984). The effect of exercise training on human hypertension: A review. *Medicine and Science in Sports and Exercise, 18*, 207–215.

Seaward, B. L. (1997a). *Managing stress: Principles and strategies for health and well-being* (2nd ed.). Boston: Jones & Bartlet.

Seaward, B. L. (1997b). *Stand like mountain—Flow like water: Reflections on stress and human spirituality.* Deerfield Beach, FL: Health Communications.

Sedula, M. K., Collins, M. E., & Williamson, D. F. (1993). Weight control practices of United States adolescents and adults. *Annals of Internal Medicine, 119*, 667–671.

Segerstrom, S. C., Taylor, S. E., Kemeny, M. E., & Fahey, J. L. (1998). Optimism is associated with mood, coping and immune change in response to stress. *Journal of Personality and Scial Psychology, 74*, 1646–1655.

Seligman, M. E. P. (2002). *Authentic happiness: Using the new positive psychology to realize your potential for lasting fulfillment.* New York: Free Press.

Selye, H. (1950). *Stress.* Montreal: Acta.

Selye, H. (1956). *The stress of life.* New York: McGraw-Hill.

Selye, H. (1975). *Stress without distress.* New York: Signet.

Sevcikova, L., Ruzanska, S., & Sablova, M. (2000). Neuroticism, physical activity, and nutritional habits in school children. *Homeostasis in Health and Disease, 40*, 143–144.

Sharp, P. A., Clark, N. M., & Janz, N. K. (1991). Differences in the impact and management of heart disease between older women and men. *Women and Health, 17,* 25–43.

Shavelson, R. J., Hubner, J. J., & Stanton, G. C. (1976). Validation of construct interpretations. *Review of Educational Research, 46,* 407–441.

Sheehan, G. (1978). *Running & being: The total experience.* New York: Simon and Schuster.

Sheehan, G. (1979). Negative addiction: A runner's perspective. *Physician and Sportsmedicine, 7,* 49.

Sheehan, G. (1984). Today's contemplative. *The Physician and Sportsmedicine, 12* (7), 37.

Sheehan, G. (1990). The ages of a runner. *Annals of Sports Medicine, 5,* 210.

Sheehan, G. (1992a). *Dr. George Sheehan on getting fit and feeling great.* New York: Wings.

Sheehan, G. (1992b). *Getting fit and feeling great.* New York: Wings Books.

Sheehan, G. (1995, September). The road to self-discovery. *Runner's World,* 18.

Shepherd, R. J. (1987). *Physical activity and aging.* London: Croom Helm.

Shepherd, R. J. (1996a). Habitual physical activity and academic performance. *Nutritional Reviews, 54,* S32–56.

Shepherd, R. J. (1996b). Habitual physical activity and quality of life. *Quest, 48,* 354–365.

Sheppard, B. H., Hartwick, J., & Warshaw, P. R. (1988). The theory of reasoned action: A meta-analysis of past research with recommendations for modification and future research. *Journal of Consumer Research, 15,* 325–343.

Silva, J. M., III, & Applebaum, M. I. (1989). Association-dissociation patterns of United States Olympic marathon trial contestants. *Cognitive Therapy and Research, 13*(2), 185–192.

Simoes, E. J., Byers, T., Coates, R. J., & Serdula, M. K. (1995). The association between leisure-time physical activity and dietary fat in American adults. *American Journal of Public Health, 85,* 240–244.

Simons-Morton, D. G., Simons-Morton, B. G., Parcel, G. S., & Bunker, J. F. (1988). Influencing personal and environmental conditions for community health: A multilevel intervention model. *Family and Community Health, 11,* 25–35.

Simons-Morton, D., Calfas, K., Oldernbuurg, B., & Burton, N. (1998). Effects of interventions in health care settings on physical activity or cardiorespiratory fitness. *American Journal of Preventive Medicine, 15,* 413–430.

Simpson, H. M., & Pavio, A. (1966). Changes in pupil size during an imagery task without motor involvement. *Psychonomic Science, 5,* 405–406.

Sinaki, M., Nwaogwugwu, N. C., Phillips, B. E., & Mokri, M. P. (2001). Effect of gender, age, and anthropometry on axial and appendicular muscle strength. *American Journal of Physical Medicine and Rehabilitation, 80*(5), 330–338.

Sinden, A. R., Ginis, K. A. M., & Angove, J. (2003). Older women's reactions to revealing and nonrevealing exercise attire. *Journal of Aging and Physical Activity, 11* (4), 445–458.

Singer, R. N. (1972). *Coaching, athletics, and psychology.* New York: McGraw-Hill.

Singer, R. N. (1996). Moving toward the quality of life. *Quest, 48,* 246–252.

Singh, N. A., Clements, K. M., & Fiatarone, M. A. (1997). A randomized controlled trial of progressive resistance training in depressed elders. *Journal of Gerontology: Series A: Biological Sciences & Medical Sciences, 52A,* M27–M35.

Sinyor, D., Golden, M., Steinert, Y., & Seraganian, P. (1986). Experimental manipulation of aerobic fitness and the response to psychosocial stress: Heart rate and self-report measures. *Psychosomatic Medicine, 48,* 324–337.

Sinyor, D., Schwartz, S. G., Peronnet, F., Brisson, G., & Seraganian, P. (1983). Aerobic fitness level and reactivity to psychosocial

stress: Physiological, biochemical, and subjective measures. *Psychosomatic Medicine, 65,* 205–217.

Slavin, L., & Lee, C. (1994). Psychological effects of exercise among adult women: The impact of menopausal status. *Psychology and Health, 9,* 297–303.

Slowikowski, S. S., & Loy, J. W. (1993). Ancient athletic motifs and the modern Olympic games. In A. G. Ingham & J. W. Loy (Eds.), *Sport in social development* (pp. 21–49). Champaign, IL: Human Kinetics.

Sluiter, J. K., Frings-Dresen, M. H. W., Meijman, T. F., & van der Beek, A. J. (2000). Reactivity and recovery from different types of work measured by catecholamines and cortisol: A systematic literature overview. *Occupational & Environmental Medicine, 57,* 298–315.

Smith, A. D. (1996). Memory. In J. E. Birren, K. W. Schaie, R. P. Abeles, M. Gatz, & T. A. Salthouse (Eds.), *Handbook of the psychology of aging* (4th ed., pp. 236–250). San Diego: Academic Press.

Smith, A. M. (1996). Psychological impact of athletic injuries. *Sports Medicine, 22(6),* 391–405.

Smith, D., & Hale, B. (2004). Validity and factor structure of the bodybuilding dependence scale. *British Journal of Sports Medicine, 38,* 177–181.

Smith, J. C. (2001). (Ed.). *Advances in ABC relaxation: Application and inventories.* New York: Springer.

Smith, P. F., & Remington, P. L. (1989). The epidemiology of drinking and driving: Results from the Behavioral Risk Factor Surveillance System, 1986. *Health Education Quarterly, 16,* 345–358.

Smith, R. A., & Biddle, S. J. H. (1995). Psychological factors in the promotion of physical activity. In S. Biddle (Ed.), *European perspectives on exercise and sport psychology.* Champaign, IL: Human Kinetics.

Smith, T. W., & Williams, P. G. (1992). Personality and health: Advantages and limitations of the five-factor model. *Journal of Personality, 60,* 395–423.

Smolak, L., Levine, M. P., & Schermer, F. (1999). Parental input and weight concerns among elementary school children. *International Journal of Eating Disorders, 25,* 263–271.

Snooks, M. K., & Hall, S. K. (2002). Relationship of body size, body image, and self-esteem in African American, European American, and Mexican American middle-class women. *Health Care for Women International, 23*(5), 460–466.

Snyder, G., Franklyn, B., Foss, M., & Rubenfire, N. (1982). Characteristics of compliers and non-compliers to cardiac exercise therapy programs [abstract]. *Medicine and Science in Sports and Exercise, 14,* 179.

Solomon, E. G., & Bumpus, A. K. (1981). The running meditation response: An adjunct to psychotherapy. In M. H. Sacks & M. L. Sachs (Eds.), *Psychology of running* (pp. 40–49). Champaign, IL: Human Kinetics Publishers.

Solomon, L. J., & Rothblum, E. D. (1986). Stress, coping, and social support in women. *Behavior Therapist, 9,* 199–204.

Song, K., & Ah, J. (2004). Premotor and motor reaction time of educable mentally retarded youths in a Taekwondo program. *Perceptual and Motor Skills, 99,* 711–723.

Sonstroem, R. J. (1984). Exercise and self-esteem. *Exercise and Sport Sciences Reviews, 12,* 123–155.

Sonstroem, R. J. (1988). Psychological models. In R. K. Dishman (Ed.), *Exercise adherence* (pp. 125–154). Champaign, IL: Human Kinetics.

Sonstroem, R. J. (1997). The physical self-system: A mediator of exercise and self-esteem. In K. Fox (Ed.), *The physical self: From motivation to well being* (pp. 3–26). Champaign, IL: Human Kinetics.

Sonstroem, R. J. (1998). Physical self-concept: Assessment and external validity. *Exercise and Sport Sciences Reviews, 26,* 133–164.

Sonstroem, R. J., Harlow, L. L., & Josephs, L. (1994). Exercise and self-esteem: Validity of model expansion and exercise associations. *Journal of Sport and Exercise Psychology, 16*, 24–42.

Sorenson, M., Anderssen, S., Hjerman, I., Holme, X., & Ursin, H. (1997). Exercise and diet interventions improve perceptions of self in middle-aged adults. *Scandinavian Journal of Medicine and Science in Sports, 7*, 312–320.

Sothmann, M. S. (1991). Catecholamines, behavioral stress, and exercise—introduction to the symposium. *Medicine and Science in Sports and Exercise, 23*, 836–867.

Sovik, R. (1997a, July). Breath awareness: When mindfulness meets concentration. *Yoga International, 36*, 51–54.

Sovik, R. (1997b, November). Breathe easy: Untie your breath. *Yoga International, 38*, 57–60.

Spalding, T. W., Lyon, L. A., Steel, D. H., & Hatfield, B. D. (2004). Aerobic exercise training and cardiovascular reactivity to psychological stress in sedentary young normotensive men and women. *Psychophysiology, 41*, 552–562.

Spielberger, C. D. (1972). *Anxiety: Current trends in theory and research* (Vol. 1). London: Academic Press.

Spilker, B., Molinek, F. R., Jr., Johnston, K. A., Simpson, R. L., & Tilson, H. H. (1990). Quality of life bibliography and indexes. *Medical Care, 28* (suppl.), DS1–DS77.

Spink, K. (1988). Facilitating endurance performance: The effects of cognitive strategies and analgesic suggestions. *The Sport Psychologist, 2*, 97–104.

Spink, K. (1992). Relation of anxiety about social physique to location of participation in physical activity. *Perceptual and Motor Skills, 74*, 1075–1078.

Spirduso, W. W. (1995). *Physical dimensions of aging.* Champaign, IL: Human Kinetics.

Spirduso, W. W., & Cronin, D. L. (2001). Exercise dose-response effects on quality of life and independent living in older adults. *Medicine & Science in Sports & Exercise, 33*, S598–S608.

Spirduso, W. W., & MacRae, P. (1991). Physical activity and quality of life in the frail elderly. In J. E. Birren, J. E. Lubben, J. C. Rowe, & D. E. Deutchman (Eds.), *The concept and measurement of quality of life in the frail elderly* (pp. 226–255). San Diego: Academic Press.

Spirduso, W. W., & MacRae, P. G. (1990). Motor performance aging. In J. E. Birren, K. W. Schaie, R. P. Abeles, M. Gatz, & T. A. Salthouse (Eds.), *Handbook of the psychology of aging* (3rd ed., pp. 184–197). San Diego: Academic Press.

Spirduso, W. W., Francis, K. L., & MacRae, P. G. (2005). *Physical dimensions of aging* (2nd ed.). Champaign, IL: Human Kinetics.

Spitzack, C. (1990). *Confessing excess: Women and the politics of body reduction.* Albany, NY: State University of New York Press.

Stainbeck, R.D. (1997) *Alcohol and sport.* Champaign, IL: Human Kinetics.

Steinberg, H., & Sykes, E. (1985). Introduction to symposium on endorphins and behavioral processes: Review of literature on endorphins and exercise. *Pharmacology, Biochemistry and Behavior, 23*(5), 857–862.

Stelter, R. (1998). The body, self, and identity: Personal and social constructions of the self through sport and movement. In R. Seiler (Ed.), *European yearbook of sport psychology* (pp.1–32). Sankt Augustin, Germany: Academia Verlag.

Stephens, T., & Craig, C. L. (1990). *The well-being of Canadians: Highlights of the 1988 Campbell's Survey.* Ottawa: Canadian Fitness and Lifestyle Research Institute.

Stephens, T., Craig, C. L., & Ferris, B. F. (1986). Adult physical activity in Canada: Findings from the Canada Fitness Survey I. *Canadian Journal of Public Health, 77*, 285–290.

Steptoe, A., & Bolton, J. (1988). The short-term influence of high and low-intensity physical exercise on mood. *Psychological Health, 2*, 91–106.

Steptoe, A., & Cox, S. (1988). Acute effects of aerobic exercise on mood. *Health Psychology, 7*, 329–340.

Steptoe, A., Kearsley, N., & Walters, N. (1993). Acute mood responses to maximal and submaximal exercise in active and inactive men. *Psychology & Health, 8*, 89–99.

Sternfeld, B. (1992). Cancer and the protective effect of physical activity: The epidemiological evidence. *Medicine and Science in Sports and Exercise, 24*, 119–125.

Steroid Trafficking Act of 1990 (1990, August). Committee of the Judiciary, 101st Congress, 2nd Session, Report No. 101–433.

Stetson, B. A., Rahn, J. M., Dubbert, P. M., Wilner, B. I., & Mercury, M. G. (1997). Prospective evaluation of the effects of stress on exercise adherence in community residing women. *Health Psychology, 16*, 515–520.

Stewart, A., Mills, K., Sepsis, P., King, A., McLellan, B., Roitz, K., & Ritter, P. (1997). Evaluation of CHAMPS, a physical activity promotion program for older adults. *Annals of Behavioral Medicine, 19*, 353–361.

Stone, E., McKenzie, T., Welk, G., & Booth, M. (1998). Effects of physical activity interventions in youth: Review and synthesis. *American Journal of Preventive Medicine, 15*, 298–315.

Stones, M. J., & Dawe, D. (1993). Acute exercise facilitates semantically cued memory in nursing home residents. *Journal of the American Geriatrics Society, 41*, 531–534.

Stones, M. J., & Kozma, A. (1988). Physical activity, age, and cognitive/motor performance. In J. E. Birren & K. W. Schaie (Eds.), *Cognitive development in adulthood: Progress in cognitive development research* (pp. 273–321). New York: Springer-Verlag.

Stones, M. J., & Kozma, A. (1996). Activity, exercise, and behavior. In J. E. Birren, K. W. Schaie, R. P. Abeles, M. Gatz, & T. A. Salthouse (Eds.), *Handbook of the psychology of aging* (4th ed., pp. 338–352). San Diego: Academic Press.

Stucky-Ropp, R., Renee, C., & DiLorenzo, T. M. (1993). Determinants of exercise in children. *Preventive Medicine, 22*, 880–889.

Stucky-Ropp, R., Vanderwal, J. S., & Gotham, H. J. (1998). Determinants of exercise among children: A longitudinal analysis. *Preventive Medicine, 27*, 470–477.

Subrahmanyam, K., Kraut, R.E., Greenfield, P.M., & Gross, E. F. (2000). The impact of home computer use on children's activities and development. *Future of Children, 10*, 123–144

Sullum, J., Clark, M., & King, T. (2000). Predictors of exercise relapse in a college population. *Journal of American College Health, 48*, 175–180.

Suls, J., & Bunde, J. (2005). Anger, anxiety, and depression as risk factors for cardiovascular disease: The problems and implications of overlapping affective dispositions. *Psychological Bulletin, 131*, 260–300.

Sutton, S. (1998). Predicting and explaining intentions and behavior: How well are we doing? *Journal of Applied Social Psychology, 28*, 1317–1338.

Swann, W. B., Jr. (1985). The self as architect of social reality. In B. Schlenker (Ed.), *The self and social life* (pp. 100–125). New York: McGraw-Hill.

Swann, W. B., Jr., & Hill, C. A. (1982). When our identities are mistaken: Reaffirming self-conceptions through social interaction. *Journal of Personality and Social Psychology, 43*, 59–66.

Swann, W. B., Jr., Hixon, J. G., Stein-Seroussi, A., & Gilbert, D. T. (1990). The fleeting gleam of praise: Behavioral reactions to self-relevant feedback. *Journal of Personality and Social Psychology, 59*, 17–26.

Swoap, R. A., & Murphy, S. M. (1995). Eating disorders and weight management in athletes. In S. M. Murphy (Ed.), *Sport psychology interventions* (pp. 307–329). Champaign, IL: Human Kinetics.

Taillefer, M. C., Dupuis, G., Roberge, M. A., & LeMay, S. (2003). Health-related quality of life models: Systematic review of the literature. *Social Indicators Research, 64*, 293–323.

Talbot, L. A., Metter, E. J., & Fleg, J. L. (2000). Leisure time physical activities and their relationship to cardiorespiratory fitness in healthy men and women 18–95 years old. *Medicine and Science in Sports and Exercise, 32*, 417–425.

Tammen, V. V. (1996). Elite middle and long distance runners associative/dissociative coping. *Journal of Applied Sport Psychology, 8,* 1–8.

Tappe, M. K., Duda, J. L., & Ehrnwald, P. M. (1989). Perceived barriers to exercise among adolescents. *Journal of School Health, 59,* 153–155.

Tappe, M. K., Duda, J. L., & Menges-Ehrnwald, P. (1990). Personal investment predictors of adolescent motivational orientation toward exercise. *Canadian Journal of Sport Sciences, 15,* 185–192.

Tarnopolsky, M. A., Zawada, C., Richmond, L. B., Carter, S., Shearer, J., Graham, T., & Phillips, S. M. (2001). Gender differences in carbohydrate loading are related to energy intake. *Journal of Applied Physiology, 91*(1), 225–230.

Tate, A. K., & Petruzzello, S. J. (1995). Varying the intensity of acute exercise: Implications for changes in affect. *Journal of Sports Medicine and Physical Fitness, 35,* 295–302.

Taylor, A. H., & Fox, K. R. (2005). Effectiveness of a primary care exercise referral intervention for changing physical self-perception over 9 months. *Health Psychology, 24*(1), 11–21.

Taylor, A. W. (1992). Aging: A normal degenerative process—with or without regular exercise. *Canadian Journal of Sport Science, 17,* 163–167.

Taylor, S. E., Pham, L. B., Rivkin, I. D., & Armor, D. A. (1998). Harnessing the imagination: Mental stimulation, self-regulation, and coping. *American Psychologist, 53,* 429–439.

Taylor, W. C. Baranowski, T., & Sallis, J. F. (1994). Family determinants of childhood physical activity: A social-cognitive model. In R. K. Dishman (Ed.), *Advances in exercise adherence* (pp. 319–342). Champaign, IL: Human Kinetics.

Taylor, W. C., Baranowski, T., & Young, D. R. (1998). Physical activity interventions in low-income, ethnic minority, and populations with disabilities. *American Journal of Preventive Medicine, 15,* 334–343.

Taylor, W. N. (1987). Synthetic anabolic-androgenic steroids: A plea for controlled substance status. *The Physician and Sportsmedicine, 15,* 140–150.

Telama, R. Yang, X., Laasko, L., & Viikari, J. (1997). Physical activity in childhood and adolescence as predictor of physical activity in young adulthood. *American Journal of Preventive Medicine, 13,* 317–323.

Telama, R., & Yang, X. (1999). Factors explaining the physical activity of young adults: The importance of early socialization. *Scandinavian Journal of Medicine and Science in Sports, 9,* 120–127.

Terry, P. C., Lane, A. M., Lane, H. G., & Kehohane, L. (1999). Development and validation of a mood measure for adolescents: POMS-A. *Journal of Sports Sciences, 17,* 861–872.

Tesser, A., & Campbell, J. (1983). Self-definition and self-evaluation maintenance. In J. Sulls & A. Greenwald (Eds.), *Social psychological perspectives on the self* (Vol. 2, pp. 1–31). Hillsdale, NJ: Erlbaum.

Thayer, R. E. (1986). Activation-Deactivation Check List: Current overview and structural analysis. *Psychological Reports, 58,* 607–614.

Thayer, R. E. (1987a). Energy, tiredness, and tension effects of a sugar snack versus moderate exercise. *Journal of Personality and Social Psychology, 52,* 119–125.

Thayer, R. E. (1987b). Problem perception, optimism, and related states as a function of time of day (diurnal rhythm) and moderate exercise: Two arousal systems in interaction. *Motivation and Emotion, 11,* 19–36.

Thayer, R. E. (1989). *The biopsychology of mood and arousal.* New York: Oxford University Press.

Thayer, R. E. (1996). *The origin of everyday moods: Managing energy, tension and stress.* New York: Oxford University Press.

Thayer, R. E. (2001). *Calm energy: How people regular mood with food and exercise.* New York: Oxford University Press.

Thayer, R. E., Newman, J. R., & McClain, T. M. (1994). Self-regulation of mood: Strategies for changing a bad mood, raising energy, and reducing tension. *Journal of Personality and Social Psychology, 67,* 910–925.

Thayer, R. E., Peters, D. P., Takahashi, P. J., & Birkhead-Flight, A. M. (1993). Mood and behavior (smoking and sugar snacking) following moderate exercise: A partial test of self-regulation theory. *Personality and Individual Differences, 14,* 97–104.

The Oxford American Dictionary and Thesaurus (2003). New York: Oxford University Press.

The, D. J., & Ploutz-Snyder, L. (2003). Age, body mass, and gender as predictors of Masters Olympic weightlifting performance. *Medicine & Science in Sports & Exercise, 35*(7), 1216–1224.

Theodorakis, Y. (1994). Planned behavior, attitude strength, role identity, and the prediction of exercise behavior. *The Sport Psychologist, 8,* 149–165.

Thompson, J. K., & Blanton, P. (1987). Energy conservation and exercise dependence: A sympathetic arousal hypothesis. *Medicine and Science in Sports and Exercise, 19,* 91–99.

Thompson, R. A. (1987). Management of the athlete with an eating disorder: Implications for the sport management team. *The Sport Psychologist, 1,* 114–126.

Thompson, R., & Sherman, R. (1993). *Helping athletes with eating disorders.* Champaign, IL: Human Kinetics.

Thornton, J. S. (1990). Feast or famine: Eating disorders in athletes. *Physician and Sportsmedicine, 18,* 116–122.

Tiggemann, M., & Lynch, J. E. (2001). Body image across the lifespan in adult women: The role of self-objectification. *Developmental Psychology, 37*(2), 243–253.

Tiggemann, M., & Ruutel, E. (2001). A cross cultural comparison of body dissatisfaction in Estonian and Australian young adults and its relationship with media exposure. *Journal of Cross-Cultural Psychology, 32*(6), 736–742.

Tiggemann, M., & Williamson, S. (2000). The effect of exercise on body satisfaction and self-esteem as a function of gender and age. *Sex Poles, 43*(1–2), 119–127.

Tillman, K. (1965). Relationship between physical fitness and selected personality traits. *Research Quarterly, 36,* 483–489.

Tinetti, M. E., & Powell, L. (1993). Fear of falling and low self-efficacy: A cause of dependence in elderly persons [special issue]. *Journal of Gerontology, 48,* 35–38.

Tinning, R. (1997). Performance and participation discourses in human movement: Toward a socially critical physical education. In J. Fernandez-Balboa (Ed.), *Critical postmodernism in human movement, physical education, and sport* (pp. 99–119). Albany, NY: State University of New York Press.

Tobar, D. A. (2005). Overtraining and staleness: The importance of psychological monitoring. *International Journal of Sport and Exercise, 4,* 455–468.

Tobar, D. A. (in press). Overtraining and staleness: The importance of psychological monitoring. *International Journal of Sport and Exercise Psychology.*

Tomporowski, P. D., & Ellis, N. R. (1986). Effects of exercise on cognitive processes: A review. *Psychological Bulletin, 99,* 338–346.

Tomporowski, P. D., Cureton, K., Armstrong, L. E., Kane, G. M., Sparling, P. B., & Millard-Stafford, M. (2005). Short-term effects of aerobic exercise on executive processes and emotional reactivity. *International Journal of Sport and Exercise Psychology, 3,* 131–146.

Tracey, J., & Elcombe, T. (2004). A lifetime of healthy meaningful movement: Have we forgotten the athletes? *Quest, 56,* 241–260.

Tracey, M. D. (2005, November). Helping people 'flourish' best boosts their mental health. *Monitor on Psychology, 36,* 64.

Treasure, D. C., & Newbery, D. M. (1998). Relationship between self-efficacy, exercise intensity, and feeling states in a sedentary population during and following an acute bout of exercise. *Journal of Sport & Exercise Psychology, 20,* 1–11.

Treasure, D. C., Lox, C. L., & Lawton, B. R. (1998). Determinants of physical activity in a sedentary, obese population. *Journal of Sport and Exercise Psychology, 20*, 218–224.

Tricker, R., & Cook, D. L. (Eds.). (1990). *Athletes at risk: Drugs and sport*. Dubuque, IA: Wm. C. Brown.

Tricker, R., Cook, D. L., & McGuire, R. (1989). Issues related to drug use in college athletics: Athletes at risk. *The Sport Psychologist, 3*, 155–165.

Trine, M. R., & Morgan, W. P. (1997). Influence of time of day on the anxiolytic effects of exercise. *International Journal of Sports Medicine, 18*, 161–168.

Triplett, N. (1898). The dynamogenic factors in pacemaking and competition. *American Journal of Psychology, 9*, 507–533.

Trudeau, F., Laurencelle, L., & Shephard, R. J. (2004). Tracking of physical activity from childhood to adulthood. *Medicine & Science in Sport & Exercise, 36*, 1937–1943.

Trumbull, R., & Appley, M. H. (1986). A conceptual model for the examination of stress dynamics. In M. H. Appley & R. Trumbull (Eds.), *Dynamics of stress: Physiological, psychological, and social perspectives* (pp. 21–45). New York: Plenum Press.

Tucker, L. A. (1985). Dimensionality and factor satisfaction of the body image construction: A gender comparison. *Sex Roles, 12*, 931–937.

Tucker, L. A. (1987). Effect of weight training on body attitudes: Who benefits most? *Journal of Sports Medicine and Physical Fitness, 27*, 70–78.

Tucker, L. A., & Mortell, R. (1993). Comparison of the effects of walking and weight training programs on body image in middle-aged women: An experimental study. *American Journal of Health Promotion, 8*(1), 34–42.

Tuckman, B. W., & Hinckle, J. S. (1986). An experimental study of the physical and psychological effects of aerobic exercise on school children. *Health Psychology, 5*, 197–207.

Tunks, T., & Bellissimo, A. (1988). Coping with the coping concept: A brief comment. *Pain, 34*, 171–174.

Turner, E. E., Rejeski, W. J., & Brawley, L. R. (1997). Psychological benefits of physical activity are influenced by the social environment. *Journal of Sport & Exercise Psychology, 19*, 119–130.

U.S. Centers for Disease Control and Prevention. (1993). Prevalence of sedentary lifestyle-behavioral risk factor surveillance system. United States, 1991. *Morbidity and Mortality Weekly Report, 42*, 576–579.

U.S. Department of Health and Human Services. (1996). *Physical activity and health: A report of the Surgeon General*. Washington, DC: U.S. Department of Health and Human Services, Centers for Disease Control and Prevention, National Center for Chronic Disease Prevention and Health Promotion.

U.S. Department of Health and Human Services. (1996). *Physical activity and health: A report of the Surgeon General*. Atlanta, GA: U.S. Department of Health and Human Services, Centers for Disease Control and Prevention, National Center for Chronic Disease Prevention and Health Promotion.

U.S. Department of Health and Human Services. (2000*). Healthy people 2010: Understanding and improving health*. Washington, DC: U.S. Government Printing Office, 017-001-00543-6, 1–70.

U.S. Department of Health and Human Services. (2000). *Healthy people 2010* (Conference edition). Washington, DC: U.S. Department of Health and Human Services.

Udry, E. (1999). The paradox of injuries: Unexpected positive consequences. In D. Pargman (Ed.), *Psychological bases of sport injuries* (2nd ed., pp. 79–88). Morgantown, WV: Fitness Information Technology.

United States Bureau of the Census. (1992). *Statistical abstract of the United States: 1992* (112th ed.). Washington, DC: US Department of Commerce.

United States National Center for Health Statistics. (1991). *Vital Statistics of the United States* (annual).

United States Olympic Committee. (1983). U.S. Olympic Committee establishes guidelines for sport psychology services. *Journal of Sport Psychology, 5*, 4–7.

University of Michigan Integrative Medicine. Retrieved December 14, 2005, from http//www.med.umich.edu/umim.

Ursin, H., & Eriksen, H. R. (2004). The cognitive activation theory of stress. *Psychoneuroendocrinology, 29*, 567–592.

Ussher, J. (1989). *The psychology of the female body*. London: Routledge.

Vallerand, R. J., & Losier, G. F. (1999). An integrative analysis of intrinsic and extrinsic motivation in sport. *Journal of Applied Sport Psychology, 11*, 142–169.

Valois, P., Shephard, R. J., & Godin, G. (1986). Relationship of habit and perceived physical ability to exercise behavior. *Perceptual and Motor Skills, 62*, 811–817.

van Eck, M., Nicolson, N., & Berkhof, J. (1998). Effects of stressful daily events on mood states: Relationship to global perceived stress. *Journal of Personality and Social Psychology, 75*, 1572–1585.

Van Mechelen, W., Twisk, J. W. R., Post, G. B, Snel, J., & Kemper, H. C. G. (2000). Physical activity of young people: Amsterdam Longitudinal Growth and Health Study. *Medicine and Science in Sports and Exercise, 32*, 1610–1616.

Van Raalte, J. L., Brewer, B. W. (Eds.). (2002). *Exploring Sport and Exercise Psychology* (2nd ed.). Washington, DC: American Psychological Association.

Vanden Auweele, Y., Boen, P., Schapendonk, W., & Dorenz, K. (2005). Promoting stair use among female employees: The effects of a health sign followed by an e-mail. *Journal of Sport and Exercise Psychology, 27*(2), 188–196.

Vanden Auweele, Y., De Cuyper, B., Van Mele, V., & Rzewnicki, R. (1993). Elite performance and personality: From description and prediction to diagnosis and intervention. In R. N. Singer, M. Murphey, & L. K. Tennant (Eds.), *Handbook of research on sport psychology* (pp. 257–287). New York: Macmillan.

Vanden Auweele, Y., Rzewnicki, R., & Van Mele, V. (1997). Reasons for not exercising and exercise intentions: A study of middle-aged sedentary adults. *Journal of Sport Sciences, 15*, 157–165.

Vann, J. (1983). Yoga. In D. E. Corbin & J. Metal-Corbin (Eds.), *Reach for it! A handbook of exercise and dance activities for older adults* (pp. 182–203). Dubuque, IA: Eddie Bowers.

Varni, J. W., Jay, S. M., Masek, B. J., & Thompson, K. L. (1986). Cognitive-behavioral assessment and management of pediatric pain. In A. D. Holzman & D. C. Turk (Eds.), *Pain management: A handbook of psychological treatment approaches* (Vol. 136, pp. 168–192). Elmsford, NY: Pergamon Press.

Vechi, H., Takenaka, K., & Oka, K. (2000). Relationship between physical activity and stress response of children. *Japanese Journal of Health Psychology, 13*, 1–8.

Verhoef, M. J., & Love, E. J. (1994). Women and exercise participation: The mixed blessing of motherhood. *Health Care for Women International, 15*, 297–306.

Verhoef, M. J., & Love, E. J. (1992). Women's exercise participation: The relevance of social roles compared to non-role related determinants. *Canadian Journal of Public Health, 83*, 367–371.

Vilhjalmsson, R., & Thorlindsson, T. (1998). Factors related to physical activity: A study of adolescents. *Social Science and Medicine, 47*, 665–675.

Viveros, O. H., Diliberto, E. J., Jr., Hazum, E., & Chang, K. (1979). Opiate-like materials in the adrenal medulla: Evidence for storage and secretion with catecholamines. *Molecular Pharmacology, 16*, 1101–1108.

Vlachopoulos, S., Biddle, S., & Fox, K. (1996). A social-cognitive investigation into the mechanisms of affect generation in children's physical activity. *Journal of Sport and Exercise Psychology, 18*, 174–193.

von Känel, R., Mills, P. J., Fainman, C., & Dimsdale, J. J. (2001). Effects of psychological stress and psychiatric disorders on blood coagulation and fibrinolysis: A biobehavioral pathway to coronary artery disease? *Psychosomatic Medicine, 63*, 531–544.

Voy, R., & Deeter, K. D. (1991). *Drugs, sports, and politics*. Champaign, IL: Human Kinetics.

Wallis, C., Galvin, R. M., & Thompson, D. (1983, June 6). Stress: Can we cope? *Time*, pp. 48–54.

Wankel, L. M. (1984). Decision-making and social support strategies for increasing exercise involvement. *Journal of Cardiac Rehabilitation, 4*, 124–135.

Wankel, L. M. (1985). Personal and situational factors affecting exercise involvement: The importance of enjoyment. *Research Quarterly for Exercise and Sport, 56*, 275–282.

Wankel, L. M. (1993). The importance of enjoyment to adherence and psychological benefits from physical activity. *International Journal of Sport Psychology, 24*, 151–169.

Wankel, L. M. (1997). "Strawpersons," selective reporting, and inconsistent logic: A response to Kimiecik and Harris's analysis of enjoyment. *Journal of Sport & Exercise Psychology, 19*, 98–109.

Wankel, L. M., & Berger, B. G. (1990). The psychological and social benefits of sport and physical activity. *Journal of Leisure Research, 22*, 167–182.

Wankel, L. M., & Kreisel, P. S. J. (1985). Factors underlying enjoyment of youth sports: Sport and age group comparisons. *Journal of Sport Psychology, 7*, 51–64.

Wankel, L. M., & Pabich, P. (1982). The minor sport experience: Factors contributing to or detracting from enjoyment. In J. T. Partington, T. Orlick, & J. H. Salmela (Eds.), *Mental training for coaches and athletes* (pp.70–71). Ottawa: Sports in Perspective.

Wankel, L. M., & Sefton, J. M. (1989). A season-long investigation of fun in youth sports. *Journal of Sport & Exercise Psychology, 11*, 355–366.

Wankel, L. M., & Thompson, C. (1977). Motivating people to be physically active: Self-persuasion vs. balanced decision making. *Journal of Applied Social Psychology, 7*, 332–340.

Ware, J. E., Jr. (2004). SF-36 health survey update. In M. E. Maruish (Ed.), *The use of psychological testing for treatment planning and outcomes assessment: Volume 3: Instruments for adults* (3rd ed.) (pp. 693–718). Mahwah, NJ: Lawrence Erlbaum.

Ware, J. E., Jr., & Sherbourne, C. D. (1992). The MOS 36-item short-form health survey (SF-36). I. Conceptual framework and item selection. *Medical Care 30*: 473–483.

Ware, J. E., Jr., Kosinski, M., & Dewey, J. E. (2000). *How to Score Version 2 of the SF-36¨ Health Survey.* Lincoln, RI: QualityMetric Incorporated.

Ware, J. E., Jr., Kosinski, M., & Gandek, B. (1993/2000). *SF-36¨ health survey: Manual and interpretation guide.* Lincoln, RI: QualityMetric Incorporated.

Washburn, R. (2000). Assessment of physical activity in older adults. *Research Quarterly for Exercise and Sport, 71*, 79–88.

Waterman, A. S. (1985). *Identity in adolescence: Process and contents.* Jossey-Bass: San Francisco.

Watkins, B. (1992). Youth beliefs about health and physical activity. *Journal of Applied Developmental Psychology, 13*, 257–269.

Watson, D. & Clark, L. A. (1994). The PANAS-X: Manual for the Positive and Negative Affect Schedule—Expanded Form. Retrieved June 16, 2005 from the University of Iowa, Psychology Faculty web site: http://www.psychology.uiowa.edu/Faculty/Watson/PANAS-X.pdf

Watson, D., & Clark, L. A. (1997). Measurement and mismeasurement of mood: Recurrent and emergent issues. *Journal of Personality Assessment, 68*, 267–296.

Watson, D., & Tellegen, A. (1985). Toward a consensual structure of mood. *Psychological Bulletin, 98*, 219–235.

Watson, D., Clark, L. A., & Tellegen, A. (1988). Development and validation of brief measures of positive and negative affect: The PANAS scales. *Journal of Personality & Social Psychology, 54*, 1063–1070.

Webster, S., & Rutt, R., & Weltman, A. (1990). Physiological effects of a weight loss regimen practiced by college wrestlers. *Medicine and Science in Sports and Exercise, 22*, 229.

Weinberg, R. S., & Gould, D. (2003). *Foundations of sport and exercise psychology* (3rd ed.). Champaign, IL: Human Kinetics.

Weinberg, R. S., Burton, D., Yukelson, D., & Weigand, D. (1993). Goal setting in competitive sport: An exploratory investigation of practices of collegiate athletes. *The Sport Psychologist, 7*, 275–289.

Weinberg, R. S., Burton, D., Yukelson, D., & Weigand, D. (2000). Perceived goal setting practices of Olympic athletes: An exploratory investigation. *The Sport Psychologist, 14*, 280–296.

Weinberg, R. S., Butt, J., & Knight, B. (2001). High school coaches' perceptions of the process of goal setting practices. *The Sport Psychologist, 15*, 20–47.

Weinberg, W. T. (1980, April). *Relationship of commitment to running scale to runners' performances and attitudes.* Paper presented at the annual convention of the American Alliance for Health, Physical Education, Recreation, and Dance, poster presentation session, Detroit.

Weiss, M. R. (2000). Motivating kids in physical activity. *President's Council on Physical Fitness and Sports Research Digest, 3*(11), 1–8.

Weiss, M. R., & Troxell, R. K. (1986). Psychology of the injured athlete. *Athletic Training, 21*(2), 104–109, 154.

Welk, G. J. (1999). The youth physical activity promotion model: A conceptual bridge between theory and practice. *Quest, 51*, 5–23.

Wells, A. J. (1988). Variations in mother's self-esteem in daily life. *Journal of Personality and Social Psychology, 55*, 661–668.

Weuve, J., Kang, J. H., Manson, J. E., Breteler, M. M., Ware, J., & Grodstein, F. (2004). Physical activity, including walking, and cognitive function in older women. *Journal of the American Medical Association, 292*(12), 1454–1461.

Whitehead, R., Chillag, S., & Elliot, D. (1992). Anabolic steroid use among adolescents in a rural state. *Journal of Family Practice, 35*, 401–405.

Widmeyer, W. N., Carron, A. V., & Brawley, L. R. (1990). The effects of group size in sport. *Journal of Sport & Exercise Psychology, 12*, 177–190.

Wiese, D. M., & Weiss, M. R. (1987). Psychological rehabilitation and physical injury: Implications for the sports medicine team. *The Sport Psychologist, 1*, 318–330.

Wiese-Bjornstal, D. M., & Smith, A. M. (1999). Counseling strategies for enhanced recovery of injured athletes within a team approach. In D. Pargman (Ed.), *Psychological bases of sport injuries* (2nd ed., pp. 125–155). Morgantown, WV: Fitness Information Technology.

Wilber, K. (1983). *A sociable god.* New York: McGraw-Hill.

Wilber, K. (1996). *A brief history of everything.* Boston: Shambhala.

Wilcox, S., & Storandt, M. (1996). Relations among age, exercise, and psychological variables in a community sample of women. *Health Psychology, 15*, 110–113.

Williams, J. M., & Andersen, M. B. (1998). Psychosocial antecedents of sport injury: Review and critique of the stress and injury model. *Journal of Applied Sport Psychology, 10*, 5–25.

Willis, J. D., & Campbell, L. F. (1992). *Exercise psychology.* Champaign, IL: Human Kinetics.

Willis, S. L. (1996). Everyday problem solving. In J. E. Birren, K. W. Schaie, R. P. Abeles, M. Gatz, & T. A. Salthouse (Eds.), *Handbook of the psychology of aging* (4th ed., pp. 287–307). San Diego: Academic Press.

Wilmore, J. H. (1992). Body weight and body composition. In K. D. Brownell, J. Rodin, & J. H. Wilmore (Eds.), *Eating, body weight, and performance in athletes* (pp. 77–93). Malvern, PA: Lea & Febiger.

Wilmore, J. H., & Costill, D. L. (2004). *Physiology of sport and exercise* (3rd ed.). Champaign, IL: Human Kinetics.

Wilson, P., & Eklund, R. C. (1998). The relationship between competitive anxiety and self-presentational concerns. *Journal of Sport and Exercise Psychology, 20,* 81–97.

Winter, D.G. (2005). Things I've learned about personality from studying political leaders at a distance. *Journal of Personality, 73*(3), 557–584.

Wister, A. (2003). It's never too late: Healthy lifestyles and aging. *Canadian Journal on Aging, 22*(2), 149–150.

Wold, B., & Anderssen, N. (1992). Health promotion aspects of family and peer influences on sport participation. *International Journal of Sport Psychology, 23,* 343–359.

Woodward, D., Green, E., & Hebron, S. (1989). The sociology of women's leisure and physical recreation: Constraints and opportunities. *International Review for the Sociology of Sport, 24,* 121–133.

Woorons, X., Mollard, P., Lamberto, C., Letournel, M., & Richalet, J. P. (2005). Effect of acute hypoxia on maximal exercise in trained and sedentary women. *Medicine & Science in Sports & Exercise, 37*(1).

World Health Organization Group. (1995). The World Health Organization Quality of Life assessment (WHOQOL): Position paper from the World Health Organization. *Social Science and Medicine, 41,* 1403–1409.

Wragg, J. (1990). The impact of adolescent development: Implications for timing. Evaluation and development of drug-education programs. *Drug Education Journal of Australia, 4,* 233–239.

Wright, J., & Cowden, J. E. (1986). Changes in self-concept and cardiovascular endurance of mentally retarded youths in a Special Olympics swim training program. *Adapted Physical Activity Quarterly, 3,* 177–183.

Wrisberg, C. A., & Anshel, M. H. (1989). The effect of cognitive strategies on the free throw shooting performance of young athletes. *Sport Psychologist, 3,* 95–104.

Wuthnow, R. (1978). Peak experiences: Some empirical tests. *Journal of Humanistic Psychology, 18,* 59–75.

Yan, J. H., & McCullagh, P. (2004). Cultural influence on youth's motivation of participation in physical activity. *Journal of Sport Behavior, 27,* 378–390.

Yates, A. (1991). *Compulsive exercise and the eating disorders: Toward an integrated theory of activity.* New York: Bruner/Mazel.

Yates. A., Leehey, K., & Shisslak, C. M. (1983). Running: An analogue of anorexia? *New England Journal of Medicine, 308,* 251–255.

Yesalis, C., & Cowart, V. (1998*). The steroids game: An expert's inside look at anabolic steroid use in sports.* Champaign, IL: Human Kinetics.

Yeung, R. R. (1996). The acute effects of exercise on mood state. *Journal of Psychosomatic Research, 40,* 123–141.

Yeung, R. R., & Hemsley, D. R. (1997). Personality, exercise and psychological well-being: Static relationships in the community. *Personality and Individual Differences, 22,* 47–53.

Yoshinaga, M., Shimago, A., Koriyama, C., Miyata, K., Hashiguchi, J., & Arima, K. (2004).

Zautra, A. J., Potter, P. T., & Reich, J. W. (1998). The independence of affects is context-dependent: An integrative model of the relationship between positive and negative affect. In K. W. Schaie & M. P. Lawton (Eds.). *Annual review of gerontology and geriatrics: Focus on emotion and adult development* (Vol. 17, pp. 75–103). New York: Springer.

Zeidner, M., & Saklofske, D. (1996). Adaptive and maladaptive coping. In M. Zeidner & N. S. Endler (Eds.), *Handbook of coping: Theory, research, applications* (pp. 505–531). New York: Wiley.

Zemva, A., & Rogel, P. (2001). Gender differences in athlete's heart: Association with 24-h blood pressure. A study of pairs in sport dancing. *International Journal of Cardiology, 77*(1), 49–59.

Zuckerman, M. (1979a). *Sensation seeking: Beyond the optimal level of arousal.* Hillsdale, NJ: Erlbaum.

Zuckerman, M. (1979b). Sensation-seeking and risk-taking. In C. E. Izard (Ed.), *Emotions in personality and psychotherapy* (pp. 163–187). New York: Plenum Press.

Zuckerman, M. (1983a). *Biological bases of sensation seeking, impulsivity, and anxiety.* Hillsdale, NJ: Erlbaum.

Zuckerman, M. (1983b). Sensation seeking and sports. *Personality and Individual Differences, 4,* 285–293.

Zuckerman, M. (1994). *Behavioral expression and biosocial bases of sensation seeking.* New York: Cambridge University Press.

Zunft, H. J. F., Friebe, D., Sppelt, B., Widhalm, K., Remaut de Winter, A. M., Vaz de Almeida, M. D., Kearney, J. M., & Gibney, M. (1999). Perceived benefits and barriers to physical activity in a nationally representative sample in the European Union. *Public Health Nutrition, 2* (Suppl.), 153–160.

INDEX

ABOUT THE AUTHORS

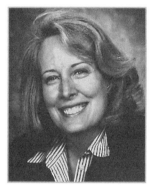

Bonnie G. Berger is professor and director of the School of Human Movement, Sport, & Leisure Studies at Bowling Green State University in Ohio. Before coming to Bowling Green, Berger was professor and associate dean in the School of Physical and Health Education and the College of Health Sciences at the University of Wyoming and a professor at Brooklyn College of the City University of New York, and Dalhousie University, Halifax Nova Scotia.

In addition to teaching undergraduate and graduate exercise and sport psychology for more than 35 years, Berger has been an active researcher. She has published more than 75 journal articles and book chapters and has delivered applied presentations and more than 90 scholarly papers at national and international conferences, as well as in business and industry. She has been a Visiting Fellow at the University of Western Australia during the fall of 1989 and 1990, and at Edith Cowan University in 2001 in Perth. Most recently, she was a visiting Research Professor at the University of Western Australia during the fall of 2006.

Dr. Berger is a charter member, fellow, and certified consultant of the Association for the Advancement of Applied Sport Psychology (AAASP), and former chairperson of its Health Psychology section and member of its Executive board. She is also a founding member of the Exercise and Sport Psychology Division (Div. 47) of the American Psychological Association and a charter member of the North American Society for the Psychology of Sport and Physical Activity from which she received the Outstanding Dissertation Award in 1971. Bonnie is a fellow of the American Academy of Kinesiology and Physical Education and a fellow of the American Alliance for Health, Physical Education, Recreation and Dance (AAHPERD) Research Consortium. She has served on editorial boards of numerous journals including *Journal of Applied Sport Psychology*, *Quest*, *The Sport Psychologist,* and the *International Journal of Sport Psychology* and also has served as the exercise and health psychology section editor of the *Journal of Applied Sport Psychology*.

Dr. Berger received a B.S. from Wittenberg University and an M.A. and Ed.D., with a specialization in exercise and sport psychology and motor learning, from Teachers College, Columbia University. She enjoys international travel, visiting family and friends, swimming, downhill skiing, and weight training.

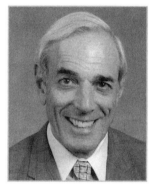

David Pargman is Professor Emeritus in the Department of Educational Psychology and Learning Systems, Florida State University, Tallahassee, Florida, where he completed 31 years of service. While at FSU he served as Program Coordinator for Educational Psychology and Coordinator of Sport and Exercise Psychology. He was also an Adjunct Professor in Florida State University's School of Music. He did his undergraduate work at the City College of New York, his Master's degree at Teachers College, Columbia University, and his Ph.D. at New York University.

Prior to coming to Florida State University he taught at Boston University and the City College of New York. He has served as major professor to approximately 50 doctoral students.

David Pargman has authored or coauthored numerous articles, book chapters, refereed abstracts, etc., and delivered approximately 200 regional, national, and international lectures at various professional forums. He is currently working on his seventh book, which focuses upon the relationship between psychology and physical activity. For nine years, he provided a weekly commentary about various issues related to sport and exercise psychology on a local affiliate of National Public Radio.

Dr. Pargman has served on the Executive Board of the Association for the Advancement of Applied Sport Psychology, was Chairman of its Health Psychology Section, and is a past Chairman of the Sport Psychology Academy of the American Alliance for Health, Physical Education, Recreation and Dance. He is a Fellow of the Association for the Advancement of Applied Sport Psychology, the Research Consortium of the American Alliance for Health, Physical Education, Recreation and Dance, and the American College of Sports Medicine. He is a member of the United States Olympic Committee Sport Psychology Registry and a Certified Consultant of the Association for the Advancement of Applied Sport Psychology.

Dr. Pargman has served as Visiting Professor at the University of Akron, Ohio, USA; Srinakharinwirot University, Bangkok, Thailand; University of San Marcos, Lima, Peru; University of the Andes, Merida, Venezuela; Lund University, Lund, Sweden; and the University of Zulia, Mariacaibo, Venezuela. He currently serves on the Editorial Board of the *Journal Studia Kinanthropologia* (Czech Republic) and Board of Directors of the Multidisciplinary Institute of Neuropsychological Development, Cambridge, Massachusetts.

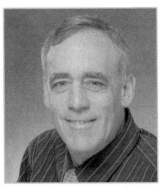

Robert S. Weinberg is a professor in the Department of Physical Education, Health, and Sport Studies at Miami University in Oxford, Ohio. Before coming to Miami University, Weinberg taught in the Department of Kinesiology at the University of North Texas where he was also regents professor, regents faculty lecturer, and a Toulouse Scholar. He was voted one of the top ten sport psychology specialists in North America by his peers.

In addition to teaching undergraduate and graduate sport/exercise psychology for over 30 years, Weinberg has written extensively on topics related to exercise and sport psychology. He has published six books related to sport/exercise psychology, over 135 refereed journal articles, and 20 book chapters. He has presented more than 300 scholarly papers at sport/exercise psychology conferences and has spoken worldwide in Israel, Spain, England, Greece, Germany, France, Portugal, Hong Kong, New Zealand, and Australia.

Dr. Weinberg served as president of the North American Society for the Psychology of Sport and Physical Activity, the Association for the Advancement of Applied Sport Psychology, and the Sport Psychology Academy of AAHPERD. He also has served as the editor-in-chief of the *Journal of Applied Sport Psychology*. Currently, Weinberg serves on the editorial boards of the *Journal of Sport and Exercise Psychology*, *The Sport Psychologist*, *International Journal of Sport Psychology*, and *Psychology of Sport and Exercise*. He is a certified consultant (AAASP), a member of the United States Olympic Committee Sport Psychology Registry, and a fellow in the prestigious American Academy for Physical Education and

Sport. Recently, Weinberg was named Distinguished Scholar at Miami University and won the Outstanding Faculty award in the School of Education and Allied Professionals at Miami University, Oxford, Ohio.

Dr. Weinberg earned his Ph.D. in sport psychology from the University of California, Los Angeles, in 1977. He recently married and moved to Cincinnati to be with his wife, Cynthia. In his free time, Dr. Weinberg enjoys tennis, basketball, jogging, and traveling.